MITRAL VALVE REGURGITATION

Collected Reprints (1961-2019)

By

William C. Roberts, MD

and

Colleagues

ISBN: 979-8-88862-156-1
Printed in the United States of America on acid-free paper.

Table of Contents

Articles are numbered based on WCR's CV.

DIFFERENTIAL DIAGNOSIS OF MITRAL REGURGITATION IN CHILDHOOD: CLINICAL PATHOLOGICAL CONFERENCE AT THE NATIONAL INSTITUTES OF HEALTH *

Moderator: Eugene Braunwald, M.D. *Discussants:* Richard S. Ross, M.D., F.A.C.P., *Baltimore, Maryland;* Andrew G. Morrow, M.D., and William C. Roberts, M.D., *Bethesda, Maryland*

Dr. Eugene Braunwald: The patient whose records form the basis of this conference taught a good deal to those of us who were involved in his care, and for this reason his case was selected for this presentation.

He was a 13-year-old colored male who was the product of a normal full term pregnancy and delivery and who weighed over six pounds at birth. His growth and development were retarded, walking occurring at 18 months and talking after the age of two years. His mother felt that he had always been small and sickly compared with his siblings.

He was not examined by a physician until the age of six years when he was hospitalized because of fever and tachypnea. Physical examination revealed a pulse of 108, and blood pressure of 120/75 mm. Hg. The lungs were clear. A grade IV, high pitched, systolic murmur was heard at the apex; there was a protodiastolic sound at the apex and a questionable presystolic murmur at the apex. Chest x-rays revealed cardiomegaly with a cardiothoracic ratio of 0.61. The left ventricle was considered to be greatly enlarged and there was slight fullness in the area of the pulmonary conus. The electrocardiogram was said to show prolongation of the PR interval when age and rate were considered. Acute rheumatic fever was diagnosed and, following discharge from the hospital, the patient was placed on oral penicillin. Examination eight months later showed a regular rhythm, a systolic thrill and loud systolic murmur at the apex, and a questionable presystolic murmur at the apex. The electrocardiogram showed a PR interval of 0.19 sec. and a heart rate of 110/min.

He convalesced slowly but was not able to resume normal activity. He was hospitalized near his home four times because of fever, with abdominal pain on one occasion, and symptoms of left and right sided heart failure on three occasions. His C-reactive protein and antistreptolysin titer were always unremarkable. Cardiac examination always revealed systolic and diastolic murmurs, and during the latter two hospitalizations he was in atrial fibrillation which converted to sinus rhythm upon

* Received for publication March 17, 1961.

This is an edited transcription of a clinical pathological conference at the Clinical Center, Bethesda, Md., by the National Heart Institute, National Institutes of Health, Public Health Service, Department of Health, Education, and Welfare.

Requests for reprints should be addressed to Eugene Braunwald, M.D., Chief, Cardiology Branch, National Heart Institute, Bethesda, Md.

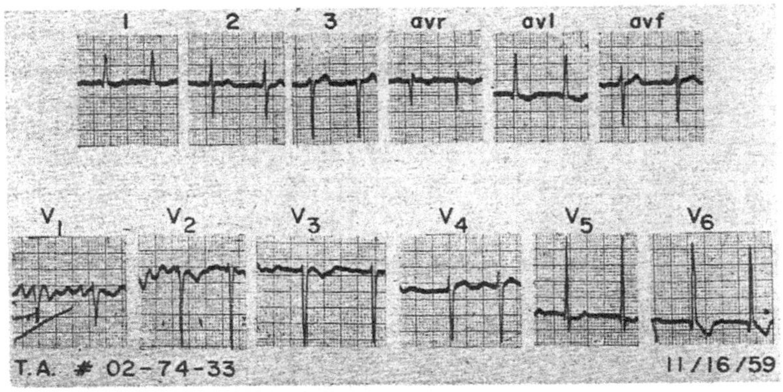

FIG. 1. Electrocardiogram of patient T. A.

administration of quinidine. The electrocardiograms showed left atrial and ventricular enlargement with a first degree heart block.

He was referred to the National Heart Institute because of persistent dyspnea and orthopnea. On physical examination the patient was a small, poorly developed, undernourished boy who appeared to be chronically ill. Blood pressure was 110/87 mm. Hg and the pulse rate was 100/min. and grossly irregular. The neck veins were dilated and pulsated vigorously when he was in the sitting position. There was a prominent precordial bulge, a striking left ventricular lift, and a modest right ventricular lift. The second heart sound was palpable along the left sternal border. On auscultation this sound was split with a loud pulmonic component. The phonocardiogram showed that P_2 remained split even after the Valsalva maneuver. A grade 3/6 pansystolic murmur was best heard at the apex but was well transmitted to the axilla and over the entire precordium. A grade 3/6 mid-diastolic, rumbling

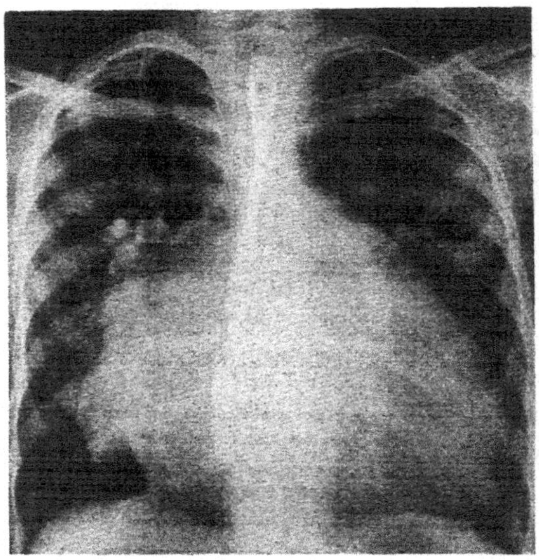

FIG 2. Chest roentgenogram of patient T. A.

murmur and an early diastolic sound were heard at the apex. The liver edge was palpable five fingerbreadths below the costal margin. The complete blood count, sedimentation rate, serology, urinalysis, CRP, ASO, blood electrolytes, and "liver chemistries" were unremarkable. The electrocardiogram is reproduced in Figure 1 and the chest roentgenograms in Figures 2 and 3.

Our discussant today is Dr. Richard S. Ross, Associate Professor of Medicine and Radiology at the Johns Hopkins University School of Medicine. Dr. Ross had only the above protocol on hand for the preparation of his initial discussion.

DR. RICHARD S. ROSS: The electrocardiogram shows left axis deviation and atrial fibrillation. There is no R wave in Lead V_1. Deep S waves are present over the right precordium. The R wave is 24 mm. in Lead V_6, and small Q

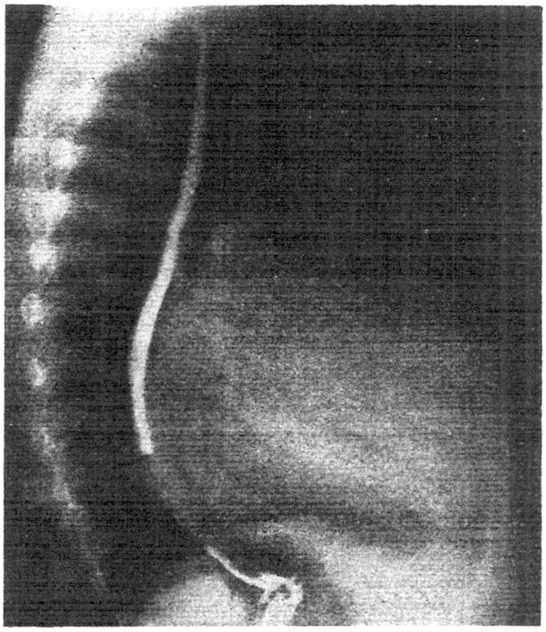

FIG. 3. Lateral roentgenogram of patient T. A.

waves are present over the left precordium. The sagging of the ST segments and inversion of T waves in Lead V_6 are characteristic of left ventricular hypertrophy or, in older terminology, "left ventricular strain." On the roentgenograms the heart is huge and there appears to be enlargement of all chambers. There is fullness in the region of the pulmonary artery and there is a double density which I believe represents the left atrium. I think the little prominence on the right border of the heart is also part of a giant left atrium. In the lateral and right oblique views, there is posterior deviation of the esophagus, which makes me feel that this individual had a greatly enlarged left atrium. In the right oblique projection, the left atrium bulges out behind the esophagus. The left oblique film shows the left ventricle to be enlarged and it is seen to project posteriorly well beyond the spine. In summary, the x-rays show enlargement of the left atrium and left ventricle and slight fullness of the right ventricular outflow tract.

There was an excellent history of retarded growth and development which can be used to support the contention that the disease was congenital. The febrile illness may or may not be significant, but it could have been either rheumatic fever or bacterial endocarditis. The most prominent physical sign was a loud apical pansystolic murmur which was noted by several observers. It was heard maximally at the apex, but also at other places on the precordium. Throughout the history there was evidence of both right and left ventricular failure. The patient was dyspneic and tachypneic, but he also had a large liver and distended neck veins.

Occasionally, the heart may be enlarged, or may function abnormally from extracardiac causes, and this possibility must always be considered first. In this case we can say, from the size of the heart and other findings, that this individual had primary heart disease. The intensity of the murmur and the coexisting thrill makes me feel certain that this patient had either valvular disease, a septal defect, or obstruction to the outflow tract in one or the other of the cardiac chambers. A murmur of this intensity, associated with a thrill, is not heard in the absence of one of these recognized causes of turbulence within the heart.

We next come to the question of whether this be congenital or acquired heart disease. The early appearance of the murmur and the retarded growth and development indicate that it was congenital heart disease. It is possible to have rheumatic fever at an early age. We have seen a patient recently with mitral insufficiency who had unequivocal chronic rheumatic valvular disease at the age of six years, but this is not the usual situation. There were no associated manifestations of rheumatic fever in the case under discussion today and the laboratory studies for detecting active rheumatic fever were negative. In difficult clinical situations such as this, the C-reactive protein and antistreptolysin titer, are most useful when they are negative. At this point, rheumatic heart disease can be eliminated from consideration, and the patient can be considered to have had congenital heart disease.

We then have to reconsider the two general categories of diseases in which murmurs of this intensity are heard—septal defects and valvular diseases. On the x-rays the lung fields did not appear to be abnormally vascular. The electrocardiogram showed no evidence of right ventricular hypertrophy or right axis deviation, and I was unable to explain the giant atrium on the basis of any of the well known septal abnormalities. I considered ventricular septal defect, atrial septal defect, a shunt from the left ventricle to the right atrium, and a patent ductus arteriosus. I did not give specific consideration to right-to-left shunts because no mention was made of cyanosis.

The ostium primum defects and the varieties of persistent common atrioventricular canal receive special attention because these defects are frequently associated with mitral valve abnormalities. The electrocardiogram in the ostium primum defects always shows some evidence of right ventricular hypertrophy, and this was lacking in today's patient. Furthermore, the left atrium is never enlarged to this degree. These two facts allowed me to eliminate ostium primum defects from this initial discussion.

The left ventriculo-right atrial communications were considered with Dr.

Braunwald's article as the reference.[1] The electrocardiogram in his patients showed right ventricular hypertrophy, combined hypertrophy, or ". . . a suggestion of left." Thus, left axis deviation and left ventricular hypertrophy were inconsistent with ventriculo-atrial shunt. Left atrial enlargement would not be expected in these patients and it was not present in the reported patients. At this point I eliminated all the common and uncommon left-to-right shunts.

The category of valvular and obstructive lesions must be considered next. Because of the massive dilatation of the left atrium and the left ventricle, attention was directed to the left side of the heart. Valvular aortic stenosis seemed an unlikely cause of this murmur. Subvalvular aortic stenosis could produce a murmur in this location. We have seen a few cases of a subvalvular obstruction in which the murmur was maximal at the apex or near the apex; in one case, there was a thrill at the apex in association with the murmur.

In favor of the diagnosis of subvalvular aortic stenosis, we might list the signs of left ventricular hypertrophy on the electrocardiogram and the large left ventricle on the x-ray. The left atrium may be enlarged in aortic stenosis but I have never seen a left atrium attain the size which our patient's did in the presence of aortic stenosis alone. Therefore, against the diagnosis of aortic

TABLE 1

Congenital Mitral Insufficiency

1. Fused fixed valve.
2. Cleft mitral leaflet.
3. Perforated mitral leaflet.
4. Double orifice of the mitral valve.
5. Anomalous insertion of chordae tendineae.
6. Corrected transposition of great vessels
    a. Anomalous insertion of chordae tendineae.
    b. Ebstein's malformation, left.
7. Fibroelastosis of left ventricle.

stenosis would be this tremendous enlargement of the left atrium and the description of the murmur as pansystolic. This is unusual even for the murmurs in subaortic stenosis which are usually confined to the early part of systole. Obstruction to left ventricular outflow did not offer an adequate explanation for all the important findings and therefore was excluded.

Mitral insufficiency, the other cause of murmurs of this type, offered the best explanation for the enlarged left atrium. The left atrium may reach this size in mitral stenosis, but the more common cause of giant atrium is mitral insufficiency. The signs of left ventricular hypertrophy on physical examination, the enlarged left ventricle on x-ray, and the electrocardiographic findings were perfectly compatible with this diagnosis. The murmur was much more compatible with mitral insufficiency than it was with aortic stenosis.

I had some reservations about the electrocardiogram because, though left axis deviation and left ventricular hypertrophy occur in mitral insufficiency, the axis is usually not much to the left of 0°. Furthermore, this particular type of ST segment is uncommon in mitral insufficiency. There were minor objections and I concluded that congenital mitral insufficiency was the best diagnosis.

This led to a consideration of the various anatomic lesions which result in mitral regurgitation (Table 1).

The literature contains descriptions of valves with fused, fixed cusps, valves with a cleft leaflet in association with the ostium primum defect and without this lesion, perforated valve leaflets, valves with a double orifice, and cusps with anomalous insertion of the chordae tendineae in such a way as to hold the valve open. This latter lesion may be associated with corrected transposition of the great vessels. Corrected transposition of the great vessels is associated with another interesting mitral valve lesion, referred to as Ebstein's malformation of the left AV valve, in which the left AV valve, which looks like the normal tricuspid valve, is displaced downward into the left ventricle and may be incompetent. Finally, fibroelastosis of the left ventricle may cause mitral regurgitation by sticking the leaflets to the wall of the ventricle and holding the valve open.

Without much difficulty, we can dispose of diagnoses 6 and 7 in Table 1. The mitral lesions associated with the corrected transpositions can be excluded by the electrocardiogram which, in our patient, has definite Q waves in Leads V_5 and V_6. This electrocardiographic pattern is almost never seen with corrected transposition.[2] There were several other points against corrected transpositions. First, when mitral insufficiency occurs in this malformation, it is usually not this severe and clinically dominant, and it is not associated with a giant left atrium. Second, there was no evidence of any of the defects commonly associated with corrected transposition, such as ventricular septal defect and pulmonary stenosis. Fibroelastosis is unlikely because patients with this disease usually die earlier and murmurs are usually not a prominent feature. Murmurs of such intensity are not heard in this disease, and the left atrium, though enlarged, is never this big.

At this point I was left with an isolated congenital mitral insufficiency, which was probably anatomically one of the first five diagnoses in Table 1. In this malformation, the left atrium may be large, there is an early history of failure, growth is retarded, and the electrocardiogram shows left ventricular hypertrophy. There is no certain way of differentiating between the first five types of congenital mitral insufficiency. In Dr. H. B. Taussig's book[3] there is a drawing of a heart exhibiting a kind of mitral insufficiency in which the mitral valve is replaced by a perforated diaphragm. The clinical course in this patient was similar to that of the subject of today's conference. There was auricular fibrillation, a huge left atrium, and an enlarged left ventricle. I thought the patient under discussion today would have a similar mitral valve.

Therefore, in summary, on the basis of the protocol, x-rays, and electrocardiogram before I received the catheterization data, my diagnosis was congenital mitral insufficiency due to a fused fixed perforated diaphragm in place of the mitral valve.

Dr. Eugene Braunwald: A right heart catheterization was carried out and the pressure in the right atrium was markedly elevated with V wave peaks of 17 mm. Hg and a mean pressure of 13 mm. Hg. The catheter crossed an atrial communication into the left atrium where the pressure pulse was found to have V wave peaks of 27 mm. Hg and the mean pressure in the left atrium was 15 mm. Hg, only slightly but distinctly higher than the mean pressure in the right atrium. The contours of the two pressure pulses were also quite different. The systolic pressure in the right ventricle was elevated to 55 mm. Hg; the end-diastolic pressure was 15 mm. Hg; the femoral arterial oxygen saturation was normal.

The krypton^{85} inhalation test[4] for the characterization of left-to-right shunts indicated a value of 46% in the right atrium. The upper limit of normal is 15%, and the value observed in our patient represents a left-to-right shunt entering the right atrium. The value of 34% in the right ventricle confirmed the fact that a left-to-right shunt existed.

Indicator dilution curves were obtained. Injection of indocyanine dye into the left atrium and sampling from the femoral artery resulted in a curve which indicated the presence of a left-to-right shunt. Injection of dye into the inferior vena cava showed no evidence of a right-to-left shunt, but showed a broad diffuse curve which was compatible with congestive heart failure and/or a left-to-right shunt. The levels of pressure in the various cardiac chambers and the results of the krypton^{85} test and of the dye dilution curves were then sent to Dr. Ross *after* he had prepared the foregoing discussion. However, we did not indicate how the left atrium was entered.

Dr. Richard S. Ross: I should have asked a question when I first got the catheterization data because I have just realized for the first time that the catheter entered the left atrium. I had assumed that the transseptal technic[5] had been employed, and I am distressed to learn that the left atrium was entered without puncture of the septum.

The catheterization report adds four important facts to the list of clinical evidence we have already considered:

1. Evidence of a left-to-right shunt into the right atrium.
2. Right ventricular systolic hypertension.
3. No right-to-left shunt.
4. Tall V waves in the left atrium.

The next step is to consider the clinical diagnosis of congenital mitral insufficiency in the light of the catheterization data. Certainly, the tall V waves support this diagnosis and the right ventricular hypertension was consistent with it. The evidence of the left-to-right shunt into the right atrium was difficult to reconcile with the large left atrium. It is difficult to see how the left atrium could have reached this size if there were an atrial septal defect, as the atrial septal defect would tend to decompress the left atrium. It is well recognized that in Lutembacher's syndrome, in which the hemodynamic situation is similar, though the mitral valve is involved in a different way, the left atrium is not huge.

We have seen three patients who have mitral insufficiency and an ostium secundum defect. These people by and large have not been severely ill, and the left atrium has not been as big as we would have expected it to be on the basis of the mitral valvular disease alone. They have not had signs of gross left ventricular hypertrophy on electrocardiogram or on x-ray. The systolic murmurs were far less impressive than the one heard in this patient.

A similar set of cases has been reported by Bashour and Simmons.[6] None of their cases of mitral insufficiency and ostium secundum atrial septal defects had a left atrium as large as did our patient. Of course, it could be said that in this particular case there was more than the usual amount of mitral insufficiency and a very small atrial defect, and that this accounted for the unusual clinical picture.

Before settling on this diagnosis, I thought I should consider some other possibilities, so I began to consider the possible sources of a left-to-right shunt of oxygenated blood into the right atrium. The various possibilities are:

1. Aorta to right atrium.
2. Left ventricle to right ventricle—tricuspid insufficiency to right atrium.
3. Left ventricle to right atrium.
4. Left atrium to right atrium.

The simple atrial defect can be excluded because of the size of the left atrium. The aorta to right atrium shunt can be excluded on the basis of physical findings; patients with this communication almost always have a continuous murmur, are usually sicker, and the disease runs a more rapid course. The possibility of the ventricular septal defect with a regurgitant tricuspid valve seemed real, but on the basis of the electrocardiogram, it was excluded. If the right side of the heart were overloaded by a ventricular septal defect and tricuspid insufficiency, there would certainly be evidence of right hypertrophy in the electrocardiogram. The absence of right hypertrophy on the electrocardiogram was also the major objection to the diagnosis of ostium primum defect. The objections were the same as those raised in the earlier discussion.

The diagnosis selected will have to provide an explanation for the following findings:

1. Oxygenated blood to right atrium.
2. Incompetent mitral valve.
3. Huge left atrium (intact atrial septum).
4. Left ventricular hypertrophy.

The large left atrium excluded the existence of a significant atrial septal defect and yet we had evidence of oxygenated blood entering the right atrium. The left ventricular hypertrophy that we saw in the EKG suggested that there might be a cause of ventricular overloading other than the mitral insufficiency.

In a search for other causes of left ventricular hypertrophy, I considered various kinds of aortic stenosis and found an illustration in Dr. Taussig's book [3] which shows an infundibular aortic stenosis with anomalous insertion of the chordae of the mitral valve. This insertion caused the aortic leaflet of the mitral valve to be pulled away from the mural leaflet. The patient died, presumably due to a combination of mitral insufficiency and an infundibular aortic stenosis. This malformation would have explained all the findings in today's case except for the shunt. From this case, I was led to a case reported by Dr. Charlotte Ferencz in 1957 which had all of the features necessary to explain the findings in the case today.

In conclusion, I believe the patient under discussion today had the malformation described by Ferencz. The x-ray findings in this malformation are almost identical with those presented today. The left atrium is equally prominent and gives the same configuration to the right heart border in the PA projection (Figure 4). The other projections show the massive dilatation of the left atrium and the enlarged left ventricle. The electrocardiogram is also similar to that of today's patient. The tall R waves over the left precordium are accompanied by similar ST segment changes.

The anatomy of the heart in Ferencz' patient can be seen in Figure 5. The chordae from the aortic leaflet of the mitral valve were attached to the ventricular septum and the mitral valve was rendered incompetent. These same anomalous chordae formed a network in the outflow tract of the left ventricle and interfered with left ventricular emptying. There was a communication between the left ventricle and the right atrium which would explain very nicely the left-to-right shunt with an intact atrial septum. Before hearing Dr. Braunwald's discussion of the catheterization I had assumed that the atrial septum was intact, and I still feel it hard to explain the large left atrium in any other way.

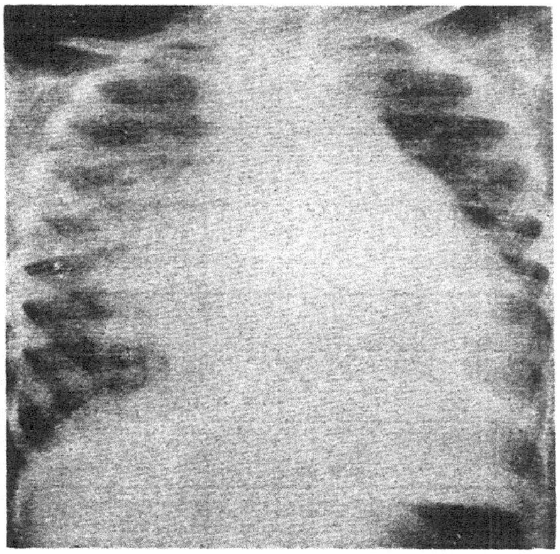

FIG. 4. Chest roentgenogram of patient described by Ferencz.[7] (Reproduced by permission of Bull. Johns Hopkins Hosp. **100**: 209, 1957.)

The diagram in Figure 6 shows how the heart in Ferencz' patient would function. If this isn't the right diagnosis, I'm quite sure that it would give an identical clinical picture. The chordae from the mitral valve are shown extending across the outflow tract of the left ventricle. There is a communication between the left ventricle and the right atrium. There is a huge left atrium, which of course has many hemodynamic factors operating to make it so large: first, there is an intact septum; second, the mitral valve is incompetent; third, there is left ventricular outflow obstruction so that the pressure in the left ventricle is very high; and fourth, there is a left-to-right shunt so that the return of blood to the left atrium from the lung would be increased.

Therefore, in conclusion, I think the correct diagnosis is left ventriculo-right atrial communication, with mitral insufficiency due to anomalous insertion of the chordae tendineae, and obstruction of left ventricular outflow due to the chordae tendineae extending across the left ventricular outflow tract.

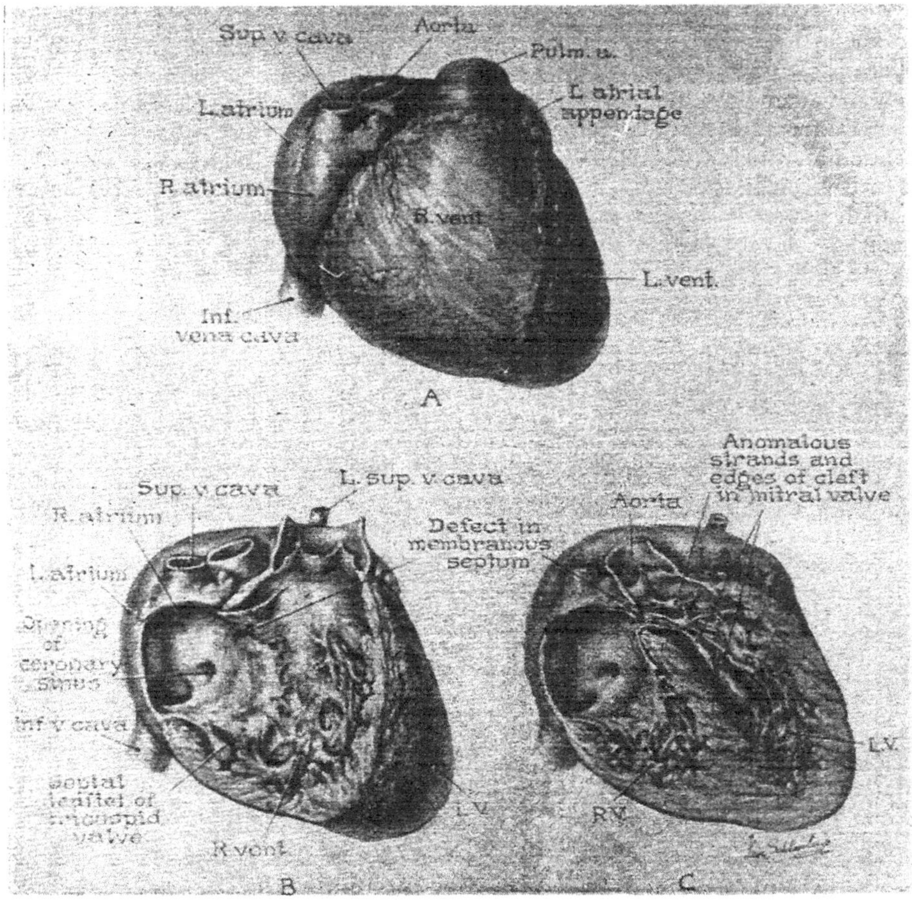

FIG. 5. Drawing of the heart in the case described by Ferencz. (Reproduced by permission of Bull. Johns Hopkins Hosp. **100**: 209, 1957.)

DR. EUGENE BRAUNWALD: Thank you very much for this most instructive discussion, Dr. Ross. In passing the catheter from the right atrium to the left, we didn't assume that it had passed across an atrial septal defect because the left atrium was so large and because there was a distinct pressure difference between the two atria. The possibility was considered that the catheter had been passed across a patent foramen ovale. Dr. Morrow operated upon this patient and I will ask him to describe the operative findings and the clinical course.

DR. ANDREW G. MORROW: I'm glad that we did not have to deal with the type of anomaly reported by Ferencz and which you discussed, Dr. Ross. Before the operation we were not certain of the exact diagnosis, but it seemed clear that mitral regurgitation was the dominant lesion and the one which should receive first consideration. For this reason we made a bilateral anterior thoracotomy so that we might approach any chamber of the heart and would also have optimal exposure of the left atrium.

The entire heart, as you might imagine, was enormous, and the left atrium was particularly prominent. It bulged out behind the right atrium and venae cavae, extending several centimeters beyond the border of the right chambers of the heart. The right atrium was also strikingly enlarged, and there was a faint systolic thrill over it. Over the exposed posterior portion of the left atrium, however, there was an intense systolic thrill.

The digital intracardiac exploration, through the right atrial appendage, was revealing. In the region of the foramen ovale I could feel no interatrial communication but low in the right atrium, immediately above the tricuspid annulus, was a tiny defect which would not admit my finger. Most strikingly, one could feel an intense systolic jet of blood impinging on the interatrial septum from the left side. There was also evidence of a moderate jet of tricuspid regurgitation.

When the cannulations and other preparations for bypass had been completed, I introduced my finger into the left atrium. I could reach the mitral valve only with some difficulty because of the size of the atrium but could easily feel an intense regurgitant jet of blood coming through it. By palpation the jet did not seem to be localized to a commissure but more to the central portion of the valve. We then went on bypass and opened the left atrium from the right side. When the blood had been evacuated we could see a small interatrial

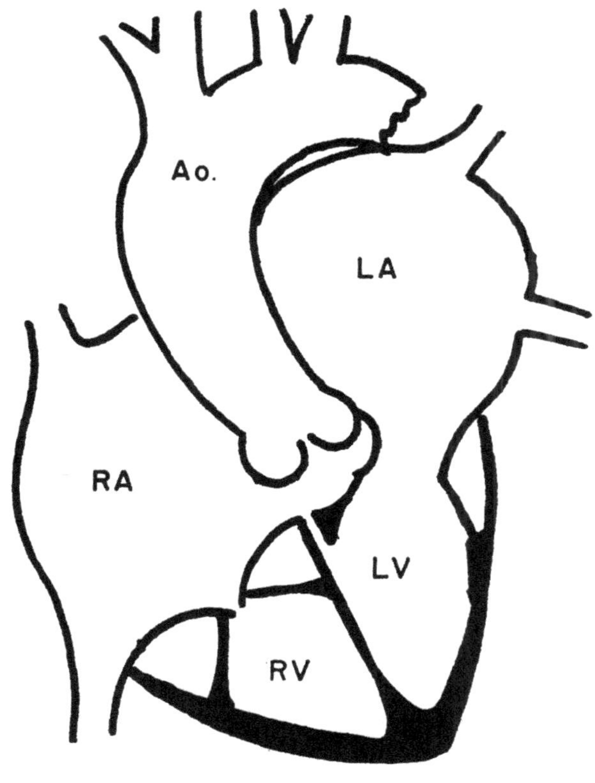

Fig. 6. Diagrammatic representation of the lesion in the case described by Ferencz.

communication which lay immediately above the atrioventricular ring. This was less than a centimeter in diameter. Coming through the opening from the right side was dark blood, the coronary return.

Inspection of the mitral valve revealed that the posterior or mural leaflet was somewhat thickened but was essentially normal. In the anterior or aortic leaflet of the mitral valve, however, there was a complete cleft which extended from the common endocardial cushion through the length of the valve to its free margin. The cleft was of the type typically seen in the partial form of persistent atrioventricular canal. We closed the interatrial septal defect from the left side

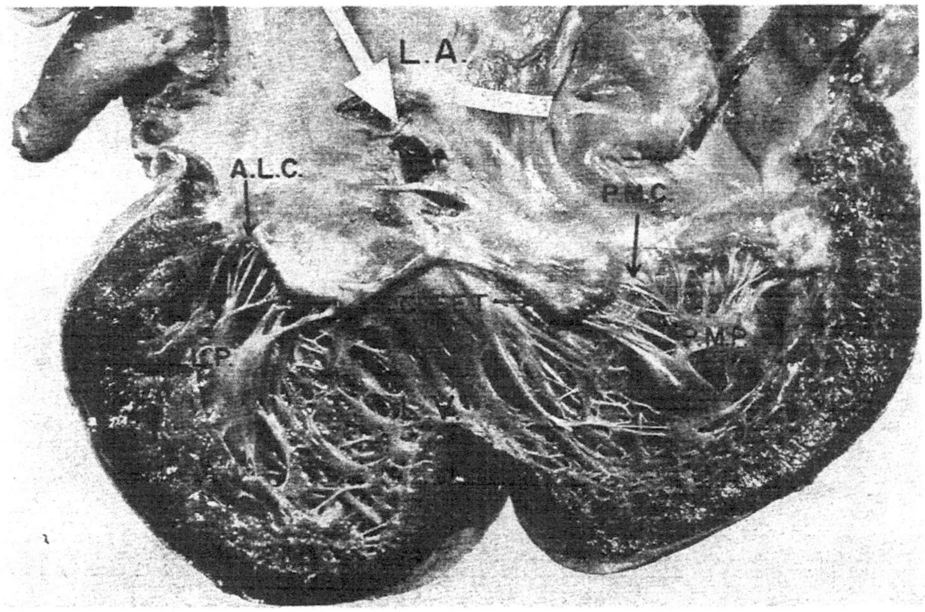

Fig. 7. The left atrium (L.A.), mitral valve, and left ventricle (L.V.) are opened. The left atrium is markedly dilated and the left ventricle is hypertrophied and dilated. The sutures closing the ostium primum defect (white arrow) have been removed. The defect is located at the apex of the cleft in the anterior mitral leaflet. The chordae tendineae extending to the anterolateral (A.L.P.) and posteromedial (P.M.P.) papillary muscles are normal. The anterolateral (A.L.C.) and posteromedial (P.M.C.) commissures are designated for orientation purposes.

with a few sutures and then approximated the valve cleft with a series of reinforced interrupted mattress sutures. After it had been repaired the valve seemed to be competent.

The left atriotomy was then closed and we opened the right atrium in order to inspect the tricuspid valve. There was obvious tricuspid regurgitation, but we could find no discrete lesion that seemed amenable to repair. There was no distinct cleft in any of the leaflets. The regurgitation through the tricuspid valve seemed to be coming from the commissure between the septal and posterior leaflets and it was felt that it might be corrected by an annuloplasty. This was performed with three or four mattress sutures placed through the annulus at the commissure described.

We then came off bypass and the child maintained his circulation well. There was still enlargement of the left atrium and it was quite tense, but we could not feel systolic thrill in the left atrium after the repair. The child did well during the day of operation and that night. On one occasion his blood pressure fell for no apparent reason, but it responded immediately to a single small dose of metaraminol. On the day following the operation, he was sitting up in bed. The nurse was having him cough to evacuate secretions. He did cough, and vigorously, and that moment he died. The resident was there and immediately

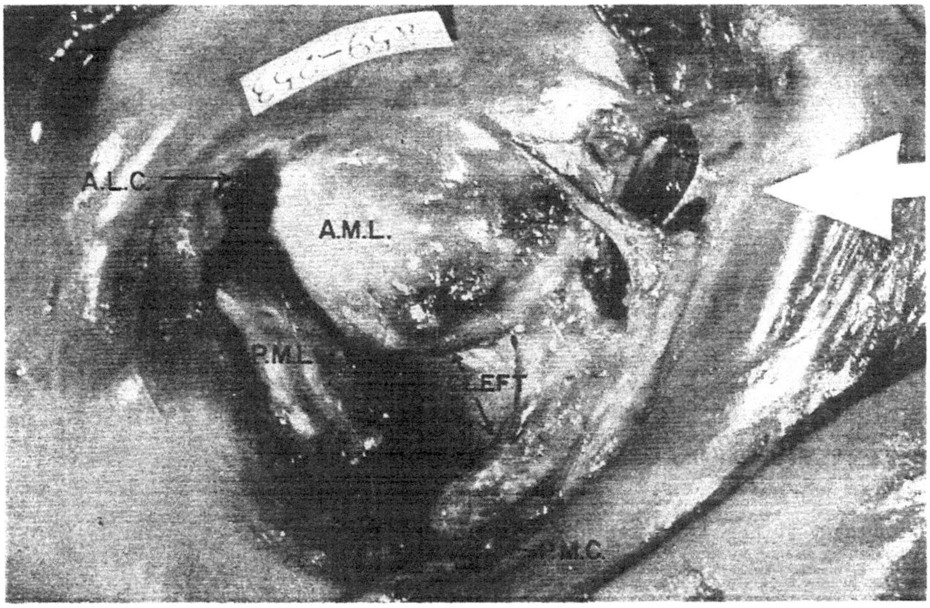

FIG. 8. The mitral valve viewed from the left atrium. The cleft in the anterior mitral leaflet (A.M.L.) is readily apparent. The small defect (white arrow) in the lowest portion of the atrial septum is located at the apex of the cleft. The posterior mitral leaflet (P.M.L.) is unremarkable. The posteromedial (P.M.C.) and the anterolateral (A.L.C.) commissures are evident.

opened the chest; the heart was found to be in arrest and could not be resuscitated.

DR. EUGENE BRAUNWALD: The pathologic findings will now be presented and discussed by Dr. Roberts.

DR. WILLIAM C. ROBERTS: The complete cleavage or cleft in the anterior or aortic leaflet of the mitral valve produced a wide-open canal between the left atrium and the left ventricle (Figures 7, 8). The mitral regurgitation led to extreme dilatation of the left atrium and to moderate hypertrophy and dilatation of the left ventricle. A small defect, measuring only 1 cm. in its largest diameter, was present in the lower portion of the atrial septum—a so-called ostium primum type atrial septal defect. In addition, the tricuspid valve was abnormal. Although there was no cleavage of its septal leaflet, the most superior portion of the septal leaflet was absent, and the remaining portion of this leaflet was shortened. These abnormalities prevented complete closure of the tricuspid valve during ventricular systole, and tricuspid regurgitation resulted. Other cardiovascular findings included anomalous chordae tendineae from the anterior leaflet of the mitral valve, a quadricuspid pulmonic valve, and moderate hypoplasia of the right coronary artery. The lungs were collapsed bilaterally; the liver and spleen showed marked changes of chronic passive congestion.

The normal mitral valve consists of two leaflets, the anterior, which is the larger and which is continuous with the aortic valve, and the posterior. Nor-

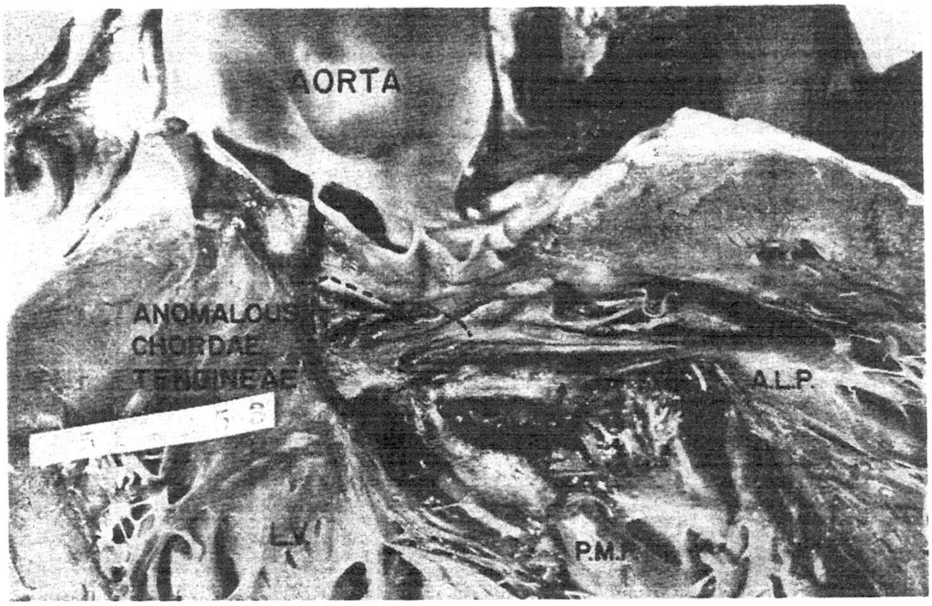

FIG. 9. The left ventricle (L.V.), aortic valve, and aorta are opened. The anomalous chordae tendineae, enclosed by the broken lines, extend from the anterior portion of the cleft anterior mitral leaflet to the crest of the ventricular septum immediately beneath the aortic valve cusps. The anterolateral (A.L.P.) and posteromedial (P.M.P.) papillary muscles are labeled.

mally, chordae tendineae from the margins of each of the two leaflets insert only into the two papillary muscles of the left ventricle. In the patient under discussion the anterior mitral leaflet was divided by the cleft into two halves, which may be designated "anterior" and "posterior." Chordae tendineae not only inserted into the two papillary muscles of the left ventricle, but chordae from the "anterior" portion of the anterior mitral leaflet also inserted into the crest of the muscular ventricular septum immediately beneath the aortic valve (Figure 9). These thickened and fused anomalous chordae, which have no counterpart in the normal heart, are always present when there is a cleft anterior mitral leaflet. They are important because, as emphasized by Edwards,[8] if they are not divided at the time the cleft is repaired, some mitral insufficiency will invariably remain. Caution must be exerted by the surgeon, however, when cutting these accessory chordae in order not to lacerate an aortic valve cusp or perforate the membranous ventricular septum. In addition, as already stressed by Dr. Ross, these anomalous chordae may interfere with the outflow of blood from the left ventricle and thus produce a form of subaortic stenosis.

A cleft anterior mitral valve and an ostium primum defect, both of which were present in this patient, are two of the components of the complex anomaly

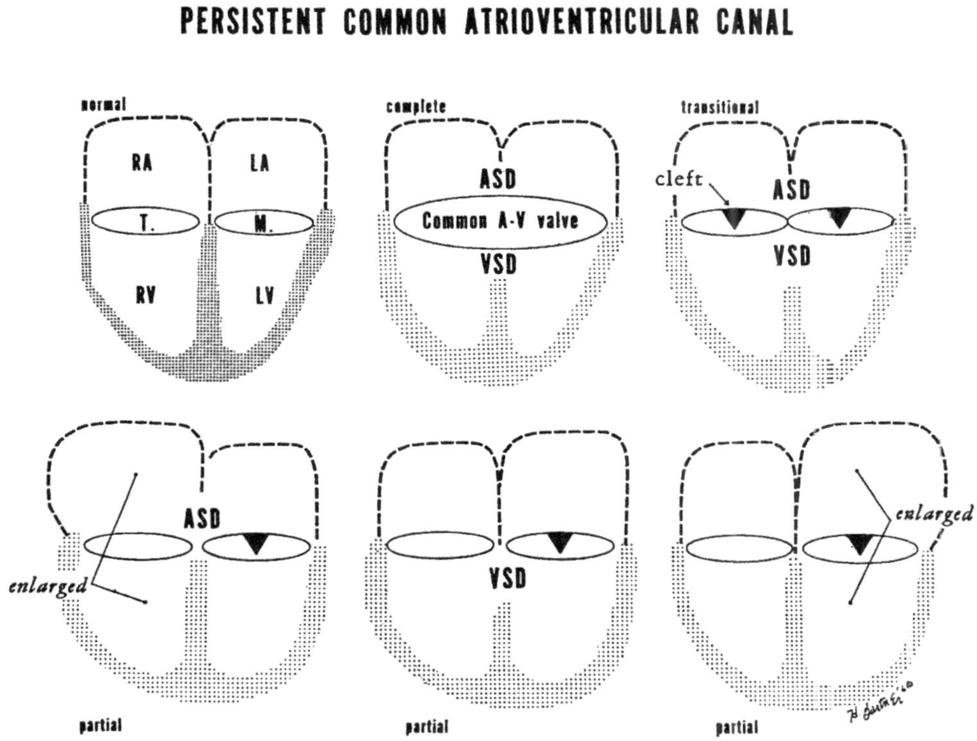

FIG. 10. Diagrammatic representation of various forms of persistent common AV canal. RA, right atrium, LA, left atrium, RV, right ventricle, LV, left ventricle; T, tricuspid valve ring; M, mitral valve ring; ASD, atrial septal defect; VSD, ventricular septal defect.

variously termed persistent common atrioventricular canal, atrioventricularis communis, and endocardial cushion defect. Persistent common atrioventricular canal has been divided by Wakai and Edwards[9,10] into three forms: complete, transitional or intermediate, and partial (Figure 10). In the complete form there is only one valve common to both sides of the heart; an atrial septal defect of the ostium primum type and a high ventricular septal defect are also present. In the transitional form (Figure 10, upper right diagram) the common valve meets in the midline, forming two atrioventricular valves. A cleft is present in the septal leaflet of the tricuspid valve as well as in the anterior leaflet of the mitral valve. The partial forms (Figure 10, lower diagrams) are characterized by the presence of a cleft in the anterior mitral valve and by the absence of a cleft in the tricuspid valve, although portions of the latter may be shortened or absent.

The patient under discussion had a cleft mitral valve and an atrial septal defect (Figure 10, lower left diagram). Since the atrial septal defect in this patient was extremely small, however, the "run-off" through the defect was likewise small, and consequently (as illustrated in Figure 10, lower right diagram) left atrial dilatation and left ventricular hypertrophy occurred, rather than right atrial and right ventricular enlargement.

In the 109 specimens with congenital malformations of the heart and great vessels in the pathologic collection of the Clinical Center, there are 12 instances of persistent common AV canal (Table 2). The subject of this conference is case 12. The age range of these 12 patients is nine months to 54 years. The partial form of AV canal was the most common. The complete type, the most frequent in most series, was absent. The anterior mitral valve was cleft in all but two patients. In contrast, the septal tricuspid valve was cleft in only one patient and normal in only two. In eight, there was either partial or total absence of the septal leaflet. When the ventricular septal defects were present, they were quite small, except in two patients. The two patients with the large ventricular septal defects had no ostium primum type atrial septal defect, but did have cleft anterior mitral valves. It is not necessary for an ostium primum type atrial septal defect to be present in order that the diagnosis of persistent common atrioventricular canal be made. The one anatomic feature noted in all patients listed in Table 2 is the presence of anomalous chordae tendineae from the mitral valve to the ventricular septum (Figure 9). I therefore consider anomalous chordae tendineae to be a hallmark of the complex anomaly of persistent common atrioventricular canal. Thus, the patient described by Ferencz[7] and discussed by Dr. Ross may perhaps be considered to have had an unusual form of the persistent common atrioventricular canal.

A patent foramen ovale was present in eight of the 12 patients whom we have examined. In three of these eight cases the valve guarding the foramen was incompetent. Of special note is the presence of right ventricular hypertrophy in all patients in this series, except case 12, the patient under discussion, who had isolated left ventricular hypertrophy.

Dr. Eugene Braunwald: The unusual anatomic features presented by this patient and discussed by Drs. Roberts and Morrow were responsible for the clinical and hemodynamic findings which are unusual for patients with the partial form of persistent AV canal. The majority of these patients have a large atrial septal defect and a mild or moderate degree of mitral regurgitation. Clinically, although they present with a loud pansystolic apical murmur they usually have only mild left atrial and left ventricular enlargement. In general the lung fields are plethoric on roentgenograms of the chest and these patients have all of the other clinical features associated with a large left-to-right shunt and increased pulmonary blood flow. The electrocardiograms usually show more marked left axis deviation of the terminal forces than our patient did. In addition, there is evidence of "right ventricular diastolic overload," i.e., an RSR′ configuration in right precordial leads. The absence of this feature in our patient may reasonably be attributed to the small left-to-right shunt and the only slightly augmented right ventricular output (Figure 1). The prolonged PR interval, which our patient exhibited on several EKGs prior to the development of atrial fibrillation, could have been a clue to the diagnosis since this finding is common in patients with AV canal.

TABLE 2

A Summary of the Anatomic Features in 12 Patients with Persistent Common Atrioventricular Canal Studied at the Clinical Center

Case	Age / Sex, Race	Type	Mitral Valve* (Ant. leaf.)	Tricuspid Valve (Septal leaf.)	VSD	Ostium Primum Defect	Patent Foramen Ovale	Cardio-megaly	Associated Anomalies
1. A54–66	9 mo. / N F	Partial	Cleft	Absent (partial)	+ (minute)	+	+	RVH	0
2. A56–111	17 mo. / W M	Partial	Short	Absent (partial)	+ (minute)	+	+	RVH	0
3. A57–117	26 / W F	Partial	Cleft	Normal	0	+	+ (valv. incomp.)	RVH	0
4. A57–184	14 / W F	Partial	Cleft	Absent (partial)	0	+	+ (valv. incomp.)	RVH	0
5. A57–195	42 / N M	Partial	Cleft	Absent (partial)	0	+	0	RVH	0
6. A57–226	2 / W F	Trans.	Cleft	Cleft	+ (small)	+	+	RVH LVH	Mongolism
7. A59–12	23 / W M	Partial	Cleft	Absent	+ (minute)	+	+ (valv. incomp.)	RVH	Rt. PV→RA† LSCV→CS‡
8. A59–207	54 / W F	Partial	Cleft (partial)	Absent	0	+	+	RVH	CS→LA§
9. A60–41	13 / W F	Partial	Cleft (partial)	Normal	+ (large)	0	+	RVH	0
10. A60–84	13 / W F	Partial	No cleft	Anomalous‖ chordae	+ (large)	0	0	RVH LVH	LSVC→CS‡ Bicuspid pul. valve
11. A60–276	31 / W F	Partial	Cleft	Absent (partial)	0	+ (small)	0	RVH LVH	0
12. A59–253	14 / N M	Partial	Cleft	Absent (partial)	0	+ (small)	0	LVH	0

*All patients had anomalous chordae tendineae from the mitral valve to the ventricular septum.

†Rt. PV→RA: The right pulmonary veins drained only into the right atrium.

‡LSCV→CS: A left superior vena cava drained into the coronary sinus.

§CS→LA: The coronary sinus drained only into the left atrium. The right atrial ostium of the coronary sinus was atretic.

‖Double orifice, tricuspid valve.

The clinical findings in this patient, and in one other patient with identical anatomic findings, were those of massive mitral regurgitation; there was a prominent apical holosystolic murmur which was transmitted well into the axilla and over the precordium. Prominent left ventricular lifts were palpable. The roentgenographic findings were of left atrial enlargement rather than of increased pulmonary blood flow. Since the atrial septal defect was very small it could not adequately decompress the left atrium, and a pressure gradient between these two chambers was present throughout the cardiac cycle, particularly during ventricular systole when a large V wave was present in the left atrial pressure pulse; the latter was related to massive mitral regurgitation and is not usually present in patients with mitral regurgitation and a large atrial septal defect.

I shall now ask Dr. Morrow to discuss some of the surgical considerations in persistent AV canal.

Dr. Andrew G. Morrow: From the standpoint of making a decision as to whether a given child or adult with a variety of AV canal should be operated upon, I think that one important consideration is whether the lesion is the complete, the transitional, or the partial form of the anomaly. In other words, if one has to deal only with a cleft anterior leaflet of the mitral valve and to close an interatrial communication, a completely corrective operation can be carried out with an acceptable risk. In a child or a young adult who presents with these findings and no other contraindications we now recommend that operation be undertaken electively, regardless of the presence or absence of symptoms. Our feeling about operation is somewhat less optimistic when the complete form of AV canal is present and there is an associated large interventricular communication. The bundle of His lies immediately under the endocardium, on top of the ventricular septum, and the difficulty in repairing a complete persistent canal is to close the interventricular communication without producing complete heart block. This complication has unfortunately occurred in a large percentage of such patients who were operated upon.

In a patient such as the one described today, i.e., one who presents with the primary problem of mitral regurgitation but in whom a shunt into the right atrium is also present, another problem presents itself. First, it is difficult, I think, to be certain before operation that the patient does not have a small atrial septal defect of the ostium secundum type and a mitral valve which is not congenitally cleft but which has been damaged in another fashion, as by rheumatic fever. The importance of this differential diagnosis is that, in general, a cleft mitral valve can be repaired without undue difficulty and a competent valve can be established. On the other hand, the problem of the treatment of rheumatic mitral regurgitation, at this time in our unenlightenment, remains an extremely difficult one.

I feel that one of the reasons this child died may have been the fact that Edwards, at the time of the operation, had not yet published his article about the abnormal chordae tendineae which are present in AV canal.[8] He points out, on morphologic grounds, that if one does not divide these abnormal chordae, although the anterior leaflet is reconstituted, the chordae may restrict the motion of the valve and hold it down in the left ventricle during ventricular systole. Thus even though the leaflet itself appears competent there still may be significant mitral regurgitation. At the time of the operation we were unaware of the existence or the importance of these structures. Perhaps if we had done a more effective repair the child might have survived.

Dr. Eugene Braunwald: It is technically simpler to close the atrial septal defect than it is to restore complete competency to the mitral valve in patients with the lesion which our patient presented. If this occurs the patient can actually be made worse by operation, since the atrial defect does serve as a type of escape valve for the distended left atrium. In the other patient with this malformation whom we have encountered, the pulmonary artery pressure prior to operation was 22/8 mm. Hg. Following operation, the defect remained closed but mitral regurgitation persisted, the pulmonary artery pressure rose to 54/20 mm. Hg, and the patient required a second operation.

Dr. Ross, do you have any further comments?

Dr. Richard S. Ross: Do you think that the anomalous chordae produced left ventricular outflow obstruction in this case? If they did, and if the mitral valve were repaired but the left ventricular outflow obstruction were allowed to remain, a satisfactory result could not be anticipated.

Dr. Eugene Braunwald: At the time of the left ventricular catheterization there was no gradient between the left ventricle and the aorta; therefore there is little hemodynamic evidence that the chordae interfered with left ventricular ejection.

Dr. Richard S. Ross: I see. I think I erred in making the categorical assumption that the atrial septum might be intact to explain the giant left atrium. In general this is true, but, as has been pointed out, the atrial size is more a function of the ratio of the magnitude of mitral regurgitation to the size of the atrial septal defect. If there is a lot of mitral regurgitation and a small atrial septal defect, there can be a large left atrium.

Question: How can one differentiate preoperatively the lesion which this patient presented from that described by Dr. Ferencz?

Dr. Eugene Braunwald: Since we have not encountered the latter anomaly I can only speculate: (1) A selective left ventricular angiocardiogram or preferably a selective cine-angiogram with left ventricular injection would show immediate opacification of both atria, while this type of study in our patient would show left atrial opacification prior to right atrial opacification. The value of selective left ventricular angiocardiography in the differential diagnosis of the various forms of persistent common AV canal and of related anomalies has recently been discussed elsewhere in detail.[11] (2) The anomalous chordae in Ferencz' patient presumably resulted in a pressure gradient between the left ventricle and the aorta. This did not occur in our patient. (3) A cardiac catheter could be passed from the right to the left atrium in our patient, but this would not be possible in Ferencz' patient, who had an intact interatrial septum.

Question: What was the cause of the diastolic rumbling murmur at the apex? There was no evidence of mitral stenosis at autopsy.

Dr. Eugene Braunwald: In patients with pure mitral regurgitation of large degree a diastolic rumbling murmur is frequently audible at the apex. This is related to the flow of abnormally large volumes of blood from the left atrium to the left ventricle during diastole.

Summario in Interlingua

Le patiente esseva un puero de 13 annos de etate in qui—al etate de sex annos, durante le curso de un maladia febril—un forte murmure systolic apical e cardiomegalia habeva essite constatate. In le curso del sequente annos, ille esseva hospitalisate repetitemente a causa de congestive disfallimento cardiac. Le examine physic monstrava pulsante venas in le collo, un allargate hepate, e un forte e findite secunde sono cardiac in le area pulmonal. Forte murmures systolic e diastolic esseva audibile al apice. Le electrocardiogramma revelava fibrillation atrial e deviation axial al sinistra. Le catheterismo cardiac monstrava hypertension systolic dextero-ventricular, un micre derivation sinistro-dextere que entrava in le atrio dextere, alte undas V in le pulso de pression sinistro-atrial, e un distincte gradiente de pression inter le duo atrios. Le diagnose differential inter iste lesion e regurgitation mitral in le pueritia es discutite in detalio.

Al operation il esseva trovate que le patiente habeva un micre defecto atrio-septal del typo de atrio prime e un complete scission in le lobo anterior del valvula mitral. Le duo lesiones esseva reparate, sed le patiente moriva le die post le operation.

Es discutite le aspectos anatomic, pathologic, e clinic de persistente canal atrio-ventricular.

BIBLIOGRAPHY

1. Braunwald, E., Morrow, A. G.: Left ventriculo-right atrial communication. Amer. J. Med. **28**: 913–920, 1960.
2. Anderson, R. C., Lillehei, C. W., Lester, R. G.: Corrected transposition of the great vessels of the heart. A review of 17 cases. Pediatrics **20**: 626–646, 1957.
3. Taussig, H. B.: Congenital malformations of the heart. Rev. Ed., Harvard University Press, Cambridge, Mass., 1960.
4. Sanders, R. J., Morrow, A. G.: The identification and quantification of left-to-right circulatory shunts: a new diagnostic method utilizing the inhalation of a radioactive gas, Kr^{85}. Amer. J. Med. **26**: 508–516, 1959.
5. Ross, J., Jr., Braunwald, E., Morrow, A. G.. Left heart catheterization by the trans-septal route. A description of the technic and its applications. Circulation **22**: 927–934, 1960.
6. Bashour, F. A., Simmons, D. H.: Atrial septal defect with mitral valvulitis: clinical and catheterization diagnosis. Ann. Intern. Med. **48**: 1194–1204, 1958.
7. Ferencz, C.: Atrioventricular defect of the membranous septum. Left ventricular-right atrial communication with malformed mitral valve simulating aortic stenosis. Report of a case. Bull. Johns Hopkins Hosp. **100**: 209–222, 1957.
8. Edwards, J. E.: The problem of mitral insufficiency caused by accessory chordae tendineae in persistent common atrioventricular canal. Proc. Mayo Clin. **35**: 299–305, 1960.
9. Wakai, C. S., Edwards, J. E.: Developmental and pathologic considerations in persistent common atrioventricular canal. Proc. Mayo Clin. **31**: 487–500, 1956.
10. Wakai, C. S., Edwards, J. E.: Pathologic study of persistent common atrioventricular canal. Amer. Heart J. **56**: 779–794, 1958.
11. Braunwald, E., Morrow, A. G., Cooper, T.: Left ventricular angiocardiography in the diagnosis of persistent atrioventricular canal and related anomalies. Amer. J. Cardiol. **4**: 802–808, 1959.

Partial persistent atrioventricular canal simulating pure mitral regurgitation

Edwin C. Brockenbrough, M.D.
Eugene Braunwald, M.D.
William C. Roberts, M.D.
Andrew G. Morrow, M.D.
Bethesda, Md.

The two principal anatomic malformations which comprise the partial or incomplete form of persistent atrioventricular (A-V) canal are an interatrial septal defect of the ostium primum variety and a cleft in the anterior leaflet of the mitral valve. The atrial septal defect is usually large, and the predominant functional abnormality is the left-to-right shunt at the atrial level. In addition, the cleft mitral leaflet generally produces valvular regurgitation of minimal to moderate severity. In such patients the interatrial defect serves to decompress the left atrium and prevents elevation of left atrial pressure and marked enlargement of this chamber. We have had the opportunity, however, to study two patients with partial persistent A-V canal who were initially considered to have mitral regurgitation of rheumatic origin, and who, only after detailed study, were shown to have small interatrial communications. A description of the clinical, hemodynamic, and pathologic findings in the patients with this unusual variant of A-V canal forms the subject of this report.

Clinical summaries

Case 1 (02-74-33). T. A. was a 13-year-old schoolboy whose growth and development had been slow throughout his life. He was not examined by a physician until he was 6 years old, at which time he was hospitalized for 4 months because of fever and tachypnea, and was found to have apical systolic and diastolic murmurs and an enlarged heart. He was considered to have acute rheumatic fever. After this illness he was unable to play actively without excessive fatigue, but he attended school. Between the ages of 11 and 13 years the patient was hospitalized on four additional occasions, once because of fever and abdominal pain and other times because of left-sided and right-sided heart failure. Determinations of C-reactive protein and antistreptolysin titers were always normal. Cardiac examinations always revealed the systolic and diastolic murmurs. Electrocardiograms taken when he was in sinus rhythm showed P-R prolongation when corrected for heart rate, but after he was 12 years old, atrial fibrillation was present. In November, 1959, he was admitted to the National Heart Institute because of persistent dyspnea and orthopnea.

Physical examination showed that the patient was a small, poorly developed, and cachectic child who weighed only 24 kilograms and appeared to be chronically ill. The blood pressure was 110/87 mm. Hg, and the pulse was grossly irregular. The neck veins were dilated and showed large systolic pulsations. There was a prominent precordial bulge, a striking left ventricular lift, and a modest right ventricular lift. The second sound over the pulmonic area was palpable, and on auscultation was split, with a loud pulmonic component. The split remained fixed, even during the Valsalva maneuver. A Grade 3/6 pansystolic murmur was best heard at the apex but was well transmitted over the entire precordium. At the lower left sternal border there appeared to

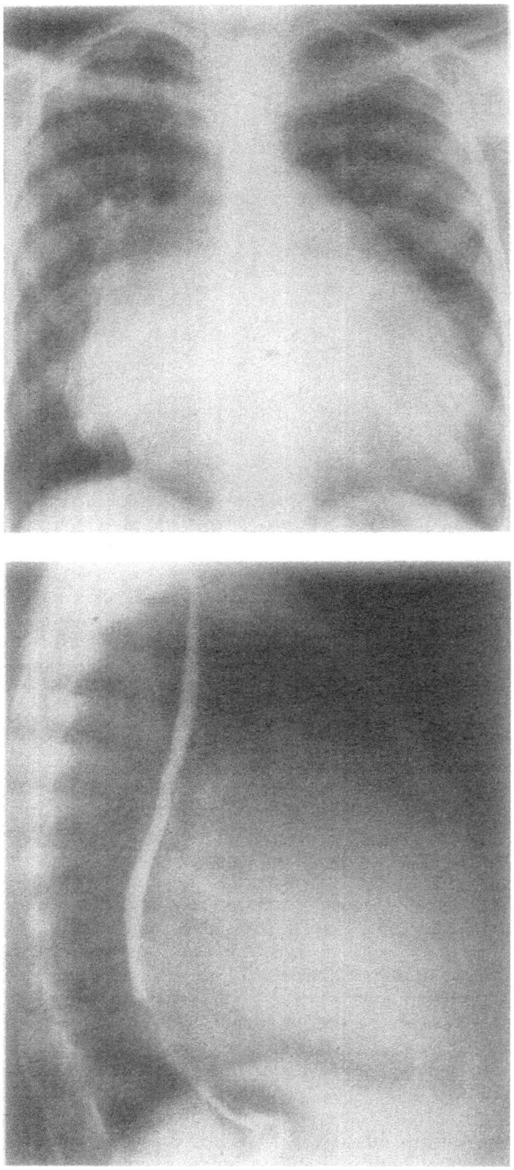

Fig. *1.* Chest roentgenograms in the posteroanterior (*top*) and lateral (*bottom*) projections in Patient T. A.

be a separate systolic murmur which increased with inspiration. An early diastolic sound, which was followed by a Grade 3/6 mid-diastolic rumbling murmur, was also heard at the apex. The liver was enlarged to below the level of the umbilicus; there was no peripheral edema.

Cardiac fluoroscopy and radiography demonstrated massive enlargement of the heart, with particular prominence of both right and left atria (Fig. 1). The pulmonary vascularity was not increased. The electrocardiogram (Fig. 2) revealed atrial fibrillation, left axis deviation, digitalis effect, and left ventricular hypertrophy. On the basis of the foregoing findings, observers considered the patient to have rheumatic mitral regurgitation.

At cardiac catheterization the right ventricular pressure was elevated to 55/15 mm. Hg, and the pulmonary artery could not be entered. The tip of the catheter repeatedly refluxed from the right ventricle into the right atrium, which indicated the presence of tricuspid regurgitation. The mean pressure in the right atrium was 13 mm. Hg, and the v waves peaked at 17 mm. Hg. Surprisingly, the catheter passed into the left atrium through an interatrial communication. The peaks of the v waves in this chamber were 27 mm. Hg, and the mean pressure was 15 mm. Hg. A Kr^{85}-inhalation test[1] demonstrated that a small left-to-right shunt entered the right atrium, and the calculated pulmonary-systemic flow ratio was 1.4/1.0. A selective left ventricular angiocardiogram demonstrated massive mitral regurgitation and, also, opacification of the right atrium from the left.

With the additional information provided by the hemodynamic studies it appeared likely that the patient had congenital heart disease—an ostium primum defect with cleft mitral and tricuspid valves. At operation there was massive enlargement of both atria and a systolic thrill in each. After the institution of cardiopulmonary bypass a left atriotomy was made (Fig. 3). There was a complete cleft in the anterior leaflet of the mitral valve, and a small ostium primum interatrial defect which was less than 1 cm. in diameter. The thickened margins of the cleft were approximated with interrupted sutures, and the defect was closed similarly. The valve appeared to be competent after the repair. Inspection of the tricuspid valve after right atriotomy revealed that regurgitation of blood was occurring between the anterior and septal leaflets. No discrete cleft in either leaflet could be discerned, and the tricuspid annulus was plicated in this area. After operation the general condition of the patient was poor, and on the day after the procedure, cardiac arrest occurred and resuscitation was unsuccessful.

PATHOLOGIC FINDINGS. The heart weighed 350 grams, and the left atrium was greatly enlarged (Fig 4). The surgically closed mitral cleft extended from the mid-portion of the free margin of the anterior leaflet to the annulus, dividing the leaflet into anterior and posterior halves. The chordae tendineae from the anterior portion of the cleft leaflet, in addition to inserting normally into the anterolateral papillary muscle of the left ventricle, also inserted into the superior ridge of the muscular ventricular septum (Fig. 5). The accessory chordae tendineae to the ventricular septum were thickened, shortened, and adherent to one another. They did not appear to interfere with the outflow of blood from the left ventricle. The chordae tendineae from the posterior portion of the anterior mitral leaflet inserted normally into the posteromedial papillary muscle. The left ventricle was hypertrophied and dilated. Although no ventricular septal defect was present, the membranous portion of the septum was thickened and malformed. The ostia of both coronary arteries were located in the sinus of Valsalva behind the right anterior aortic cusp; the right coronary artery was markedly hypoplastic but the left was normal. Both the aortic ring and

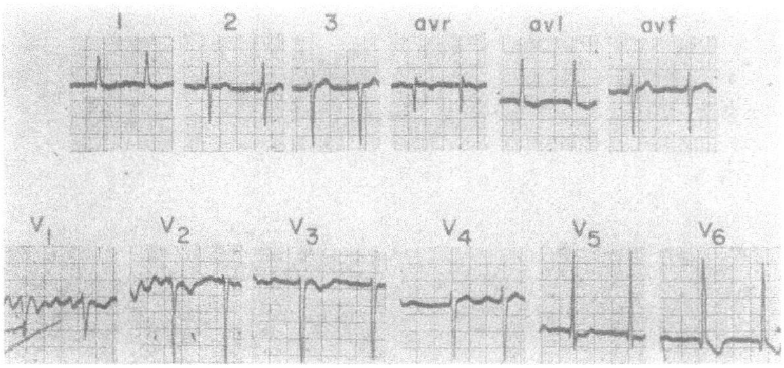

Fig. 2. Electrocardiogram of Patient T. A.

the ascending aorta were small. The right atrium was moderately dilated, and the foramen ovale was closed. The tricuspid chordae tendineae, although delicate, were extremely short and few in number. There was no cleft in any tricuspid leaflet, but a portion of the septal leaflet adjacent to the anterior leaflet was absent. This malformation probably accounted for the tricuspid regurgitation which had been present. The small interatrial communication was located immediately above the absent portion of the septal leaflet. The pulmonic valve, in addition to three normal cusps, contained a fourth rudimentary one.

Case 2 (00-98-43). N. R., a 31-year-old woman, was known to have had heart disease since the age of 12 years, when she was thought to have had acute rheumatic fever. She was given digitalis in her late teens because of recurrent episodes of paroxysmal atrial tachycardia. Aside from mild exertional dyspnea, however, she felt well and completed a pregnancy at the age of 19 years without difficulty. When she was 27 years old, she developed atrial fibrillation and experienced exertional dyspnea and fatigability. Over the next 4 years these symptoms progressed and she developed signs of congestive heart failure.

On admission to the National Heart Institute she was found to be thin and anxious and appeared to be dyspneic at rest. Her blood pressure was 110/60 mm. Hg, and the peripheral pulse was grossly irregular. The jugular venous pulse exhibited prominent v waves. Both right and left ventricular lifts were present. In addition to an apical systolic thrill there was a Grade 4/6 pansystolic murmur, loudest at the apex and transmitted well into the axilla. A prominent third heart sound was followed by a short low-pitched apical diastolic rumbling murmur. At the left sternal border there was a Grade 4/6 pansystolic murmur accompanied by a high-pitched mid-diastolic murmur, which increased in intensity with inspiration. In the pulmonic area there was a short ejection murmur, and the second sound was accentuated and maintained a fixed split throughout the respiratory cycle. The liver was enlarged to 5 cm. below the right costal margin and expanded with cardiac systole. Mild pitting edema of the ankles was present.

The sedimentation rate was normal and the C-reactive protein was negative. Roentgenologic examinations demonstrated moderate cardiac enlargement with prominence of the left atrium and left ventricle (Fig. 6). The pulmonary vascularity appeared to be normal and no valvular calcifications were seen. The electrocardiogram revealed atrial fibrillation, left ventricular hypertrophy, and digitalis effect (Fig. 7). The patient was considered to have rheumatic heart disease with mitral and tricuspid regurgitation. At cardiac catheterization the pulmonary arterial (22/8 mm. Hg) and right ventricular (24/5 mm. Hg) pressures were normal. The catheter unexpectedly crossed from the right atrium to the left, and the mean pressure in each chamber was 4 mm. Hg. A Kr^{85}-inhalation test confirmed the presence of a left-to-right shunt which entered the right atrium, and the calculated pulmonary-systemic flow ratio was 1.7/1. Indicator-dilution curves demonstrated that the shunt originated from the left ventricle. In order to exclude the possibility of an associated ventricular septal defect, a selective angiocardiogram with left ventricular injection was

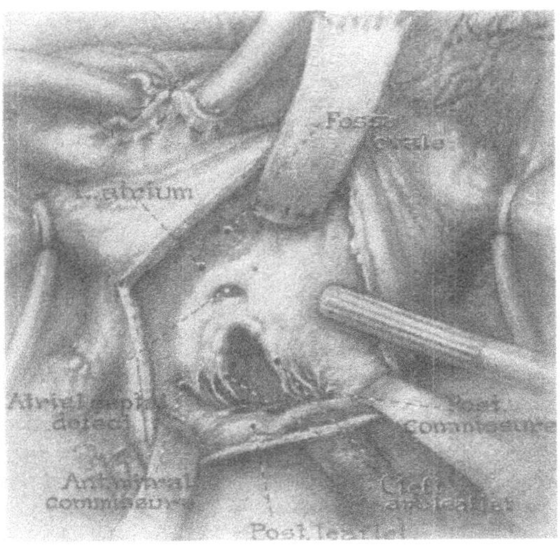

Fig. 3. The completely cleft anterior mitral valve leaflet and small interatrial communication encountered after cardiotomy.

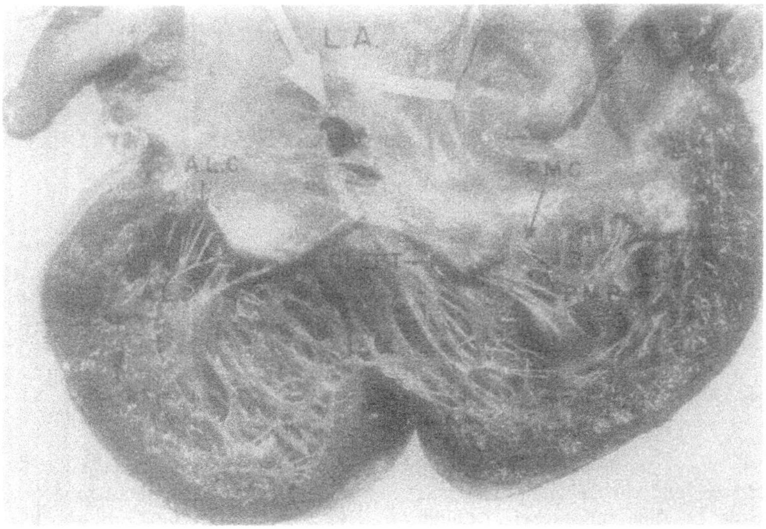

Fig. 4. Autopsy appearance of the heart of Patient T. A. The left atrium (*L. A.*), mitral valve, and left ventricle (*L. V.*) are shown. The left atrium is markedly dilated, and the left ventricle is hypertrophied and dilated. The sutures which close the small ostium primum defect (*white arrow*) have been removed. The defect is located at the apex of the cleft in the anterior mitral leaflet. The chordae tendineae which extend to the anterolateral (*A. L. P.*) and posteromedial (*P. M. P.*) papillary muscles are normal. The anterolateral (*A. L. C.*) and posteromedial (*P. M. C.*) commissures are designated for orientation purposes.

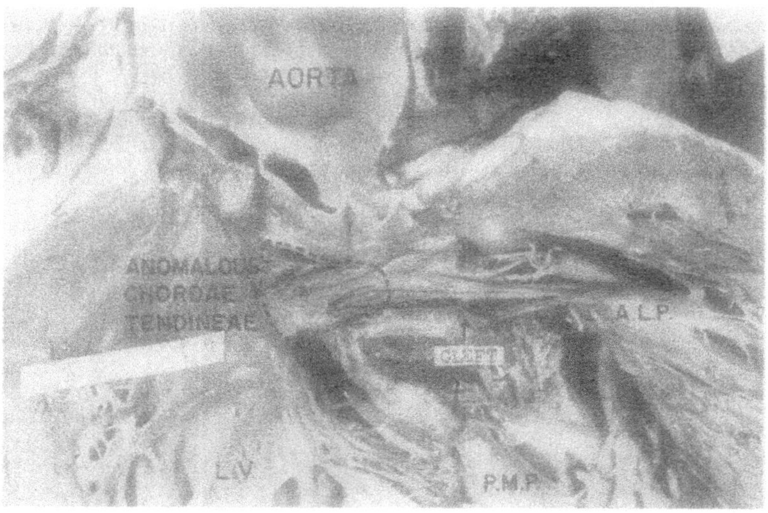

Fig. 5. The left ventricle (*L. V.*), aortic valve, and aorta of Patient T. A. Anomalous chordae tendineae (*demarcated by the broken line*) are seen to extend from the anterior portion of the cleft anterior mitral leaflet to the crest of the ventricular septum immediately beneath the aortic valve cusps. The anterolateral (*A. L. P.*) and posteromedial (*P. M. P.*) papillary muscles are labeled.

carried out.[2] This demonstrated severe mitral regurgitation into an enlarged left atrium, opacification of the right atrium through an interatrial septal defect, and an intact ventricular septum (Fig. 8). These findings were considered to support the diagnosis of ostium primum defect with a cleft mitral valve, although the possibility of an ostium secundum defect with rheumatic mitral regurgita-

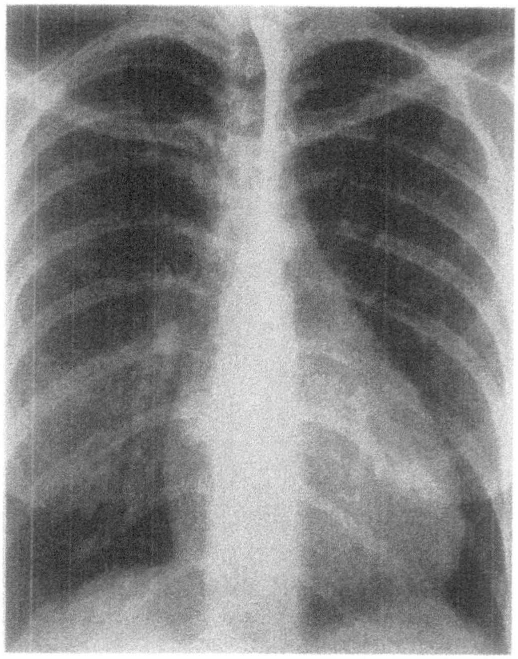

Fig. *6*. Preoperative chest roentgenogram in the posteroanterior projection in Patient N. R.

tion could not be excluded. At operation a right atriotomy was made and a small crescent-shaped defect, which measured 1 by 2 cm. in diameter, was found in the lowermost portion of the interatrial septum. When the superior margin of the defect was retracted upward, a complete cleft in the anterior leaflet of the mitral valve was revealed. This was repaired with continuous sutures in two layers. The interatrial defect was then closed with a prosthetic patch. The patient tolerated the operation well and made a satisfactory recovery.

After discharge the patient felt that she was improved and was able to return to part-time employment in a sedentary job. After 3 months, however, she began to develop increasingly severe exertional dyspnea and was again troubled with retention of fluid. Signs of congestive heart failure progressed over the next several months and she was rehospitalized in July, 1959. The systolic murmur in the tricuspid area now had a loud, cooing quality and became strikingly accentuated with inspiration. The pulmonic second sound moved normally with respiration. The other auscultatory findings were similar to those of her preoperative examination. The liver, which had become further enlarged to 12 cm. below the right costal margin, was firm and pulsatile, and a small amount of ascitic fluid was present. The chest roentgenogram revealed a considerable increase in the size of the left atrium (Fig. 9). The electrocardiogram again showed atrial fibrillation, left ventricular hypertrophy, and digitalis effect.

The patient underwent right heart and transbronchial left heart catheterization. The pulmonary arterial pressure was now elevated to 54/20 mm. Hg, and the right atrial pressure tracing exhibited the contour characteristic of tricuspid regurgitation. The right atrial mean pressure was 12 mm. Hg. There was no evidence of a residual shunt. The left atrial mean pressure was 27 mm. Hg, and the v waves were 55 mm. Hg (Fig. 10). There was a mean diastolic gradient of 10 mm. Hg across the mitral valve.

Because of the deterioration in the condition of the patient, and the evidence of significant mitral and tricuspid regurgitation, it was thought that a second attempt at surgical correction was indicated. At operation there was an intense systolic thrill within the left atrium, which was large and tense. Inspection, through a left atriotomy, revealed that the cleft in the anterior leaflet had been incompletely repaired. The residual valvular cleft, which was about 2.5 cm. in length, was closed with interrupted mattress sutures. After completion of the repair the valve appeared to be competent but somewhat stenotic. The anterolateral commissure, which was apparently fused, was incised to yield an orifice which would accept two fingers with ease.

The patient's convalescence was complicated by a massive hemorrhage from the upper gastrointestinal tract on the sixth postoperative day. After a partial gastrectomy for a bleeding prepyloric ulcer, she recovered satisfactorily. She continued to have evidence of mitral regurgitation, however, and remained severely limited after her discharge. Eight months later she died in chronic congestive heart failure.

PATHOLOGIC FINDINGS. At necropsy the heart was found to be enlarged; it weighed 470 grams. All chambers were dilated and hypertrophied. The

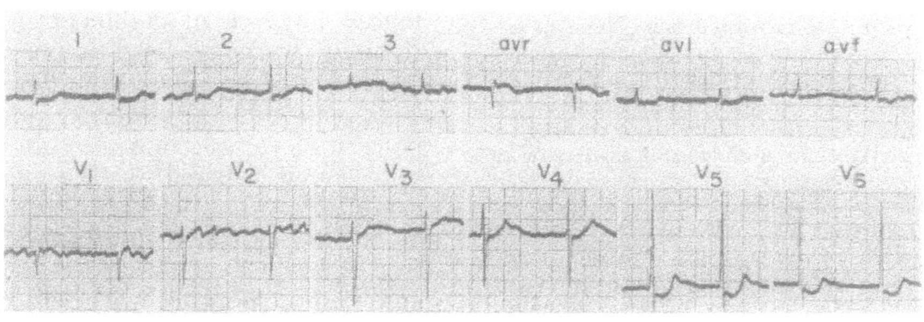

Fig. 7. The electrocardiogram of Patient N. R.

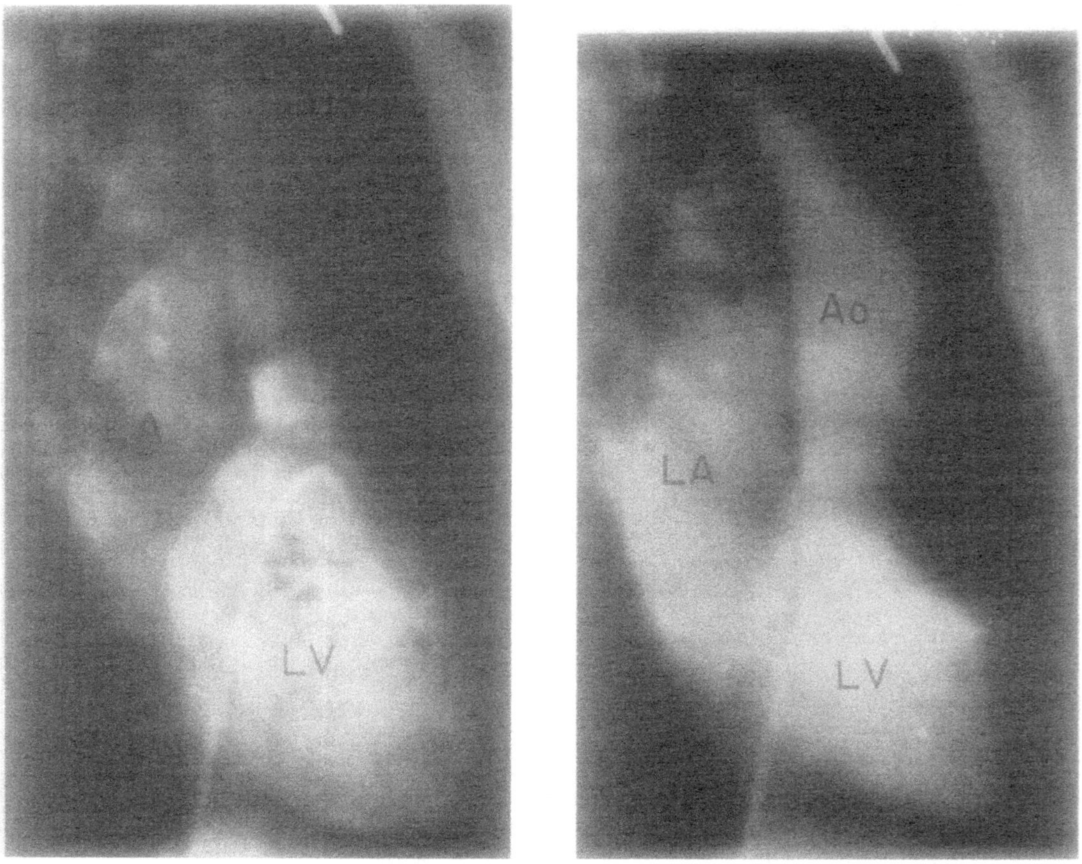

Fig. *8*. Selective left ventricular angiocardiogram of Patient N. R. which demonstrates gross mitral regurgitation. Lateral views exposed during ventricular diastole (*left*) and ventricular systole (*right*) are shown. During systole the left atrium (*LA*) increases strikingly in size, whereas the left ventricle (*LV*) diminishes in size. *Ao:* Aorta.

right ventricle measured 7 mm. in thickness, and the left, 12 mm. The prosthetic patch, covered by opaque endocardium, occupied and completely closed a crescent-shaped defect in the lowermost portion of the interatrial septum. Although the tricuspid valve was not cleft, and its chordae tendineae were normal, a portion of the septal leaflet was absent, and, as in Patient T. A., it was believed that this abnormality had been responsible for the tricuspid regurgitation. The pulmonic valve and pulmonic trunk were mildly dilated. There was a jet lesion on the posterior wall of the left atrium. The mitral valve ring measured only 7 cm. in circumference, compared to 12 cm. for the tricuspid valve ring. There was no evidence of a remaining cleft in the anterior leaflet of the mitral valve, and the silk sutures in its mid-portion were covered by endocardium. Although both mitral leaflets were thickened, their appearance did not resemble rheumatic valvulitis. Anomalous chordae tendineae, which were thickened and fused, extended from the ventricular aspect of the most distal margin of the anterior mitral leaflet to the superior crest of the muscular ventricular septum. These accessory chordae did not apparently cause any obstruction to outflow of blood from the left ventricle. The chordae tendineae which inserted into the left ventricular papillary muscles were normal.

Comment

Prior to cardiac catheterization both of the patients described were considered by most observers to have rheumatic heart disease with predominant mitral regurgitation. Both patients had had febrile illnesses in childhood which were thought to have been acute rheumatic fever. On physical examination each had left ventricular prominence and a loud pansystolic apical murmur; an early diastolic sound ushered in the mid-diastolic rumbling murmur which is so characteristic of massive mitral regurgitation. The electrocardiograms showed atrial fibrillation and were compatible with left ventricular hypertrophy. Neither patient had an RSR′

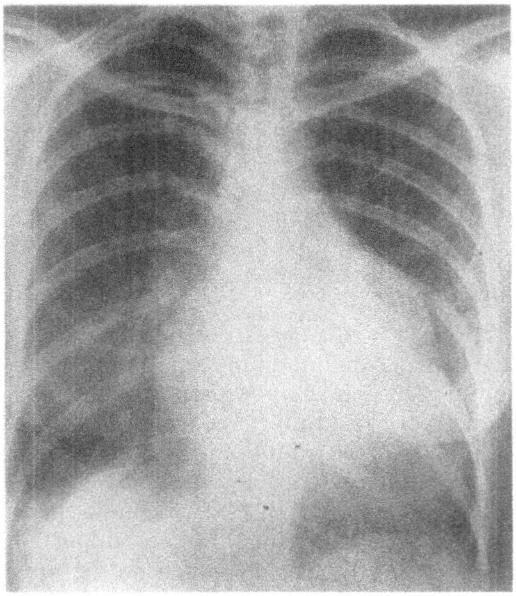

Fig. *9*. Chest roentgenogram of Patient N. R. taken 6 months after closure of the atrial septal defect and incomplete repair of the mitral valve. The posteroanterior projection demonstrates striking enlargement of the left atrium and ventricle in comparison to preoperative films (see Fig. 6).

pattern in leads from the right precordium. Patient N.R. had a normal electrical axis, and, although Patient T.A. exhibited left axis deviation of the terminal electrical forces, this deviation was less than that usually encountered in patients with A-V canal. The roentgenograms revealed gross left atrial and left ventricular enlargement without evidence of increased pulmonary vascularity.

Cardiac catheterization in each patient revealed a left-to-right shunt into the right atrium, and an interatrial communication which was crossed by the catheter. The unusually small size of the defects was predicted from the finding of a small shunt in the presence of striking left atrial enlargement. In Patient T. A. there was, in addition, a pressure gradient between the atria.

Retrospectively, the presence of fixed splitting of the second heart sound in the pulmonary area in both patients should have suggested the presence of an interatrial septal defect; prolongation of the P-R interval, repeatedly seen in Patient T. A., has frequently been observed in patients with A-V canal,[3] but in this instance was mistakenly attributed to active rheumatic fever.

Burchell and co-workers,[3] in a recent comprehensive review of the electrocardiographic findings in patients with endocardial cushion defects, concluded that the presence of the typical vector loop in a young individual with a large left-to-right interatrial shunt was almost pathognomonic of a defect of the ostium primum type. Although all of the patients with the complete form of persistent A-V canal studied by these authors had the characteristic electrocardiographic pattern, superior orientation and counterclockwise rotation of forces in the frontal plane, occasionally a patient with the partial form failed to show this configuration. It would seem correct to conclude, therefore, on the basis of their report and the two patients described herein, that the absence of the typical electrocardiographic features does not necessarily exclude the presence of an ostium primum type of atrial septal defect.

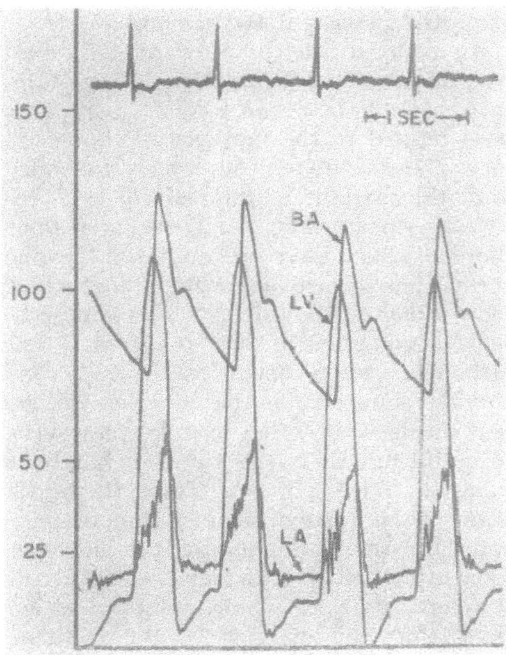

Fig. *10*. Simultaneous left atrial (*LA*), left ventricular (*LV*), and brachial arterial (*BA*) pressure pulses obtained 6 months after the initial operation in Patient N. R. The left atrial pressure was obtained by transbronchial puncture, and the left ventricular pressure by percutaneous puncture of this chamber.

The primary surgical problem in the type of malformation presented by the patients described is the correction of the mitral regurgitation. In Patient N.R. the mitral cleft was not completely repaired by the first operation, and closure of the interatrial defect eliminated the vent through which the left atrium was being decompressed. After this procedure her condition deteriorated rapidly. Within 6 months the mean left atrial pressure had risen from 4 to 27 mm. Hg, the left atrium had become massively enlarged, and severe pulmonary hypertension had developed. Although at the time of the second operation the cleft was completely repaired, she continued to have evidence of considerable mitral regurgitation. In Patient T. A. the cleft in the anterior mitral leaflet was also completely closed, but the loud murmur of mitral regurgitation persisted during the postoperative period. Residual regurgitation probably contributed to his death. Other authors have also stressed the hazard of closing an atrial septal defect without correcting associated mitral regurgitation in patients with the usual form of partial persistent A-V canal.[4,5]

As demonstrated by Edwards,[6] the persistence of mitral regurgitation after surgical repair in these two patients may have been related to the presence of the accessory chordae tendineae which extended from the margins of the cleft to the ventricular septum (Fig. 5). These anomalous chordae, which have no counterpart in the normal heart, are a constant feature of endocardial cushion defects and appear to be pathognomonic of these malformations.[7] Although prior to operation these chordae provide support for the margins of the cleft during ventricular systole, they serve no useful function after the cleft has been repaired. Indeed, by restraining the apposition of the anterior against the posterior leaflet they may actually produce incompetence of the valve. Edwards has suggested, therefore, that all of the chordae which insert into the margins of the cleft be divided. Failure to appreciate the significance of these structures in the two patients reported on herein probably accounted for the persistent mitral regurgitation which each demonstrated.

Both patients also had tricuspid regurgitation, but no cleft of the tricuspid valve could be recognized either at operation or at postmortem examination. A portion of the septal leaflet in each case, however, was absent. This malformation does not lend itself so readily to surgical correction as does a discrete cleft; plication of the septal portion of the annulus in Patient T.A. was of questionable value.

Summary

Patients with persistent partial atrioventricular canal and only small interatrial communications may present the clinical features of pure mitral regurgitation. Two such individuals, who on clinical examination were mistakenly considered to have rheumatic mitral regurgitation, are described. The roentgenographic findings supported this diagnosis, and the electrocardiograms did not exhibit the vector loop characteristic of an endocardial cushion defect. Cardiac catheterization made possible the correct diagnosis, however, and at operation each patient was found to have a cleft anterior mitral leaflet and an unusually small interatrial defect of the ostium primum type. Problems which relate to the diagnosis and surgical management of this unusual variant of persistent A-V canal are discussed.

REFERENCES

1. Sanders, R. J., and Morrow, A. G.: The identification and quantification of left-to-right circulatory shunts: a new diagnostic method utilizing the inhalation of a radioactive gas, Kr^{85}, Am. J. Med. **26**:508, 1959.
2. Braunwald, E , Morrow, A. G., and Cooper, T.: Left ventricular angiocardiography in the diagnosis of persistent atrioventricular canal and related anomalies, Am. J. Cardiol. **4**:802, 1959.
3. Burchell, H. B., DuShane, J. W., and Brandenburg, R. O.: The electrocardiogram of patients with atrioventricular cushion defects (defects of the atrioventricular canal), Am. J. Cardiol. **6**:575, 1960.
4. Watkins, E., Jr., and Gross, R. E.: Experiences with surgical repair of atrial septal defects, J. Thoracic Surg. **30**:469, 1955.
5. Gerbode, F., Johnston, J. B., Robinson, S., Harkins, G. A., and Osborn, J. J.: Endocardial cushion defects: diagnosis and technique of surgical repair, Surgery **49**:69, 1961.
6. Edwards, J. E.: The problem of mitral insufficiency caused by accessory chordae tendineae in persistent common atrioventricular canal, Proc. Staff Meet. Mayo Clin. **35**:299, 1960.

7. Braunwald, E., Ross, R. S., Morrow, A. G., and Roberts, W. C.: Differential diagnosis of mitral regurgitation in childhood: clinical pathological conference at the National Institutes of Health, Ann. Int. Med. **54**:1223, 1961.
8. Wakai, C. S., and Edwards, J. E.: Pathologic study of persistent common atrioventricular canal, Am. Heart J. **56**:779, 1958.
9. Wakai, C. S., and Edwards, J. E.: Developmental and pathologic considerations in persistent common atrioventricular canal, Proc. Staff Meet. Mayo Clin. **31**:487, 1956.
10. Rogers, H. M., and Edwards, J. E.: Incomplete division of the atrioventricular canal with patent interatrial foramen primum (persistent common atrioventricular ostium), Am. Heart J. **36**:28, 1948.
11. Campbell, M., and Missen, G. A. K.: Endocardial cushion defects: common atrioventricular canal and ostium primum, Brit. Heart J. **19**:403, 1957.
12. Paul, M. H.: Endocardial cushion defects: persistent common atrioventricular canal and persistent ostium primum, Pediat. Clin. North America 1011, 1958.
13. Kiely, B., Adams, P., Jr., Anderson, R. C., and Lester, R. G.: The ostium primum syndrome, A.M.A. J. Dis. Child. **96**:381, 1958.
14. Toscano-Barboza, E., Brandenburg, R. O., and Burchell, H. B.: Electrocardiographic studies of cases with intracardiac malformations of the atrioventricular canal, Proc. Staff Meet. Mayo Clin. **31**:513, 1956.
15. Beregovich, J., Bleifer, S. Donoso, E., and Grishman, A.: The vectorcardiogram and electrocardiogram in persistent common atrioventricular canal, Circulation **21**:63, 1960.
16. Ellis, F. H., Jr., McGoon, D. C., and Kirklin, J. W.: Surgical management of persistent common atrioventricular canal, Am. J. Cardiol. **6**:598, 1960.
17. Cooley, D. A.: Results of surgical treatment of atrial septal defects, Am. J. Cardiol. **6**:605, 1960.
18. McGoon, D. C., DuShane, J. W., and Kirklin, J. W.: The surgical treatment of endocardial cushion defects, Surgery **46**:185, 1959.

Acute Severe Mitral Regurgitation Secondary to Ruptured Chordae Tendineae

Clinical, Hemodynamic, and Pathologic Considerations

By WILLIAM C. ROBERTS, M.D., EUGENE BRAUNWALD, M.D., AND ANDREW G. MORROW, M.D.

THE MAJORITY of patients with severe mitral regurgitation have enlarged left atria, atrial fibrillation, a history of acute rheumatic fever, and a gradual onset of symptoms of cardiac decompensation that may persist for many years. This report describes 10 patients with severe mitral regurgitation caused by rupture of one or more chordae tendineae, and contrasts the clinical, radiographic, hemodynamic, and pathologic findings in these patients with those commonly noted in patients with the more usual form of mitral regurgitation. Thus, the majority of the patients with ruptured chordae tendineae had little left atrial enlargement, were in sinus rhythm, and had not had a history of acute rheumatic fever. The symptoms of cardiac decompensation generally appeared abruptly, and were usually present for only several months before they led to the patient's death or necessitated operative treatment. An appreciation of this relatively pure, acute form of mitral regurgitation is important in the understanding of the wide range of physiologic, pathologic, and clinical findings that may accompany this valvular lesion.

Description of Patients

A summary of the clinical, electrocardiographic, hemodynamic and pathologic findings in the individual patients is presented in table 1.

History. The 10 patients ranged in age from 17 to 54 years. Six were women. Only one patient (L. L.) had a history suggestive of acute rheumatic fever, and none had a history of chorea or chest trauma. Six patients had a definite history of bacterial endocarditis, and each had been asymptomatic and fully active prior to the onset of the infection. Pregnancy appeared to have played a role in the appearance of the bacterial endocarditis in three patients; A. L. and A. A. developed the infection shortly after parturition, while patient R. H. developed pyogenic endometritis after an abortion which in turn was followed by bacterial endocarditis. In two patients each *alpha streptococcus* and *staphylococcus aureus* were the organisms responsible for the endocarditis, and in one patient each the causative organisms were *streptococcus faecalis* and *staphylococcus albus.* The onset of cardiac decompensation was abrupt in nine patients and was progressive thereafter, while in patient V. C., who did not have a history of bacterial endocarditis, symptoms developed more slowly. In seven patients the period of time from the onset of symptoms of cardiac failure to autopsy or operation was less than 16 months, while in the other three patients the interval ranged from 5 to 8 years. Seven patients had no knowledge of heart murmurs before the onset of bacterial endocarditis or cardiac failure. Three patients, two of whom had a history of bacterial endocarditis, were known to have had precordial murmurs for periods ranging from 12 to 43 years before operation or death. In one of these patients, the murmur may have resulted from the presence of associated partial anomalous pulmonary venous connection and a small atrial septal defect.

Each of the patients complained of easy fatigability, exertional and nocturnal dyspnea, and all but one had pedal edema. All were treated with digitalis and salt restriction, but despite these measures they were severely disabled and considered to be in functional classes III or IV.

Physical Examination. Each of the 10 patients had prominent right ventricular and less prominent left ventricular lifts as well as easily papable apical systolic thrills. The sound of pulmonic valve closure was accentuated in all patients, and a third heart sound was almost always audible. In every patient, a blowing pansystolic murmur of at least grade IV/VI intensity was heard over the entire precordium, loudest over the cardiac apex, with radiation to the left axilla. In two patients the murmur at the cardiac apex was of whistling or

From the Clinic of Surgery and the Cardiology Branch, National Heart Institute, National Institutes of Health, Bethesda, Maryland.

cooing quality, and in two others the systolic murmur was also audible over the entire vertebral column.[1] In five patients the systolic murmur along the lower left sternal border became louder during inspiration. Seven patients had short, low-pitched, mid-diastolic flow murmurs at the apex, and two patients had high-pitched, blowing, diastolic murmurs along the left sternal border. The liver was palpable and tender in the majority of the patients, and pulsated during systole in three of them.

Electrocardiograms (Fig. 1). Eight patients had sinus rhythm, and two had atrial fibrillation; in one of the latter this arrhythmia appeared shortly before death. Right axis deviation was present in five patients, and left axis deviation in one. Four patients had first-degree atrioventricular block. Right ventricular hypertrophy was present in seven patients and left ventricular hypertrophy as well in three. Seven patients exhibited the peaked P waves characteristic of right atrial enlargement, and one had left atrial enlargement.

Roentgenograms (Fig. 2). Some degree of cardiac enlargement was evident on the chest roentgenograms of all 10 patients. The left atrium was mildly or moderately enlarged in eight patients, and markedly enlarged in only the two patients who had been symptomatic for the longest times, 5 and 8 years. Both ventricles were considered to be enlarged in all 10 patients. Calcification in the region of the mitral valve was detected in only one patient (L. L.). Angiographic studies with left ventricular injection in each of two patients (A. F. and L. S.) showed near-normal sized left atria which expanded strikingly during ventricular systole, but there was no evidence of prolapse of a mitral valve leaflet into the left atrium.

Hemodynamic Findings (Fig. 3). All nine patients who underwent right heart catheterization had markedly elevated pulmonary arterial and right ventricular systolic pressures, ranging from 61 to 110 mm. Hg. The mean left atrial pressures were elevated to between 15 and 32 mm. Hg in eight patients, and within normal limits (11 mm. Hg) in the ninth. The v-wave peaks were abnormally elevated in all nine patients and ranged from 23 to 66 mm. Hg (average, 45 mm. Hg). The left ventricular end-diastolic pressure was normal ($\leqq$ 12 mm. Hg) in six of the eight patients in whom it was measured, and was markedly elevated (20 and 27 mm. Hg) in two. The

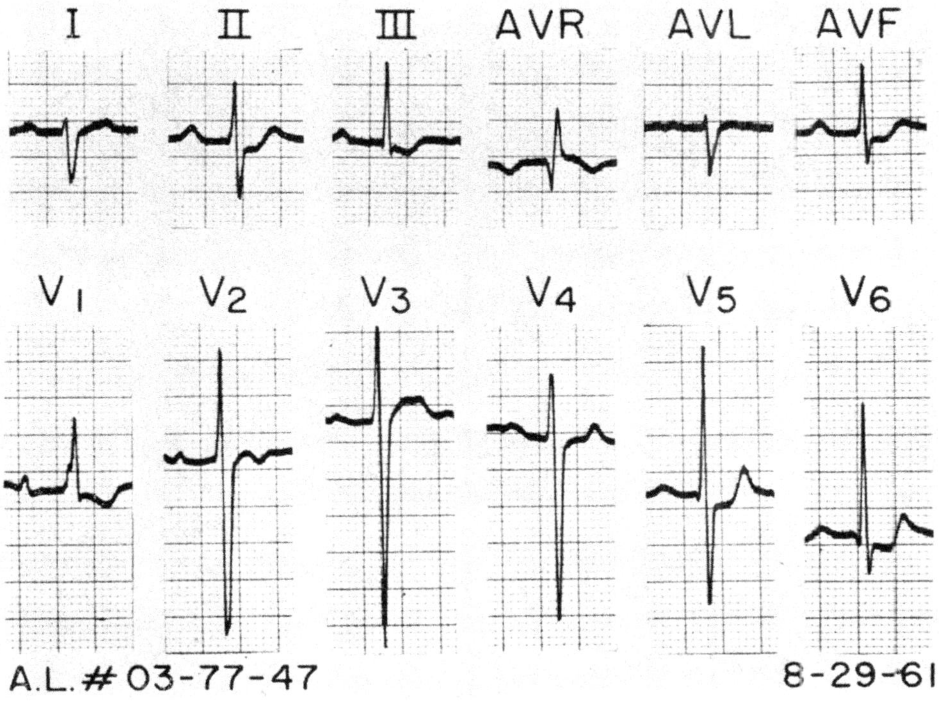

Figure 1

Electrocardiogram of patient A.L. Right axis deviation, right atrial enlargement, right ventricular hypertrophy, and possible left ventricular hypertrophy are present, although mitral regurgitation had been present for only 16 months.

Table 1

Clinical, Electrocardiographic, Hemodynamic, and Pathologic Data from the 10 Patients with Ruptured Mitral Chordae Tendineae

				Hemodynamic data					
Patient no. (sex)	Age at death or at operation / Length of symptoms	History of bacterial endocarditis (organism)	Electro-cardiogram	PA s/d (mean) (mm. Hg)	LA mean—v wave (mm. Hg)	LV s/d (mm. Hg)	Cardiac index (L./min./M.²)	Pulmonary vascular resistance (dynes sec. cm.⁻⁵)	LA size at operation (O) at autopsy (A)
1. V.C. 01-21-66 (M)	41 yr. / 5 yr.	—	AF, RAD, RAE, RVH, LVH	110/40 (67)	32—39*		1.4	1217	Dilated (A)
2. A.A. 01-71-62 (F)	37 yr. / 7 mo.	—	NSR, RAE, RVH		24—52	92/27			"Normal" (A)
3. A.L. 03-77-47 (F)	19 yr. / 16 mo.	+ Streptococcus Group D	NSR, RAD, RAE, RVH, First-degree HB	70/30 (45)	15—36	100/10	1.7	950	"Normal" (A)
4. R.H. 03-99-19 (F)	24 yr. / 5 mo.	+ Enterococcus	NSR, RAE, First-degree HB	72/32 (54)	27—66	108/11	1.5	1000	"Normal" (A)
5. P.H. 04-94-07 (F)	29 yr. / 5 yr.	+ Staphylococcus albus	NSR, RAD, RAE, RVH, LVH	105/40 (70)	15—35		1.6	2000	"Normal" (A)
6. B.F. 04-85-25 (F)	21 yr. / 13 mo.	+ Staphylococcus aureus	NSR, RAD, RAE, RVH, LVH	65/28† ↓ 32/11 (16)‡	11—23† ↓ 6—11‡	100/9†	1.4† ↓ 3.0‡	1100† ↓ 179‡	"Normal" (O)
7. J.W. 04-87-16 (M)	54 yr. / 8 yr.	+ Alpha strepto-coccus	NSR, RVH, LAE, First-degree HB	70/27 ↓(37)† 44/20 (28)‡	15—32† ↓ 7—10‡	90/11† ↓ 95/5‡	2.8‡	382‡	Dilated (O)
8. L.L. 05-45-40 (M)	53 yr. / 9 mo.	—	AF, LAD	61/25† ↓(39) 29/10 (17)‡	22—56† ↓ 10—21‡	81/9† ↓ 119/9‡	0.9† ↓ 3.2‡	1070† ↓ 94‡	"Normal" (O)
9. A.F. 05-78-22 (M)	48 yr. / 7 mo.	—	NSR, Nonspecific T-wave changes	84/30	25—65	100/20	1.8	609	"Normal" (O)
10. L.S. 05-99-23 (F)	17 yr. / 5 mo.	+ Staphylococcus aureus	NSR, RVH, RAE, RAD, First-degree HB	71/41 (51)	24*	86/12			"Normal" (A)

*Pulmonary arterial wedge pressures.
†Before operation.
‡Several months after operation.

Abbreviations: PA, pulmonary arterial pressure; LA, left atrial pressure; LV, left ventricular pressure; s/d (mean), systolic/diastolic (mean) pressures; AF, atrial fibrillation; RBBB, right bundle-branch block; NSR, normal sinus rhythm; RVH, right ventricular hypertrophy; RAE, right atrial enlargement; LVH, left ventricular hypertrophy; LAE, left atrial enlargement; LAD, left axis deviation; HB, heart block. "Normal," near normal size or only moderately dilated.

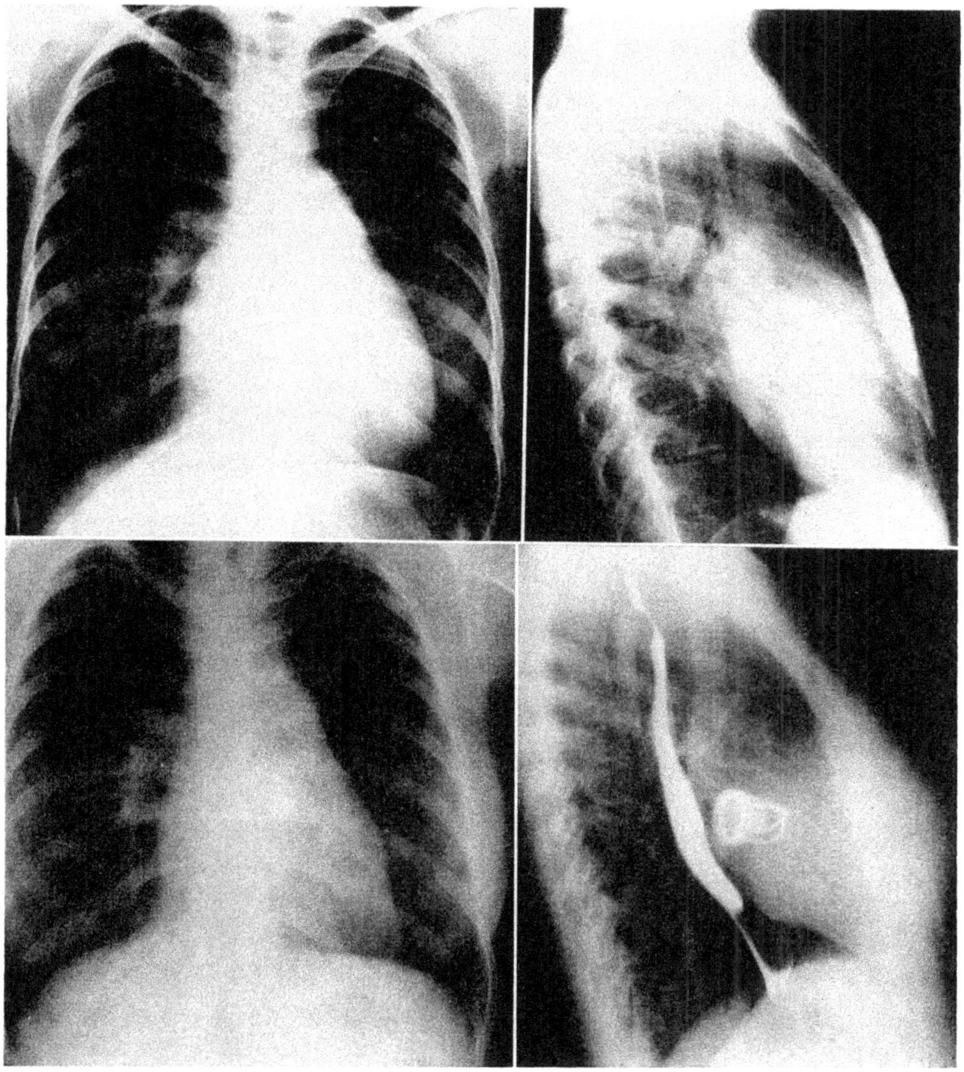

Figure 2

Roentgenograms obtained preoperatively (upper) *and 7 months postoperatively* (lower) *in patient B.F. This patient had had severe mitral regurgitation for 13 months before operation, but there was only minimal left atrial enlargement.*

cardiac output was markedly reduced in each of the seven patients in whom it was measured, and ranged from 0.9 to 1.8 L./min./M.^{2}, with an average of 1.5 L./min./M.^{2}. Pulmonary vascular resistance was calculated in seven patients and ranged from 609 to 2,000 with an average of 1135 dynes sec. cm.$^{-5}$. Indicator-dilution curves recorded from a systemic artery following injection into the left ventricle or left atrium in seven patients showed the prolonged descending limb characteristic of severe mitral regurgitation.

Pathologic Findings (Figs. 4-11). The mitral valves and chordae tendineae were examined in six patients at necropsy. In the other four patients the mitral valve was examined after it had been surgically excised with the chordae tendineae and papillary muscles intact. One patient died of heart failure, one from a complication of cardiac catheterization, three following mitral annuloplasty, and one following Starr-Edwards mitral valve replacement.

Ruptured chordae tendineae were responsible for mitral regurgitation in every patient, and in six of them the rupture was clearly the result of bacterial endocarditis. Active endocarditis was present in two patients (R. H. and L. S.); it involved the posterior half of the aortic leaflet of the mitral valve in one (fig. 6); and both anterior and posterior leaflets in the other patient. All chordae that had inserted into these portions of the valve had been destroyed. Organisms, however, were not found in sections of the valves of either of these patients. In six patients most or all of the chordae to one half of the anterior leaflet of the mitral valve were ruptured, in one patient all of the chordae that had been attached to the posterior leaflet were involved, and in three patients several chordae from both leaflets were destroyed. With the exception of the two patients with active endocarditis, there were no essential differences between the pathologic findings in the patients with and those without a history of bacterial endocarditis. Although some fibrous thickening of the mitral leaflet adjacent to the ruptured chordae was usually evident, the remaining mitral valve leaflets, commissures, and remaining chordae showed no apparent abnormalities. The aortic valve was normal in the six autopsied patients. In the other four patients, no abnormalities of the aortic valve were detected at the time of operation. The tricuspid and pulmonic valves also were normal in the hearts examined at necropsy.

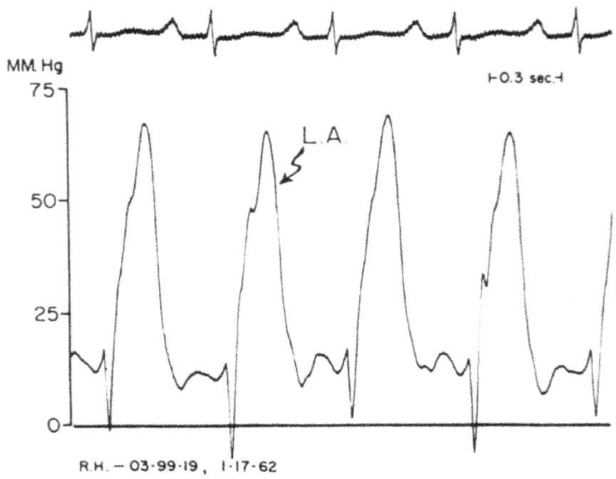

Figure 3

Left atrial pressure tracing in patient R.H., who had had mitral regurgitation for only 5 months.

The left atrial chamber was near normal size, or only moderately enlarged, in the six autopsied patients, and in each of them the left atrial wall was considerably thickened. In two of the patients, who had had symptoms for 5 and 8 years, the left atrium was severely dilated. Jet lesions were present on the endocardial surface of the left atrium in all 10 patients, their location depending upon the position of the ruptured chordae. The right

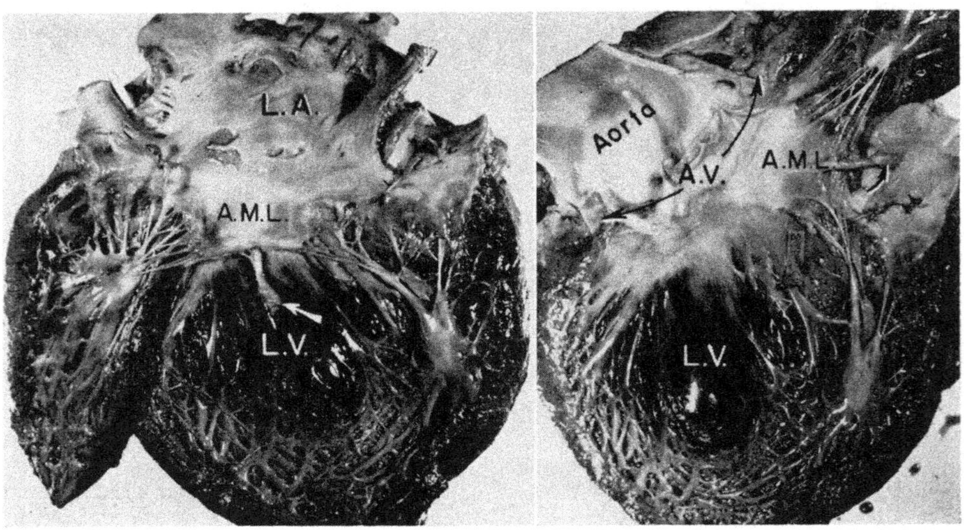

Figure 4

Photographs of heart of patient 2 (A.A.). Left. *The left atrium (L.A.), mitral valve, and left ventricle (L.V.) are seen. The ruptured chorda* (arrow), *which is club-shaped, arises from the midportion of the anterior mitral leaflet (A.M.L.). The nonruptured chordae are normal. The left atrium is not dilated, but the left ventricle is considerably dilated.* Right. *The anterior mitral leaflet (A.M.L.) is now seen from the ventricular aspect. The aortic valve (A.V.) is normal.*

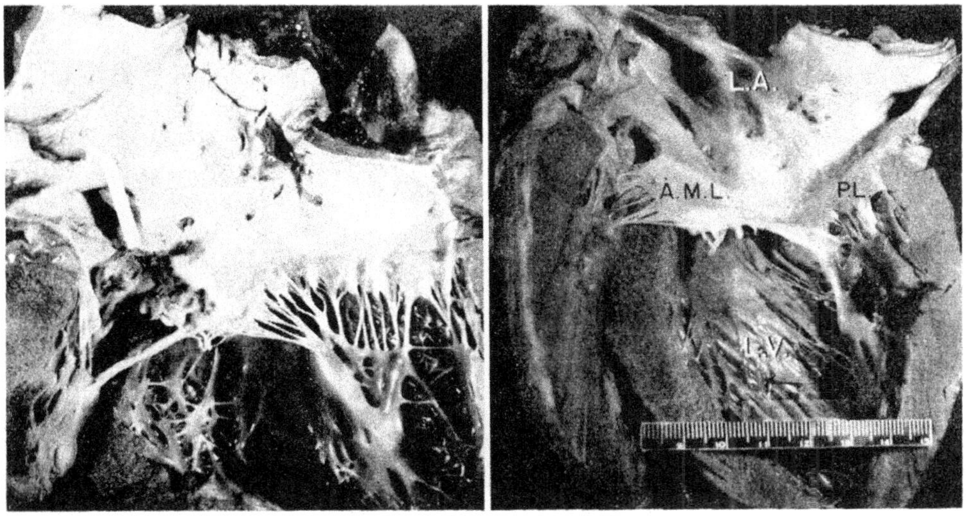

Figure 5

Photographs of opened left atrium (L.A.), mitral valve, and left ventricle (L.V.) of patient 3 (A.L.) left, *and patient 5 (P.H.)* right. *Chordae tendineae that had attached to the anterior (A.M.L.) and posterior (P.L.) mitral leaflets adjacent to the anterolateral commissure are absent in the heart of patient 3* (left). *The arrow points to the site of jet lesion in the left atrium in this patient. All chordae tendineae from the posterior portion of the anterior mitral leaflet (A.M.L.) are severed in patient 5* (right). *The nonruptured chordae in each patient are normal, and in neither is the left atrium dilated.*

ventricle was dilated and hypertrophied in the six patients studied at necropsy.

On microscopic examination, there were no Aschoff bodies in sections of the heart from any of the six autopsied patients, and sections of the left atrial walls disclosed severe hypertrophy of the myocardial fibers and marked thickening of the endocardium (fig. 8). Histologic examination of sections from the lungs of the six autopsied patients disclosed grade 3/6 hypertensive pulmonary vascular changes in each (classification of Heath and Edwards[2]). Three patients had ossific nodules scattered in the lungs. Examples of microscopic changes in the lungs of two patients are shown in figures 9 and 10. The pulmonary vascular changes in patients R. H. and A. A. were particularly noteworthy, since these patients had had clinical evidence of mitral regurgitation for only 5 and 7 months, respectively, before death. There was severe centrolobular hepatic congestion in each of the six autopsied patients, an example of which is shown in figure 11.

Discussion

In the past, the conditions considered to be responsible for ruptured chordae tendineae of the mitral valve included rheumatic fever,[3–5] trauma,[6] so-called spontaneous rupture,[7] and bacterial endocarditis involving either diseased or normal valves.[5, 8–10] Most authors have considered that chordal rupture occurs predominantly in previously diseased valves. In the National Institutes of Health collection of almost 150 hearts with acquired mitral valvular disease, there are only two with ruptured mitral chordae, and in both patients this was clearly of secondary importance in the resultant regurgitation. On the other hand, we have encountered the 10 patients, described in this report, who had ruptured mitral chordae involving a valve that otherwise appeared not to be grossly diseased. Critical review of earlier reports, including published photographs of ruptured mitral chordae, indicated numerous instances of ruptured mitral chordae in valves that also did not appear grossly abnormal,[4, 5, 7, 10–17] although some of the authors had considered that rheumatic heart disease was the underlying process. Although bacterial endocarditis tends to affect obviously malformed or previously diseased valves most often, and chronic rheumatic involvement might thus predispose to chordal rupture, it seems entirely possible that the marked thickening and shortening of the chordae tendineae of a rheumatic valve may actually serve to protect these structures from rupture. On the basis of the experience with the patients described in this report, as well as the many published illustrations of ruptured chordae in valves that do not appear grossly abnormal, it is suggested that bacterial endocarditis occurring in hearts without detectable anatomic valvular abnormalities is an important cause of chordal rupture.

Immediately following rupture of a single chorda in the dog, the left atrial pressure, particularly the v-wave peak, rises abruptly, a systolic thrill and murmur become detectable in this chamber, and the left atrial appendage begins to balloon during each ventricular systole.[18, 19] The animals rapidly develop congestive cardiac failure, and their course is usually one of rapid progression. From the hemodynamic point of view, the

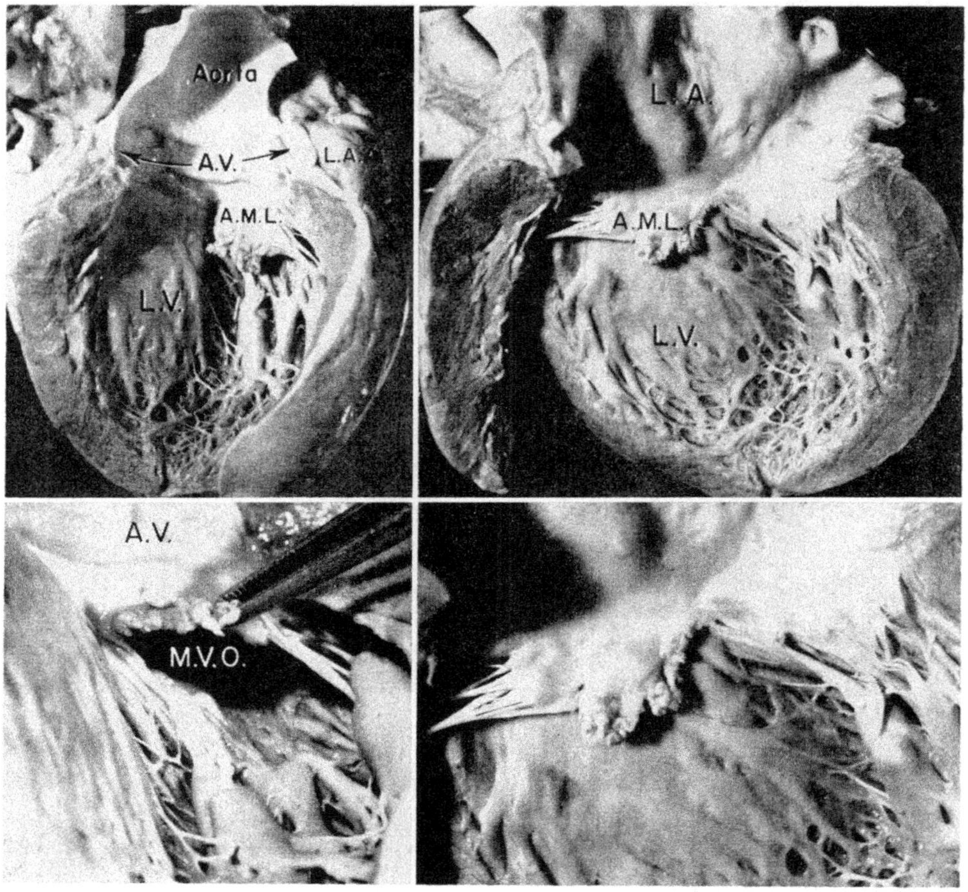

Figure 6

Photographs of heart of patient 4 (R.H.). Upper left. *The mitral valve is exposed by opening the left ventricle (L.V.), aortic valve (A.V.), and aorta. All chordae tendineae that had attached to the posterior portion of the anterior mitral leaflet (A.M.L.) are severed. The endocarditis that ruptured the chordae is active. The aortic valve is normal. L.A.A., left atrial appendage.* Lower left. *The size of the incompetent mitral valve orifice (M.V.O.) is apparent from this view. A.V., aortic valve cusps.* Upper right. *The left atrium (L.A.), mitral valve, and left ventricle (L.V.) are opened. The nonruptured mitral chordae are normal. A.M.L., anterior mitral leaflet.* Lower right. *Close-up of the ruptured mitral chordae of the anterior leaflet.*

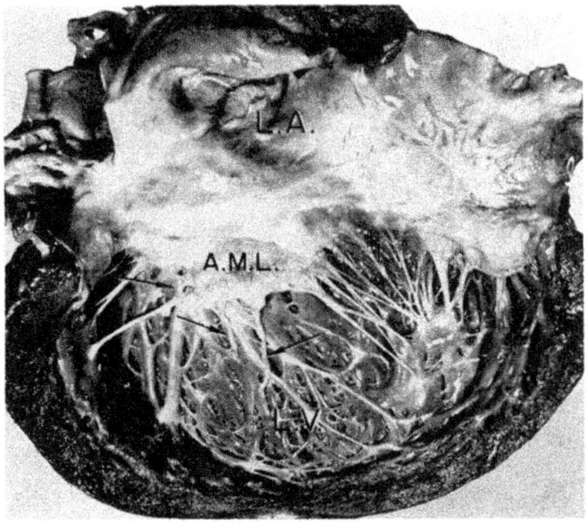

Figure 7

Photograph of heart of patient 1 (V.C.). The left atrium (L.A.), mitral valve, and left ventricle (L.V.) are opened. Both chambers are considerably dilated as is the mitral valve annulus. This patient had known mitral regurgitation for at least 5 years. At least three chordae tendineae (arrows) from the anterior mitral leaflet (A.M.L.) are severed and each of these is thickened as is a portion of this leaflet. The nonruptured chordae are elongated, but otherwise normal. The posterior leaflet is normal.

regurgitation produced suddenly in experimental animals more closely resembles the mitral regurgitation that developed acutely in the patients described herein than the regurgitation observed in patients with chronic rheumatic mitral regurgitation. In the latter condition, the regurgitation usually develops gradually, and sufficient time is available for the usual adjustments to this lesion to take place. In addition, the myocardium of the left atrium and of the left ventricle may also be affected by the rheumatic process. In the present group of patients with ruptured mitral chordae tendineae, however, the myocardium and pulmonary vascular bed were presumably normal at the time the chordae ruptured, and the resultant clinical, hemodynamic, and anatomic abnormalities may be attributed entirely or almost entirely to the mechanical defect.

The unusual hemodynamic and clinical features of the majority of patients described herein may be emphasized by comparing them with other groups of patients having severe mitral regurgitation. Patients with se-

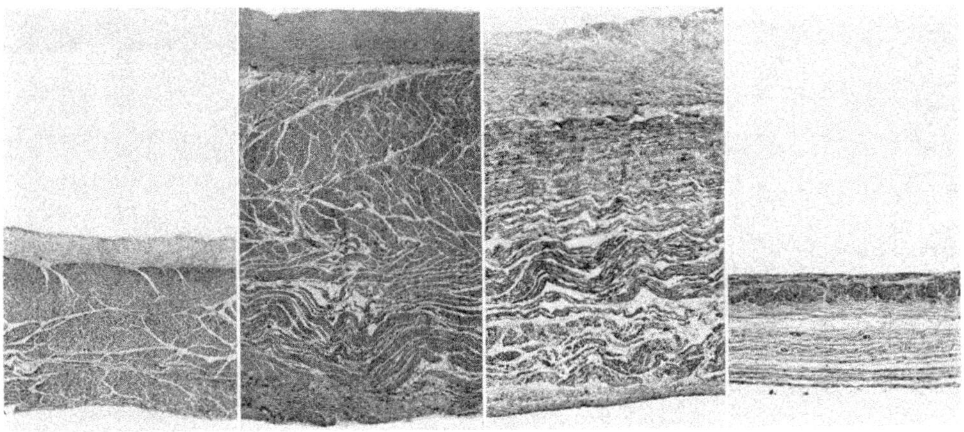

Figure 8

Photomicrographs of sections of posterior wall of left atrium in four patients each taken from a site approximately 3 cm. above the mitral annulus. Left. *Left atrial wall in 30-year-old woman dying of acute leukemia (for control). The endocardium is above, the epicardium, below.* Mid-left. *Left atrial wall in patient 4 (R.H.) showing marked thickening. This patient died 5 months after the onset of cardiac decompensation.* Mid-right. *Left atrial wall in patient 5 (P.H.) who lived for 5 years after the onset of cardiac decompensation. The endocardium is thicker, but the myocardium is thinner than in patient R.H.* Right. *Left atrial wall of a patient with mitral regurgitation, a giant left atrium, and normal left atrial pressures. The myocardial fibers are extremely elongated and thinned. The smooth muscle immediately beneath the endocardium is hypertrophied. Hematoxylin and eosin stains, original magnification in each × 20.*

vere mitral regurgitation were previously separated into three major groups on the basis of obvious differences in atrial compliance.[20] I. A group with the sudden development of mitral regurgitation in whom there was mild to moderate enlargement of the left atrium, striking elevation of the mean left atrial pressure, of the left atrial v wave, the pul-

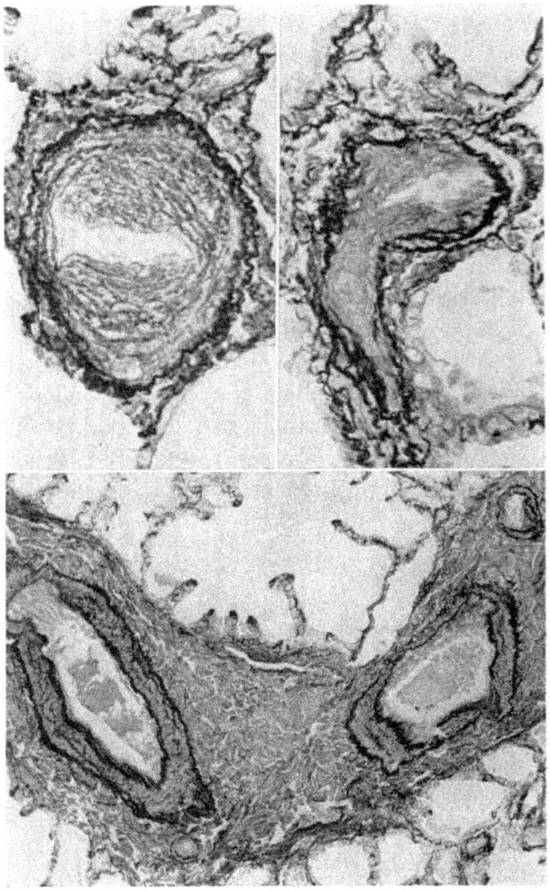

Figure 9

Photomicrographs of sections of pulmonary blood vessels in patient 4 (R.H.) who lived for only 5 months after the onset of mitral regurgitation. Upper left. *Pulmonary vein showing severe intimal proliferation and luminal narrowing.* Upper right. *Small muscular pulmonary artery with arteriolar branch showing severe intimal proliferation in each and luminal obliteration in the arteriole.* Lower. *Larger muscular pulmonary arteries showing medial hypertrophy and mild intimal proliferation. An adjacent small pulmonary artery is markedly narrowed by intimal fibrosis. Elastic tissue stains; original magnification × 340 (two upper), × 125 (lower).*

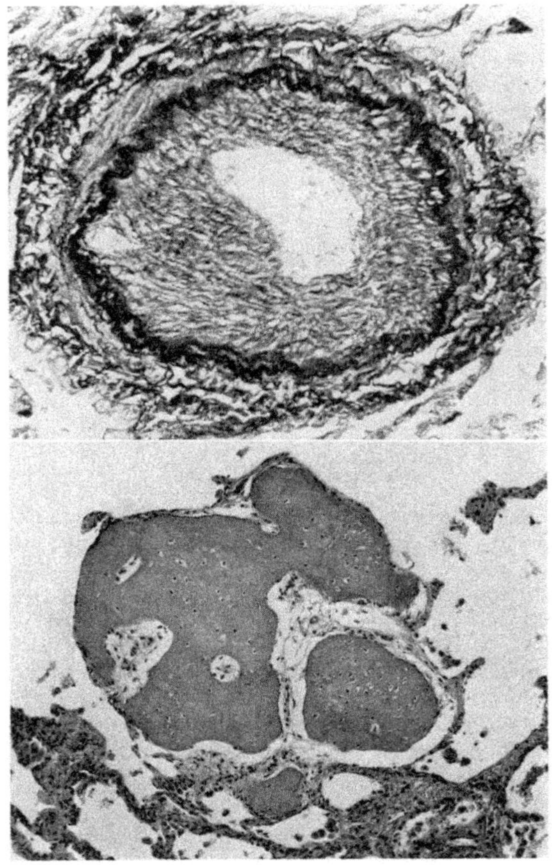

Figure 10

Photomicrographs of sections of lung in patient 2 (A.A.), who survived 7 months after the onset of mitral regurgitation. Upper. *Pulmonary vein showing severe intimal fibrosis.* Lower. *Ossific nodule. These "lung bones" were seen in sections of lungs in three of the six autopsied patients. Elastic tissue stain (upper), hematoxylin and eosin stain (lower); original magnification × 210 (upper), × 135 (lower).*

monary vascular resistance, and in whom severe right heart failure was often present. II. A group who had normal left atrial and pulmonary arterial pressures, normal pulmonary vascular resistance, a low cardiac output, huge left atria, atrial fibrillation, a history of acute rheumatic fever, and a long-standing history of heart failure (the syndrome of severe mitral regurgitation with normal left atrial pressure).[20] III. The largest number of patients with severe mitral regurgitation lies between these two extremes, and they exhibit both gross left atrial enlargement and an

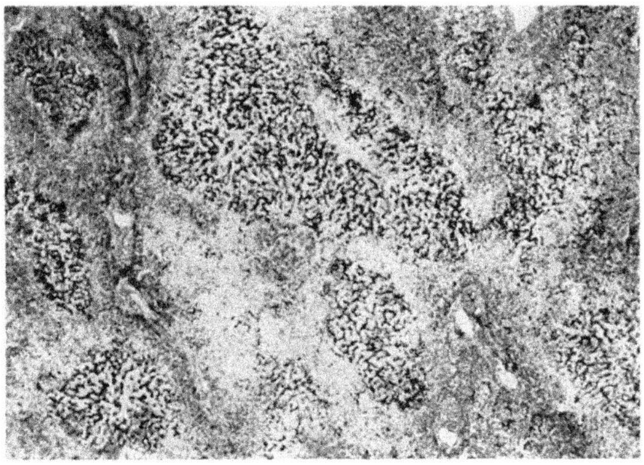

Figure 11

Photomicrograph of section of liver in patient 4 (R.H.), showing massive centrolobular necrosis (dark areas). The few remaining hepatic cells are located adjacent to the portal areas. Similar degrees of hepatic congestion and necrosis were seen in each of the six autopsied patients in this series. Phosphotungstic-acid hematoxylin stain, original magnification × 32.

elevated left atrial pressure. Thus, the patients with the syndrome of severe mitral regurgitation with normal left atrial pressure represent one end of the spectrum of mitral regurgitation, and the seven patients described in this report whose cardiac failure progressed rapidly represent the opposite end.

The severe pulmonary vascular changes observed in these patients with ruptured chordae tendineae are interpreted as anatomic expressions of the markedly elevated left atrial and pulmonary arterial pressures. The advanced pulmonary vascular changes, in association with little or no left atrial enlargement, contrasts sharply with the absence of these changes in patients with huge left atria secondary to long-standing mitral regurgitation.[20] As a consequence of the abnormalities in the pulmonary vascular bed, right ventricular hypertrophy was always present in the patients with acute mitral regurgitation and relatively small left atria, whereas right ventricular hypertrophy is rare in the patients with extremely dilated left atria.[21]

It is likely that the rapidity with which regurgitation develops is the primary determinant of hemodynamic, pathologic, and clinical changes observed in patients with severe mitral insufficiency. It is apparent that the walls of the left atria, and of the pulmonary vessels, were far less compliant in the nine patients with ruptured chordae tendineae who developed heart failure rapidly than in the group of patients with severely dilated left atria and normal left atrial pressures described previously.[20] Long-standing, gradually developing mitral regurgitation would appear, in some instances, to alter the elastic properties of the left atrial wall and, thereby, displace the atrial pressure-volume curve to make this chamber more compliant, so that a normal pressure may exist in a greatly enlarged atrium. Mitral regurgitation was present for only 5 to 16 months in seven of the eight patients in this series with normal or only moderately enlarged left atria. In contrast, symptoms of cardiac decompensation had been present for 5 to 8 years in the two patients with ruptured chordae tendineae who had very large left atria. Additional support for the view that the atrial compliance may increase as a late development in the course of mitral regurgitation was gained from observations in a 9-year-old patient with congenital mitral regurgitation in whom serial catheterization studies were carried out.[22] He was in sinus rhythm and exhibited slight disability at the time his left atrial pressure was grossly elevated (mean, 25; v peak, 45 mm. Hg). Subsequently, the patient developed cardiac failure, atrial fibrillation, and roentgenographic evidence of further increase in size of the left atrium. These changes were accompanied by a decline of left atrial pressure (mean, 15; v peak, 24 mm. Hg). Thus, in this patient a decrease in the mean left atrial pressure and the atrial v-wave peak pressure occurred in the face of an increase in the left atrial size, further substantiating the notion that the elastic properties of the left atrial wall had been altered.

In other reports of patients with ruptured mitral chordae tendineae, the left atrial chamber is usually described as being quite dilated. This finding was present in the six patients with ruptured mitral chordae reported by Menges et al.,[12] and the five described in detail by Osmundson et al.[5] These patients had been symptomatic for a number of years and, in general, the size of the left atrium correlated with the duration of the illness. In contrast, the heart of the first reported patient with ruptured mitral chordae, described by Corvisart in 1812,[23] was not grossly enlarged, but this patient survived for only 10 days after the onset of cardiac symptoms. Similarly, in the patient with ruptured mitral chordae reported by Frothingham and Hass,[7] who had been symptomatic for only 8 months, the left atrium was apparently not enlarged. In the patients described in these reports and others,[4, 10, 11, 13–16] a good correlation existed between left atrial size and the presence or absence of atrial fibrillation. The patients with atrial fibrillation were generally those with symptoms of cardiac disease for several years and very large left atria. The presence of atrial fibrillation in all of the patients with markedly dilated left atrial chambers, but normal atrial pressures,[20] and the absence of this arrhythmia in the patients with ruptured chordae tendineae, as well as in the child with congenital mitral regurgitation discussed above, suggest the possibility that the process that increases atrial compliance may be related to the development of atrial fibrillation.

Operative treatment was undertaken in seven of the 10 patients described herein. Mitral annuloplasty, with or without insertion of artificial chordae, which was originally utilized in this clinic for repair of ruptured chordae, was attempted in two patients, but each of them died in the immediate postoperative period. Mitral valve replacement with a Starr-Edwards prosthesis was carried out in the other five patients, and four have shown considerable improvement. The fifth died 2 weeks after operation of severe pulmonary infection including pulmonary abscess and empyema. Total valve replacement appears to be the most effective operative method for correcting ruptured chordae, although others[12, 15, 16, 17, 24] have reported good results with mitral plication and insertion of artificial chordae tendineae.

Since, with any given magnitude of regurgitant flow, the atrial pressure varies inversely with the compliance of the atrium, the extent to which the atrial pressure can be expected to decline following a corrective operation will also vary inversely with atrial compliance. Accordingly, the clinical and hemodynamic benefits of operation may be expected to be greatest in patients with relatively small left atria and high left atrial pressures. This may be illustrated by two patients in this series who have had postoperative catheterization following mitral valve replacement. B. F., a 21-year-old woman, was completely bedridden immediately before operation, although she had been well until 13 months earlier, when bacterial endocarditis was soon followed by the development of mitral regurgitation. At the time of the operation she weighed only 33 Kg. Preoperatively, the left atrial (mean, 11; v peak, 23 mm. Hg) and pulmonary arterial (65/28, mean 38 mm. Hg) pressures were elevated, roentgenographically the left atrium was only mildly enlarged, and on a standard oral sodium tolerance test she was unable to excrete any sodium.[25] Following replacement of the mitral valve with a Starr-Edwards prosthesis, she has been entirely asymptomatic. Seven months after operation she weighed 50 Kg. and the pulmonary arterial wedge (mean, 6; v peak, 11 mm. Hg) and pulmonary arterial (32/11, mean 16 mm. Hg) pressures were normal, the heart was smaller roentgenographically (fig. 2), and her sodium tolerance had become normal. J. W., a 54-year-old man, also was incapacitated before operation. He was emaciated, in severe cardiac failure, and the mean left atrial pressure was 15 with v waves of 32 mm. Hg, and the pulmonary arterial pressure was 70/27 mm. Hg. Twelve months after replacement of his mitral valve, the left atrial mean pressure had fallen to 7, the v waves to 10 mm. Hg, and the pulmonary arterial pressure to 44/20 mm. Hg. This patient has improved symptomatically, but he continues to accumulate fluid despite diuretic therapy, presumably consequent to persistent "relative" tricuspid regurgitation, and his heart had remained enlarged. Although this man also developed severe mitral regurgitation following rupture of chordae tendineae as a consequence of bacterial endocarditis, 8 years had elapsed from the onset of the valvular regurgitation until the valve was replaced, and the left atrium dilated during this interval. It is suspected that the left atrial pressures were greatly elevated immediately following the mitral chordal rupture, but as the left atrial chamber dilated the left atrial pressures decreased to levels approaching normal.

Summary and Conclusions

This report describes the clinical, radiographic, hemodynamic, and pathologic findings in 10 patients, in each of whom ruptured mitral chordae tendineae were responsible for severe mitral regurgitation. In six patients, the chordal rupture was the result of proved bacterial endocarditis, and in the other four, although the cause was not determined, it is considered that bacterial endocarditis may have been the etiologic factor in them as well. Only one of the patients had a history suggestive of acute rheumatic fever. From examination of the mitral valves at autopsy, or after operative excision, no gross abnormalities of the valves were apparent, other than the ruptured chordae and mild thickening of the adjacent leaflet. The signs and symptoms of mitral regurgitation appeared abruptly in all but one patient and were unrelenting thereafter. Eight patients had sinus rhythm and two had atrial fibrillation. Each of the latter had had symptoms of cardiac decompensation for several years, and their left atria were markedly enlarged. The left atrial chamber in the other eight patients was of near normal size or only moderately enlarged. The interval from the onset of symptoms of mitral regurgitation to operation in the two patients with dilated left atria averaged 6½ years, whereas the interval in the eight patients with near normal or only moderately dilated left atria averaged 15 months. In all patients the pulmonary arterial and the left atrial pressures, particularly the v-wave peak, were elevated. The cardiac index was low, and the calculated pulmonary vascular resistance was elevated in the seven patients in whom it was measured. Mitral annuloplasty was performed in two patients, with insertion of artificial chordae, but both died in the early postoperative period. Replacement of the mitral valve with a Starr-Edwards prosthesis was performed in five patients, with considerable improvement in four. The fifth died of a pulmonary complication 2 weeks after operation.

The distinctive clinical and hemodynamic findings in the majority of these patients, i.e., the rapid progression of heart failure, sinus rhythm, normal-sized or only moderately enlarged left atria, and the greatly elevated pressures in the pulmonary artery and left atrium are attributed to the sudden onset of the mitral regurgitation. These findings are contrasted to those in patients with chronic rheumatic mitral regurgitation, whose disability progresses slowly and who exhibit atrial fibrillation, marked left atrial enlargement, and sometimes normal pulmonary arterial and left atrial pressures. It is proposed that the majority of patients with ruptured chordae cannot sustain the acutely imposed hemodynamic burden for periods of time sufficient to allow the increase in left atrial compliance so frequently observed in patients with chronic rheumatic mitral regurgitation.

References

1. Perloff, J. K., and Harvey, W. P.: Auscultatory and phonocardiographic manifestations of pure mitral regurgitation. Progr. Cardiovas. Dis. **5**: 172, 1962.
2. Heath, D., and Edwards, J. E.: The pathology of hypertensive pulmonary vascular disease. A description of six grades of structural changes in the pulmonary arteries with special reference to congenital cardiac septal defects. Circulation **18**: 533, 1958.
3. Frew, H. W. O.: Rupture of the chordae tendineae following scarlet fever. Glasgow M. J. **115**: 195, 1931.
4. Bailey, O. T., and Hickman, J. B.: Rupture of mitral chordae tendineae. Clinical and pathologic observations on seven cases in which there was no bacterial endocarditis. Am. Heart J. **28**: 578, 1944.
5. Osmundson, P. J., Callahan, J. A., and Edwards, J. E.: Ruptured mitral chordae tendinae. Circulation **23**: 42, 1961.
6. Barber, H.: The effects of trauma, direct and

indirect, on the heart. Quart. J. Med., n.s., **13:** 137, 1944.

7. Frothingham, C., and Hass, G. M.: Rupture of normal chordae tendineae of the mitral valve. Am. Heart J. **9:** 492, 1934.
8. Libman, E., and Friedberg, C. K.: Subacute Bacterial Endocarditis. London, Oxford University Press, 1941, 108 pp.
9. Saphir, O.: Endocarditis. *In* Gould, S. E., Editor: Pathology of the Heart. Springfield, Illinois, Charles C Thomas Publisher, 1953, p. 707.
10. Hepper, N. G. G., Burchell, H. B., and Edwards, J. E.: Cardiac Clinic CXLVI. Mitral insufficiency in healed, unrecognized bacterial endocarditis. Proc. Staff Meet., Mayo Clinic **31:** 659, 1956.
11. Perrin, A., Froment, R., and Pasquier, J.: Insuffisances mitrales par luxation de la petite valve et rupture de cordages. (A propos de 5 observations anatomo-cliniques simulant le retrecissement aortique). Arch. mal. coeur **54:** 82, 1961.
12. Menges, H., Jr., Ankeney, J. L., and Hellerstein, H. K.: The clinical diagnosis and surgical management of ruptured mitral chordae tendineae. Circulation **30:** 8, 1964.
13. Miller, R., Jr., and Pearson, R. J., Jr.: Mitral insufficiency simulating aortic stenosis. Report of an unusual manifestation of Marfan's syndrome. New England. J. Med. **260:** 1210, 1959.
14. Shapiro, H. A., and Weiss, D. R.: Mitral insufficiency due to ruptured chordae tendineae simulating aortic stenosis. New England J. Med. **261:** 272, 1959.
15. January, L. E., Fisher, J. M., and Ehrenhaft, J. L.: Mitral insufficiency resulting from rupture of normal chordae tendineae. Report of a surgically corrected case. Circulation **26:** 1329, 1962.
16. Wolnisty, C., and Freidman, S. L.: Mitral insufficiency secondary to ruptured chordae tendineae. Report of surgically corrected case. J.A.M.A. **188:** 687, 1964.
17. Morris, J. D., Penner, D. A., and Brandt, R. L.: Surgical correction of ruptured chordae tendineae. J. Thor. & Cardiov. Surg. **48:** 772, 1964.
18. Haller, J. A., Jr., and Morrow, A. G.: Experimental mitral insufficiency. An operative method of chronic survival. Ann. Surg. **142:** 37, 1955.
19. Haller, J. A., Jr., and Morrow, A. G.: Experimental mitral insufficiency. Surgery **38:** 518, 1955.
20. Braunwald, E., and Awe, W. C.: The syndrome of severe mitral regurgitation with normal left atrial pressure. Circulation **27:** 29, 1963.
21. Best, P. V., and Heath, D.: The right ventricle and small pulmonary arteries in aneurysmal dilatation of the left atrium. Brit. Heart J. **26:** 312, 1964.
22. Carney, E. K., Braunwald, E., Roberts, W. C., Aygen, M., and Morrow, A. G.: Congenital mitral regurgitation. Clinical, hemodynamic, and angiocardiographic findings in nine patients. Am. J. Med. **33:** 223, 1962.
23. Corvisart, J. N.: An Essay on the Organic Diseases of the Heart and Great Vessels. (Translated by Jacob Gates) Boston, Bradford and Read, 1812, 344 pp.
24. McGoon, D. C.: Repair of mitral insufficiency due to ruptured chordae tendineae. J. Thor. & Cardiov. Surg. **39:** 357, 1960.
25. Braunwald, E., Plauth, W. H., Jr., and Morrow, A. G.: A method for the detection and quantification of impaired sodium excretion: Results of an oral sodium tolerance test in normal subjects and in patients with heart disease. Circulation **32:** 223, 1965.

CHRONIC MITRAL REGURGITATION OF UNRESOLVED ETIOLOGY IN THE ELDERLY

A Clinico-pathologic Study of Two Patients

WILLIAM C. ROBERTS, RICHARD S. ROSS, JOSEPH C. EGGLESTON, AND RASHID A. MASSUMI

The Section of Pathology, Clinic of Surgery, National Heart Institute, National Institutes of Health, Bethesda, Maryland; the Departments of Medicine, Radiology and Pathology, The Johns Hopkins University School of Medicine and Hospital; and the George Washington University Division of Medicine and the Cardiopulmonary Laboratory, District of Columbia General Hospital, Washington, D. C.

Received for publication July 10, 1967

Of the various hemodynamic lesions of the cardiac valves, mitral regurgitation and tricuspid regurgitation are the ones most likely to be compatible with a long existence. Chronic mitral regurgitation is most frequently rheumatic in origin. Recently, we studied two patients, aged 60 and 84 years, respectively, and each had known mitral regurgitation for 25 years or more. Neither had a history of acute rheumatic fever, chorea, or infective endocarditis, or other clinically recognized causes of mitral regurgitation. This report describes the clinical and pathologic observations in these two subjects.

REPORT OF PATIENTS

1. M.K. (J.H.H. #312579), a 60-year-old Negro woman, died on March 20, 1966. She had been well until 1939 (age 34) when signs and symptoms of cardiac failure developed during the third month of pregnancy and a therapeutic abortion was performed. In each of the years 1935, 1937, and 1940 she had a baby without difficulty. From 1944 (age 39) until her death in 1966 (age 60) she was admitted to The Johns Hopkins Hospital on 11 occasions and was seen in the outpatient clinic numerous times. When first seen in 1944, because of a threatened abortion, she gave a history of having had mild dyspnea on exertion for four years. She never had acute rheumatic fever or chorea, nor was there a history of cardiac disease in her family. Physical examination showed a mildly enlarged heart, no precordial murmurs or thrills, and normal cardiac sounds. The blood pressure was 180/100 mm Hg, weight 223 pounds, and height 69 inches. Electrocardiogram showed only atrial fibrillation. Chest roentgenograms disclosed slight cardiomegaly without definite evidence of left atrial enlargement. At this time she received pelvic irradiation (for sterilization), was digitalized, and remained on this drug for the rest of her life.

In 1946 the thyroid gland was noted to be enlarged, and subtotal thyroidectomy disclosed a colloid adenoma. Preoperatively, she had no symptoms of hyperthyroidism, and her serum cholesterol was 245 mg per 100 ml. The blood pressure was 170/105 mm Hg. Attempted conversion of the atrial fibrillation with quinidine was unsuccessful. Except for mild dyspnea on exertion and occasional headaches, she was well until March 1949, when she developed sudden transient right-sided numbness and weakness with dysphasia. The blood pressure was 180/110 mm Hg and she weighed 208 pounds. From that time until 1961 the blood pressure on most occasions was elevated (up to 190/110 mm Hg), but on rare occasions was normal (<140/90 mm Hg). The weight from 1950 to 1961 ranged from 150 to 200 pounds. After 1961 the blood pressure was always less than 140/90 mm Hg.

Also in 1949 she had the sudden appearance of dyspnea, pleuritic pain and hemoptysis associated with cardiac failure and a diagnosis of pulmonary embolus was made. In 1949 (age 43) a precordial murmur was heard for the first time; it was a "soft" systolic blowing murmur heard over the cardiac apex and in the left axilla. A chest roentgenogram taken in 1949 is shown in Figure 1.

In February 1956, the thyroid gland again was enlarged; at this time she was nervous, bothered

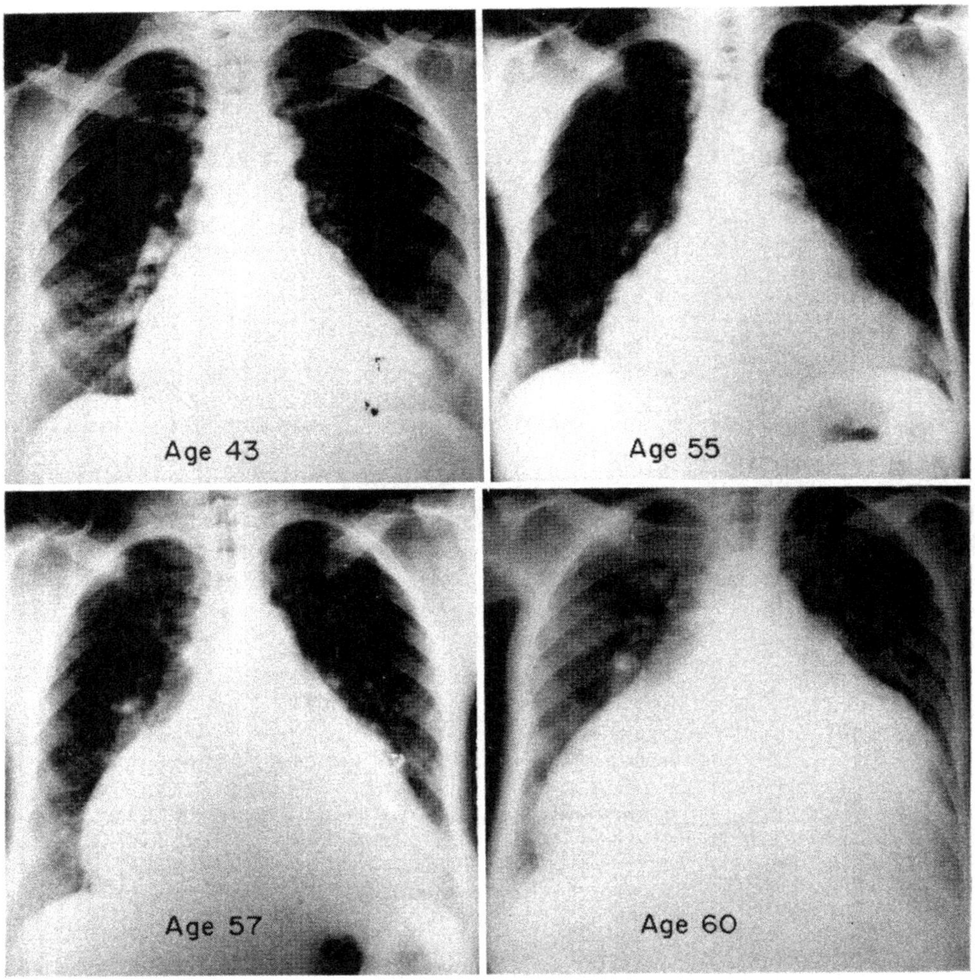

FIG 1. Patient #1. Chest roentgenograms showing progressive cardiac enlargement from age 43 to 60. The right lower radiograph was taken two months before death.

by heat, had smooth skin and a fine tremor of the hands. The serum cholesterol was 173 mg per 100 ml, the serum protein bound iodine was 13.9 micrograms per 100 ml, and she was treated with radioactive iodine[131] (7 millicuries). Following this therapy the signs and symptoms of hyperthyroidism disappeared, and during the next three years she gained 30 pounds (to 185 pounds).

Except for one episode of acute pulmonary edema in 1958, she was able to carry on her activities fairly well until 1961 although she was dyspneic on walking uphill and upstairs and had occasional edema and right upper quadrant pain. In 1961 she had signs and symptoms interpreted as resulting from a pulmonary embolus (Fig 1). A cholecystectomy also was performed because of gallstones and signs of cholecystitis during this year. The heart failure progressively worsened during her last five years of life.

Examination in February 1963 (Fig 1), showed that the systolic murmur had increased to grade 4/6 intensity, was pansystolic, and loudest over the cardiac apex and left axilla. In addition, a grade 3/6 systolic murmur, which became louder with inspiration, was heard over the left sternal border. The liver was enlarged and pulsatile. She weighed 173 pounds, and the blood pressure was 100/70 mm Hg.

In January 1964, she had another pulmonary embolus associated with marked right-sided

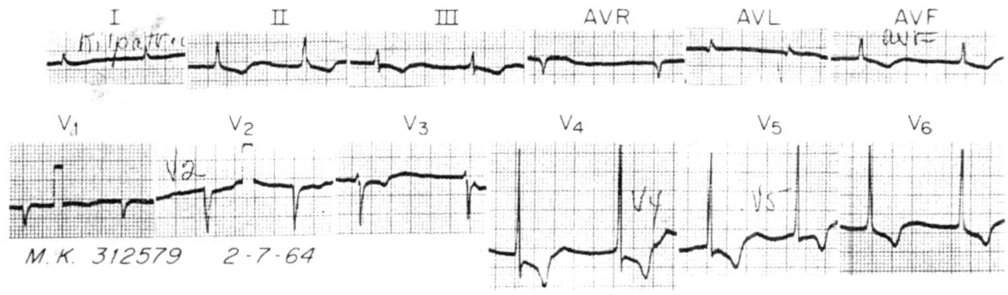

FIG 2. Patient ※1. Electrocardiogram two years before death.

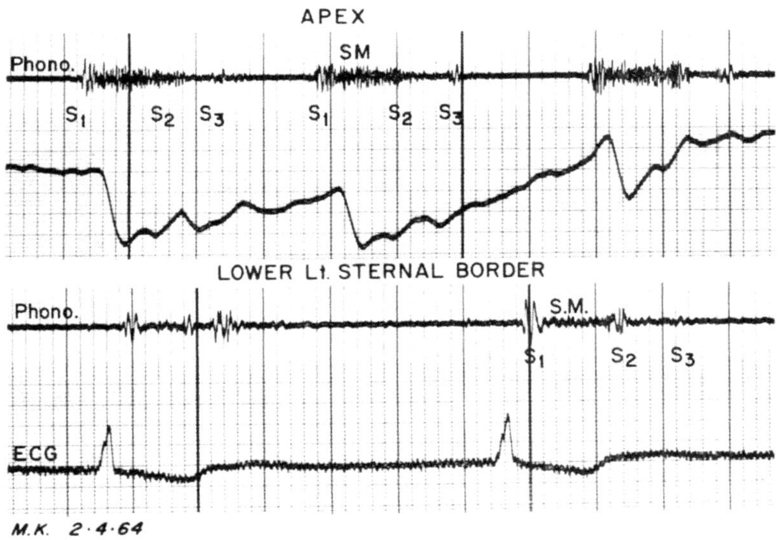

FIG 3. Patient ※1. Phonocardiogram recorded over the cardiac apex (upper) and over the lower left sternal border (lower). The murmur (SM) extends throughout systole. A ventricular gallop (S_3) is recorded. S_1 = first heart sound and S_2 = second heart sound.

cardiac failure. The chest roentgenogram showed massive cardiomegaly, and the electrocardiograms (Fig 2), atrial fibrillation with ST-T wave changes consistent with digitalis effect and/or ischemia. A phonocardiogram recorded in February 1964 is shown in Figure 3. In March 1964 she had a transient unilateral hemiparesis without residua presumedly due to a cerebral embolus. In November 1964 she was again hospitalized because of persistent cardiac failure, and although there was transient precordial pain, there was no electrocardiographic or serum enzyme evidence of acute myocardial infarction. She had occasional attacks of precordial pain thereafter and these were sometimes relieved by nitroglycerin.

In January 1966 she was awakened because of tightness in her chest associated with severe dyspnea and was hospitalized for the last time. The blood pressure was 120/70 mm Hg, and she weighed only 110 pounds (in July 1964 she had weighed 150 pounds). During this admission myocardial infarction was never documented by serial electrocardiograms or by serum enzyme studies. The hematocrit was 37%. She died of intractable cardiac failure (Fig 1).

At necropsy (J.H.H. ※34488), there was evidence of severe right- and left-sided cardiac failure, old and recent pulmonary emboli, congestion of both lungs and viscera with cardiac sclerosis. Death was due to bleeding from a large acute gastric ulcer.

The heart weighed 440 gms, and both atria were severely dilated (Fig 4). The walls of both atria were thin, and antemortum thrombus was present in each. A 4 × 4 cm area of endocardial thickening was present in the left atrium just above the posterior mitral leaflet. The tricuspid,

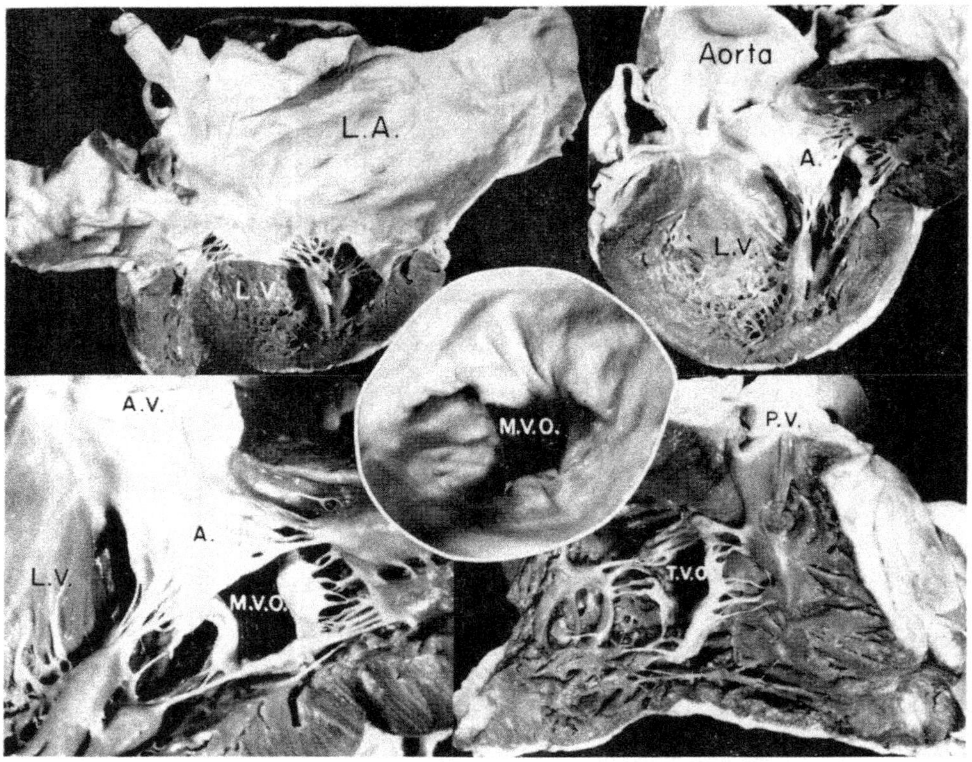

FIG. 4. Patient #1. Opened heart. *Upper left:* Open left atrium (L.A.), mitral valve and left ventricle (L.V.). The left atrium is greatly dilated and its wall is thin. A close-up of the opened mitral valve is shown in Figure 8. *Upper right:* Opened left ventricle, normal aortic valve and ascending aorta. No scars are present in the left ventricular wall which is midly hypertrophied. *Lower left:* Close-up view of the ventricular aspect of the mitral orifice (M.V.O.) before it was opened. The orifice is incompetent. *Lower right:* Opened right ventricle and pulmonic valve (P.V.) showing the tricuspid valve orifice (T.V.O.). The valvular leaflets and chordae are normal, but its annulus is dilated and its orifice is incompetent. The right ventricular wall is not hypertrophied. *Center insert:* Mitral valvular orifice (M.V.O.) as seen from the left atrium.

aortic and pulmonic valves were normal. There was slight focal thickening of the mitral leaflets and the "posterior" leaflet was trilobed. The circumference of the tricuspid valve ring was 13.5 cm and that of the mitral 14 cm. The right ventricular wall was 0.4 cm thick and its cavity dilated. The left ventricular wall was 1.6 cm thick; its chamber was mildly dilated. No myocardial scars were seen. The ostia and courses of the coronary arteries were normal. Focal yellow streaks, fibrous plaques and complicated calcified lesions were present in the walls of all three major coronary arteries, but their lumens throughout were widely patent and never compromised more than 25%.

2. C. D. (D.C.G.H. #226434), an 84-year-old Negro man, died on November 5, 1966. He had known of the presence of cardiac disease since age 40 years when a precordial murmur was heard for the first time. During his last 40 years he was dyspneic, and during his last 20 years this symptom was often severe and frequently accompanied by recurrent pedal edema. He had many episodes of congestive cardiac failure and digitalis intoxication during his last 10 years; with the exception of one hospitalization for cardiac failure in 1961, each episode was treated at home by his private physician. During his hospitalization (Freedman's Hospital, Washington, D. C.) in 1961 the patient apparently aroused considerable interest among medical students and house officers because of the loud intensity of his precordial murmur. He was first hospitalized at District

of Columbia General Hospital in February 1966 because of severe congestive cardiac failure. Questioning at that time disclosed that the patient had never had acute rheumatic fever or chorea, chest pain, or systemic hypertension. He had never smoked.

He had to sit up to breathe easily. The neck veins were markedly distended with large v waves. The point of maximal impulse of the heart was in the sixth left intercostal space in the anterior axillary line. A systolic thrill was palpable over the cardiac apex. A grade 4/6 pansystolic blowing murmur was heard over the cardiac apex and in the left axilla. In addition, a different pitch, grade 3/6, blowing, systolic murmur which increased in intensity with inspiration was audible over the lower left sternal border. A short, grade 1/6 diastolic rumble and a ventricular gallop were audible over the cardiac apex. Rales were heard in the lung bases bilaterally. The blood pressure was 135/80 mm Hg. He weighed 110 pounds and stood 70 inches in height. The liver was tender and enlarged, its anteroinferior edge being 5 cm below the costal margin. There was no subcutaneous edema. Electrocardiogram showed atrial fibrillation with a slow ventricular response, premature ventricular contractions from multiple foci, prolonged P-R interval (0.28 sec), and myocardial ischemia and/or digitalis effect. Chest roentgenogram showed cardiomegaly and pulmonary congestion. The hematocrit was 39%.

During his ten days in the hospital he lost 10 pounds; with discontinuation of digitalis for several days the number of premature contractions decreased, and he was discharged. He was readmitted in September 1966 again because of worsening of the cardiac failure, but, in addition, he was severely dehydrated. The physical findings, chest roentgenogram (Fig 5) and electrocardiogram (Fig 6) were unchanged when compared to those seven months earlier, except that he now had fewer premature contractions. On the twenty-third hospital day, while awaiting disposition to a nursing home, he suddenly developed acute pulmonary edema and died.

At necropsy, the heart (Figs 7–10) weighed 400 gm. All chambers were dilated; the right ventricular wall was 0.4 cm thick, the left ventricular wall, 1.3 cm thick, and the right atrial wall was translucent. An organized thrombus was present in the left atrium. The tricuspid valve leaflets and chordae were normal; its annulus measured 14.5 cm and the mitral annulus, 14.0 cm in circumference. The margins of the mitral leaflets were focally thickened, and the chordae tendineae, although of normal caliber, were shorter than normal. The "posterior" mitral leaflet was trilobed. The anterolateral papillary muscle was severely scarred as was the adjacent free wall of the left ventricle (Figs 7–9) and the posteromedial papillary muscle was slightly scarred. The semilunar valvular cusps were normal, but the valve "rings" were dilated; each measured 9 cm in circumference. The coronary arteries and ostia were widely patent and virtually free of atheroma (Fig 9).

COMMENTS

The cause of the mitral regurgitation in these two patients is uncertain. The mitral valve in each was mildly deformed in that there were three small posterior cusps rather than one large one, but this minor deviation from normal would not appear to account for mitral regurgitation. The mitral leaflets in each patient were thickened, and their chordae tendineae shortened, but these changes were also mild and would not appear to cause severe regurgitation. The fact that the mitral leaflets were not diffusely thickened and that the chordae tendineae were of normal caliber is strong evidence against rheumatic disease being the underlying etiology. In addition, no Aschoff bodies were present in either heart and neither patient had a history of acute rheumatic fever or chorea. In patient #1 no chorda tendina was attached to one portion of the posterior leaflet, but there was no indication that one had ever been attached in this area. The possibility remains, although remote, that one or more chorda tendina could have been present at this site (Fig 8) and subsequently ruptured and healed. In patient #2 there was localized left ventricular scarring involving only the papillary muscles, mainly the anterolateral one, and the adjacent free walls. The lumens of the coronary arteries, both extra- and intramural ones, however, in this patient were wide open, and thus

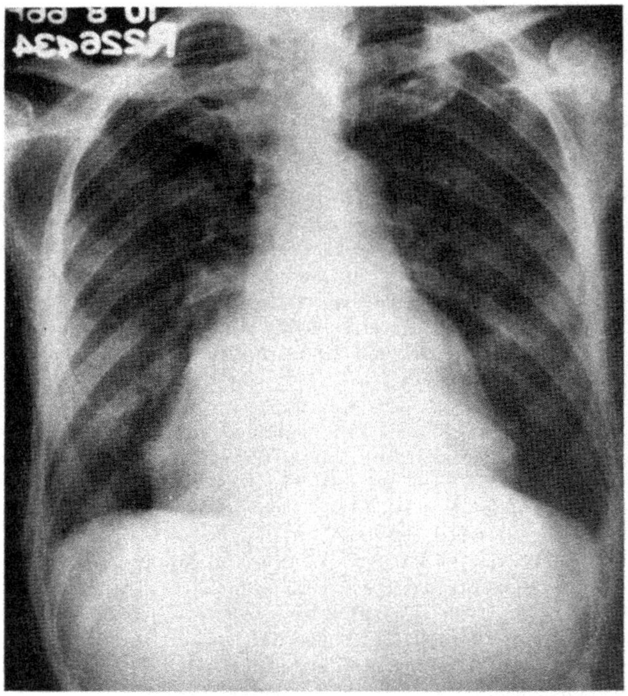

FIG. 5. Patient #2. Chest roentgenogram taken 27 days before death.

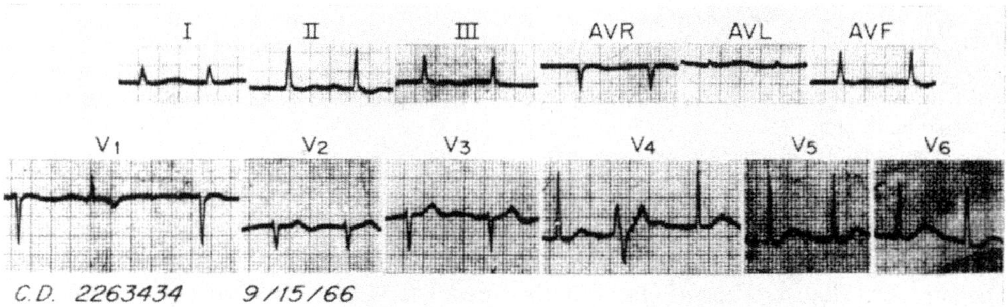

FIG. 6. Patient #2. Electrocardiogram 50 days before death.

the scarring cannot be the result of coronary arterial disease. The papillary muscle scarring could account for the mitral regurgitation in this patient, but the cause of the focal myocardial fibrosis is speculative. Focal myocarditis, which healed many years earlier, could possibly have been the cause. In each of these two patients the mitral annuli were dilated, and this dilatation almost certainly contributed to the regurgitation, but probably was not the initial event. When mitral regurgitation results from dilatation of the base of the left ventricle, which includes the mitral annulus, the precordial murmur produced by this mechanism is rarely of the intensity demonstrated in either of the patients described. Infective endocarditis may cause mitral regurgitation at any age, but for it to initiate incompetence which persists for over 25 years, as in the two patients presented, would be rare.

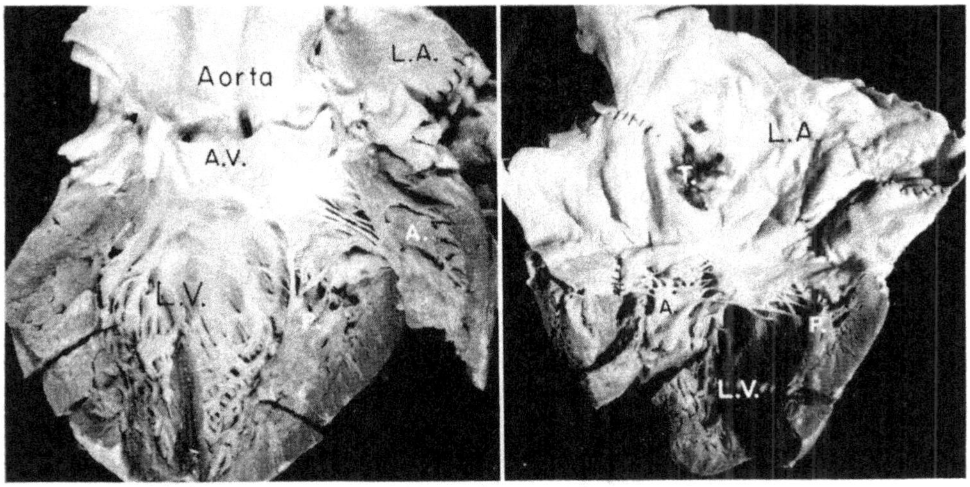

FIG 7. Patient #2. Opened left side of the heart. *Left:* Left ventricle (L.V.), normal aortic valve (A.V.), and aorta. There is slight opacification of the left ventricular endocardium and extensive fibrous scarring with flattening of the anterolateral (A.) papillary muscle. P. = posteromedial papillary muscle. *Right:* Left atrium (L.A.), mitral valve, and left ventricle. The left atrial cavity is markedly dilated and its wall is thin. A small flat thrombus (T.) is present.

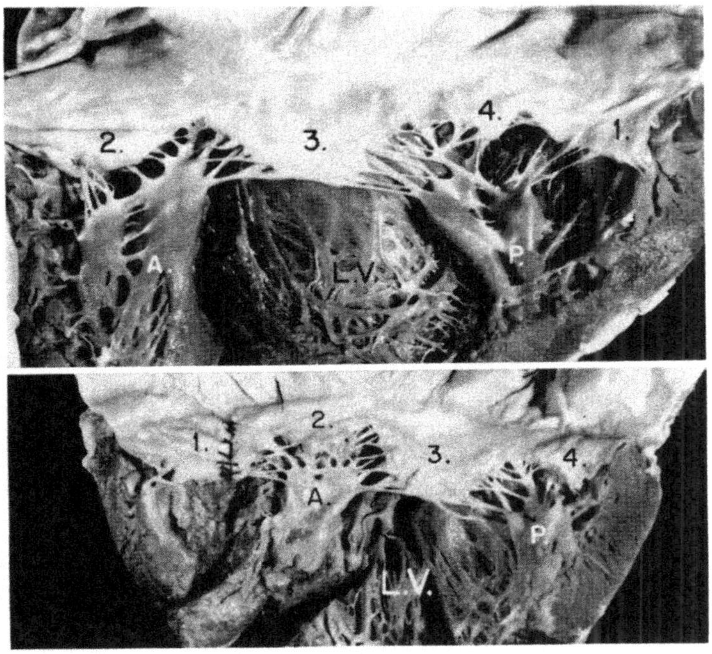

FIG 8. The mitral valves and papillary muscles in each of the two patients. Each of the mitral valves contains four leaflets. The anterior leaflet in each is No. 3. There is mild focal fibrous thickening of the leaflets and shortening of the chordae tendineae in each. *Upper:* Patient #1. The papillary muscles are hypertrophied, but free of scars. *Lower:* Patient #2. The papillary muscles, particularly the anterolateral (A.) one, are scarred and the anterolateral one is flattened. P. = posteromedial papillary muscle.

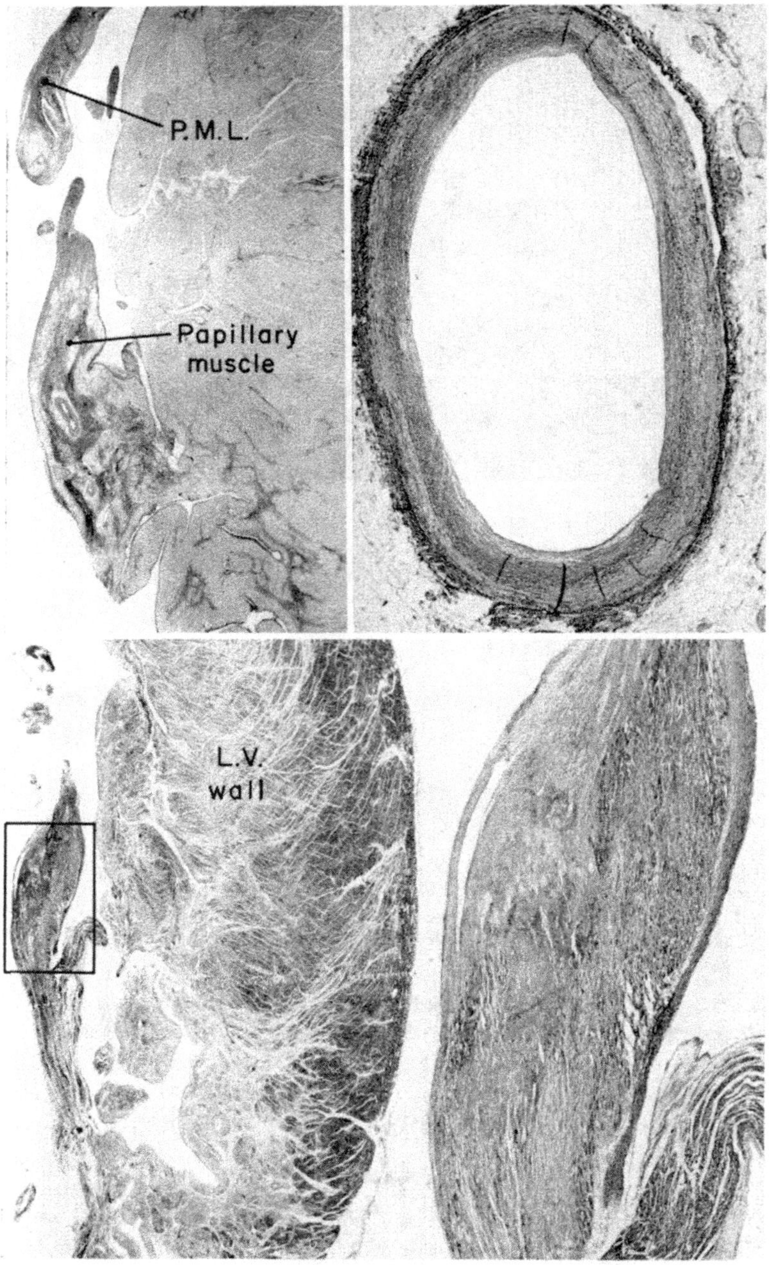

FIG 9. Patient #2. Anterolateral papillary muscle and left main coronary artery. *Upper left:* Elastic tissue stain (× 4.5) showing extensive scarring in this papillary muscle. P.M.L. = posterior mitral leaflet. *Lower left:* Another section (H and E; × 4) showing not only fibrosis of the anterolateral papillary muscle, but also extensive fibrosis of the left ventricular free wall at the base of the papillary muscle. *Lower right:* A close-up of the area in brackets of the papillary muscle. The myocardium is 90% replaced by fibrous tissue (H and E; × 18). *Upper right:* Left main coronary artery showing that its lumen was wide open. There was no narrowing of either the extra- or intramural coronary arteries in this patient. (Elastic tissue stain; × 21.)

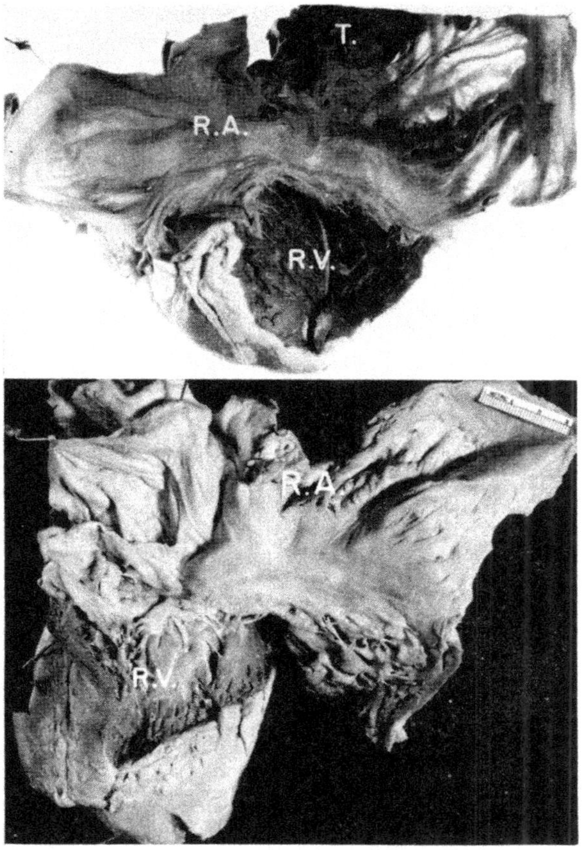

FIG 10. Opened right atrium (R.A.), tricuspid valve, and right ventricle (R.V.) in each of the two patients. The right atrium is markedly dilated in each, and in patient #1 (upper) its wall is translucent, and ante mortum thrombus (T.) is present. The right ventricular wall is not hypertrophied in either subject.

The etiology of mitral regurgitation in older individuals has been the subject of debate for some time. Friedberg and Tartakower (1), Sprague and Carmichael (2), and Graham and associates (3) have all emphasized that rheumatic valvular disease is by no means uncommon in patients over age 50 years. Bedford and Caird in their monograph, "Valvular Disease of the Heart in Old Age," stated that rheumatic heart disease occurs in 2 to 3% of individuals 65 years of age and over (4). These authors apparently considered any scarring of the mitral leaflets and chordae to be of rheumatic etiology. In our experience, focal scarring of the mitral leaflets is common in the elderly, but these focal lesions rarely lead to left ventricular and left atrial dilatation and rarely produce a precordial murmur. Diffuse scarring of the mitral leaflets and chordae and a positive history of acute rheumatic fever or chorea is most unusual in elderly patients in our experience. Possibly, some of the authors mentioned above would have attributed a rheumatic etiology to the diseased hearts of the two patients described here, but in our judgment there is no evidence for this etiology. We have found no reports describing incompetent mitral valves similar to those in our two subjects.

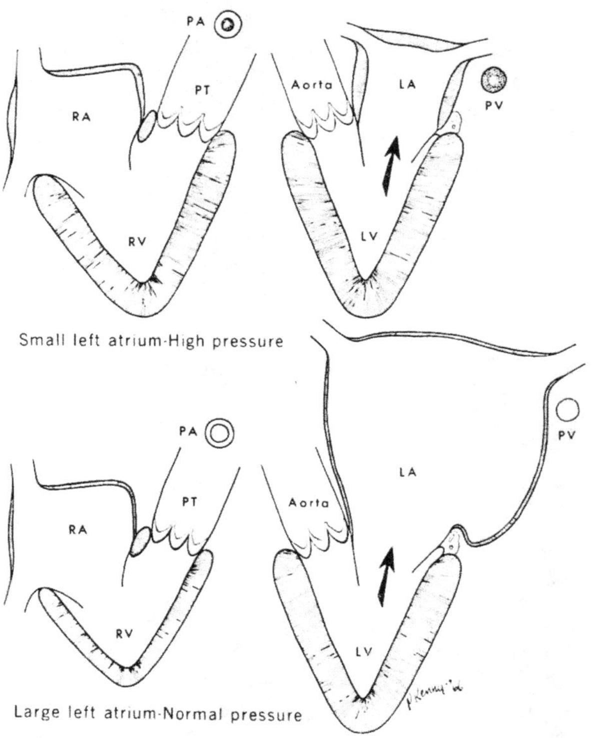

FIG 11. Diagrammatic representation of the two extremes of the spectrum of mitral regurgitation. The two subjects described in this report represent one end of the gamut, that is, large left atrium (LA), but normal left atrial and pulmonary arterial (PA) pressures. These pressures justifiably may be assumed to have been normal in the two subjects described since there was no medial hypertrophy or intimal proliferation of the pulmonary arteries and the right ventricular (RV) wall was not hypertrophied. When severe mitral regurgitation appears suddenly in individuals with previoulsy normal or near-normal hearts the left atrium is relatively small and the high pressure within it is reflected back into the pulmonary vessels and finally to the right ventricle. The anatomic indicator of this latter physiologic event is severe hypertrophy of the left atrial and right ventricular walls and marked intimal proliferation and medial hypertrophy of the pulmonary arteries, arterioles, and veins (PV). PT = pulmonary trunk; LV = left ventricle; and R. A. = right atrium.

Another intriguing aspect of each of the two patients described is the severe left atrial dilatation, the lack of right ventricular hypertrophy, and the absence of changes in the pulmonary arterial blood vessels. Best and Heath have made similar observations in patients with aneurysmal dilatation of the left atrium (5). Thus, these patients represent one end of the spectrum of mitral regurgitation, that is, those subjects with large left atrial chambers but no left atrial, pulmonary venous, pulmonary arterial or right ventricular hypertension (Fig 11). This syndrome of normal left atrial and pulmonary arterial pressures but, nevertheless, severe mitral regurgitation was initially described by Braunwald and Awe (6). The left atrial walls in these subjects are thin, and thus readily compliant and able to "absorb" the volume of blood regurgitated into the left atrium during ventricular systole without elevating the intraatrial pressure. Since the thin left atrial walls are capable of expanding easily, the pressure in the pulmonary veins and, thus, the pulmonary arteries and right ventricle, does not become elevated. The other extreme of the syndrome of mitral regurgitation occurs in individuals in whom the regurgitation appears suddenly and involves a previously normal or nearly normal mitral valve (7). With the acute onset of regurgitation in these individuals the left atrial walls resist expansion (noncompliant), and thus, the high left ventricular pressure is not "absorbed" by the left atrium, but is reflected backwards into the pulmonary veins and thereafter into the pulmonary arteries and right ventricle. These individuals consequently develop severe changes of pulmonary hypertension in the pulmonary vasculature and severe thickening of the right ventricular wall. Obviously, the majority of patients with mitral regurgitation fall physiologically and anatomically somewhere between these two extreme groups.

SUMMARY

The clinical and necropsy features of each of two older patients with mitral regurgitation are described. The etiology of the incompetence in them is uncertain, and descriptions of similar valves have not been found. Each had a precordial murmur typical of mitral regurgitation for over 25 years and both had severely dilated left atria, without pulmonary vascular changes or right ventricular hypertrophy.

REFERENCES

1. Friedberg, C. K. and Tartakower, T.: Ueber den guenstigen Verlauf der endokarditischen Herzklappenfehler (Mit besonderer Berucksichtigung des Alters under der Schwangerschaft). Z. Klin. Med., **116:** 759, 1931.
2. Sprague, H. B. and Carmichael, D. B.: Rheumatic valvular disease in the aged. Geriatrics, **5:** 239, 1950.
3. Graham, G. K., Taylor, J. A., Ellis, L. B., Greenberg, D. J. and Robbins, S. L.: Studies in mitral stenosis II: A correlation of post-mortem findings with the clinical course of the disease in 101 cases. Arch. Intern. Med., *88:* 533, 1951.
4. Bedford, P. D. and Caird, F. I.: Valvular disease of the heart in old age. Little, Brown and Co., Boston, 1960, pp. 194.
5. Best, P. V. and Heath, D.: The right ventricle and small pulmonary arteries in aneurysmal dilatation of the left atrium. Brit. Heart J., **26:** 312, 1964.
6. Braunwald, E. and Awe, W. C.: The syndrome of severe mitral regurgitation with normal left atrial pressure. Circulation, **27:** 29, 1963.
7. Roberts, W. C., Braunwald, E. and Morrow, A. G.: Acute severe mitral regurgitation secondary to ruptured chordae tendineae. Clinical, hemodynamic, and pathologic considerations. Circulation, **33:** 58, 1966.

The Mitral Apparatus

Functional Anatomy of Mitral Regurgitation

By Joseph K. Perloff, M.D., and William C. Roberts, M.D.

SUMMARY

This review deals with the functional anatomy of the six components of the mitral apparatus, namely, the left atrial wall, annulus, leaflets, chordae tendineae, papillary muscles, and left ventricular wall. Each component is considered individually, in the context of the apparatus as a whole, in relation to the mode of closure of the normal mitral valve, and in the light of many acquired and congenital disorders that disturb the harmony of the finely coordinated mitral mechanism and render it incompetent.

The left atrium is related to mitral valve competence in terms of contraction and relaxation and in terms of dilatation of its posterior wall. The annulus not only serves as a fulcrum for the leaflets but exhibits sphincteric contraction in systole that decreases the size of the orifice. The two leaflets differ in shape but are nearly identical in area, and together are about two and one half times the area of the orifice that they are required to close. Leaflet abnormalities causing acquired or congenital mitral regurgitation result from deficient leaflet tissue, excessive leaflet tissue, or restricted leaflet mobility. Chordae tendineae are considered according to their leaflet attachments, ventricular attachments, thicknesses, lengths, and arborization patterns. Mitral regurgitation due to chordal abnormalities results from chordae that are abnormally long, abnormally short, ectopically inserted, or ruptured. In this context, systolic clicks and late systolic murmurs are discussed, and severe *acute* mitral regurgitation is contrasted with severe *chronic* mitral regurgitation. The papillary muscles and the left ventricular wall represent the two muscular components of the mitral apparatus. An appraisal of papillary muscle dysfunction includes dysfunction with loss in continuity (rupture) and dysfunction without loss in continuity (fibrosis, ischemia, replacement). Finally, the role of altered left ventricular shape is discussed in the context of mitral regurgitation, and the effect of dilatation is ascribed chiefly to alterations in the position of papillary muscles and their directional axes of tension.

Additional Indexing Words:
Left atrial wall   Mitral annulus   Leaflets   Chordae tendineae
Papillary muscles   Left ventricular wall   Systolic clicks
Late systolic murmurs

Our current conceptions as to the dynamic consequences of a leaking mitral valve . . . are still at variance. It is pertinent, therefore to discuss a few of the supposed consequences of mitral regurgitation.—Carl J. Wiggers, 1922[1]

THE MITRAL APPARATUS is a complex, finely coordinated mechanism that can be deranged by a multiplicity of acquired and congenital disorders and requires for its competence the functional integrity of six anatomic elements working in delicate concert. These anatomic elements are: (1) posterior left atrial wall, (2) annulus, (3)

From the Department of Medicine, Georgetown University School of Medicine, Division of Cardiology, Georgetown University Hospital, Washington, D.C., and the Section of Pathology, National Heart and Lung Institute, Bethesda, Maryland.

Supported in part by the Eric T. Paglin Memorial Fund for Cardiovascular Teaching and Research.

Address for reprints: Dr. Joseph K. Perloff, Hospital of the University of Pennsylvania, 3400 Spruce Street, Philadelphia, Pennsylvania 19104.

Received January 28, 1972; revision accepted for publication March 3, 1972.

leaflets, (4) chordae tendineae, (5) papillary muscles, and (6) left ventricular wall.

The exact mode of closure of the normal mitral valve is still uncertain.[2,3] Left ventricular systole begins with contraction of the papillary muscles. The vertical forces exerted by the contracting papillary muscles move the leaflets into apposition. As the intraventricular pressure rises, the free edges of the cusps firmly coapt, mutually supporting each other along a comfortable margin of their atrial surfaces, and firmly sealing the orifice. The remainder of each leaflet bulges like a parachute toward the left atrium.[4] The annulus not only serves as a fulcrum for the leaflets, but during ventricular systole decreases its circumferential size, thus reducing the area that the leaflets are required to bridge.[5,6] Even so, the surface area of the leaflets is about two and one half times the area of the orifice, thus providing a comfortable reserve. As the left ventricle ejects, its apex and the mitral orifice approach each other. Shortening of the vertical axis of the left ventricle is accompanied by synergistic contraction of the papillary muscles and adjacent left ventricular wall so that an appropriate vertical anchoring force is applied to the chordae tendineae, that prevents eversion of the leaflets. Let us now turn attention to the six anatomic components of the mitral apparatus which when faulty can disturb the harmony of the valvular mechanism and render it incompetent. Coordinated interaction among these elements—which are interdependent—usually means that more than one, or even several, are deranged at any one time although with varying degrees of importance.

Left Atrial Wall

Two contributions of the left atrium have been related to competence of the mitral valve: (1) contraction and relaxation[7–9] and (2) atrial dilatation.[4] Even recently, it has been affirmed that atrial contraction and relaxation result in mitral valve closure in man.[8] Contractility rather than flow has been considered the chief determinant of mitral valve closure as a result of atrial activity.[7] Vigorous atrial systole followed by a rapid decline in atrial pressure has been held responsible for substantial changes in the rate of development of ventriculoatrial pressure gradients before the onset of ventricular systole.[7] Although atrial contraction and relaxation seem capable of closing the mitral valve in man, the *absence* of such activity does *not* cause mitral regurgitation.[9] Competence of the mitral apparatus depends in part on a normal sequence of *ventricular activation* (see below) but not on a normal sequence of atrial and ventricular contraction. Loss of effective atrial contraction (atrial fibrillation, complete heart block, and others) does not necessarily result in regurgitation.[9]

Left atrial enlargement itself can contribute to mitral regurgitation[4] (fig. 1). Dilatation of the left atrium does not affect the anterior leaflet since that leaflet is anchored to the root of the aorta.[4] The posterior leaflet, however, can be directly affected[4] (figs. 1 and 2). As the left atrium enlarges, its posterior wall is displaced posteriorly and downward. Because of the continuity of the atrial endocardium and posterior mitral leaflet, this displacement exerts tension on the posterior leaflet.[4] The displacement may prevent that cusp from contacting its mate or may aggravate preexisting leaflet malapposition. Thus, as mitral regurgitation provokes left atrial enlargement,

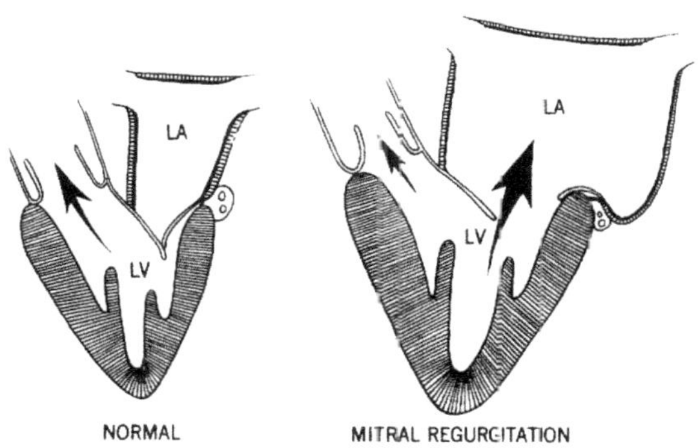

Figure 1

As the left atrium dilates, its posterior wall tends to hang over the atrioventricular sulcus. The dilatation pulls the posterior mitral leaflet cephalad since this leaflet is continuous with the left atrial endocardium.

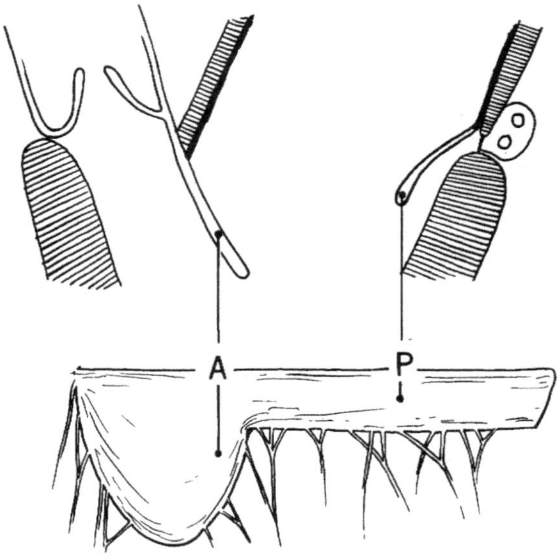

Figure 2

Diagrams of anterior (A) and posterior (P) mitral leaflets. The anterior leaflet is continuous with the aortic valve cusps and aorta. The posterior leaflet is primarily a continuation of the mural endocardium of the left atrium.

the enlargement itself may aggravate regurgitant flow. As Edwards and Burchell[10] aptly put it, "mitral insufficiency begets mitral insufficiency," irrespective of the initiating cause.

Mitral Annulus

The annulus forms an important part of the basal attachment or fulcrum of the mitral leaflets.[4, 10] A traditional point of view states that if the atrioventricular ring dilates sufficiently, the cusps are unable to meet and mitral regurgitation results.[11] This explanation is an oversimplification.[4] Left ventricular dilatation—an undoubted cause of mitral incompetence—may exert its effects independently of dilatation of the mitral ring (see below). Nevertheless, the size of the ring does play a role in preserving competence of the mitral valve, albeit a role that relates less to dilatation than to failure to decrease its circumference during systole. The tissue at the basal attachments of the mitral leaflets is tough but pliable. Toughness opposes dilatation; pliability permits sphincter-like contraction of the annulus during systole, which reduces the area that the apposing leaflets must bridge by an estimated 20 to 50%.[2, 6] Left ventricular dilatation may exert an unfavorable effect on the annulus chiefly by applying a distending pressure that opposes systolic annular contraction.[5] With calcification of the annulus—in itself a cause of mitral regurgitation[12]—the mechanism of regurgitation is believed to stem from a loss of sphincteric action of the basal attachments of the mitral cusps. In such patients, calcific deposits commonly coexist on the aortic surfaces of otherwise normal trileaflet aortic valves;[13] the resulting obstruction to left ventricular outflow augments incompetence associated with the calcified mitral ring. Calcification of the annulus is found not only in the elderly but occasionally in young patients with the Marfan syndrome,[14] and represents one of the two organic causes of mitral regurgitation in such individuals (see below). In addition, mitral annular calcification also occurs in children with Hurler's syndrome.[15]

Leaflets

Proper closure of the leaflets represents an ultimate goal of the entire mitral mechanism. The areas of the two leaflets are nearly identical, but the basal to free edge length of the anterior leaflet is two or more times that of the posterior (fig. 2). Consequently, the anterior leaflet is more mobile, while the posterior leaflet fulfills a secondary or supporting role.[11] Although the mitral leaflets, like other cardiac valves, have been looked upon as passive connective tissue structures, recent investigations have found within their substance striated muscle bundles to which an active function has been assigned.[16] It is uncertain whether such muscle fibers have physiologic significance in promoting closure of the valve.

Leaflet abnormalities can be acquired or congenital, with regurgitation resulting from deficient leaflet tissue, excessive leaflet tissue, or restricted leaflet mobility. Inadequate leaflet tissue results from a number of causes, the best known of which is rheumatic endocarditis which provokes scarring and contractures. Clefts which penetrate a leaflet from its free edge can be acquired (infective endocarditis[4]) or congenital (cleft anterior leaflet of endocardial cushion defect[17]). Acquired clefts lack chordal support so that mitral regurgitation is obligatory. Congenital clefts differ in that chordae tendineae attach to their margins and can offer support that is adequate for valve competence, or if too short, can restrict mobility of the cleft leaflet and cause regurgitation. Inadequate leaflet tissue can also result from perforations or holes within a leaflet remote from its free edge.[4] Such perforations are typically acquired (infective endocarditis[4]). Double-orifice mitral valve is, strictly speaking, *not* a congenital perforation, but rather two mitral valves equipped with supporting chordae.[18] Left atrial myxoma—correctly looked upon as a cause of obstruction at the mitral orifice—causes mitral regurgitation by destructive traumatic impact on the leaflets.

Excessive leaflet tissue may result in a hoodlike deformity in which the unsupported segment of leaflet (ruptured chordae tendineae or abnormally long chordae) balloons upward as ventricular systolic pressure is exerted against its undersurface.[19] Perhaps akin to interchordal hooding is the disorder known as the billowing or floppy mitral valve[19, 20] or the systolic click-late systolic murmur syndrome.

An occasional patient exhibiting this disorder has complete or partial stigmata of the Marfan syndrome with fibromyxomatous changes in valve tissue, marked redundancy of leaflets, and elongated chordae[19–21] (fig. 3). More recently, systolic clicks with the late systolic murmur have been found in patients with isolated thoracic bony abnormalities.[22] As a rule, however, the patient, usually female, otherwise judged as normal presents with systolic clicks and a late systolic murmur, and on angiography or echocardiography shows billowing mitral cusps, generally posterior, and relatively mild late systolic regurgitation.[23] In the latter half of ventricular systole the redundant leaflet, poorly anchored by its

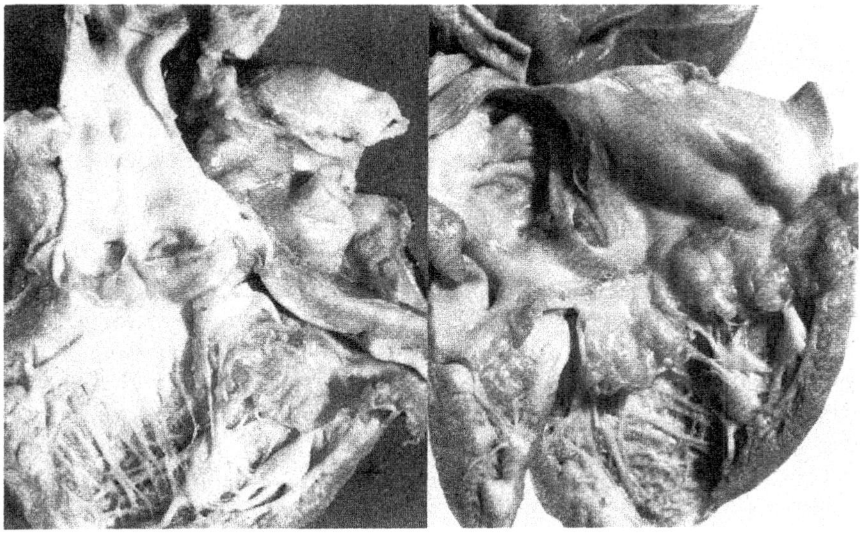

Figure 3

Opened left heart of a 2-day-old infant with features of the Marfan syndrome and auscultatory evidence of mitral regurgitation. **(Left)** *Opened aorta, aortic valve, and left ventricle. The wall of the aorta was abnormal and consistent with cystic medial necrosis. The aortic valve appears normal.* **(Right)** *Opened dilated left atrium, mitral valve, and dilated left ventricle. The mitral leaflets are floppy, i.e., elongated in both longitudinal and transverse dimensions.*

long chordae, becomes slack and prolapses into the left atrium. A late systolic murmur and occasionally bizarre musical late systolic whoops or honks[24] may accompany late systolic regurgitation.

Osler's account of the systolic whoop or honk is apt.[25] He wrote, "As she [a 12-year-old girl] sits upright in the chair, the heart sounds at apex and base loud and clear; no murmur. When she stands, a loud systolic murmur is heard at apex, high-pitched, somewhat musical. . . . It disappeared quite suddenly, and could not be detected on most careful examination. The child then suggested that she heard it most frequently when in the stooping posture; and on causing her to lean forward and relax the chest, the murmur was at once heard, and with greatly increased intensity."

Clicks, single or multiple, occur alone, may introduce the murmur, may be intermittent, persistent, or absent, and are believed to be due to tensing of the elongated chordae (chordal snaps) or the billowing leaflet.[20] Migration of the click (or clicks) toward the first heart sound is known to occur during inspiration and after amyl nitrite inhalation.[26] Recently, *persistent* early timing, i.e., *early* systolic clicks due to mitral valve prolapse, has been identified.[27] When such early clicks introduce mitral regurgitation, the accompanying murmur *sounds* holosystolic although a small gap exists between first heart sound and click. When a pressor agent is administered to subjects with isolated systolic clicks, the clicks move toward the second sound, and the rise in left ventricular systolic pressure occasionally produces a late systolic murmur presumably identifying the clicks as intracardiac and associated with potential mitral regurgitation.[28] Accordingly, subjects with clicks alone, clicks and a late systolic murmur, or a late systolic murmur alone are at risk of infective endocarditis[29] and should be so managed even though some systolic clicks may prove to be extracardiac. Patients with clicks and late systolic murmurs often have abnormal electrocardiograms, especially T-wave inversions in diaphragmatic leads.[20, 21] These auscultatory and electrocardiographic patterns are occasionally familial.[20] An increased incidence of ectopic rhythms[30] and an unknown incidence of sudden death occur in such patients.[20] One who died suddenly had a markedly redundant posterior leaflet and thin elongated chordae at necropsy.[20] Recently systolic clicks and late systolic murmurs or whoops with billowing posterior leaflets have been found in ostium secundum atrial septal defect[24, 31] and in Ebstein's anomaly of the tricuspid valve.[32] In addition, an abnormality of the inferior wall of the left ventricle has been proposed as a contributory factor in rendering the posterior leaflet slack.[21] It is not known whether the bifid apical systolic impulse in these patients relates to such an abnormality of left ventricular wall, to abrupt midsystolic decompression of the left ventricle by the prolapsing mitral leaflet, or to an unidentified cause.[33]

Not all whoops or honks are confined to late systole, and the etiology is not always a floppy mitral leaflet.[24] Furthermore, late systolic murmurs without clicks occasionally occur in rheumatic mitral regurgitation,[34] and systolic clicks may introduce the late systolic murmur of papillary muscle dysfunction in ischemic heart disease[35] (see below).

Mitral regurgitation due to restricted leaflet mobility has already been related to abnormally short chordae. Peculiarities of mitral commissural fusion following rheumatic endocarditis also keep the leaflets apart and contribute to incompetence,[4] but most patients with fused commissures have some degree of stenosis as well. In pure rheumatic mitral regurgitation, the chordae tendineae are generally not shortened. At other times, leaflet mobility may be restricted by abnormal attachments to the endocardium of the left ventricle. Fusion of the posterior cusp to the underlying ventricular endocardium has been related to organization of vegetations of infective endocarditis located in the angle formed by the posterior leaflet and left ventricular wall.[4] Occasionally leaflet motion may be restrained because of the abnormal directional pull exerted by chordae tendineae with ectopic ventricular attachments.[4] Another type of leaflet restriction accompanies congenitally corrected L-transposition of the great vessels (ventricular inversion).[4, 36] In this anomaly, the mitral orifice is equipped with a tricuspid valve (inversion, i.e., right-to-left interchange). The left-sided tricuspid valve is often the site of an Ebstein-like anomaly in which the basal portion of a leaflet is attached to the left ventricular endocardium.[4] Restricted cusp mobility is a chief cause of mitral regurgitation in this anomaly.

Chordae Tendineae

Abnormally long chordae, abnormally short chordae, and ectopically inserted chordae have been discussed. This section deals with ruptured chordae.

Chordae tendineae must be considered according to their leaflet attachments, their ventricular attachments, and their individual thicknesses, lengths, and arborization patterns. Several different orders of chordae are recognized. The physiologic consequences and clinical signs of rupture depend to a large extent on where in the chordal pattern discontinuity occurs.

The majority of chordae that attach to the leaflets form a fine network of delicate threads that spring from larger chords near the papillary muscles (fig. 4). Some chords run as single nonbranching bundles of collagen from papillary muscle to leaflet. Each papillary muscle gives rise to chordae that cross to and support both anterior and posterior cusps (fig. 4). The etiology of chordal rupture is often unclear (spontaneous). Infective endocarditis is one established cause,[4, 37] but rupture of chordae tendineae is *not* a complication of myocardial infarction.[19] Rupture of one or

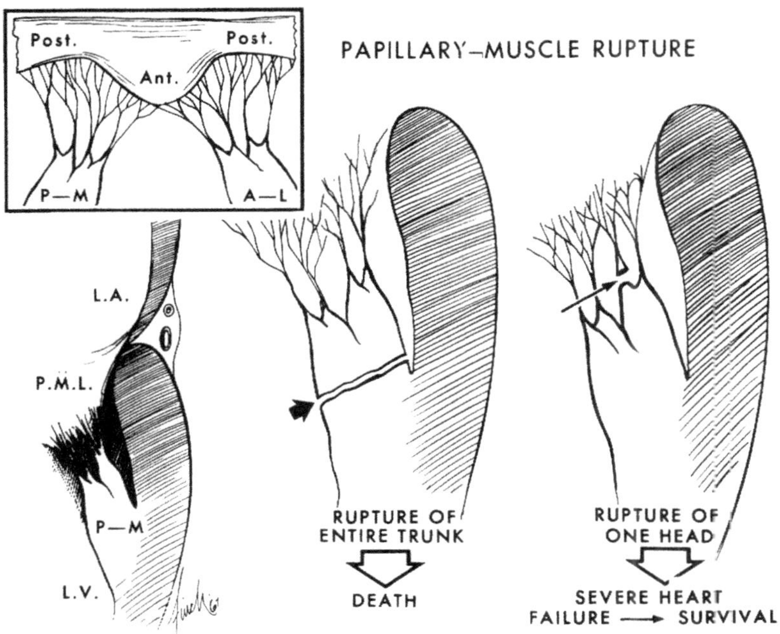

Figure 4

Schematic diagrams. **(Left upper)** *Showing that the posterior (P-M) and anterior (A-M) papillary muscles each gives rise to branching chordae that lend support to both anterior and posterior leaflets.* **(Left lower)** *Showing the posterior papillary muscle with its multiple heads. P.M.L. = posterior mitral leaflets, L.A. = left atrium, L.V. = left ventricle.* **(Right and center)** *Showing that rupture of the central body (entire trunk) results in overwhelming regurgitation, and rupture confined to one head of a papillary muscle results in regurgitation analogous to that following rupture of major chords.*

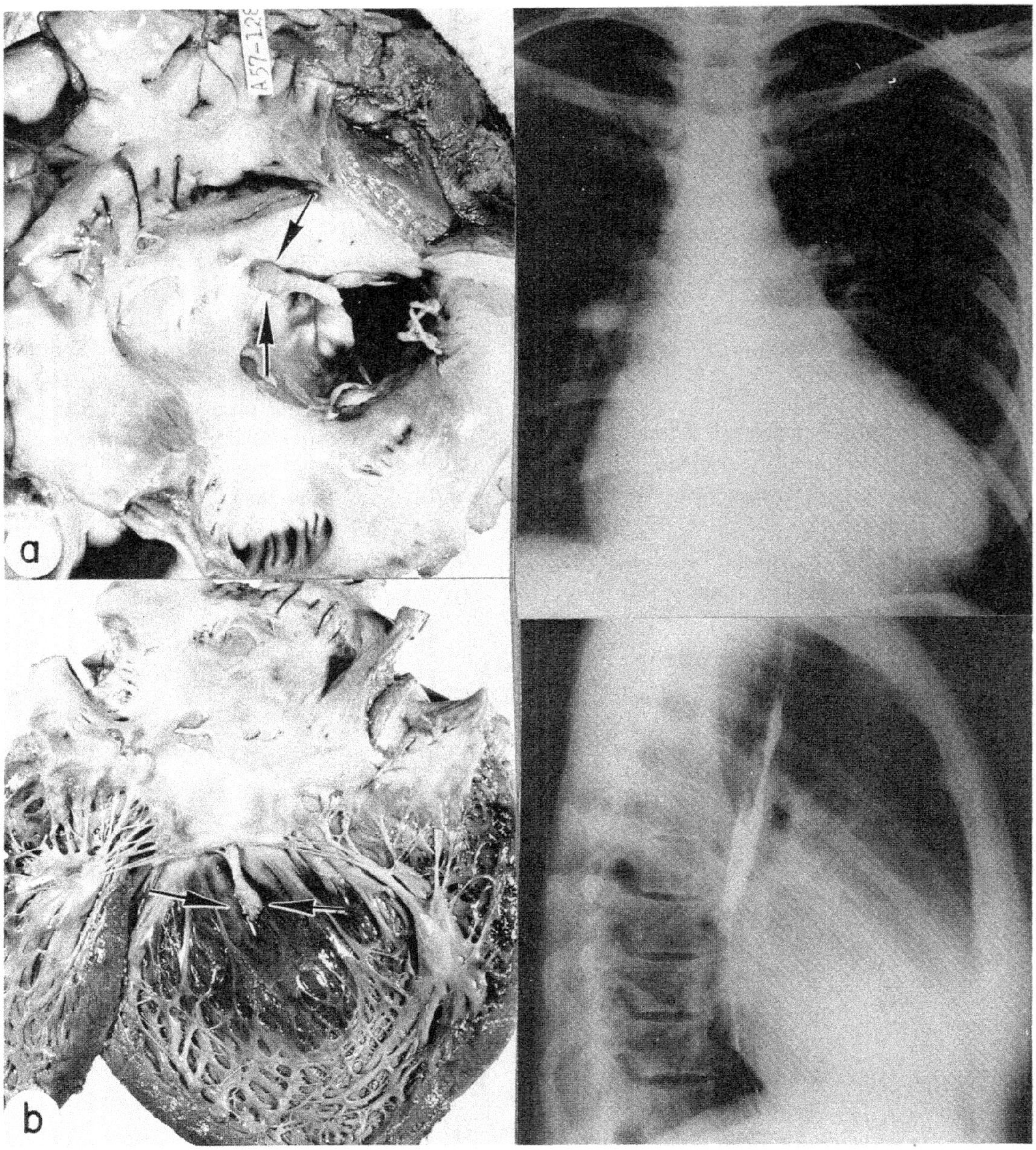

Figure 5

Opened left atrium (a) *and opened left heart* (b) *of a 37-year-old woman who developed sudden severe mitral regurgitation 7 months earlier. The left atrium is of normal size. A club-shaped ruptured chorda tendinea (arrows) from the anterior mitral leaflet was responsible for acute severe mitral regurgitation. The nonruptured chordae are normal. The chest X-rays show cardiomegaly due to left ventricular dilatation, but the left atrium is not enlarged. The left atrial* v *wave was 52 mm Hg.*

more chordae results in acute loss of leaflet support and in the abrupt onset of appreciable mitral regurgitation[37, 38] (fig. 5). Nevertheless, in contrast to papillary muscle rupture (see below) patients with chordal rupture tend to survive for months[38] or even years.[39] Such patients present in sinus rhythm with a history of sudden heart failure and are found to have a decrescendo apical systolic murmur that tends to radiate to the left sternal edge and base; both third *and* fourth heart sounds are present with presystolic distention of the left ventricle, physical and electrocardiographic signs of pulmonary hypertension, but little or no radiologic evidence of left atrial enlargement[37, 38] (fig. 5). The key to the physiologic disturbance and clinical picture is the *sudden* development of *severe* regurgitation into a

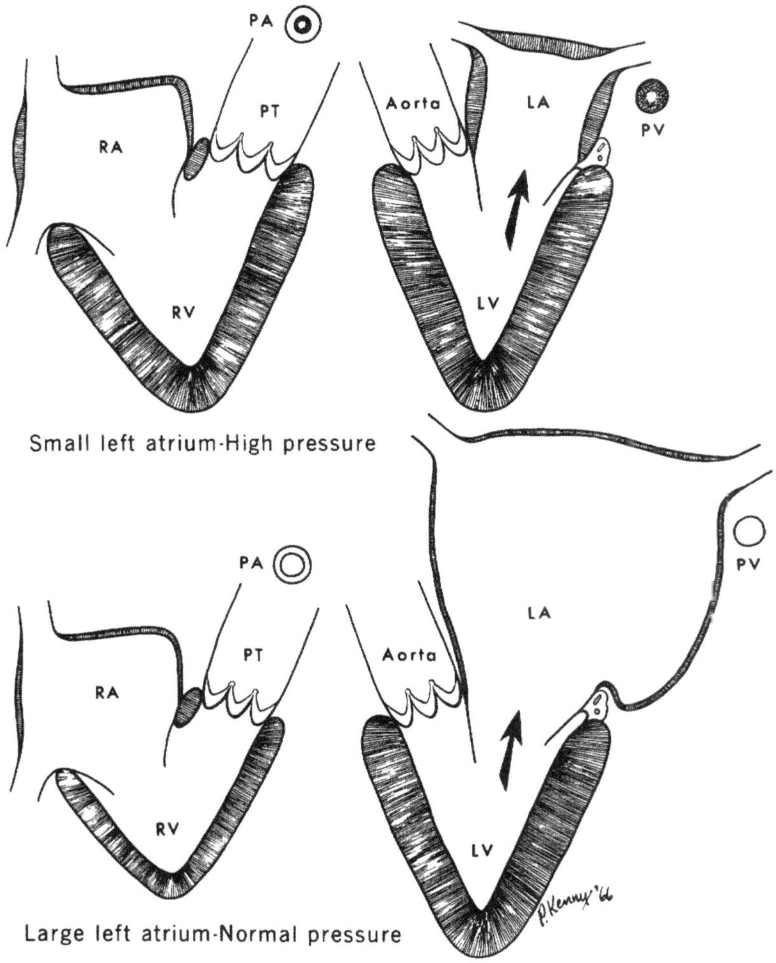

Figure 6

Diagrammatic representation of the two extremes of severe mitral regurgitation, i.e., acute, with small high-pressure left atrium, and chronic with large low-pressure atrium. **(Upper panel)** *When severe mitral regurgitation appears suddenly in individuals with previously normal or near normal hearts, the left atrium (LA) is relatively small, and the high pressure within it is transmitted into the pulmonary vessels and the right ventricle (RV). The anatomic indicator of these physiologic events is severe hypertophy of the left atrial and right ventricular walls and marked intimal proliferation and medial hypertrophy of the pulmonary veins (PV) and arteries (PA).* **(Lower panel)** *Severe mitral regurgitation also is present, but the regurgitation is chronic. The left atrium is enormously dilated and is therefore capable of "absorbing" the regurgitant flow without elevating the pressure in the pulmonary vessels and right heart. Consequently, there is no intimal proliferation or medial hypertrophy of the pulmonary veins or arteries and the right ventricular wall is not hypertrophied. PT = pulmonary trunk.*

previously *normal, small,* and therefore relatively *noncompliant* left atrium (figs. 5 and 6). The steeply rising left atrial v wave approaches left ventricular pressure in the latter part of systole, resulting in late systolic decline in both regurgitant flow and murmur intensity (holosystolic but decrescendo). The previously normal left atrium responds by increasing its wall thickness (fig. 6) and its contractile force and thus causing presystolic distention of the left ventricle and a fourth heart sound.[40] The direction of the regurgitant jet may be forward and medial toward the atrial septum adjacent to the aortic valve, so that radiation of the murmur is toward the left sternal edge and base;[10] this pattern accounts for "mitral incompetence simulating aortic stenosis."[41] In other patients, the direction of the jet is posterior or lateral.[41]

Chronic severe mitral incompetence[42] stands in contrast to acute severe mitral regurgitation (fig. 6). In chronic severe mitral incompetence, there is a long history of a murmur which is holosystolic but not decrescendo; radiation is to the axilla and back; atrial fibrillation is the rule with a prominent third heart sound; physical signs of pulmonary hypertension are absent because a distensible left atrium enlarges strikingly and "absorbs" the regurgitant flow[42] (fig. 6).

Papillary Muscles and Left Ventricular Wall

These two elements represent the muscular components of the mitral apparatus. The papillary muscle, as a functional unit, includes a portion of the adjacent left ventricular wall.

Although rupture of a papillary muscle has been known since 1803,[2] the term "papillary muscle dysfunction" was not introduced until 1963.[43] Dysfunction can occur either with loss in continuity (rupture) or without loss in continuity (fibrosis, ischemia, replacement[19]; table 1).

The papillary muscles emerge as single bodies from the left ventricular wall and divide into a variable number of heads, each of which serves as an anchor for chordae tendineae[44, 45] (fig. 4). Rupture of a papillary muscle typically results from infarction of the posteromedial segment.[19] Traumatic rupture is rare. Sudden loss in continuity results in acute severe regurgitation. The specific anatomic site at which papillary muscle rupture occurs is an important determinant of the magnitude of regurgitation and the subsequent clinical course[44] (fig. 4). If rupture is confined to one papillary muscle head, the physiologic derangement is quantitatively similar to rupture of major chordae. If rupture involves the entire papillary muscle, i.e. its central body, approximately half of the support of each leaflet is lost so that regurgitation is overwhelming and rapidly fatal[44] (fig. 4). In either case, the mitral incompetence of papillary muscle rupture is superimposed upon an acutely *infarcted* left ventricle, whereas acute regurgitation from chordal rupture usually occurs in an otherwise normal or nearly normal heart.

The papillary muscles contract before the left ventricular wall, bracing the leaflets and chordae for the ensuing abrupt rise in intraventricular pressure. When this sequence is reversed by a ventricular ectopic beat, a whiff of mitral regurgitation occurs (this is a common observation during left ventricular angiography). Papillary muscle contraction normally continues synchronously with left ventricular contraction, and thereby supports the chordae tendineae and prevents overshoot of the leaflets during ventricular systole.[46] If papillary muscle contraction is absent or ineffective, i.e., papillary muscle dysfunction is present, then, as the left ventricular apex moves toward the annulus in systole, the chordae slacken, the leaflets are not held in

Table 1

Papillary Muscle Dysfunction

1. With loss in continuity (rupture):
   a. Infarction
   b. Trauma (rarely)
2. Without loss in continuity:
   a. Infarction — persistent mitral incompetence
   b. Ischemia without infarction (angina) — transient mitral incompetence mild to severe

place, and prolapse into the left atrium occurs.

The anatomic basis of papillary muscle dysfunction without loss in continuity is still not completely settled. Burch and co-workers[43] originally called attention to the effect of coexisting aneurysm of the adjacent left ventricular wall from which the infarcted papillary muscle took origin. Subsequently, Shelburne and associates[47] commented on the role of infarction of the portion of left ventricular wall that forms the base of the papillary muscle. These authors believed that infarction at that site resulted in failure to provide an adequate anchor for the contiguous papillary muscle or, by forming an aneurysm, changed the directional axis of the papillary muscle itself. Infants with severe congenital valvular aortic stenosis exhibit atrophy of one or both papillary muscles, with mitral regurgitation ascribed to that cause.[48] Yet many older patients with valvular aortic stenosis have papillary muscles that are small in comparison with the hypertrophied left ventricular wall, but the mitral valve remains competent.[49] Mittal and co-workers[46] and Tsakiris and associates[50] have clarified these discordant views by showing that experimental damage *confined* to a canine papillary muscle does *not* necessarily render the mitral valve incompetent unless the damage extends to the adjacent left ventricular wall (fig. 7). Accordingly, the papillary muscle as a functional unit is now believed to include its muscular foundation in the contiguous left ventricular wall.[19, 46, 50]

Papillary muscle dysfunction without loss in continuity can result in either persistent mitral incompetence of varying severity[43, 51] or in intermittent mitral incompetence during episodes of ischemia (angina) without infarction (table 1).[2, 52] Occasionally, intermittent, severe mitral regurgitation (table 1) is accompanied by precipitious elevations of left atrial *v* waves and pulmonary edema due to transient ischemic papillary muscle dysfunction.[52]

Mitral regurgitation occurs not only with a classic holosystolic murmur but also with an early systolic decrescendo murmur, a late

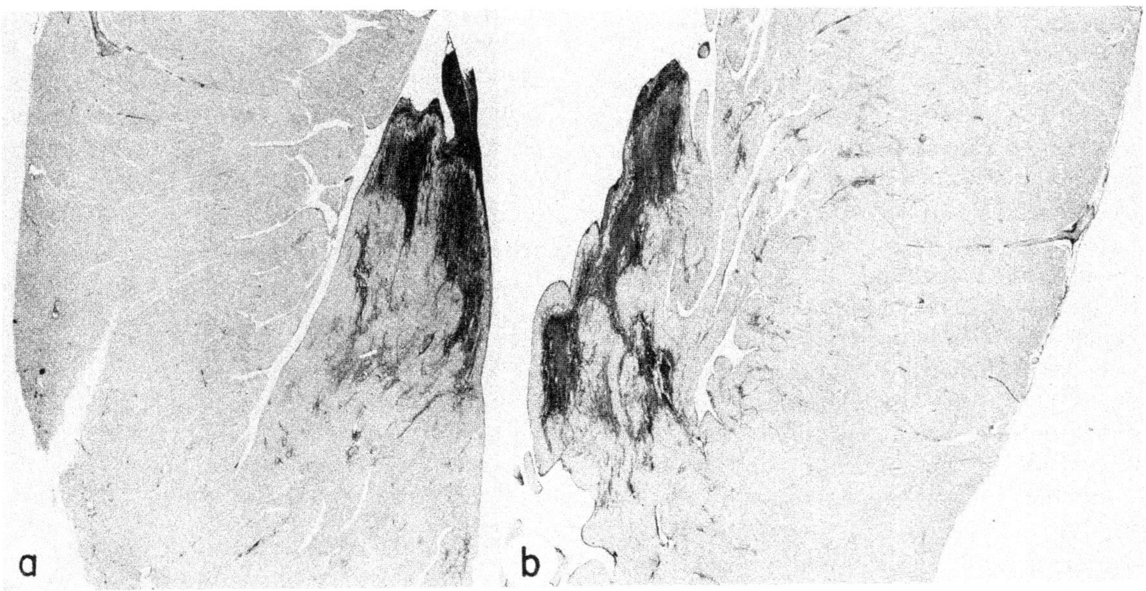

Figure 7

Histologic sections of anterolateral (a) *and posteromedial* (b) *left ventricular papillary muscles in a 51-year-old man with type II hyperlipoproteinemia and two myocardial infarcts who died suddenly. At no time was a murmur heard. Each papillary muscle is focally scarred, but the left ventricular free walls beneath them are normal.*

systolic murmur, or a midsystolic murmur. The mitral incompetence of papillary muscle dysfunction encompasses all of these types.[2, 43, 47] In fact, the configuration sometimes changes from beat to beat.[2] Variations in the functional state of the papillary muscle and left ventricular wall and in the alignment (directional tension) exerted by the papillary muscle on its chordae are likely to influence the timing of the murmur.[47] Some late systolic murmurs of papillary muscle dysfunction have recently been shown to follow one or more midsystolic clicks.[35] Accordingly, the systolic click-late systolic murmur syndrome must now be extended to include ischemic heart disease.[2, 35]

Now let's turn attention to those aspects of the left ventricular free wall related to the shape of the ventricle per se. It is axiomatic that enlargement of the left ventricle may be accompanied by mitral regurgitation. The explanation generally offered is dilatation of the annulus, but this appears to be inadequate[4] even though admittedly the mitral orifice can dilate. How then might left ventricular enlargement render the mitral valve incompetent? In part, dilatation may prevent the annulus from decreasing its circumferential size during ventricular systole. The answer, however, seems to lie chiefly in the effect of altered left ventricular shape on the position of the papillary muscles and their directional axes of tension.[2–4, 47] The papillary muscles normally arise from the left ventricular wall at its apical and middle thirds[11] (fig. 1). This position permits the contracting papillary muscles to exert a desirable *vertical* force on the chordae tendineae, effectively moving the leaflets together during isovolumetric contraction and restraining them during ventricular ejection.[4, 47] In contrast, when the papillary muscles are *not* vertically aligned with the annulus (lateral migration due to spherical dilatation of the left ventricle), the systolic forces exerted on the leaflets via the chordae are in a *lateral* as opposed to a vertical direction.[3, 4] This lateral tension, especially on the anterior leaflet, opposes apposition, and renders the valve incompetent. Lateral enlargement of the left ventricle is a feature of mitral regurgitation itself, so that once initiated, "regurgitation begets regurgitation."[10] On the other hand, lesions such as aortic incompetence result principally in downward elongation of the left ventricle. If the papillary muscles are pulled in the same direction, the distance between the mitral annulus and the apex increases so that chordae become too short to permit leaflet closure.[4] Compensatory elongation of the chordae under these circumstances serves to preserve mitral valve competence, but if the annular-apical distance subsequently decreases (correction of aortic regurgitation), these elongated chordae might result in leaflet overshoot.

A different alteration in left ventricular shape has been held responsible for another variety of mitral regurgitation, namely, the late regurgitation of idiopathic hypertrophic subaortic stenosis.[53, 54] Echocardiography has shown that in this disorder the anterior mitral leaflet reopens in midsystole after normal initial closure.[54] This reopening times with the onset of outflow obstruction as the anterior leaflet and septum approach each other.[54] It has been postulated that the abnormal systolic movement of the hypertrophied interventricular septum alters the axis of the anterolateral papillary muscle by pulling it from its closed position.[53] Such movement may not only provoke late systolic mitral regurgitation but may also contribute to obstruction to ventricular outflow.

References

1. Wiggers C, Feil H: The cardiodynamics of mitral insufficiency. Heart **9:** 149, 1922
2. Cheng TO: Some new observations on the syndrome of papillary muscle dysfunction. Amer J Med **47:** 924, 1969
3. Moller JH, Lucas RV, Adams P, Anderson RC, Jorgens J, Edwards JE: Endocardial fibroelastosis. Circulation **30:** 759, 1964
4. Levy MJ, Edwards JE: Anatomy of mitral insufficiency. Progr Cardiovasc Dis **5:** 119, 1962
5. Brolin I: The mitral orifice. Acta Radiol Diagn **6:** 273, 1967

6. Davis PKB, Kinmouth JB: The movements of the annulus of the mitral valve. J Cardiovasc Surg 4: 427, 1963
7. Sarnoff SJ, Gilmore JP, Mitchell JH: Influence of atrial contraction and relaxation on closure of mitral valve: Observations on effects of autonomic nerve activity. Circ Res 11: 26, 1962
8. Shah PM, Kramer DH, Gramiak R: Influence of the timing of atrial systole on mitral valve closure and on the first heart sound in man. Amer J Cardiol 26: 231, 1970
9. Vandenberg RA, Williams JCP, Sturm RE, Wood EH: Effect of varying ventricular function by extra systolic potentiation on closure of the mitral valve. Amer J Cardiol 28: 43, 1971
10. Edwards JE, Burchell HB: Endocardial and intimal lesions (jet impact) as possible sites of origin of murmurs. Circulation 18: 946, 1958
11. Brock RC: The surgical and pathological anatomy of the mitral valve. Brit Heart J 14: 489, 1952
12. Korn D, DeSanctis RW, Sell S: Massive calcification of the mitral annulus. New Eng J Med 267: 900, 1962
13. Roberts WC, Perloff JK, Costantino T: Severe valvular aortic stenosis in patients over 65 years of age. Amer J Cardiol 27: 497, 1971
14. Grossman M, Knott AP Jr, Jacoby WJ Jr: Calcified annulus fibrosis with mitral insufficiency with Marfan's syndrome. Arch Intern Med (Chicago) 121: 561, 1968
15. Krovetz LJ, Lorincz AE, Schiebler GL: Cardiovascular manifestations of the Hurler syndrome. Circulation 31: 132, 1965
16. Montiel MN: Muscular apparatus of the mitral valve in man and its involvement in left-sided cardiac hypertrophy. Amer J Cardiol 26: 341, 1970
17. Edwards JE: The problem of mitral insufficiency caused by accessory chordae tendineae in persistent common atrioventricular canal. Mayo Clin Proc 35: 299, 1960
18. Rosenberg J, Roberts WC: Double orifice mitral valve. Arch Path (Chicago) 86: 77, 1968
19. Edwards JE: Mitral insufficiency resulting from "overshooting" of leaflets. Circulation 43: 606, 1971
20. Barlow JB, Bosman CK, Pocock WA, Marchand P: Late systolic murmurs and non-ejection ("mid-late") systolic clicks: An analysis of 90 patients. Brit Heart J 30: 203, 1968
21. Ehlers KH, Engle MA, Levin AR, Grossman H, Fleming RJ: Left ventricular abnormality with late mitral insufficiency and abnormal electrocardiogram. Amer J Cardiol 26: 333, 1970
22. deLeon AC, Ronan JA: Thoracic bony abnormalities with the click and late systolic murmur. (Abstr) Circulation 44 (suppl II): II-157, 1971
23. Dillon JC, Haine CL, Chang S, Feigenbaum H: Use of echocardiography in patients with prolapsed mitral valve. Circulation 43: 503, 1971
24. Rizzon P, Giusppina B, Maselli-Campagna G: The praechordial honk. Brit Heart J 33: 707, 1971
25. Osler W: On a remarkable heart murmur, heard at a distance from the chest wall. Med Times Gaz 2: 432, 1880
26. Ronan JA, Perloff JK, Harvey WP: Systolic clicks and the late systolic murmur. Amer Heart J 70: 319, 1965
27. Hutter AM, Dinsmore RE, Willerson JT, DeSanctis RW: Early systolic clicks due to mitral valve prolapse. Circulation 44: 516, 1971
28. Ronan JA, Waters TJ, Escorcia E: Effect of simple bedside maneuvers on the isolated systolic click. (Abstr) Circulation 44 (suppl II): II-31, 1971
29. LeBauer J, Perloff JK, Keliher T: The isolated systolic click with bacterial endocarditis. Amer Heart J 73: 534, 1967
30. Kriesman K, Kleiger R, Schad N, Aker V, Parker B: Arrhythmia in prolapse of the mitral valve. (Abstr) Circulation 44 (suppl II): II-44, 1971
31. McDonald A, Harris A, Jefferson K, Marshall J, McDonald L: Association of prolapse of posterior cusp of mitral valve and atrial septal defect. Brit Heart J 33: 383, 1971
32. Roberts WC, Glancy DL, Epstein SE: Prolapse of the posterior leaflet of the mitral valve (floppy mitral valve) in Ebstein's anomaly of the tricuspid valve. In preparation
33. Lindgren KM, Groves BM, Ronan JA: Abnormal precordial movements in the systolic click, late systolic murmur syndrome. (Abstr) Circulation 44 (suppl II): II-32, 1971
34. Steinfeld L, Dimich I, Park SC: The late systolic murmur of rheumatic mitral regurgitation. (Abstr) Circulation 44 (suppl II): II-106, 1971
35. Steelman RB, White RS, Hill JC, Nagle JP, Cheitlin MD: Midsystolic clicks in arteriosclerotic heart disease: A new facet in the clinical syndrome of papillary muscle dysfunction. Circulation 44: 503, 1971
36. Dekker A, Mehrizi A, Vengsarker AS: Corrected transposition of the great vessels with Ebstein's anomaly of the left atrioventricular valve. Circulation 31: 119, 1965

37. ROBERTS WC, BRAUNWALD E, MORROW AG: Acute severe mitral regurgitation secondary to ruptured chordae tendineae: Clinical, hemodynamic and pathologic considerations. Circulation **33**: 58, 1966

38. RONAN JA, STEELMAN RB, DELEON AC, WATERS JA, PERLOFF JK, HARVEY WP: The clinical diagnosis of acute severe mitral insufficiency. Amer J Cardiol **27**: 284, 1971

39. CHENG TO, BASHOUR T, LINDSAY J: Chronic mitral regurgitation resulting from ruptured chordae tendineae. (Abstr) Circulation **44** (suppl II): II-150, 1971

40. COHEN LS, MASON DT, BRAUNWALD E: Significance of an atrial gallop sound in mitral regurgitation: Clue to the diagnosis of ruptured chordae tendineae. Circulation **35**: 112, 1967

41. PERLOFF JK, HARVEY WP: Auscultatory and phonocardiographic manifestations of pure mitral regurgitation. Progr Cardiovasc Dis **5**: 172, 1962

42. BRAUNWALD E, AWE WC: The syndrome of severe mitral regurgitation with normal left atrial pressure. Circulation **27**: 29, 1963

43. BURCH GE, DEPASQUALE NP, PHILLIPS JH: Clinical manifestations of papillary muscle dysfunction. Arch Intern Med (Chicago) **112**: 112, 1963

44. MORROW AG, COHEN LS, ROBERTS WC, BRAUNWALD NS, BRAUNWALD E: Severe mitral regurgitation following acute myocardial infarction and ruptured papillary muscle: Hemodynamic findings and results of operative treatment in four patients. Circulation **37** (suppl II): II-124, 1968

45. ESTES EH, DALTON FM, ENTMAN MC, DIXON HB, HACHEL DB: The anatomy and blood supply of the papillary muscles of the left ventricle. Amer Heart J **71**: 356, 1966

46. MITTAL AK, LANGSTON M, COHN KE, SELZER A, KERTH WJ: Combined papillary muscle and left ventricular wall dysfunction as a cause of mitral regurgitation. Circulation **44**: 174, 1971

47. SHELBURNE JC, RUBENSTEIN D, GORLIN R: A reappraisal of papillary muscle dysfunction. Amer J Med **46**: 862, 1969

48. MOLLER JH, NAKIB A, EDWARDS JE: Infarction of papillary muscles and mitral insufficiency in association with aortic stenosis. Circulation **34**: 87, 1966

49. FALCONE MW, ROBERTS WC, MORROW AG, PERLOFF JK: Congenital aortic stenosis resulting from a unicommissural valve. Circulation **44**: 272, 1971

50. TSAKIRIS AG, RASTELLI GC, AMORIN DDES, TITUS JL, WOOD E: Effect of experimental papillary muscular damage on mitral valve closure in intact anesthetized dogs. Mayo Clin Proc **45**: 275, 1970

51. BAVE AW, BAUM A, BLAKEMORE WS, ZINSER HF: A later stage of anomalous coronary circulation with origin of the left coronary artery from the pulmonary artery. Circulation **36**: 878, 1967

52. BRODY W, CRILEY JM: Intermittent severe mitral regurgitation. New Eng J Med **283**: 673, 1970

53. ADELMAN AG, MCLOUGLIN MJ, MARQUIS Y, AUGER P, WYLE ED: Left ventricular cineangiographic observations in muscular subaortic stenosis. Amer J Cardiol **24**: 689, 1969

54. OAKLEY CM: Hypertrophic obstructive cardiomyopathy—patterns of progression. *In* Hypertrophic Obstructive Cardiomyopathy. Ciba Foundation Group Study No. 37, edited by EG Wolstenholme and M O'Connor. London, J. & A. Churchill, 1971, p 9

Mitral Valvular Disease

A Clinicopathologic Survey of the Conditions Causing the Mitral Valve To Function Abnormally

WILLIAM C. ROBERTS, M.D., and JOSEPH K. PERLOFF, M.D., Bethesda, Maryland

The mitral valve is the most complex of the cardiac valves. Its leaflets are unequal in size: one is continuous with the left atrial endocardium and the other with the aorta. The valve contains about 120 chordae tendineae connecting the leaflets to myocardial pillars (papillary muscles), which in turn are continuous with the left ventricular free wall. It has only a partial anulus fibrosis (only at the base of the posterior mitral leaflet). Since the mitral valve connects with the left atrial wall via the mural endocardium, conditions affecting this chamber also may affect mitral function. This review surveys conditions involving the mitral anulus, leaflets, chordae tendineae, papillary muscles, and left ventricular free wall that may cause this valvular orifice to be either stenotic or incompetent, or both.

DR. WILLIAM C. ROBERTS*: This conference concerns the mitral apparatus or complex. Dr. Joseph K. Perloff will discuss clinical features. I shall present pathologic features of several conditions affecting mitral leaflets, chordae tendineae, papillary muscles, anulus, and free walls of both the left atrium and left ventricle. But first a note on the origin of the term (Figure 1) and some comments on the structure of the normal mitral valve.

The mitral valve is, in comparison with the semilunar valves, a complex structure consisting of four major components: leaflets, chordae tendineae, papillary muscles, and anulus (Figure 2). Unlike the other three cardiac valves, each of which has three cusps, the mitral valve consists of only two leaflets. The anterior leaflet has a much longer basal-to-margin length than does the posterior leaflet, but the length of anular attachment of the posterior leaflet is about twice that of the anterior leaflet (Figure 3). The posterior leaflet is attached for about 6 cm, and the anterior leaflet, approximately 3 cm. Although the basal-to-margin lengths and the lengths of the basal attachments of each mitral leaflet are quite different, the surface area of each leaflet is virtually identical. The posterior leaflet has a true bundle of fibrous tissue (the anulus) separating the myocardium of left atrium from the myocardium of left ventricle. The posterior leaflet, in a large sense, is simply an extension of mural endocardium from the posterior and lateral walls of the left atrium (Figure 3). In contrast to the posterior mitral leaflet, the anterior leaflet does not have a true anulus but is continuous with the wall of the ascending aorta, aortic valve, and membraneous ventricular septum (Figure 3). The area of the leaflets is approximately 2.5 times that of the area of the primary mitral orifice—that is, the area at the level of the mitral anulus (1). The mitral leaflets are connected with each other at the commissures. In contrast to the semilunar cusps, which are independent or discontinuous of each other, the two mitral leaflets are continuous with

* Chief, Section of Pathology, National Heart and Lung Institute.

► An edited transcription of a Combined Clinical Staff Conference at the Clinical Center, Bethesda, Md., by the National Heart and Lung Institute, National Institutes of Health, U.S. Department of Health, Education, and Welfare.

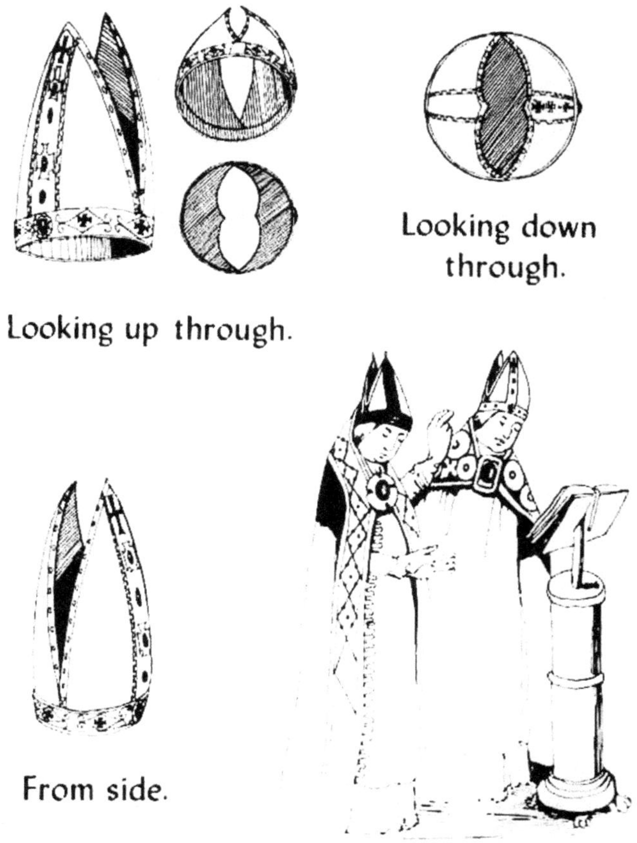

Figure 1. The miter of the mitral valve. The term "mitral" is derived from the Latin term "mitra," meaning cap, which in turn was derived from the Greek word "mitra," meaning turban or headdress. Bishops of the Christian Church wore headdresses, which they called "miters," fashioned after those of ancient Hebrew high priests. Vesalius is recorded as having compared the shape of the bishop's miter with that of the mitral valve. Disease of this valve, namely mitral stenosis, was first recorded by John Mayow in 1969.

each other.

The chordae tendineae of the mitral valve are even more complex than its leaflets. Chordae from each leaflet insert into both papillary muscles (Figure 2). About five times as many chordae are attached to leaflets as to papillary muscles (2). On an average, 24 chordae tendineae are attached to the papillary muscles (12 to each), and 120 chordae are attached to mitral leaflets (2) (Figure 4). The chordae insert onto the undersurfaces—that is, the ventricular surfaces—of both leaflets. The chordae subdivide as they progress from papillary muscle to leaflet. The subdivisions may be viewed as primary (first order), secondary (second order), and tertiary (third order) chordae. The spaces between the chordae serve as secondary orifices between left atrium and left ventricle. Obviously, the major orifice is the area between the leaflets, but much blood passes between the interchordal spaces (Figure 5). Therefore, fusion of chordae tendineae narrows the mitral inlet.

The two left ventricular papillary muscles are preferably designated anterolateral and posteromedial. There is considerable variation in the appearances of these two structures in the same person. When corresponding structures are compared in different persons, considerable variation is apparent (2). The anterolateral papillary muscle is generally the more uniform of the two. It usually consists of a single trunk that protrudes more into the cavity than the posteromedial one. The posteromedial papillary muscle is generally smaller than the anterolateral structure and often consists of two or three smaller pillars

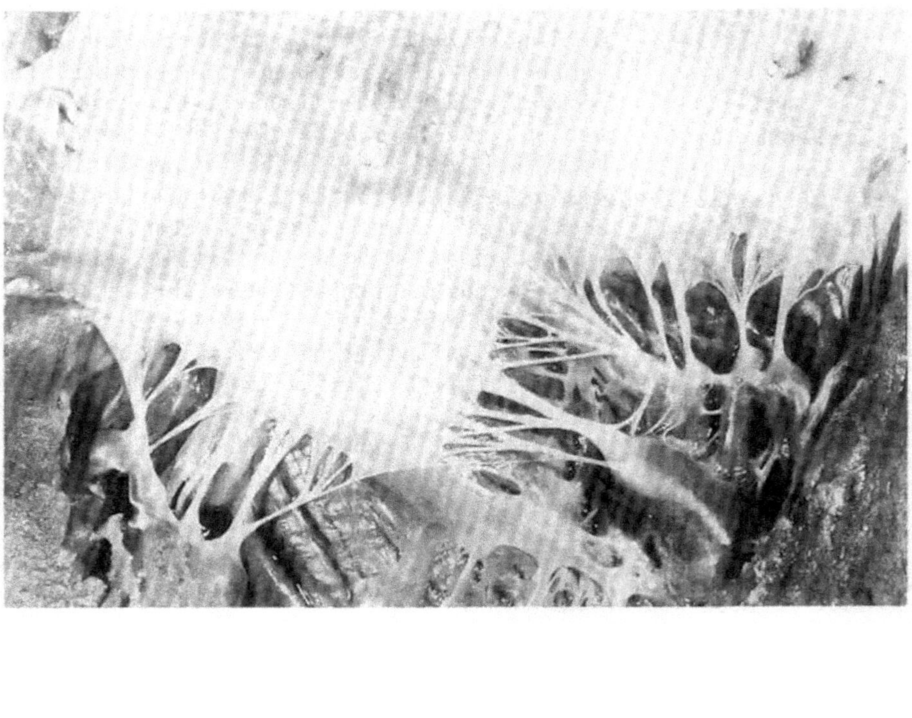

Figure 2. Opened normal mitral valve. Each papillary muscle receives chordae tendineae from both leaflets. The chordae insert on the ventricular or under-surface of the leaflets. The leaflets are continuous with one another, in contrast to the semilunar valve cusps, each of which is a separate independent unit. The mural endocardium of left atrium above the posterior leaflet is similar in appearance to the posterior leaflet; this is to be expected, since one presumably is derived from the other. The mural endocardium above the anterior leaflet, however, is not as white as this leaflet, and the leaflet is not an extension of left artrial endocardium, as is the posterior leaflet.

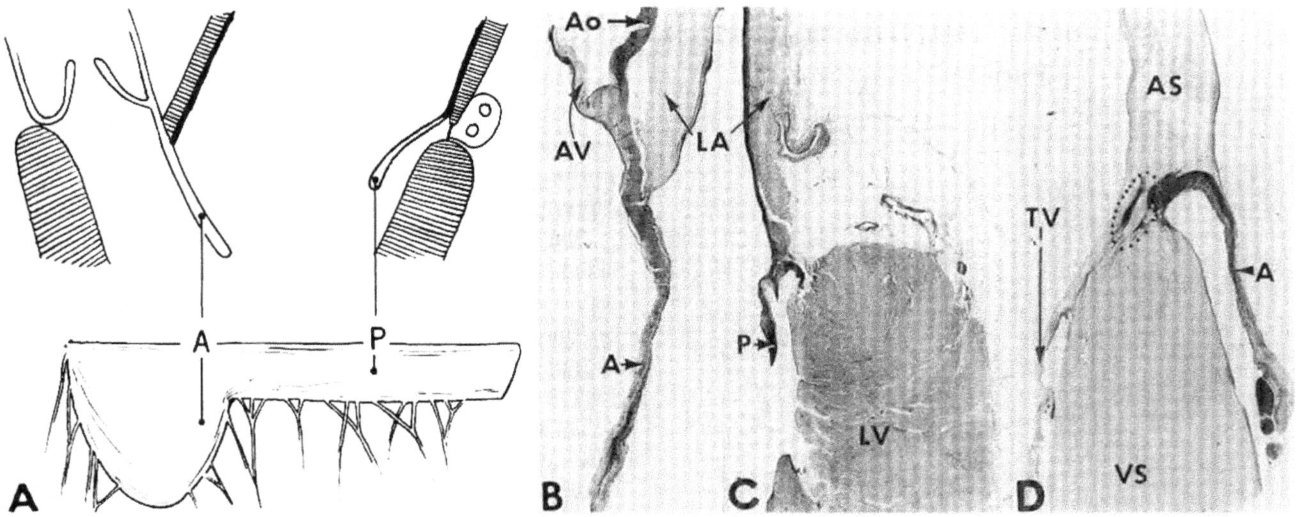

Figure 3A. Diagram of mitral valve showing that the anterior (*A*) leaflet is continuous with the ascending aorta and aortic valve and that the posterior (*P*) leaflet is continuous with left atrial endocardium. The inflow and outflow tracts of the left ventricle are divided by the anterior leaflet. The basal attachment of the posterior leaflet is twice as long as that of the anterior leaflet, although the basal-to-margin length of the anterior leaflet is twice that of the posterior leaflet. **B-D.** Histologic sections of mitral valve confirming the observations depicted in Figure 3A. **B.** This section includes anterior (*A*) mitral leaflet, aortic valve cusp (*AV*), wall of aorta (Ao), and left atrial (*LA*) wall. **C.** This section includes posterior (*P*) mitral leaflet and walls of left atrium and left ventricle (*LV*). **D.** This section extends through atrial septum (*AS*) and ventricular septum (*VS*) and includes portions of anterior (*A*) mitral leaflet and septal tricuspid leaflet (*TV*). Between the bases of these two leaflets is the penetrating portion of the atrioventricular bundle (*outlined by dots*). Thus, it is easy to see how calcific deposits from the mitral valve might extend into the conduction system and cause heart block. (Elastic van Gieson; Original magnifications: **B.** × 4.5; **C** and **D,** × 3.)

rather than a single pillar. The posteromedial muscle usually has several connections to the left ventricular wall in addition to the base of the major trunk. Both papillary muscles are attached to the lower or caudal third of the left ventricular free wall. Both papillary muscles have relatively poor blood supplies, and both are located at considerable distances from the orifices of the coronary arteries. The major supplier of the anterolateral muscle is the left anterior descending coronary artery, and the major supplier of the posteromedial muscle is the right coronary artery (3). The left circumflex contributes blood to both. To oxygenate the apexes of the papillary muscles, blood from the epicardial coronary arteries must penetrate the entire thickness of the left ventricular free wall, turn uphill, so to speak, and ascend a distance equivalent to about two more full thicknesses of left ventricular wall. Thus, it is no mystery that the papillary muscles, and particularly their apical portions, are sensitive indicators of minor deficiencies of myocardial oxygenation.

The Mitral Valve and Aging

With aging, this valve, like other tissues, may show wear and tear changes, mainly in leaflet and chordal thickening (4). The left ventricular cavity gets smaller, presumably because the cardiac output decreases as we grow older (Figure 6, *Top*). As the cavity gets smaller, less area is available in the left ventricle to accommodate the leaflets and chordae. As a consequence, the leaflets contact one another abnormally during ventricular systole and focal fibrous thickening results. Since the left ventricular cavity diminishes with age, the mitral anulus does also (Figure 6, *Bottom*). The latter change further increases the abnormal contact of the mitral leaflets with each other and furthers the leaflet scarring.

Functions of Normal Mitral Apparatus

Dr. Joseph K. Perloff*: The mitral apparatus is a complex, finely coordinated mechanism that can be deranged by a multiplicity of acquired and congenital disorders; its competency depends on the functional integrity of six anatomic components acting in delicate concert. These are posterior and lateral left atrial wall, anulus, leaflets, chordae tendineae, papillary muscles, and left ventricular free wall (5).

The exact mode of closure of the normal mitral valve is still uncertain (6-7). Left ventricular systole begins with contraction of the papillary muscles. The vertical forces exerted by this contraction move the leaflets into apposition. As the intraventricular pressure rises, the edges of the cusps coapt and mutually support each other along a comfortable margin of their atrial surfaces, firmly sealing the orifice. The

* Chief, Section of Cardiology, University of Pennsylvania School of Medicine, Philadelphia, Pa.

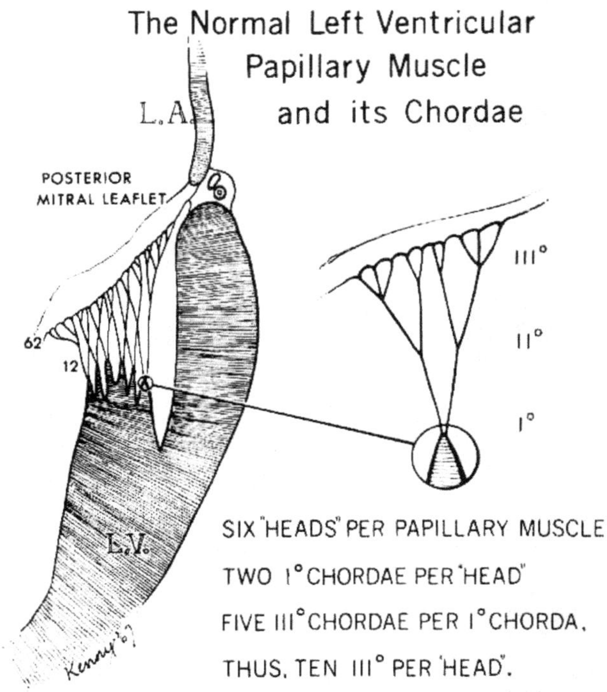

Figure 4. Diagram of the average number of chordae tendineae normally originating from each left ventricular papillary muscle. Although great variation exists, each left ventricular papillary muscle contains about six "heads," each of which contains two primary or first-order chordae tendineae. Each primary cord subdivides into two secondary chordae, each of which divides into two or three tertiary or third-order chordae. The number of chordae attached to each left ventricular papillary muscle thus averages 12, and the number of chordae inserting directly into the mitral leaflets from a single papillary muscle averages 62. (These numbers were found by counting chordae and papillary muscle heads in 12 normal hearts.) L.A. = left atrium; L.V. = left ventricle.

free edges do not merely touch; they coapt along a considerable area of their atrial surfaces. The rest of each leaflet bulges like a parachute toward the left atrium (8).

The anulus, long considered inert, not only serves as a fulcrum on which the leaflets move but also, during ventricular systole, decreases its circumference, reducing the area that the leaflets are required to seal (9, 10). As the left ventricle ejects, its apex and base approach each other. The shortening of the vertical axis of the left ventricle is accompanied by synergistic contraction of the papillary muscles and contiguous portions of left ventricular free wall, so that an appropriate vertical anchoring force is applied to the chordae tendineae, preventing eversion of the leaflets into the left atrium.

When any of its six anatomic components are faulty, the harmony of the mitral mechanism may be altered. Because of coordinated interplay among these elements, which are interdependent, more than one are usually disturbed at any given time, although with various degrees of significance. Regurgitation or stenosis, or both, is the functional consequence of derangement of the mitral complex; stenosis is the simpler of the two.

Obstruction at the mitral orifice can either be acquired (commonest), congenital, or caused by the interposition of nonleaflet tissue within the left atrial cavity.

The essential hemodynamic fault caused by obstruction at the mitral orifice is the inability of the left atrium to empty normally (11). In sinus rhythm an increased force of left atrial contraction serves to augment its emptying. This mechanical advantage is lost in atrial fibrillation, causing the mean left atrial pressure to rise or the mitral flow (and cardiac output) to fall. The obstruction, represented by a pressure gradient across the valve, is the basic mechanical disturbance of rheumatic (common) (12) or congenital (rare) (13) mitral stenosis. The consequences of obstruction at the mitral orifice can be seen most graphically in plain films of the chest (14). The posteroanterior X ray shows vascular redistribution to the upper lobes—that is, prominent upper lobe pulmonary veins, loss of the normal angle between the right upper pulmonary vein and the right pulmo-

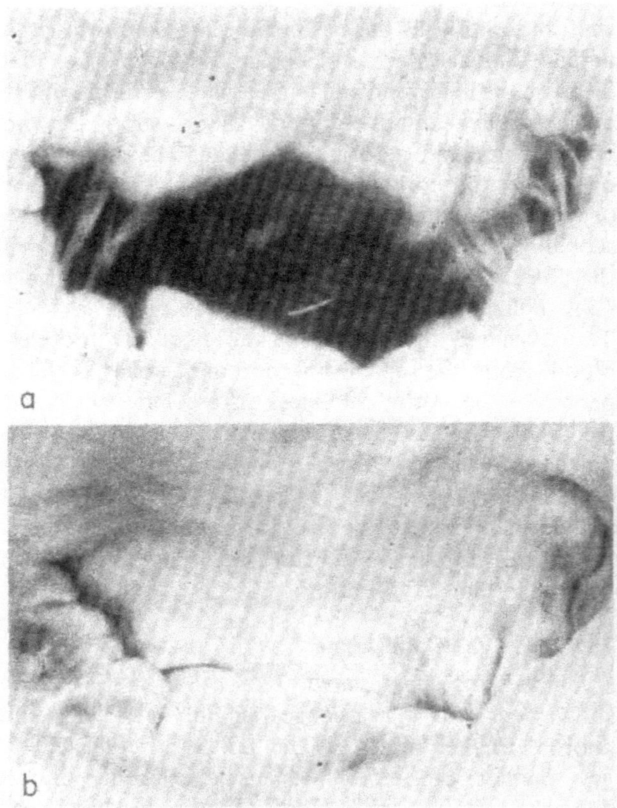

Figure 5. Normally functioning mitral valve during ventricular diastole (*a*) and systole (*b*). The valve closes over a large surface area (*b*) and not just at its margins.

nary artery, costrophrenic Kerley B lines (thickened interlobular septae), peribronchial cuffing (best seen end-on), and a general haze of interstitial pulmonary edema.

Thus, stenosis of the mitral orifice due to rheumatic endocarditis is conceptually a relatively simple anatomic fault that is translated into the mechanical problem of pulmonary venous obstruction.

Dr. Roberts: Of the nine single or combined cardiac valve lesions (excluding tricuspid regurgitation and papillary muscle dysfunction) severe enough to be fatal, mitral stenosis, in my experience, ranks second (15-17) (Table 1). Of 543 patients over age 14 years with functionally severe (classes III or IV) valvular cardiac disease whom I studied at necropsy, 206 (37%) had mitral stenosis. Only valvular aortic stenosis was commoner. Mitral stenosis occurred alone in 94 patients and in combination with other functional valvular lesions in the other 112 patients. Mitral stenosis was rheumatic in origin in all 206 patients.

Although a functional classification of valvular heart disease, as shown in Table 1, is most useful from physiologic and therapeutic standpoints, an anatomic classification is most helpful from an etiologic standpoint. Five anatomic categories have proved useful (15): isolated mitral, isolated aortic, combined mitral and aortic, combined tricuspid and mitral with or without aortic, and tricuspid with or without pulmonic. Isolated aortic valve disease is virtually never rheumatic in origin (15). Isolated mitral disease causing stenosis is, with rare exception, rheumatic in origin, but isolated mitral disease causing pure regurgitation is nonrheumatic nearly as often as it is rheumatic (Table 2). Combined valve disease is usually rheumatic in origin. Isolated anatomic disease of the tricuspid or pulmonic valves, or both, is usually congenital in origin or is associated with the carcinoid syndrome (17).

A valve may function normally and yet be anatomically abnormal. Only 57% of the 94 patients with isolated mitral stenosis (with or without mitral regurgitation) had anatomic involvement limited to the mitral valve. In contrast, 87% of the 182 patients with clinically isolated aortic stenosis (with or without regurgitation) had anatomic disease of the aortic valve only.

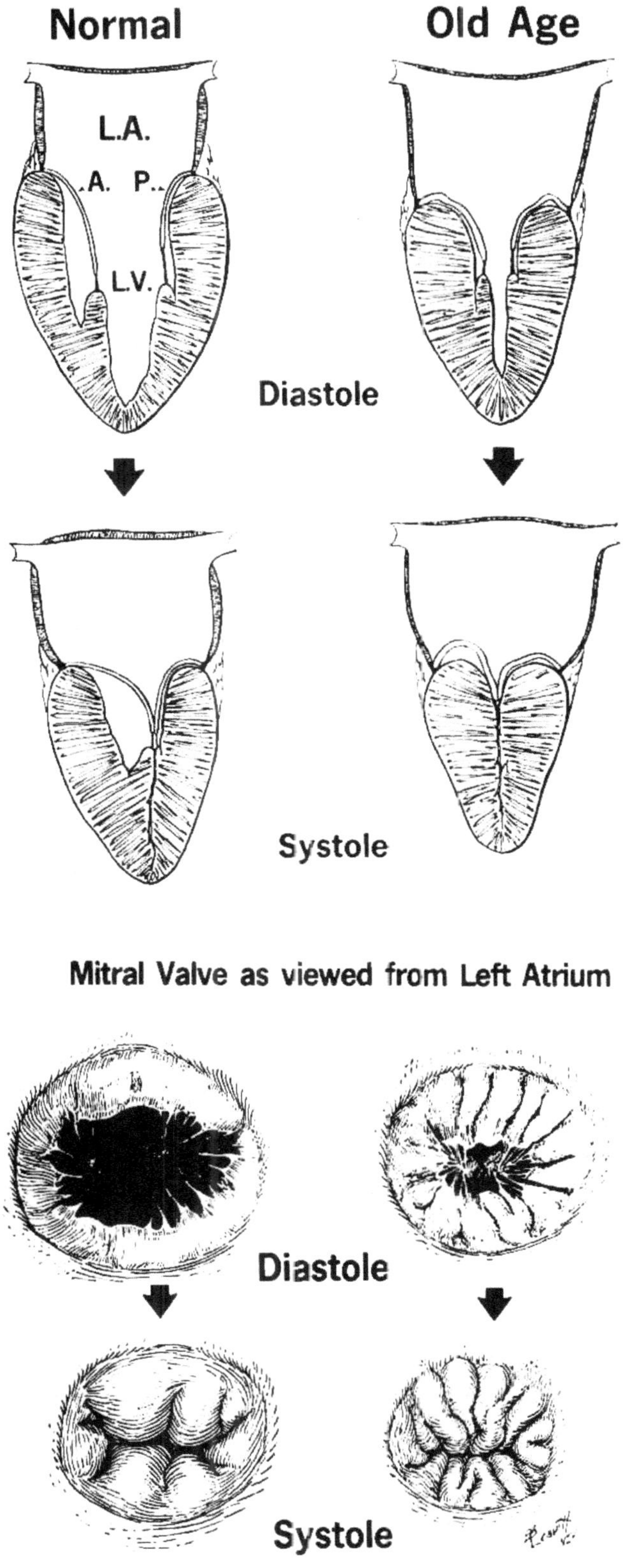

Figure 6 Top. Changes in left atrium (*LA*), anterior (*A*) and posterior (*P*) mitral leaflets, and left ventricle (*LV*) with aging. Because the left ventricular cavity is smaller, the left ventricular wall appears thicker and is probably less compliant. As a result, the left atrium has to work harder to fill the left ventricle; because of this increased effort the atrium dilates, and its wall becomes thinner. Finally, when it reaches a certain degree of dilation, atrial fibrillation occurs (idiopathic atrial fibrillation of the elderly). **Bottom.** Mitral valve viewed from left atrium in youth, compared with in the elderly. In the older person the left ventricular cavity is smaller, and since the mitral leaflets do not become smaller, there is now relatively more leaflet than cavity. The leaflets consequently contact one another abnormally and thicken. In the elderly the mitral valve during ventricular systole has the appearance of dilated hemorrhoids.

Table 1. Functional Classification of Valvular Heart Disease Data on 543 Autopsy Patients More Than 14 Years of Age

Functional Valve Lesion	Number of Patients (%)
Aortic stenosis (AS)	182 (34)
Mitral stenosis (MS)	94 (17)
Aortic and mitral stenosis	66 (12)
Pure aortic regurgitation (AR)	60 (11)
Pure mitral regurgitation (MR)	55 (10)
MS + AR	34 (6)
MR + AR	24 (5)
AS + MR	16 (3)
Tricuspid stenosis + MS ± AS	12 (2)
Total	543 (100)

Rheumatic heart disease may be viewed as a disease of the mitral valve; other valves may also be involved both anatomically and functionally, but anatomically the mitral valve is always involved. To my knowledge, Aschoff bodies have never been found in hearts without anatomic disease of the mitral valve. Twelve of the 543 patients with severe valvular heart disease whom I studied at necropsy had Aschoff bodies, and all had mitral valve disease both anatomically and functionally.

Rheumatic heart disease not only is a disorder of the cardiac valves but also affects mural endocardium, pericardium, and myocardium. Histologically, the atrial walls virtually always show interstitial myocardial fibrosis, atrophy of some myocardial cells, and hypertrophy of the smooth muscle cells of the mural endocardium (15).

Anatomic Features of Rheumatic Mitral Stenosis

The anatomic features of rheumatic mitral stenosis are illustrated in Figure 7. In all patients with rheumatic mitral stenosis the leaflets are diffusely thickened, either by fibrous tissue or calcific deposits, or both; the commissures are usually fused, and the chordae tendineae are shortened and usually fused to some degree. The greatest obstruction to this funnel-shaped valve occurs at its apex, which is within the left ventricular cavity. The primary orifice, located at the level of the anulus, is far less narrowed. Fusion may involve one or both commissures. When only one is fused or one is fused more than the other, the stenotic orifice is eccentrically located. A centrally located orifice indicates symmetrical commissural fusion. In rheumatic mitral stenosis the chordae tendineae are occasionally so retracted that the leaflets appear to insert directly into the papillary muscles. When this occurs, the stenosis is always severe because the interchordal spaces are virtually entirely obliterated. Sometimes chordae inserting into one papillary muscle are well preserved, whereas those inserting into the other papillary muscle are completely fused. Mitral commissurotomy on a valve in which the leaflets insert almost directly into the papillary muscle(s) usually must include a splitting of the papillary muscle(s) as well as the leaflet commissure(s). If there are normally about 120 third-order chordae and about 24 first-order chordae, in mitral stenosis these numbers are usually halved and, on occasion, even reduced to just 1, for practical purposes.

The amount of calcium in the leaflets of stenotic mitral valves varies considerably. Generally, men have more calcium than women, and older patients have more calcium than younger patients. The rapidity with which calcification progresses also varies considerably. Figure 7, for example, shows a heavily calcified stenotic mitral valve excised from a 26-year-old man who had had acute rheumatic fever at age 12 years. The same figure shows another stenotic mitral valve from a 62-year-old woman who also had had acute rheumatic fever when she was 12 years old. Virtually no calcific deposits are present in her valve despite a mitral commissurotomy 14 years earlier. Gross calcific deposits generally preclude mitral commissurotomy and necessitate valve replacement. Previous commissurotomy, however, does not necessarily preclude a second commissurotomy, since the first procedure does not necessarily predispose the leaflets to the deposition of calcium.

A new, acquired cause of mitral stenosis, the rigid-frame prosthetic valve, was introduced in 1960. Since the natural mitral valve is within the left ventricle, a prosthetic mitral valve is also located within this cavity. The prosthesis must be small enough for the contracting left ventricular wall not to interfere with the prosthetic poppet or disk. When the prosthesis is too large for the cavity into which it was inserted, the poppet may be prevented from moving adequately and may therefore obstruct left atrial emptying (Figure 8) (18). The latter state is far commoner than obstruction to left ventricular emptying by the prosthesis (19). Thrombus formation on a mitral prosthesis also may obstruct left atrial emptying (19).

Some Congenital Causes of Mitral Obstruction

Dr. Perloff: Congenital obstruction to left atrial flow falls into three categories (13): [1] congenital mitral stenosis (obstruction at valvular level caused by congenitally abnormal leaflets and chordae), the parachute mitral valve, or supravalvular stenosing ring; [2] cor triatriatum; and [3] congenital pulmonary-vein stenosis. Congenital mitral stenosis means that the obstruction is at the orifice itself—that is, within the leaflets or their chordal support. Cor

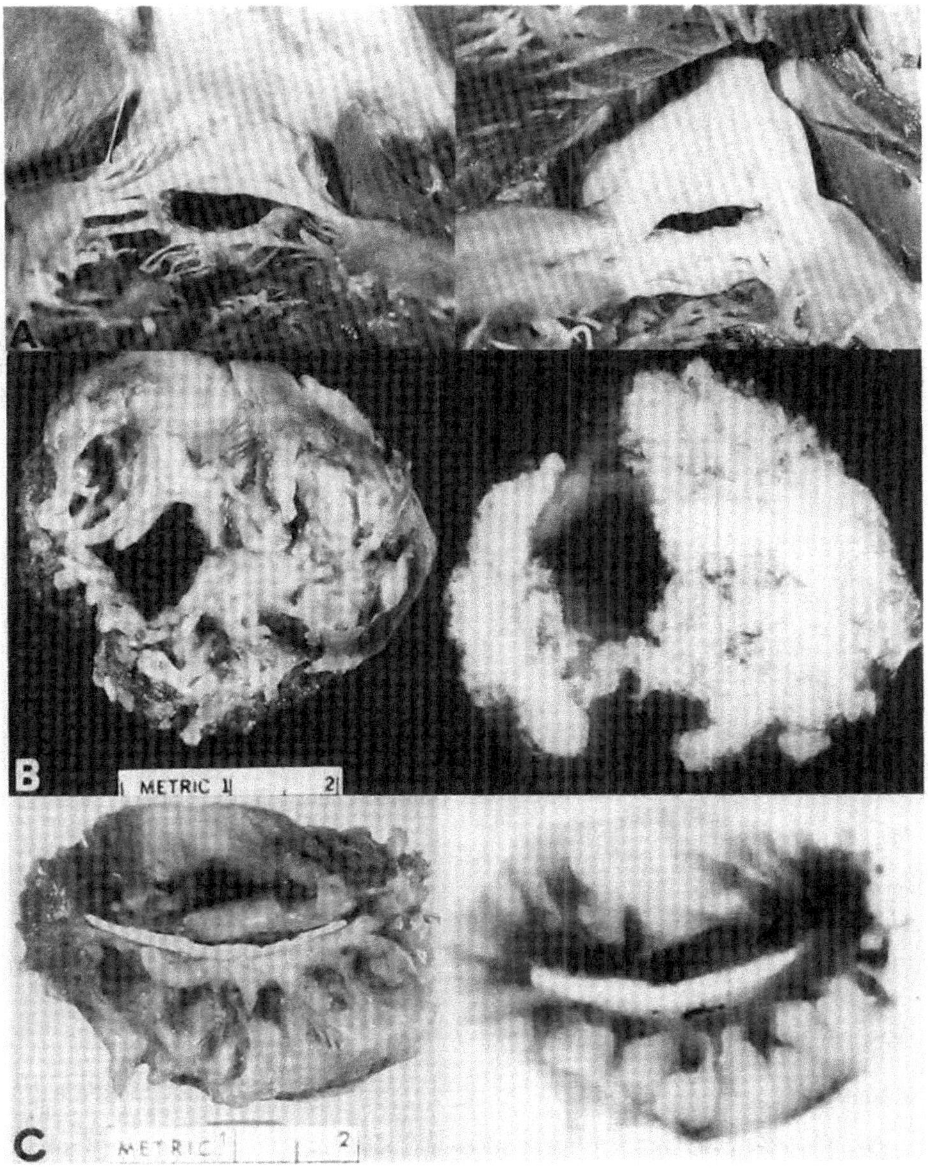

Figure 7A. Mitral valves viewed from left ventricle in two patients with mitral stenosis. **Left.** Valve in a 41-year-old woman who died of mesenteric vascular insufficiency 3 years after mitral commissurotomy (98). This orifice has the typical so-called "fish-mouth" appearance. The leaflets are separated from the papillary muscles by chordae that are thicker than normal. **Right.** Valve in a 39-year-old woman who died during induction of anesthesia for mitral commissurotomy. At catheterization several days earlier the left atrial-left ventricular mean diastolic gradient was 23 mm Hg. The left atrial pressures were mean, 35 and V wave, 43 mm Hg, and left ventricular pressure, 110/7 mm Hg. In this valve, as contrasted to the one on the left, the leaflets appear to insert directly into the papillary muscles. In other words, all chordae have fused, and commissurotomy, if carried out, probably would have required splitting of the papillary muscles as well as of the mitral commissures. **B** and **C.** Operatively excised mitral valves from two patients with mitral stenosis, showing striking differences in degrees of leaflet calcification. On the left are the valves as they would have appeared from the left ventricle, and on the right are roentgenograms of the excised valves. **B.** Valve from a 26-year-old man who died 3 days after mitral replacement. This patient, who had had acute rheumatic fever at age 12 years, preoperatively had a 15 mm Hg mean diastolic gradient between left atrium and left ventricle. This valve is massively calcified 14 years after the presumed initial attack of rheumatic fever. **C.** Valve from a 62-year-old woman who had had acute rheumatic fever at age 12 years and a mitral commissurotomy at age 48. Fourteen years later there was still only a trace of calcium in the valve.

triatriatum is caused by a partition within the left atrial cavity; the mitral valve and its chordal apparatus are normal. Pulmonary vein stenosis (very rare) is remote from the mitral orifice and left atrium.

Congenital mitral stenosis has a characteristic phonocardiogram. No opening snap is present because the mitral leaflets, even though not calcified, are not pliant. Nevertheless, a mid-diastolic or presystolic murmur may occur. With severe pulmonary hypertension murmurs may be absent (silent congenital mitral stenosis), principally because the hypertrophied right ventricle displaces the left ventricle from the apex (20, 21).

PARACHUTE MITRAL VALVE

Dr. Roberts: The commonest cause of congenital mitral stenosis is the parachute mitral valve, or single papillary muscle syndrome (22) (Figure 9). In addition to mitral stenosis, these patients usually have other cardiovascular anomalies: supravalvular mitral ring, which in itself may cause stenosis; subaortic stenosis; valvular aortic stenosis, usually superimposed on a congenitally malformed valve; and coarctation of the aortic isthmus. Other anomalies are also frequent (23).

Congenital mitral stenosis also may occur in individuals with two well-formed left ventricular papillary muscles. Probably the most frequent valve observed is one with an arcade configuration (24, 25). In this situation the chordae tendineae are extremely short.

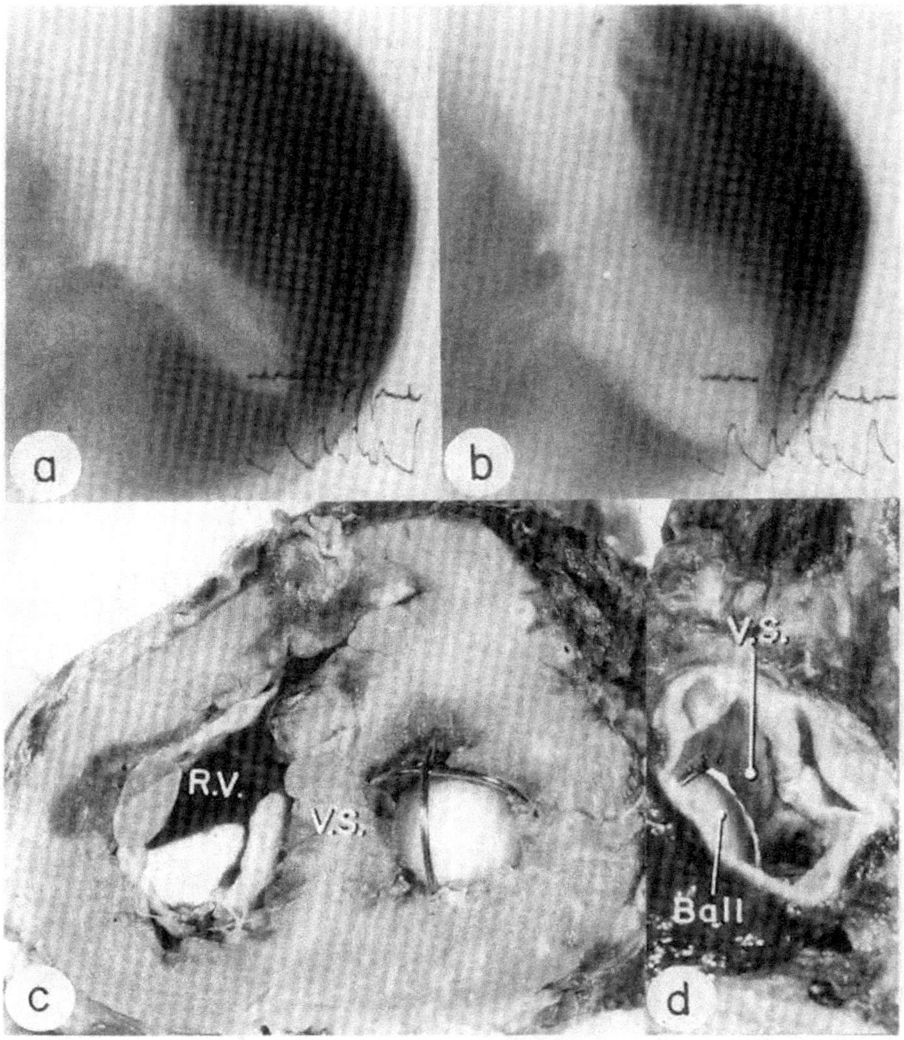

Figure 8. Stenosis of a prosthetic mitral valve in a 57-year-old man who had a small left ventricular cavity that was evident preoperatively on the cineangiocardiogram. a. Angiographic appearance of the left ventricular cavity at peak systole. b. At end-diastole. The diameter of the left ventricular outflow tract, even during diastole, is smaller than the diameter of the ascending aorta. In both angiographic frames the electrocardiogram and brachial arterial pressure pulse, recorded simultaneously, also are shown. c. Valve replacement was performed, but, after insertion of the prosthesis, bleeding from the right ventricular (*R.V.*) cannulation site occurred, and he died. At necropsy it was clear that the mitral poppet was immobile, because the prosthesis was too large for the left ventricular cavity into which it was inserted. Poppet immobility was caused by protrusion of the ventricular septum (*V.S.*) into the cage. Thus, there was no outlet for left atrial blood, and this led to severe elevation of pulmonary arterial and right ventricular pressures with rupture at the cannulation site. d. The poppet also caused narrowing of the left ventricular outflow tract.

Myxomas

Dr. Perloff: Still another form of obstruction to left atrial flow is the left atrial myoxma. A cineangiocardiogram (retrograde catheter in the left ventricle) will show a radiolucent area (negative contrast), typical of left atrial myxoma. Left atrial myxoma may present as a systemic (noncardiac) disease before symptoms of obstruction at the mitral orifice become evident (26). Some patients have systemic emboli, fever, anemia, and high erythrocyte sedimentation rates. The sex distribution is the same as it is with other forms of mitral obstruction—that is, the female predominates 2 or 3 to 1. In myxoma of the left atrium the mitral orifice is not only obstructed by the intracavitary mass, but, as a rule, the valve is also incompetent. Accordingly, it is diagnostically useful to inject contrast material into the left atrium to outline the myoxoma.

Dr. Roberts: Two left atrial myxomas are illustrated in Figure 10 (27). These myxomas may be small, thus not interfering with left atrial emptying, and may be found incidentally at necropsy. On the other hand, they may completely obstruct left atrial outflow, causing sudden death or a variety of other symptoms. Tumors of similar sizes may cause symptoms in some patients and none in others, depending on the location of the stalk. Small tumors may cause symptoms in some patients, and large tumors may not in others, again depending on the location of the stalk. The key is the site of attachment of the tumor to the atrial wall. If the left atrial tumor contacts the mitral leaflets too vigorously for too long, the leaflets may become thickened.

Although some early writers described difficulties in distinguishing left atrial myxoma from left atrial thrombus, the differences between them are great; there are many more differences than similarities between the two (27). The myxoma is attached to the atrial wall by a pedicle, the diameter of which

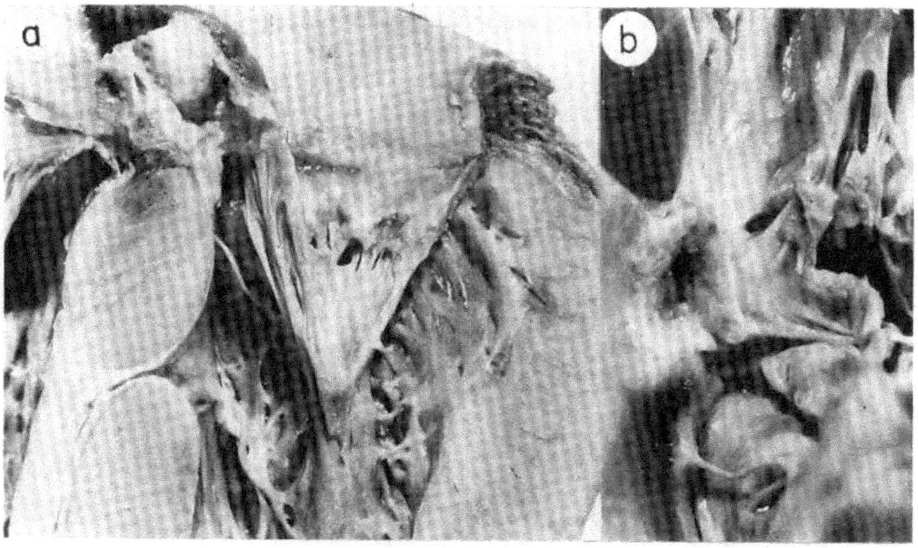

Figure 9. Parachute mitral valve (single papillary muscle) in a 14-year-old boy who presented clinically with left ventricular outflow tract obstruction. The peak systolic gradient between left ventricle and a systemic artery was 80 mm Hg. Obstruction was caused by a small aortic "anulus" with a bicuspid aortic valve and by discrete obstruction just below the aortic valve (*b*). At necropsy the mitral valve showed a parachute configuration, and all of its chordae inserted into a single left ventricular papillary muscle (*a*). Preoperatively, the left atrial mean pressure was 30 mm Hg, and the pulmonary arterial systolic pressure was 50 mm Hg. It was not realized while he was alive, however, that the mitral valve was stenotic. In addition, a functionally insignificant coarctation of the aorta was present. A ventricular septal defect had closed spontaneously (*a*).

is far smaller than the largest diameter of the myxoma. A thrombus is virtually never attached by a pedicle but is instead attached to atrial endocardium over a large area. The myxoma resembles a ping-pong ball floating in a glass of water; as the water level drops (blood descending from left atrium to left ventricle), the ping-pong ball descends. Since the myxoma more or less floats in the atrial cavity, injection of contrast material into the cavity "lights up" the entire surface of the tumor. Contrast material in a left atrial cavity containing a thrombus in its body shows an area of no filling, and the borders of the thrombus are usually not well outlined. The surface of the myxoma is smooth and shiny; that of the thrombus is often ragged. With rare exception, neither thrombus nor myxoma in left atrium interferes

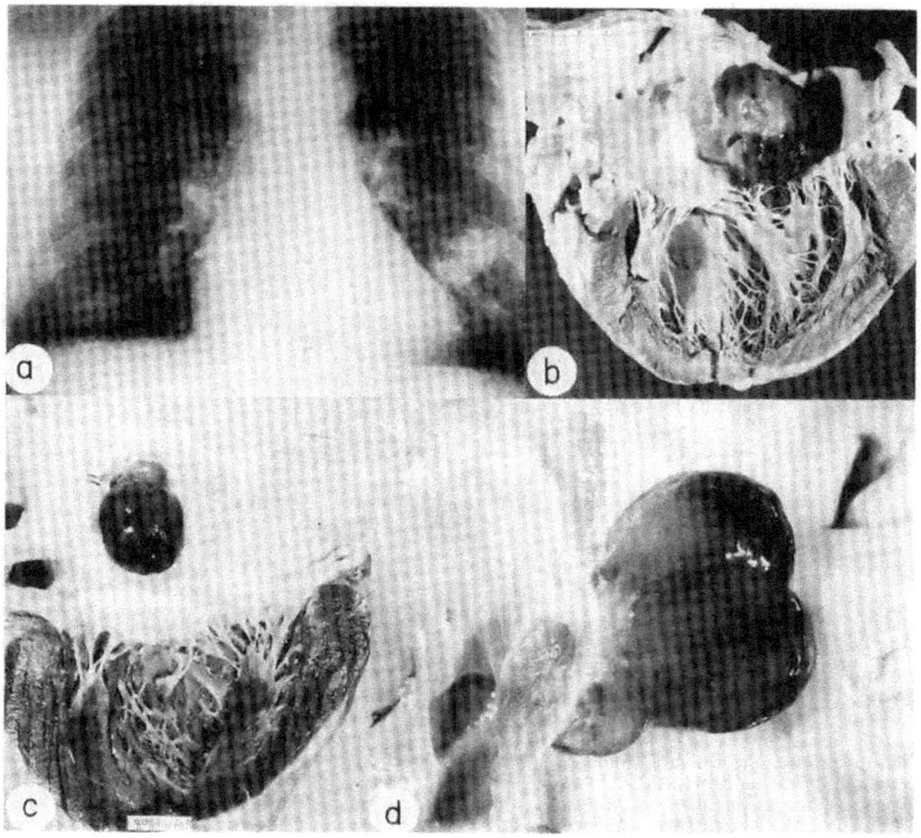

Figure 10. Left atrial myxomas in two patients. **a** and **b.** Chest radiograph and opened left atrium and ventricle in a 54-year-old man who died suddenly 2 weeks after lobectomy for carcinoma of the bronchus. Myxoma was an unexpected necropsy finding, but he had had evidence of congestive cardiac failure for 48 months before death. The myxoma (*b*) weighed 95 g and clearly partially obstructed left atrial outflow. **c** and **d.** Two views of a left atrial myxoma in a 60-year-old man who died of the carcinoid syndrome. This tumor weighed only 30 g and did not prolapse into the mitral orifice. Thus, this patient never had evidence of cardiac dysfunction. The tumor arises from the atrial septum (*d*).

with pulmonary venous drainage. Although thrombi occur in left atrial appendages in a variety of conditions (usually those associated with severely depressed cardiac output), thrombi occur in the body of the atrium only in patients with mitral stenosis. In other words, relatively severe stasis of blood is required for thrombus formation in the atrial body. Thrombi virtually never occur in the bodies of left atria in patients with pure mitral regurgitation, presumably because their atrial cavities are constantly being "washed out" during both phases of the cardiac cycle, thus preventing stasis. In contrast, myxomas occur entirely within the bodies of atria, never in atrial appendages, and the "valvular obstruction" totally disappears after excision of the neoplasm. Both thrombi and myxomas tend to form in atria that are of normal size or, at most, are moderately dilated. The huge left atrium rarely contains a thrombus.

Although thrombi and myxomas are the common-

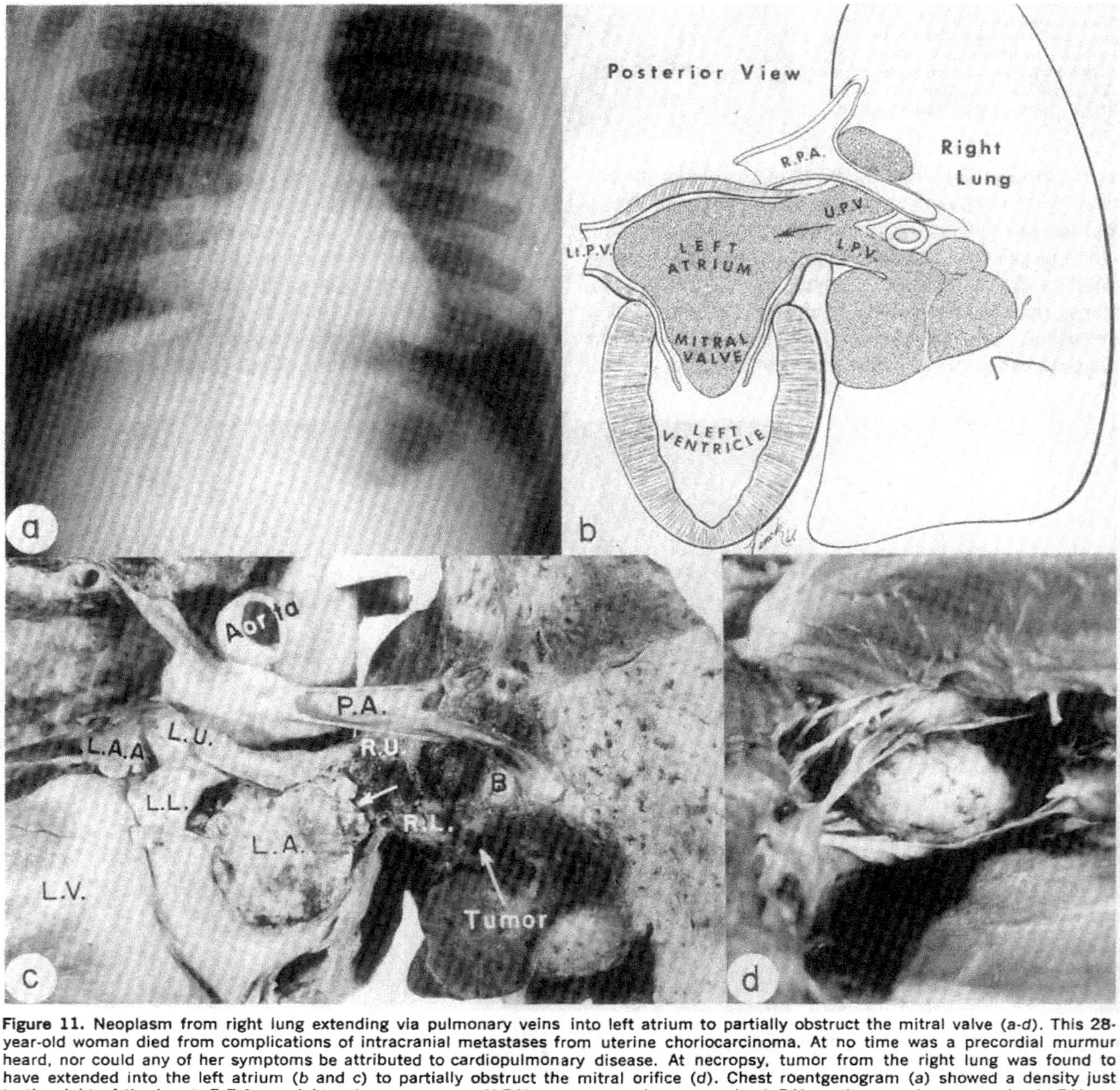

Figure 11. Neoplasm from right lung extending via pulmonary veins into left atrium to partially obstruct the mitral valve (*a-d*). This 28-year-old woman died from complications of intracranial metastases from uterine choriocarcinoma. At no time was a precordial murmur heard, nor could any of her symptoms be attributed to cardiopulmonary disease. At necropsy, tumor from the right lung was found to have extended into the left atrium (*b* and *c*) to partially obstruct the mitral orifice (*d*). Chest roentgenogram (*a*) showed a density just to the right of the heart. R.P.A. = right pulmonary artery; U.P.V. = upper pulmonary vein; L.P.V. = lower pulmonary vein; Lt.P.V. = left pulmonary vein; P.A. = pulmonary artery; L.V. = left ventricle; L.A. = left atrium; L.A.A. = left atrial appendage; B = bronchus; R.U. and L.U. = right and left upper pulmonary veins; R.L. and L.L. = right and left lower pulmonary veins.

est cause of filling defects in the left atrium, neoplasms (28, 29) and infected masses (30) may occur in this chamber and interfere with left atrial emptying (Figure 11). In contrast to thrombus and myxoma, however, the other filling defects also usually interfere with pulmonary venous return.

Mitral Regurgitation

Dr. Perloff: Remember that normal coordinated function of the left atrial wall, mitral anulus, leaflets, chordae tendineae, papillary muscles, and left ventricular free wall is required for competence of the mitral orifice.

First, we will consider the leaflets and chordae tendineae. The leaflets in mitral regurgitation may function abnormally because they are too small or too large or because they are tethered or immobilized by short chordae. A common cause of inadequate leaflet tissue is the scarring and contracture after rheumatic endocarditis. A rare but interesting feature in some patients with recurrent active rheumatic fever is Jaccoud's arthritis (Figure 12) (31). Appreciable mitral regurgitation generally coexists.

Now let us contrast two types of severe mitral regurgitation, one chronic and the other acute. In severe chronic (rheumatic) mitral regurgitation, the left atrium can be immense. Despite the large volume of regurgitant flow, the left atrial pressure may rise little, if at all, because the large left atrium is remarkably compliant (32). Accordingly, this form of severe mitral regurgitation occurs with normal or nearly normal left atrial pressure, without pulmonary hypertension, and with typical physical signs—namely, atrial fibrillation, an apical holosystolic murmur with axillary radiation, a prominent third heart sound, an apical left ventricular impulse, and anterior displacement of the heart due to systolic expansion of the large left atrium (33). In chronic severe mitral regurgitation the posterior wall of the large left atrium is displaced downward and posteriorly (8). Because of the continuity between left atrial endocardium and posterior mitral leaflet, the posterior cusp is pulled across its anulus, so that the cusp functionally shortens as the left atrium enlarges. Thus mitral regurgitation is augmented by atrial enlargement, or, as Edwards and Burchell (34) said, "mitral incompetence begets mitral incompetence."

In contrast to the chronic variety, acute severe regurgitation enlarges the left atrium hardly at all (35, 36). As a rule, the cause of the sudden regurgitation is rupture of chordae tendineae. Patients have normal sinus rhythm, as opposed to atrial fibrillation in those with chronic severe mitral regurgitation (32). Their history shows the recent onset of a systolic murmur and congestive heart failure. The apical murmur tends to be decrescendo and often radiates to the left sternal edge and base. The third heart sound of mitral regurgitation is present, but there is also a prominent fourth heart sound (37), which is not a feature of chronic mitral regurgitation. The fourth heart sound is accompanied by presystolic distention of the left ventricle. Physical signs of pulmonary hypertension develop rapidly because there is a large volume of regurgitant flow into a small, noncompliant left atrium in which the pressure

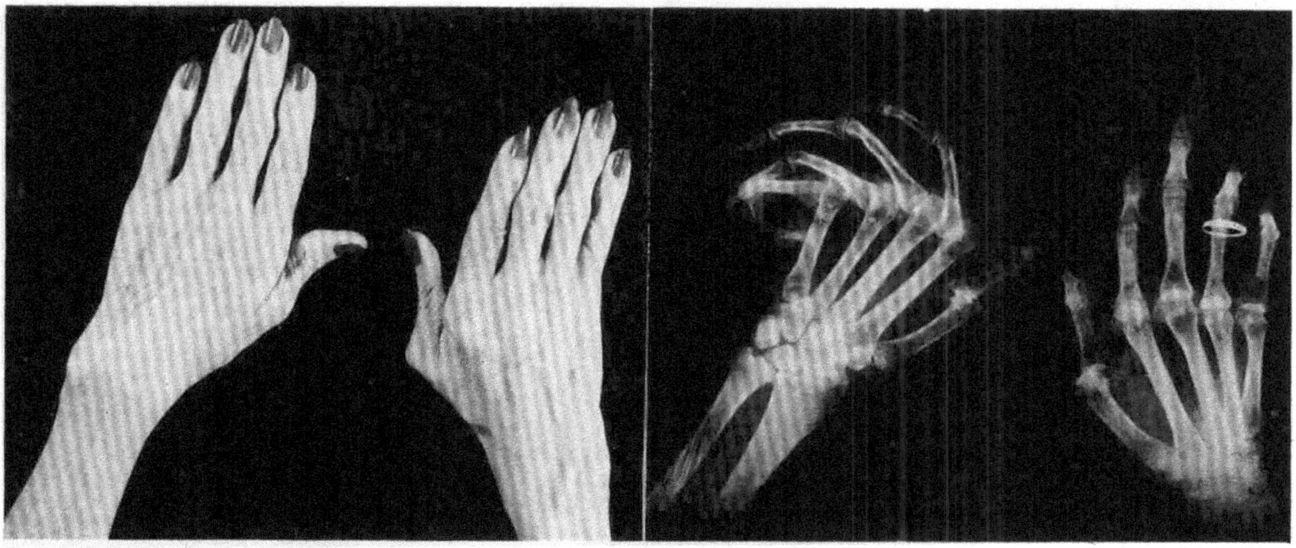

Figure 12. Hands of two patients with Jaccoud's arthritis. The inner photograph and X ray show deformities caused by subluxation of metacarpophalangeal joints. The outer photographs (hand and X ray) show that the patient can voluntarily "correct" the deformity. (With kind permission of Dr. Nathan T. Zvaifles, University of California, San Diego.)

Table 2. Cause of Clinically Isolated Fatal Pure Mitral Regurgitation in 55 Necropsy Patients More Than 14 Years of Age

Cause	Number of Patients	
Rheumatic	30	
Rupture of chordae tendineae in previously normal valve	15	
Floppy valve	4	
Congenital	4	
Corrected transposition		1
Partial A-V canal		1
Endocardial fibroelastosis		1
Parachute valve		1
Possible anular calcification	1	
Uncertain	1	
Total (20 males, 35 females)	55	

rises steeply, in striking contrast to chronic severe mitral regurgitation with a large compliant left atrium and a normal or near-normal left atrial pressure. The decrescendo systolic murmur is a useful feature in the clinical recognition of acute severe mitral regurgitation. The proposed mechanism is as follows: the left ventricular and left atrial pressure pulses and a phonocardiogram will show tall left atrial V waves and a decline in the left ventricular pressure pulse at the end of ejection; the steeply rising left atrial V wave approaches the left ventricular pressure in later systole, with the result that there is a late systolic decline in regurgitant flow and in murmur intensity (holosystolic but decrescendo). Occasionally, the decrescendo murmur ends before the second heart sound (early systolic).

An increased force of left atrial contraction accompanies acute severe mitral regurgitation. Palpation of the cardiac apex detects presystolic distention of the left ventricle, and on auscultation an accompanying fourth heart sound is heard. These two physical signs distinguish acute severe from chronic severe mitral regurgitation. The reason is evident. The previously normal left atrium in acute severe mitral regurgitation responds to an increase in volume and pressure by increasing its wall thickness and its contractile force. This force is delivered into the left ventricular cavity, resulting in presystolic distension and a fourth heart sound.

Dr. Roberts: In contrast to mitral stenosis, which has mainly one cause (rheumatic), pure mitral regurgitation has numerous causes (Table 2). Of the 543 patients with functionally severe valvular heart disease whom I studied at necropsy, 55 had pure mitral regurgitation. Cases of papillary muscle dysfunction were excluded. Rheumatic heart disease accounted for over half the cases.

Why the mitral valve affected by acute rheumatic fever becomes stenotic in some patients and why it becomes purely incompetent in others is unknown. Although the cause may be similar (rheumatic), the structural alterations in the purely incompetent mitral valve are quite different from those in the stenotic valve. The purely incompetent rheumatic valve infrequently contains calcific deposits; its commissures are virtually never fused; its chordae tendineae are only mildly thickened, if at all; and chordal fusion

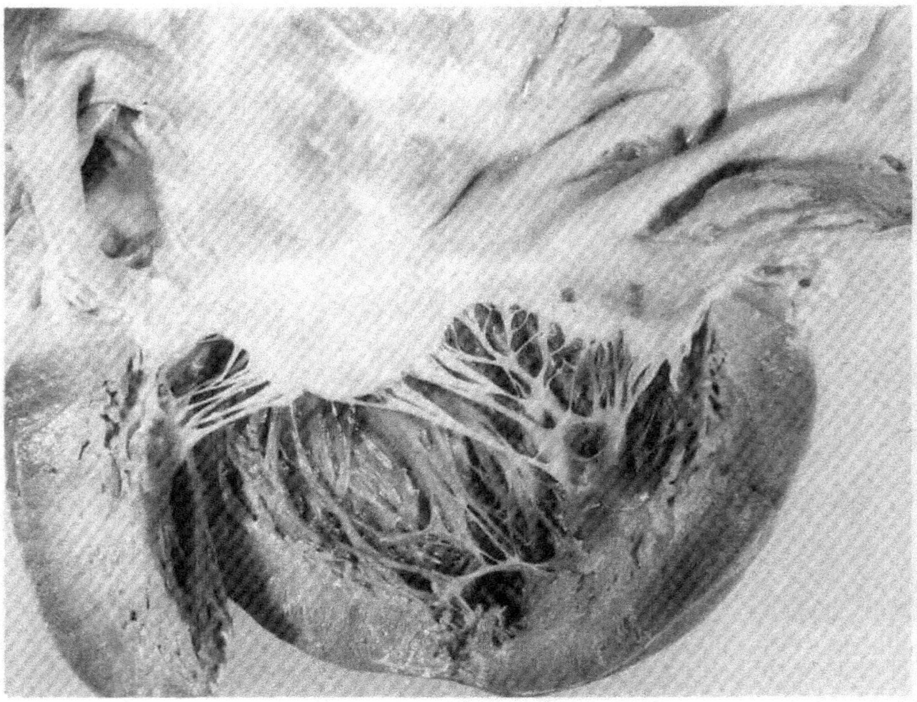

Figure 13. Pure mitral regurgitation of rheumatic cause. This 42-year-old man was said to have had acute rheumatic fever at age 7 years, with a precordial murmur since then. At age 39 years he developed congestive cardiac failure, and a grade 4/6 systolic murmur typical of mitral regurgitation was heard. Catheterization at age 40 years showed the following pressures (in mm Hg): pulmonary artery, 44/19; left atrium—V wave, 28 and mean, 16; left ventricle, 148/13; and brachial artery, 150/84. Left ventricular cineangiogram showed 4+/4+ mitral regurgitation, and aortic root cine showed no aortic regurgitation. He died of progressive congestive cardiac failure 2 years after the catheterization. At necropsy the mitral valve leaflets were diffusely but mildly thickened; the chordae were not shortened, and only a few were thickened; neither commissure was fused. The left atrium was severely dilated. This is the type of valve that is purely incompetent, presumably from damage initiated by rheumatic fever.

is infrequent (Figure 13). It is often difficult to explain the mechanism of mitral regurgitation in a valve made purely incompetent by consequences of rheumatic fever. The mitral anuli in these patients are also usually dilated, but this mechanism in and of itself rarely appears to be an adequate explanation for the regurgitation.

Rheumatic disease is never limited to endocardium. Inflammatory cells are always found in atrial walls of patients dying with acute rheumatic fever (38). The inflammation appears to weaken the walls, and superimposed mitral regurgitation tends to dilate the chamber out of proportion to the dilation that would occur with similar degrees of mitral regurgitation into a left atrium with previously normal walls. What causes the left atrium to dilate enormously in some patients with rheumatic mitral regurgitation is uncertain. Possibly, the patients with so-called giant atria have had more frequent or more severe attacks of acute rheumatic fever, with particularly severe destruction of atrial myocardial fibers. When the left atrium in pure mitral regurgitation is giant in size, intimal proliferation is rarely found in the pulmonary veins or arteries, and the right ventricular walls are not hypertrophied (39) (Figure 14). The anatomy of pure mitral regurgitation in this context thus follows the physiologic alterations outlined by Dr. Perloff. The larger the left atrial cavity in pure mitral regurgitation, the lower its intracavity pressure. Since the right ventricular walls in these patients are

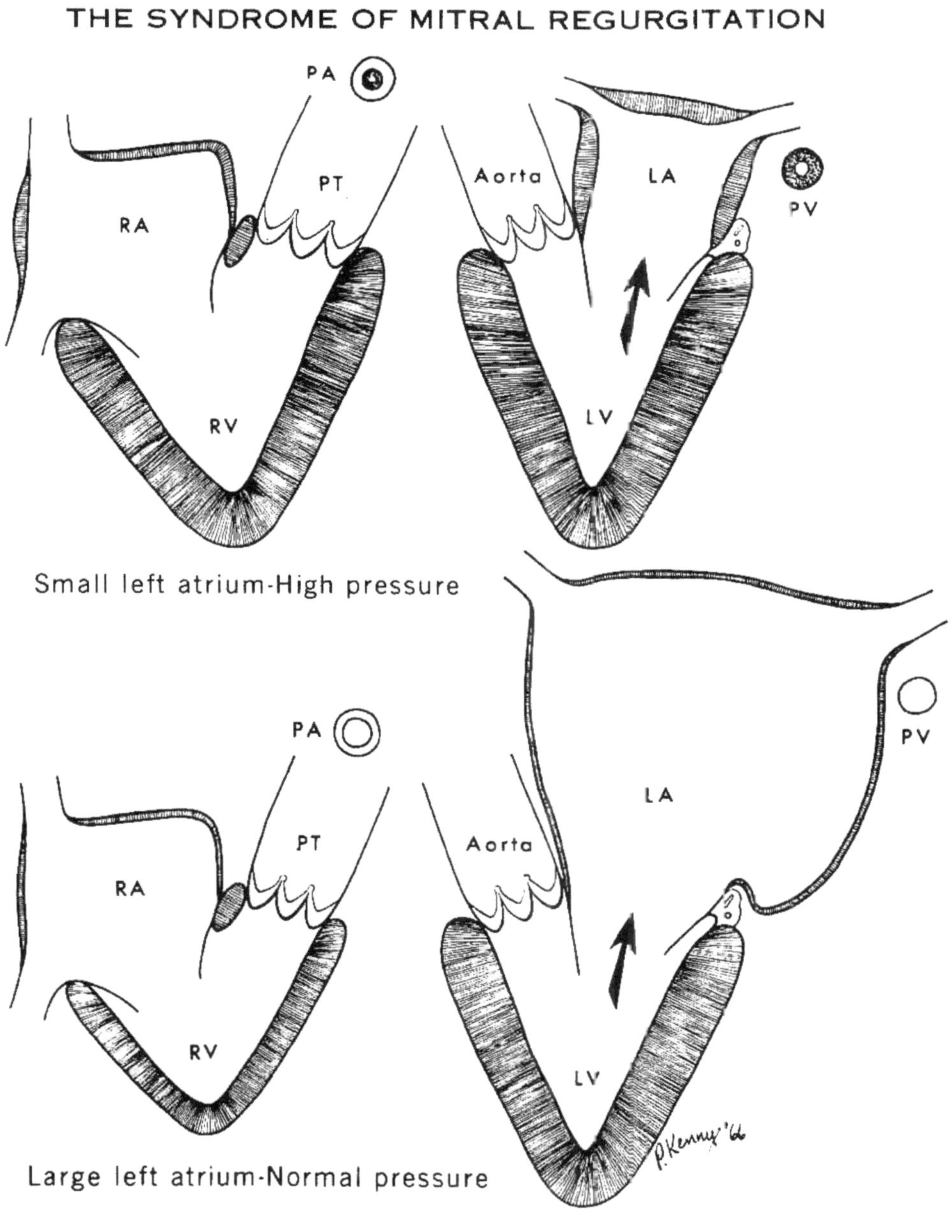

Figure 14. The two extremes of the spectrum of pure mitral regurgitation. When severe mitral regurgitation appears suddenly in individuals with previously normal or near-normal hearts, the left atrium (*LA*) is relatively small, and the high pressure within it is reflected back into the pulmonary vessels and right ventricle (*RV*). The anatomic indicator of this latter physiologic event is severe hypertrophy of the left atrial and right ventricular walls and marked intimal proliferation and medial hypertrophy of the pulmonary arteries (*PA*), arterioles, and veins (*PV*). In the other extreme, the left atrial cavity is of giant size, and its wall is thin. It is thus able to "absorb" the left ventricular (*LV*) pressure without reflecting it back into the pulmonary vessels or right ventricle. As a consequence, the pulmonary vessels remain normal, and the right ventricular wall does not thicken. PT = pulmonary trunk; RA = right atrium.

usually not hypertrophied (because the right ventricular systolic pressures are normal or near normal), tricuspid regurgitation is infrequent. In contrast, patients with large left atria from mitral stenosis or combined mitral stenosis and regurgitation have elevated left atrial, pulmonary venous, pulmonary arterial, and right ventricular pressures, and the right ventricular walls are therefore hypertrophied. Thus, tricuspid regurgitation is a common consequence.

Rupture of mitral chordae tendineae is the second commonest cause of fatal pure mitral regurgitation in patients studied by me at necropsy (35) (Table 2). The normal chordae tendineae are the ones most likely to rupture, not the previously thickened ones. Thus, rupture of one or several thick chordae tendineae in patients with mitral stenosis is extremely rare. The cause of the rupture varies. Infective endocarditis is the commonest cause of acute rupture. However, of 42 patients with healed ruptured mitral chordae tendineae studied by Buchbinder, Roberts, and Morrow (40), only 14 had had infective endocarditis. Infective endocarditis causes acute severe mitral regurgitation by chordal rupture and not, with rare exception, by leaflet perforation (41). The syndrome of acute severe mitral regurgitation associated with normal- or near-normal-sized left atria and severe elevations of left atrial, pulmonary venous, pulmonary arterial, and right ventricular pressures is usually the result of rupture of chordae tendineae by infective endocarditis involving previously normal valves (35). The left atrial myocardial fibers in these patients, as contrasted to those in patients with chronic rheumatic mitral regurgitation, have not been previously damaged by rheumatic fever, and therefore the left atrial wall is capable of responding to the sudden elevation of left atrial pressure by vigorous contractions, leading to fiber hypertrophy. The ventricular systolic pressures in these patients are reflected quickly into the vasculature of the lungs, and severe medial hypertrophy and intimal proliferation of the pulmonary arteries and veins progress rapidly. The already diseased left atrium, in contrast, appears to respond to volume load by dilating, not by contracting. Thus, the smaller the left atrial cavity in pure mitral regurgitation, the thicker the right ventricular wall, and, conversely, the larger the left atrial cavity, the thinner the right ventricular wall.

How many mitral chordae tendineae must rupture for severe regurgitation to occur? Haller and Morrow (42) ruptured only one or two primary chordae in dogs, by inserting fishhooks into left ventricles, and severe mitral regurgitation developed immediately, as evidenced by prominent expansions of the left atria during each ventricular systole.

A newly discovered cause of acquired pure mitral regurgitation is fistulas around bases of prosthetic valves (19). Small peribasilar leaks around mitral prostheses are difficult to diagnose clinically without injecting contrast material into left ventricle (43).

Dr. Perloff: The chordae, like the leaflets, can be too short, too long, or partially destroyed (ruptured) (44). First, we will discuss the chordae that are too long and the leaflets that are too long for their mitral orifices. Mid- to late-systolic clicks, single or multiple,

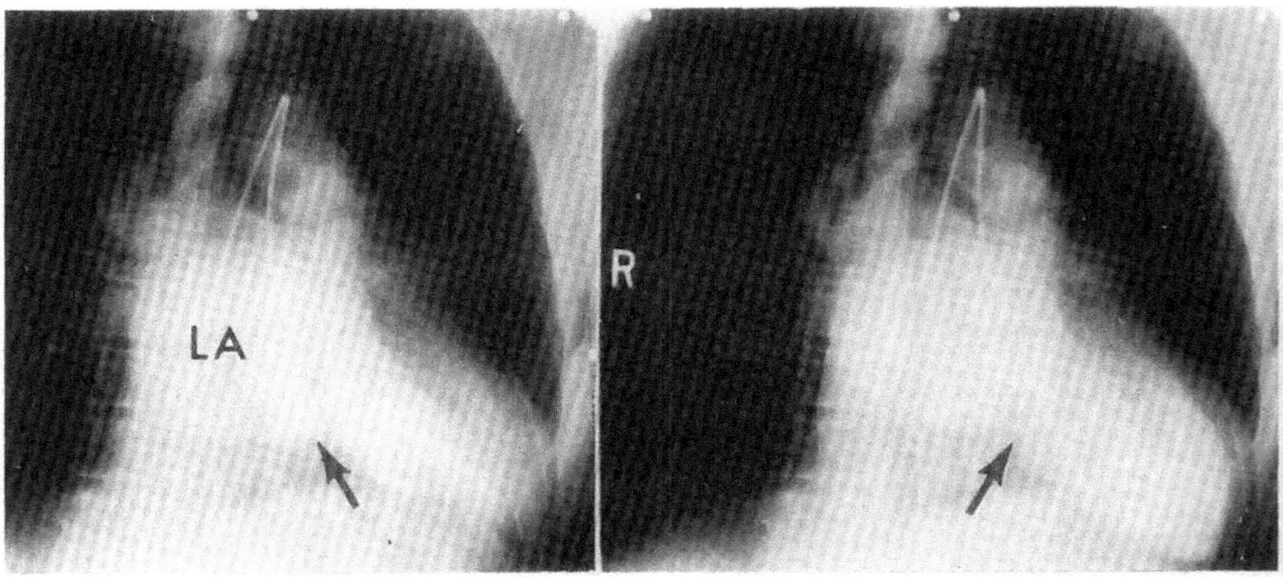

Figure 15. Right anterior oblique left ventricular angiocardiograms from a 49-year-old asymptomatic man with clicks and a late systolic murmur. **Left.** Systolic frame shows lip-like prolapse of the posterior leaflet (*arrow*). **Right.** Diastolic frame shows absence of prolapse (*arrow*). Note opacification of left atrium (*LA*) caused by late systolic mitral regurgitation.

alone or introducing a late systolic murmur, have been recognized for many years. Formerly, these auscultatory signs were believed to be extracardiac (pericardial), especially the clicks alone. Let us examine the evidence that clicks and late systolic murmurs can—and generally do—originate in the mitral apparatus, specifically in redundant posterior cusps and elongated chordae (45-47). When systemic pressure is acutely elevated (pharmacologically) in a patient with a click and a late systolic murmur, the left atrial V wave promptly rises, and the late systolic murmur becomes much louder (48). The converse effect is seen during an acute decrease in systemic pressure induced by inhalation of amyl nitrite (48). Both responses are similar to those in mitral regurgitation (33). Occasionally, during the postamyl nitrite inhalation period, the murmur becomes holosystolic, resembling that of typical mitral regurgitation (48). We can get still closer by examining the intracardiac source of clicks and late systolic murmurs. If an intracardiac phonocardiogram is recorded from the left atrium, systolic clicks and late systolic murmurs can be recovered from just above the mitral valve, a site appropriate for mitral regurgitation (48).

The best clinical evidence of mitral valve origin is the angiocardiogram, as shown in Figure 15, a right oblique left ventricular angiocardiogram. In the systolic frame the arrow points to a lip-like herniation of the redundant posterior cusp into the left atrium, which is opacified because of mitral regurgitation.

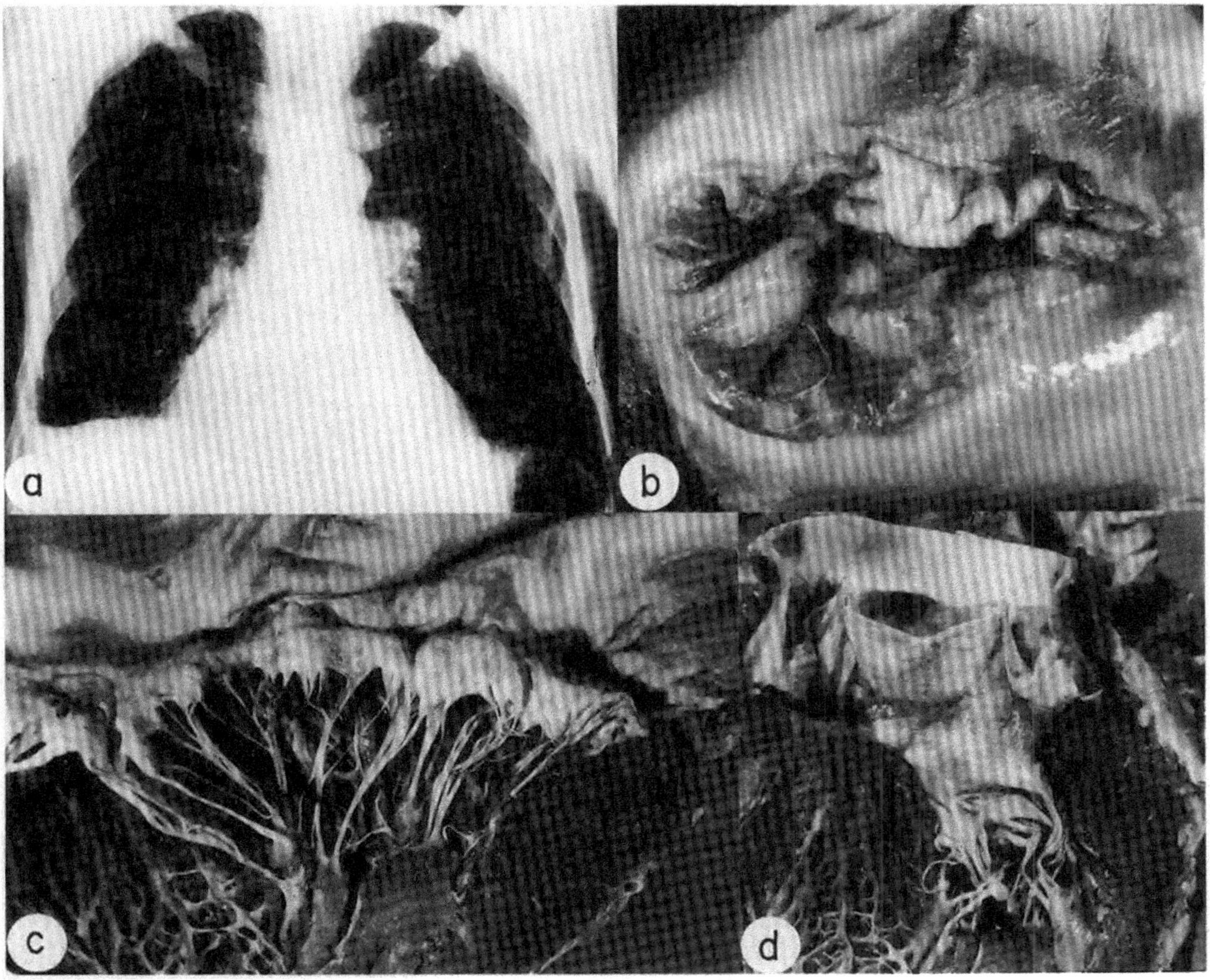

Figure 16. Floppy mitral valve in a 70-year-old man who died of gastric carcinoma. During life a grade 3/6 pansystolic blowing murmur was heard, loudest over the apex, with radiation to the left axilla. The rhythm was atrial fibrillation. He never had symptoms of cardiac dysfunction. Radiograph showed that the heart was enlarged (*a*), but at necropsy it weighed only 310 g. Both atria were quite dilated. The mitral leaflets protruded toward the left atrium (*b*) because the chordae tendineae were too long. A portion of opened mitral valve showing the elongated chordae is shown in c. The opened left ventricle and aortic valve are shown in *d*, again showing excessively long chordae. It is possible that the chordal elongation in the older patients, particularly those with debilitating diseases, results from shortening or atrophy of the ventricles.

In the diastolic frame the posterior cusp falls back into the left ventricular cavity and is not seen. Systolic prolapse of the posterior cusp is a common accompaniment of clicks and late systolic murmurs (45-47, 49). In later systole, as the apex of the left ventricle approaches the mitral anulus, the redundant chordae and posterior leaflet are too long to prevent cuspal eversion. Early in systole the leaflets coapt and seal the mitral orifice; in later systole they give way to late systolic regurgitation. The clicks are believed to

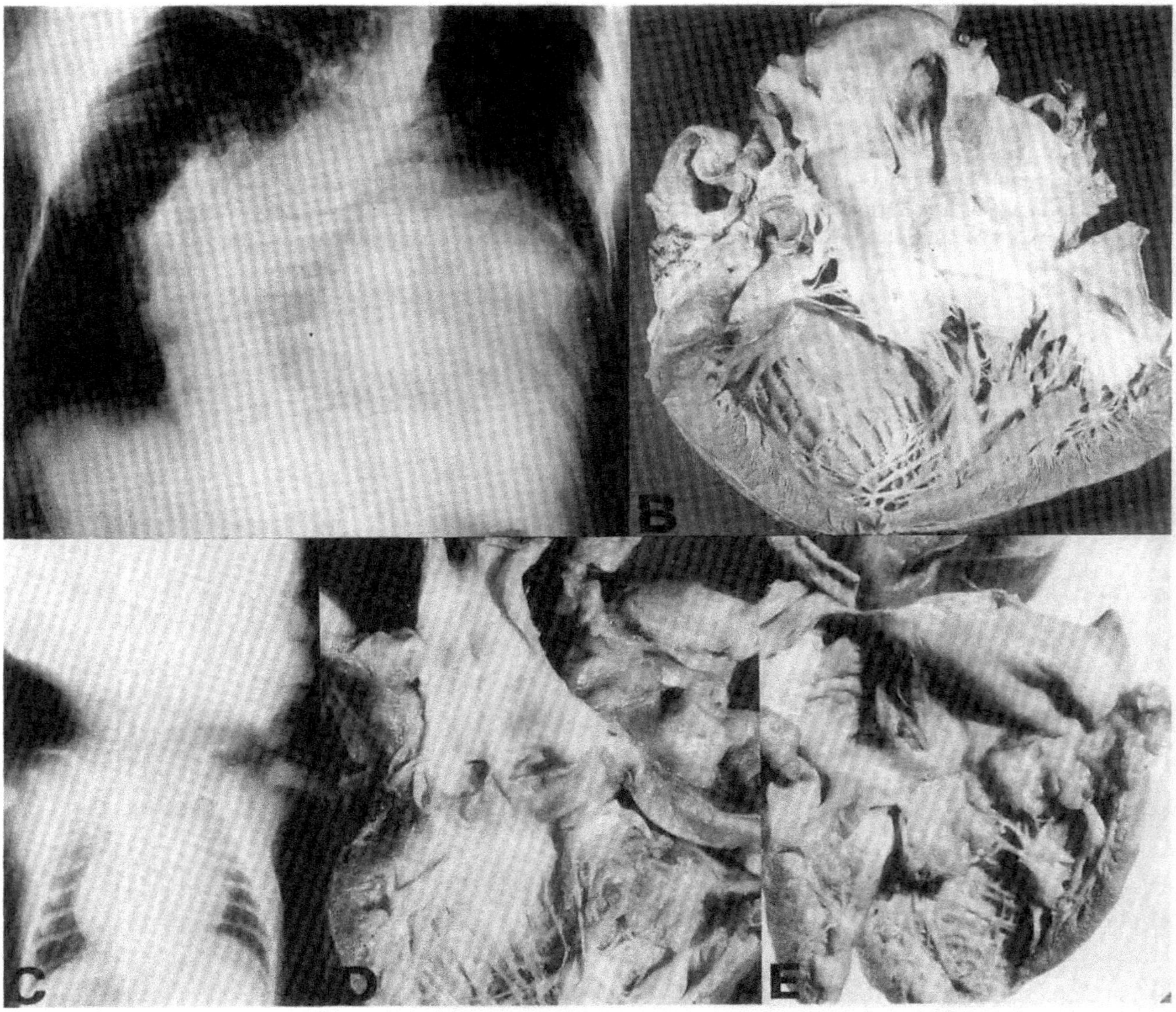

Figure 17A and B. Chest roentgenogram and opened left atrium, mitral valve, and left ventricle in a 28-year-old man with typical (arachnodactyly, myopia, kyphoscoliosis, high-arched palate and arch, and pectus excavatum) features of Marfan's syndrome and severe mitral regurgitation. He had been well until age 24 years, when he developed exertional dyspnea and hemoptysis and was found to have cardiomegaly. Catheterization was performed at age 25 years, and the pressures (in mm Hg) were as follows: pulmonary artery, 19/10; right ventricle, 19/5; right atrial mean, 5; pulmonary arterial wedge mean, 10; and systemic artery, 130/80. The cardiac output was 2.3 litres/min. He remained functionally class II for the next 3 years, but during his last year of life the congestive heart failure worsened, and he became class IV. On examination (7 days before death) he was quite ill. A grade 5/6 pansystolic precordial murmur, loudest over the apex, was audible. No diastolic murmur was present. The chest radiograph showed a big heart and severe kyphoscoliosis (*A*). Electrocardiogram showed sinus rhythm and left ventricular hypertrophy. He died of progressive heart failure. At necropsy, the heart was large (weight, 850 g). The mitral leaflets were mildly thickened and elongated, and the mitral anulus was severely dilated (15 cm) (*B*). Calcific deposits were present in the anulus behind the posterior mitral leaflet. The left atrium was quite dilated, as was the left ventricle. The aortic valve and ascending aorta were normal on both gross and histologic examinations. Thus, this patient represents pure mitral regurgitation without aortic disease in Marfan's syndrome. **C-E.** Floppy mitral valve in a 2-day-old boy who had long toes and fingers, a high-arched palate, and a grade 3/6 precordial systolic murmur typical of mitral regurgitation. The heart was enlarged (*C*). He died of congestive cardiac failure. At necropsy the intima of the ascending aorta was wrinkled (*D*), suggesting that the underlying media was abnormal at this early stage. Shown here is the opened aorta, aortic valve, and left ventricle. **E.** The opened left atrium, mitral valve, and left ventricle. The mitral leaflets are considerably elongated in both longitudinal and transverse dimensions. The left atrium is dilated. This case is particularly important because it shows that the floppy mitral valve and abnormalities in the aorta may be present from birth.

result from abrupt tautening of the chordae tendineae or the redundant leaflet and have been called "chordal snaps" (45).

Another interesting concept regarding clicks and late systolic murmurs concerns abnormal movement of the wall of the left ventricle at the site of origin of the posterior papillary muscle (50). This movement takes the form of a rather striking ventricular contraction band that is believed to prevent proper tautening of posterior leaflet support. Accordingly, during later systole the posterior papillary muscle and its supporting chordae tendineae are thrown into a slack position, and mitral regurgitation follows (50). We thus have three points of view regarding the origin of clicks and late systolic murmurs: redundant leaflet tissue, elongated chordae, and abnormal left ventricular free wall.

In 1880 William Osler published an article (51) with the engaging title "On a Remarkable Heart Murmur Heard at a Distance from the Chest Wall." He described what is now known as systolic whoops or honks (52). These very loud honking or whooping systolic events occur intermittently in some patients who have isolated clicks and late systolic murmurs (53). Redundant leaflets, elongated chordae tendineae, left ventricular contraction bands, systolic clicks, late systolic murmurs, and occasional high-frequency whoops or honks may all be variations of the same theme.

Another interesting feature in such patients—generally healthy young women—are abnormal electrocardiograms (T-wave inversions in diaphragmatic or left chest leads [50], and ectopic rhythms [54]). Sudden death has occurred in such patients, but the frequency of this complication—probably small—is unknown.

One other point regarding systolic clicks and late systolic murmurs. Patients with Marfan's syndrome are traditionally regarded as having aortic root disease. Three causes of mitral regurgitation in Marfan's syndrome are recognized, two of which we shall touch on later. In passing, I mention the third, the long redundant chordae and leaflets.

Dr. Roberts: Fortunately, patients with systolic clicks and late systolic murmurs infrequently have mitral regurgitation severe enough in itself to be fatal. As a consequence, relatively few mitral valves have been examined at necropsy in patients known to have systolic clicks and late systolic murmurs unequivocally documented during life. Several "floppy" mitral valves, the type believed responsible for the ausculatory syndrome, are illustrated in Figures 16 and 17. The posterior mitral leaflet unassociated with ruptured chordae tendineae or necrotic or fibrotic papillary muscles may prolapse abnormally toward the left atrium during ventricular systole because the chordae or the leaflets, or both, are too long. What causes the chordae to elongate in the absence of severe left ventricular dilation is unknown. Prolapsed posterior mitral leaflets are nearly always thickened, but they are nearly always devoid of calcific deposits. Despite their thickening, the leaflets are usually elongated in their basal-to-margin lengths, and usually the amount of leaflet tissue also is increased transversely. The accordion-like buckling of the posterior leaflet causes the floppy mitral valve to appear as dilated hemorrhoids when viewed intact from the left atrium (Figure 16). All floppy mitral valves have increased amounts of acid mucopolysaccharide material in them. Although normally present in all cardiac valves, the amount of acid mucopolysaccharide is greatly increased when the valve has the "floppy" appearance. Most patients with Marfan's syndrome have floppy mitral (Figure 17) and tricuspid valves. Pure mitral regurgitation without aortic regurgitation in them, however, is unusual. The floppy atrioventricular valves seen in Marfan's syndrome are almost certainly present at birth, not something acquired later in life. Evidence for this is the occurrence of floppy mitral and tricuspid valves in a 2-day-old boy studied clinically by Dr. Perloff several years ago (Figure 17*C-E*).

Various cardiovascular findings in Marfan's syndrome are summarized in Figure 18. The major lesion in the aorta in this condition is great loss of elastic fibers. Acid mucopolysaccharide is increased in the aorta in patients with Marfan's syndrome, but the accumulation of this material is not the explanation for weakening of the aortic wall. The latter results from degeneration of its elastic fibers. The smooth muscle cells in the aortic media also show evidence of degeneration by electron-microscopic examination, but this may be a secondary rather than a primary event.

Dr. Perloff: We have discussed chordae tendineae that are too long and leaflets that are too mobile. Now to mitral regurgitation caused by restricted leaflet mobility—namely, abnormally short or ectopically inserted chordae tendineae, as in endocardial cushion defect and congenitally corrected transposition of the great arteries.

Patients with endocardial cushion defects characteristically have cleft anterior mitral cusps and abnormal chordal arrangements (13). The anterior leaflet is almost invariably anatomically faulty but not always functionally incompetent. Mitral regurgitation in partial endocardial cushion defect probably depends more on the abnormally inserting chordae than on the cleft anterior leaflet. When contrast material is injected into the left ventricle in such patients, a peculiar "swan's neck" or "gooseneck" deformity of the outflow tract is seen in diastole (55). The deformity results from a combination of cleft anterior leaflet and abnormally inserting chordae and is present whether the mitral valve is functionally competent or not. The chordae arise from the margins of the cleft and insert directly into the crest of the ventricular septum just below the aortic valve. Such chordae have no counterpart in the normal heart.

A second form of congenital "mitral" regurgitation due to restricted leaflet mobility is congenitally corrected levo-type transposition of the great vessels or ventricular inversion (Figure 19). Normally, right atrial blood crosses a tricuspid valve, enters an anatomic right ventricle, and is ejected into the pulmonary trunk. Left atrial blood crosses a mitral valve, enters an anatomic left ventricle, and flows into the aorta. The pulmonary trunk is anterior to the aortic root. In congenitally corrected transposition the ventricles and their respective atrioventricular (A-V) valves are inverted—that is, right to left interchange (Figure 19). Right atrial blood crosses an anatomic mitral valve and enters an anatomic left ventricle that communicates with a pulmonary trunk. Left atrial blood crosses an anatomic tricuspid valve and enters an anatomic right ventricle that connects with the aorta. Because of this arrangement, the left A-V valve is "tricuspid" and has a relatively

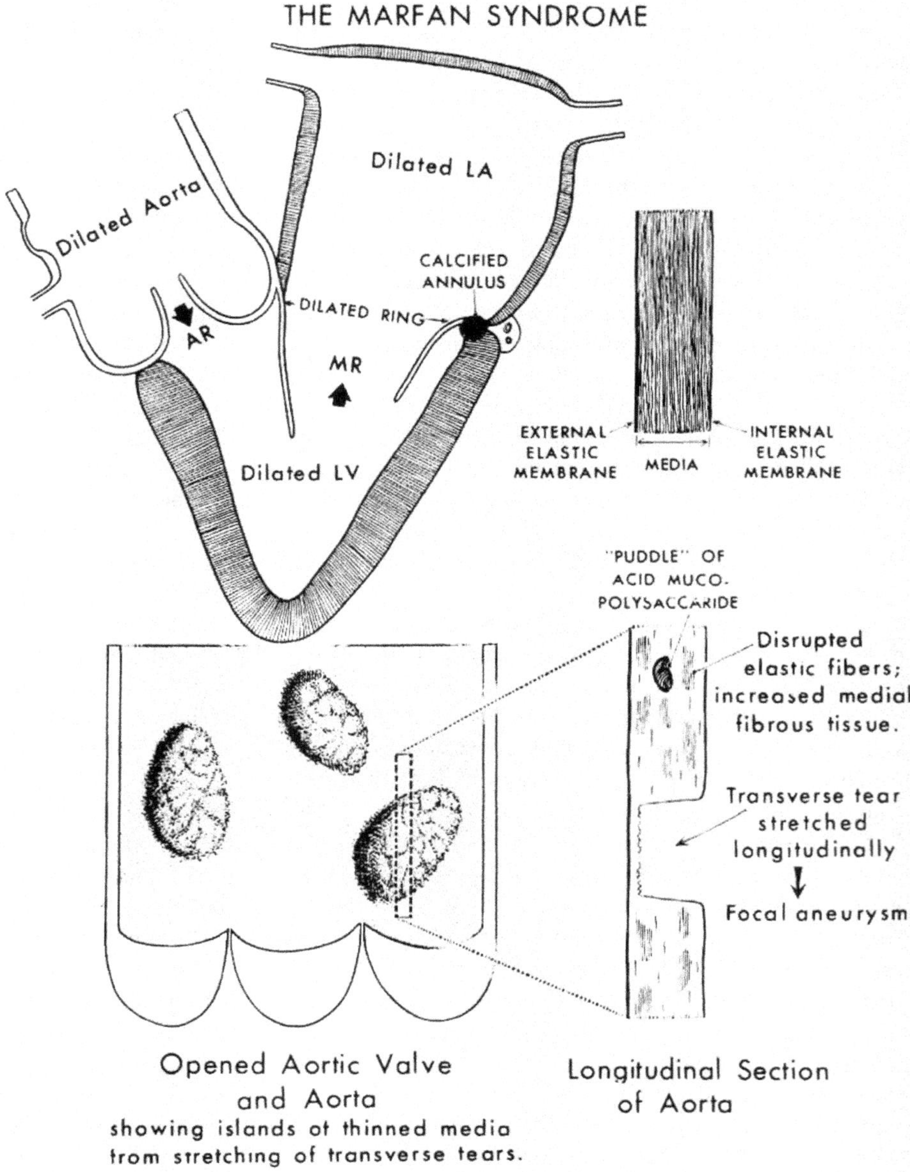

Figure 18. The various cardiovascular abnormalities in Marfan's syndrome. The aortic regurgitation (*AR*) appears to be related primarily to dilation of the aorta. The mitral regurgitation (*MR*) probably results from a combination of factors: dilation of the left ventricular cavity (*LV*) altering the papillary muscle-mitral leaflet angle; dilation of the mitral anulus; calcification of the mitral anulus; and elongation of the mitral leaflets and chordae, allowing prolapse of the leaflets into left atrium during ventricular systole. At top right is a longitudinal section of normal aorta. At bottom right is a longitudinal section in a patient with Marfan's syndrome. There is marked loss of elastic fibers, deposition of abnormal amounts of acid mucopolysaccharide material, and tears in the wall, which later expand to cause the islands of thinning noted in the view of the opened aortic valve and aorta.

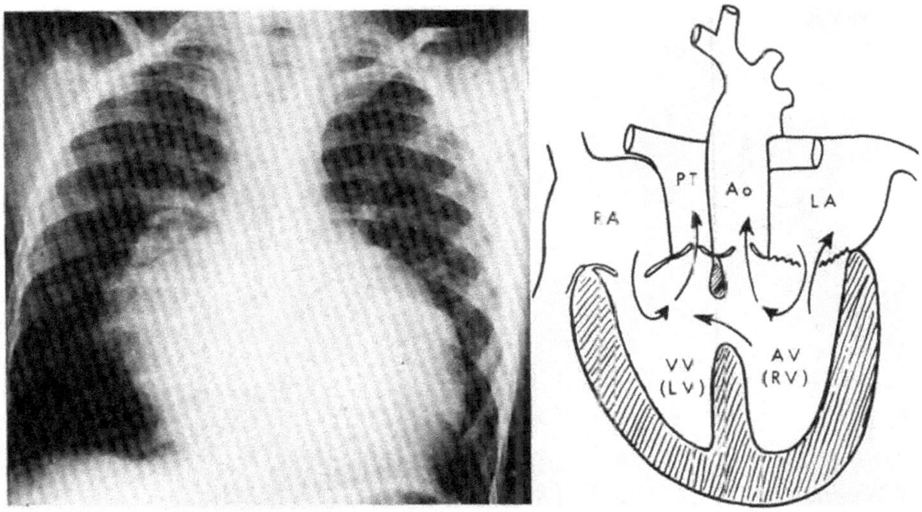

Figure 19 Left. X ray from a 2-year-old girl with congenitally corrected transposition and marked "mitral" regurgitation due to Ebstein's anomaly of the left atrioventricular valve, which was anatomically tricuspid. The vascular pedicle is narrow because the aorta courses vertically upward. A double density of left atrial enlargement is seen to the right of the vertebral column. **Right.** The aorta (*Ao*) and pulmonary trunk (*PT*) arise parallel to each other and do not cross as in the normal heart. Right atrial (*RA*) blood flows across a morphologic mitral valve into an anatomic left ventricle (*LV*) and into the pulmonary trunk. Left atrial (*LA*) blood flows across a morphologic tricuspid valve into an anatomic right ventricle (*RV*) and into the aorta. The left atrioventrioventricular valve may be incompetent (*reversed arrows*) because of an Ebstein-like deformity, and there is often a defect in the ventricular septum. VV = venous ventricle; AV = arterial ventricle. From Perloff (13); reproduced by permission of W. B. Saunders Co.

high frequency of an Ebstein-type anomaly—that is, leaflet tissue is tethered directly to ventricular endocardium below the anulus (56). Ebstein's anomaly of the tricuspid valve in its normal location causes right A-V valve incompetence; Ebstein's anomaly of a left-sided tricuspid valve (ventricular inversion) causes incompetence of the left A-V valve that may be mistaken for "mitral" regurgitation (57).

Dr. Roberts: Congenital mitral regurgitation is usually associated with other anomalies (58). "Isolated" congenital mitral regurgitation is usually accompanied by endocardial fibroelastosis of the left ventricle (Figure 20). However, it is sometimes difficult to determine what causes the mitral valve to be incompetent in this circumstance.

Neither is it always clear why the mitral valve is frequently incompetent in partial atrioventricular canal (endocardial cushion defect). As Dr. Perloff indicated, nearly all patients with partial A-V canal have a cleft, either partial or complete, in the anterior mitral leaflet. It would be easy to attribute the regurgitation to this cleft, but the regurgitation usually disappears after operative closure of the associated defect in the lowermost portion of the atrial septum (ostium primum defect), irrespective of whether the cleft in the anterior mitral leaflet is closed by suture (59). For the same reason, it is unlikely that the anomalous chordae tendineae that insert onto the crest of the ventricular septum play a significant role in the production of mitral regurgitation. It is well to think of a partial A-V canal as a syndrome consisting of five components: [1] defect in the lowermost portion of atrial septum; [2] cleft in the anterior mitral leaflet; [3] absence of tissue, either partial or complete, in the septal tricuspid valve leaflet; [4] anomalous chordae tendineae from the anterior mitral leaflet to the crest of ventricular septum; and [5] ventricular septal defect. The syndrome may include all five components or may have as few as two; most commonly, the first four components are present. A cleft in the anterior mitral leaflet may occur, however, in the absence of a defect in the lowermost portion of the atrial septum. These individuals usually present with evidence of isolated mitral regurgitation or with features of isolated ventricular septal defect. Occasionally, the ostium primum defect may be so small that the shunt through it is missed or is only trivial, and these patients also may present with essentially pure mitral regurgitation (60, 61) (Figure 21).

Corrected transposition is an entity that has produced much confusion. Corrected transposition and complete transposition are quite different; the only thing they have in common is the word "transposition." Complete transposition is essentially one defect: the great arteries are transposed, so that the aorta arises from the right ventricle and the pulmonary trunk from the left ventricle. In corrected transposition also the great arteries are transposed, but, in addition, the ventricles, atrioventricular valves, coronary arteries, and conduction system are inverted. Patients with complete transposition die because they have inadequate communications between the two circuits. Patients with corrected transposition theoretically should be able to live a full life-span, but usually this is not the case because associated defects—namely, ventricular septal defect or incompetency of the left-sided A-V valve, or both—cause the heart to function abnormally. Abnormalities of the left-sided A-V valve, a systemic valve but

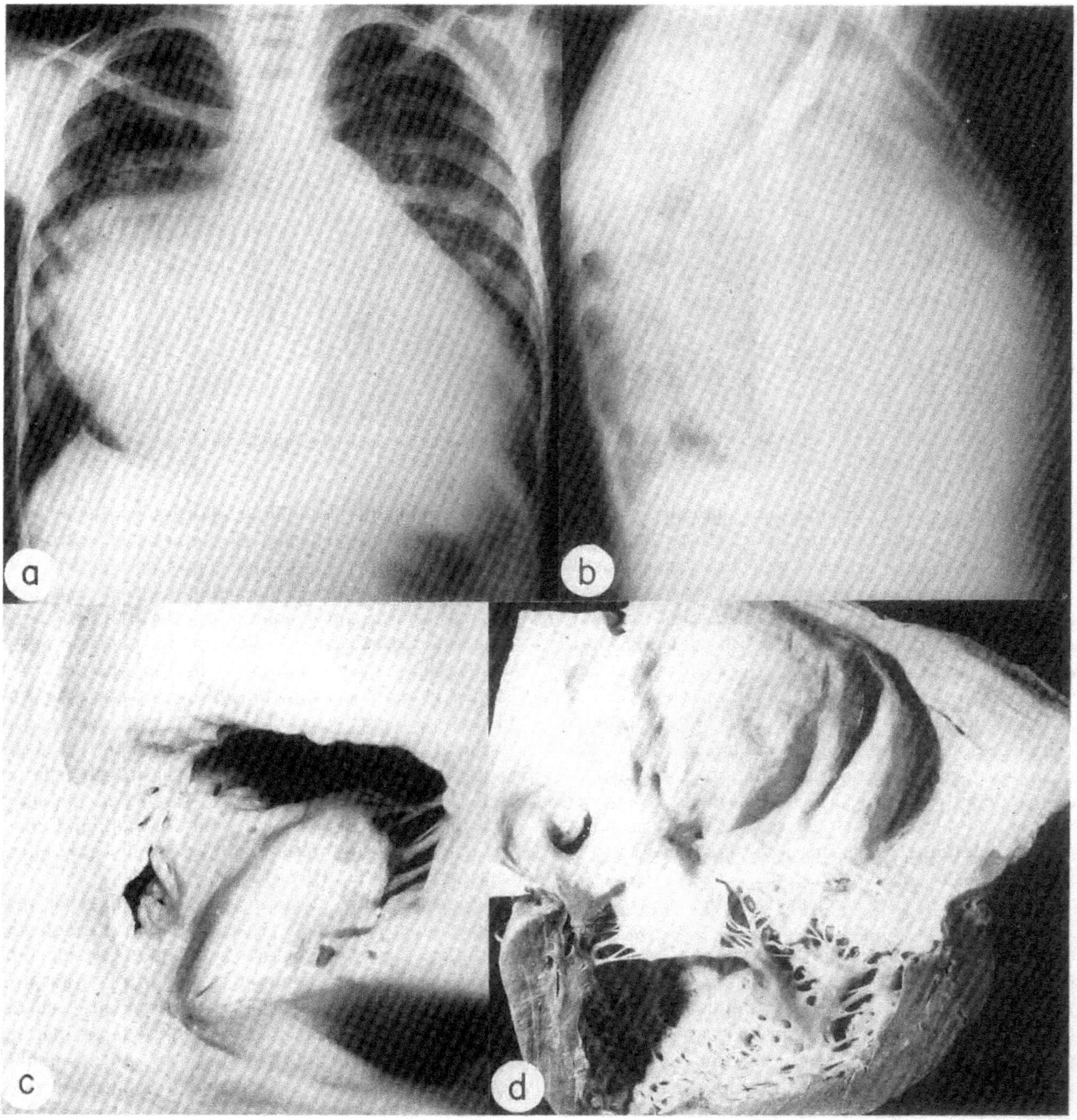

Figure 20. Congenital mitral regurgitation associated with diffuse fibroelastosis of the left ventricle in a 9-year-old boy. He was believed to be normal at birth. At age 3 years peripheral edema was noted, and examination showed generalized cardiomegaly and a grade 3/6 systolic murmur of mitral regurgitation. Electrocardiogram showed sinus rhythm and left ventricular hypertrophy. Catheterization at age 4 years showed the pulmonary arterial pressure to be 42/24 and pulmonary arterial wedge pressure mean to be 24 mm Hg. He had progressive congestive failure over the next 4 years. Examination 5 months before death showed severe cardiomegaly (*a* and *b*), atrial fibrillation, and a grade 5/6 systolic precordial murmur. On repeat catheterization the pressures (in mm Hg) were as follows: pulmonary artery, 66/36; right ventricle, 66/8; right atrium, mean 9; left atrium, mean 9; left atrium—mean, 21 and V wave, 32; left ventricle, 102/12; and brachial artery, 116/72. At operation (4 months before death) severe mitral regurgitation was found. Mitral valvuloplasty and anuloplasty was carried out. During his entire 4-month postoperative period he had evidence of progressive congestive cardiac failure. At necropsy the mitral valve orifice was severely incompetent, as viewed from the left atrium (*c*). Both left atrium and left ventricle were severely dilated, and the endocardium of both chambers (*d*) was diffusely thickened by fibroelastosis. The mitral anulus was also considerably dilated.

anatomically a tricuspid valve, are the commonest associated anomalies in corrected transposition (56). Of the anomalies the most frequent is the Ebstein-type malformation (Figure 22). These valves are intrinsically incompetent because the chordae are short and the leaflets are closely adherent to the ventricular endocardium.

A mitral valve may be abnormal anatomically and yet function entirely normally. A congenital malformation illustrating this point is the entity "double-orifice mitral valve" (62) (Figure 23), which looks like a double-barreled shotgun. Generally, both orifices are totally competent, and the patient should be asymptomatic.

PAPILLARY MUSCLE DYSFUNCTION

Dr. Perloff: Now to the muscular apparatus of the mitral valve, namely, the papillary muscles and left

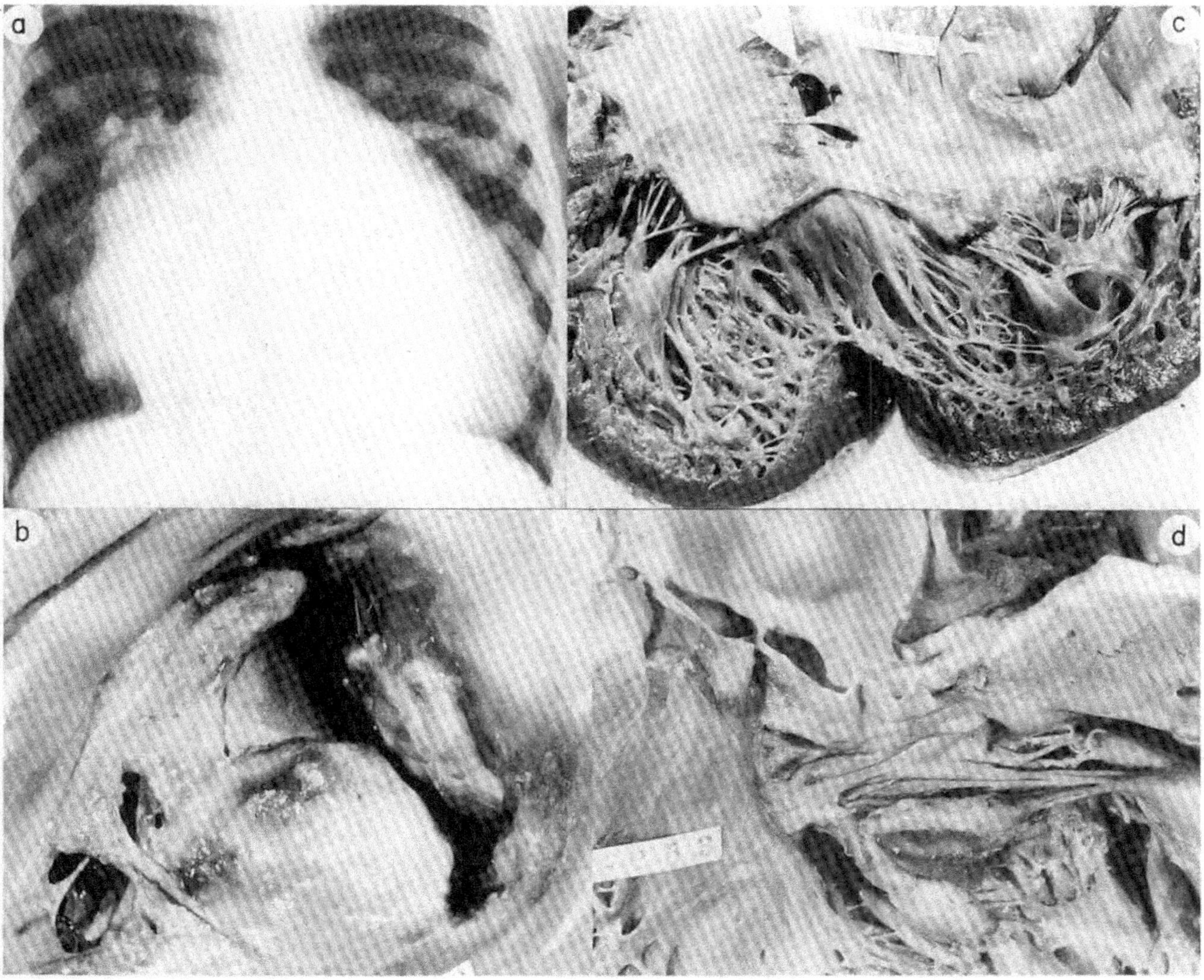

Figure 21. Congenital mitral regurgitation secondary to partial atrioventricular canal (endocardial cushion defect) in a 13-year-old boy. At age 6 years he was found to have a systolic precordial murmur and mitral regurgitation. He limited his activities because of fatigue but at age 11 years developed overt right- and left-sided congestive cardiac failure. At age 12 years atrial fibrillation appeared. On examination during his last month of life he was cachetic. A grade 3/6 pansystolic precordial murmur, loudest over the apex, and a grade 3/6 mid-diastolic rumble at the apex were audible. Electrocardiogram showed atrial fibrillation, left axis deviation, and left ventricular hypertrophy, and chest radiograph showed a large heart (*a*). At catheterization the pressures (in mm Hg) were as follows: right ventricle, 55/15; right atrium—mean, 13 and V wave, 17; and left atrium—mean, 15 and V wave, 27. Surprisingly, the catheter passed into the left atrium via an atrial septal defect. The calculated pulmonary to systemic flow ratio was 1.4/1.0. The child died 1 day after operative closure of a cleft in the anterior mitral leaflet and of a small, 1.0-cm defect in the lowermost portion of the atrial septum. At necropsy, a large cleft was found in the anterior mitral leaflet (*b* and *c*), and at the apex of the cleft there was a tiny atrial septal defect. **c.** The cleft and defect with the mitral valve, left atrium, and left ventricle opened. The left atrium is quite dilated. **d.** The opened aorta, aortic valve, and left ventricular outflow tracts, showing anomalous chordae tendineae extending from the apex of the anterior mitral leaflet to the crest of the ventricular septum. These anomalous chordae tendineae are universally found in partial atrioventricular canal and are responsible for the gooseneck deformity seen on the left ventricular angiography.

ventricular wall. First, there is papillary muscle dysfunction with loss in continuity, that is, rupture (63). The cause is almost always myocardial infarction. Rupture of chordae is unrelated to myocardial infarction. The clinical picture of ruptured papillary muscle is acute overwhelming mitral regurgitation (*see* above), although the consequences depend in part on just where in the papillary muscle structure the discontinuity occurs.

Dr. Roberts: Rupture of a portion of a papillary muscle is really an old entity, but it was not appreciated until less than 5 years ago (63). The original concept of papillary muscle rupture was rupture of its entire trunk, caused either by myocardial infarction from coronary narrowing or by trauma. Complete transsection of a left ventricular papillary muscle is incompatible with life because about 60 chordae tendineae are thus disrupted (2) (Figure

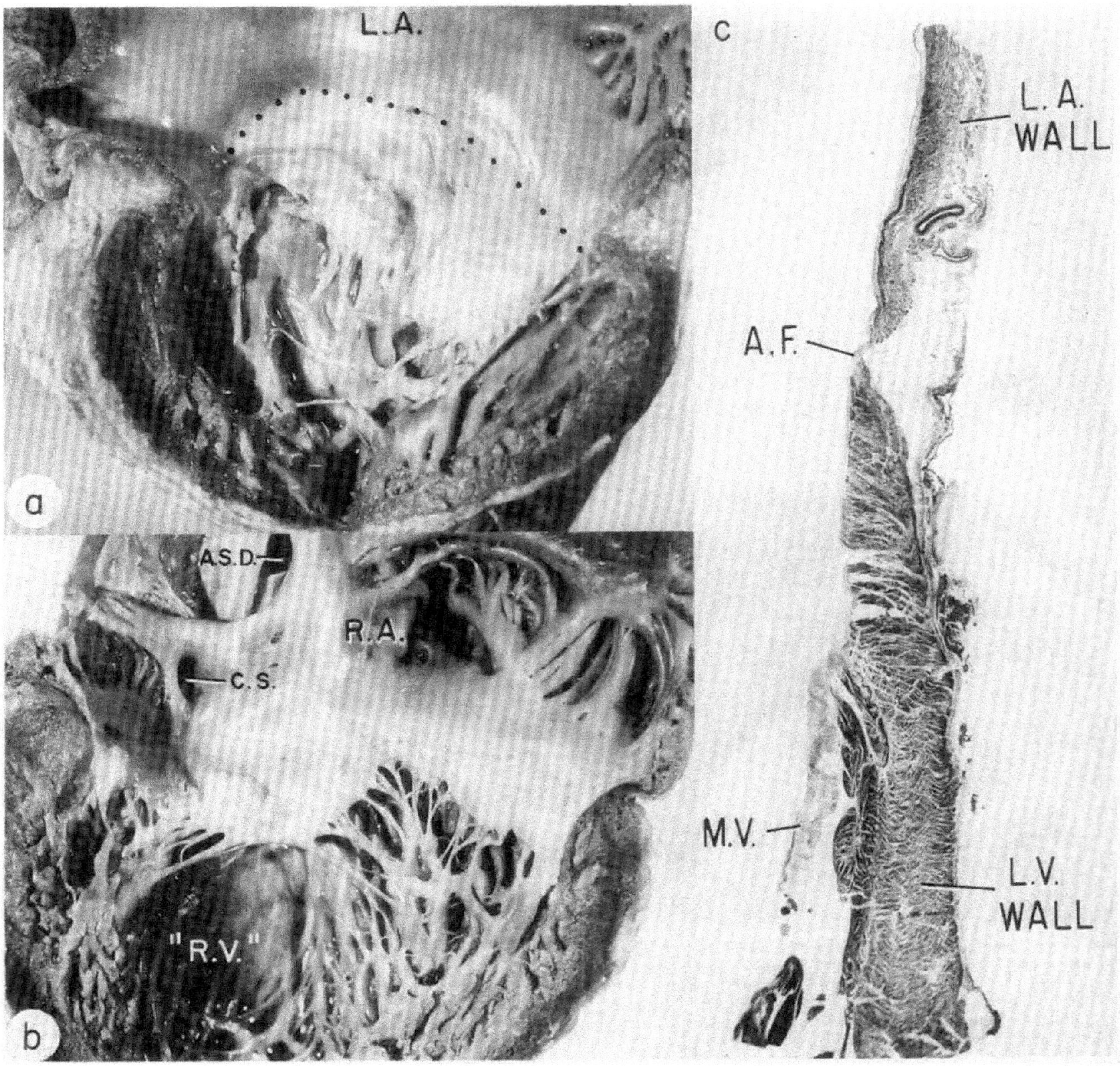

Figure 22. Congenital "mitral" regurgitation in corrected transposition of the great vessels with Ebstein-type malformation. **a.** The opened left atrium (*L.A.*), "tricuspid" valve—showing an Ebstein-type malformation—and left ventricle in a 38-year-old man who also had subvalvular pulmonic stenosis and a small atrial septal defect (*A.S.D.*). Ebstein's malformation is a downward displacement of the left-sided (anatomic tricuspid) valve. **c.** A longitudinal histologic section of the anulus fibrosis (*A.F.*), left ventricle (*L.V.*), and mitral valve (*M.V.*) (anatomically the tricuspid valve). The valve leaflet normally arises from the left ventricular wall below the anulus. The true anulus is shown by dots in *a.* **b.** The opened right atrium (*R.A.*), right-sided atrioventricular valve (anatomically the mitral valve), and the right-sided ventricle ("*R.V.*", anatomically a left ventricle). C.S. = ostium of the coronary sinus.

24*A*). More frequent is rupture of a portion of a papillary muscle (Figure 24*A*). In this situation the largest amount of regurgitation is probably caused by the rupture, but all these patients have severe necrosis of the remaining portion of the papillary muscle, and the latter probably contributes to the regurgitation (Figure 24*B*). When 1 head of a papillary muscle is ruptured, about 10 third-order chordae tendineae are disrupted (Figure 4).

Dr. Perloff: Rupture of a papillary muscle can be considered papillary muscle dysfunction with loss in continuity (44). Burch, DePasquale, and Phillips (64-66) popularized the idea that the papillary muscles may function abnormally without loss in continuity, and we now know that this is clinically the commoner form of papillary muscle dysfunction. Contraction of the papillary muscles initiates ventricular systole, pulling the two leaflets into apposition. As the left ventricle continues to contract, there must be synergistic contraction of the papillary muscles so that the mitral leaflets do not evert into the left atrium as the apex of the left ventricle approaches the anulus. If a papillary muscle cannot perform that function, the mitral leaflets evert, and regurgitation occurs.

I shall now comment briefly on certain current

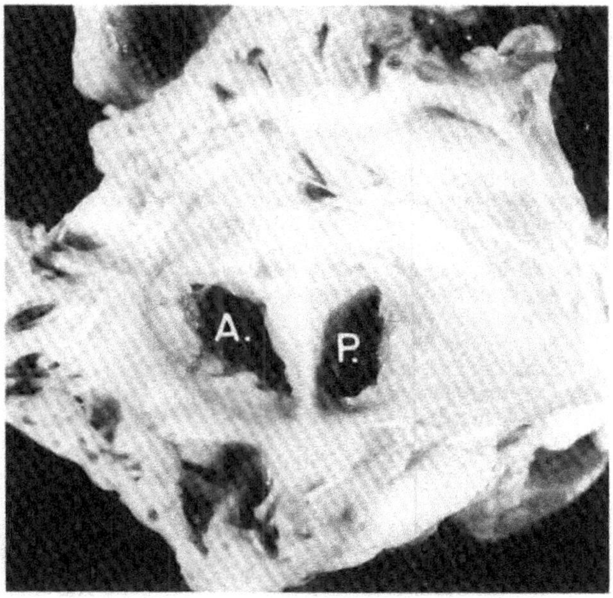

Figure 23. Congenital malformation of the mitral valve, namely, double orifice, causing no cardiac dysfunction. The two orifices, anterior (*A.*) and posterior (*P.*), have the appearance, from the left atrium, of a double-barrelled shotgun. This heart belonged to a cow killed for other reasons, but similar valves have been observed in humans.

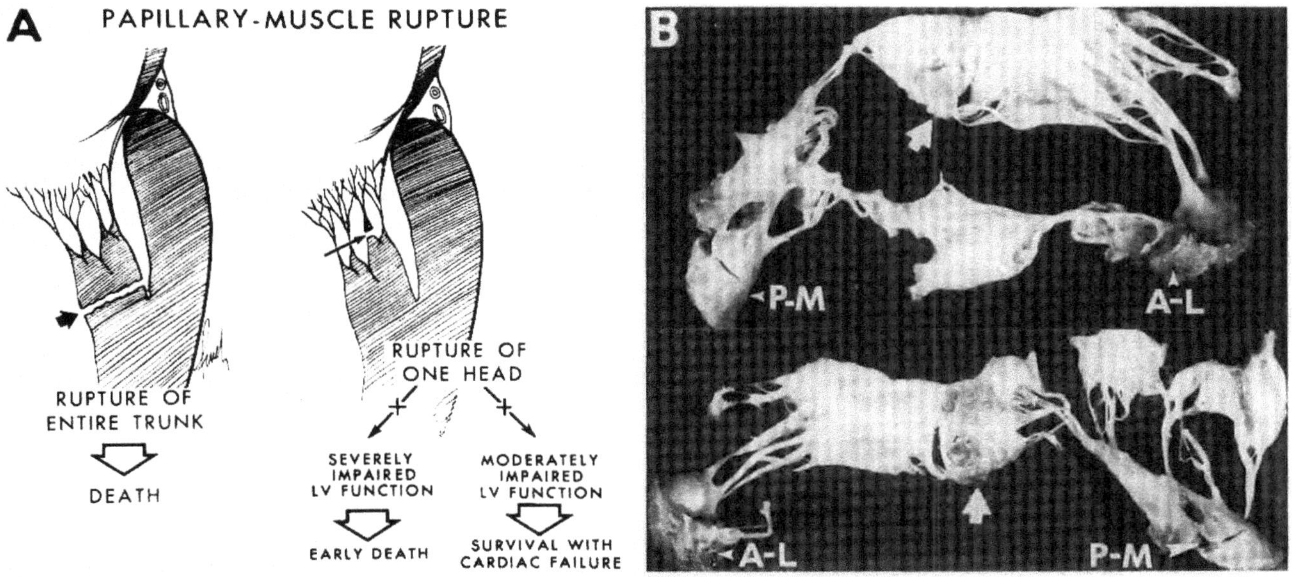

Figure 24A. Diagrammatic representation of the types, and possible consequences, of papillary muscle rupture during acute myocardial infarction. Rupture of the entire trunk (*left*) is probably incompatible with survival in any patient, since a major portion of the support to both valve leaflets is destroyed. With rupture of an apical head (*right*), survival would appear to depend on the extent to which the function of the left ventricle has been impaired by the infarct. With severely impaired ventricular function the additional burden of even modest mitral regurgitation may be intolerable, and death will ensue. If the left ventricle is less severely compromised, survival is possible for weeks or months, but congestive cardiac failure will almost invariably develop. **B.** Rupture of a portion of one papillary muscle during acute myocardial infarction in a 51-year-old man who underwent mitral valve replacement 3 months after the onset of the infarction. Preoperatively, the pulmonary arterial pressure was 60/28 mm Hg (mean, 40 mm Hg); pulmonary arterial wedge pressure —mean, 28 and V wave, 42 mm Hg; left ventricular pressure, 74/17 mm Hg; and cardiac index, 1.7 litres/min·m^2 body surface area. Shown is the excised (by Dr. Andrew G. Morrow) mitral valve. The leaflets are normal but the posteromedial (*P-M*) papillary muscle is necrotic and fibrotic, and a portion (*arrow*) of it is intwined in chordae tendineae at the margin of the anterior mitral leaflet. **Top.** Ventricular aspects of the leaflets. **Bottom.** Opened valve, showing the atrial aspects of the leaflets. A-L = anterolateral papillary muscle.

Table 3. Spectrum of Left Ventricular Papillary Muscle Disease

- Anatomically normal papillary muscles but papillary muscle dysfunction
  - Transient ischemia
  - Left ventricular dilation from any cause
    - Generalized
    - Localized
  - Necrosis or fibrosis in adjacent left ventricular free wall
    - With coronary arterial narrowing
    - Without coronary arterial narrowing
  - "Small" left ventricular cavity (hypertrophic cardiomyopathy)
- Necrosis or fibrosis of papillary muscle(s) without rupture
  - With coronary arterial narrowing
    - Acute myocardial infarction
    - Healed myocardial infarction
  - Without coronary arterial narrowing
    - Acute
      - Shock
      - Acute valvular regurgitation (infective endocarditis)
    - Chronic
      - Anemia
      - Left ventricular outflow obstruction
        - Valvular aortic stenosis
        - Discrete and diffuse subaortic stenosis
        - Supravalvular aortic stenosis
      - Systemic hypertension
      - Origin of left coronary artery or of both coronary arteries from pulmonary trunk
      - Primary endocardial fibroelastosis of left ventricle
      - Endomyocardial disease and eosinophilia
        - Löffler's fibroplastic parietal endocarditis
        - Endomyocardial fibrosis of Davies
      - Idiopathic cardiomegaly (primary or diffuse myocardial disease)
      - Focal myocardial disease
        - Idiopathic
        - "Neurogenic" heart disease
          - Progressive muscular dystrophy
          - Friedreich's ataxia
          - Myotonic muscular dystrophy
- Necrosis or fibrosis of papillary muscle(s) with rupture
  - Acute myocardial infarction from coronary heart disease
  - Trauma
  - Miscellaneous
- Infiltrative diseases of papillary muscles
  - Pyogenic abscess
  - Granulomas
    - Aschoff's bodies
    - Sarcoid
  - Amyloid
  - Neoplasm
  - Calcium
  - Iron
  - Other
- Congenital malformations of papillary muscle(s)
  - Single papillary muscle (parachute mitral valve syndrome)
  - Accessory papillary muscle
  - Abnormally large and malpositioned papillary muscles
  - Abnormally small and malpositioned papillary muscle
  - Insertion of papillary muscle directly into mitral leaflet
- Miscellaneous afflictions of papillary muscle(s)
  - Excision, partial or complete, during mitral valve replacement
    - Atrophy of nonexcised portion of papillary muscle after valve replacement
    - Left ventricular aneurysm at site of papillary muscle excision
  - Disuse atrophy after excision of mitral leaflets and chordae without excision of papillary muscle(s)

concepts of papillary muscle dysfunction without loss in continuity. In the early 1950s the murmur of mitral regurgitation was considered holosystolic. It is now well established that regurgitant flow across the mitral orifice can be accompanied not only by a holosystolic murmur but also by midsystolic, late systolic, or early systolic murmurs. I have already mentioned the click and the late systolic murmur. In papillary muscle dysfunction, lack of synergistic control of the chordae and leaflets may allow regurgitation early in systole, late in systole, throughout systole, or chiefly in midsystole. All variations occur, and all may be related to dysfunction of papillary muscle without loss in continuity (6, 64, 67).

An interesting variety of papillary muscle dysfunction gives rise to severe intermittent mitral regurgitation (68). It is well known that during angina, mild mitral regurgitation may transiently appear because of ischemic papillary muscle dysfunction without infarction. It has now been shown that transient severe regurgitation occasionally occurs during bouts of ischemic pain (68). Such an event can be looked on as the transient counterpart of acute severe persistent mitral regurgitation after chordal or papillary muscle rupture.

Ischemic papillary muscle dysfunction also occurs in congenital coronary arterial disease, namely, anomalous origin of the left coronary artery from the pulmonary trunk (69). In this disorder mitral regurgitation is common in patients surviving infancy.

Papillary muscle dysfunction without loss of continuity has, since first described by Burch, DePasquale, and Phillips (64), been related to the papillary muscle per se. More recent information indicates that the contiguous portion of left ventricular free wall—that is, the segment of left ventricle from which papillary muscle springs—is functionally a part of the papillary muscle (70-72). In experimentally induced infarction confined to a canine papillary muscle, the mitral valve is not necessarily rendered incompetent (70-72). However, if the base of the papillary muscle—the segment of left ventricle from which the papillary muscle springs—is infarcted, then the valve becomes incompetent (70-72).

Dr. Roberts: Necrosis or fibrosis of a papillary muscle without rupture is far commoner than rupture. Table 3 lists conditions frequently associated with papillary muscle dysfunction, particularly necrosis or fibrosis (2). Although coronary arterial luminal narrowing is the most frequent cause of papillary muscle necrosis or fibrosis, many other conditions may be accompanied by papillary muscle lesions. The papillary muscles are fibrotic or necrotic in so many conditions because they are the last structures in the heart to be perfused by arterial blood (73). Of the two left ventricular papillary muscles, the posteromedial one has the poorer blood supply, and, consequently, lesions are more frequent in it than in the anterolateral muscle. The posteromedial muscle receives its oxygen mainly from blood passing through the right coronary artery. The mouth of this artery may be more than 15 cm from the apex of the posteromedial muscle. To perfuse it, blood must pass through the entire thickness of left ventricular wall, turn uphill, and ascend a distance equivalent to two more full thicknesses of left ventricular wall. Thus, the apexes of the papillary muscles are the sites furthest from the coronary ostia, and they receive oxygen only after the other myocardium has had an opportunity to extract its oxygen needs. Although the entire surfaces of the papillary muscles are bathed by intracavitary ventricular blood, only a small amount of oxygen diffuses into these structures from the intracavitary blood (Figure 25).

The commonest cause of papillary muscle necrosis or fibrosis is narrowing of the coronary arterial lumen by atherosclerosis (Figure 26). The posteromedial papillary muscle is usually involved in acute posterior myocardial infarction. In anterior wall infarction, however, the anterolateral papillary muscle may be spared, presumably because its blood supply is better than that of the posteromedial muscle. Since infarction limited to the ventricular septum or to the lateral portion of the left ventricular free wall (that is, the portions of the left ventricular wall unassociated with papillary muscles) is rare, the papillary muscles are usually involved when myocardial infarction occurs. It is, therefore, surprising that papillary muscle dysfunction is not more frequent during or after acute myocardial infarction (74).

In patients with left ventricular outflow obstruction, lesions often occur in the papillary muscles. Valvular aortic stenosis, whether in infants or in adults, when superimposed on a congenitally malformed valve, either unicuspid or bicuspid, is nearly always associated with fibrosis and atrophy of at least the posteromedial papillary muscle (75-79) (Figure 27). Rheumatic valvular aortic stenosis combined with organic mitral stenosis or regurgitation, however, infrequently is associated with papillary muscle fibrosis or atrophy. Nearly all adult patients with discrete subaortic stenosis or hypertrophic cardiomyopathy with or without diffuse subaortic stenosis have small fibrous scars in both left ventricular papillary muscles, but atrophy of one or both muscles is uncommon (80).

Foci of necrosis are also common in patients with fatal severe valvular regurgitation of recent onset. Among 47 patients dying of active valvular infective endocarditis, 34 (72%) had necrotic lesions in one or both left ventricular papillary muscles, and none had significant narrowing of the extramural coronary arteries (41, 81). Most patients had pure aortic regurgitation, but some had pure mitral regurgitation secondary to the active infective endocarditis. Severely diminished cardiac output resulting in poor myocardial perfusion was believed to be the cause of the papillary muscle necrosis in these patients.

Small fibrous scars in the papillary muscles are common in patients with systemic hypertension, but atrophy of these muscles is infrequent in this condition, unless coronary heart disease also is present. In left ventricular hypertrophy of any cause, the hypertrophy of the papillary muscles should probably be proportional to that of the left ventricular free wall or ventricular septum. This proportional hypertrophy usually exists in patients with systemic hypertension but is infrequent in patients with left ventricular outflow obstruction.

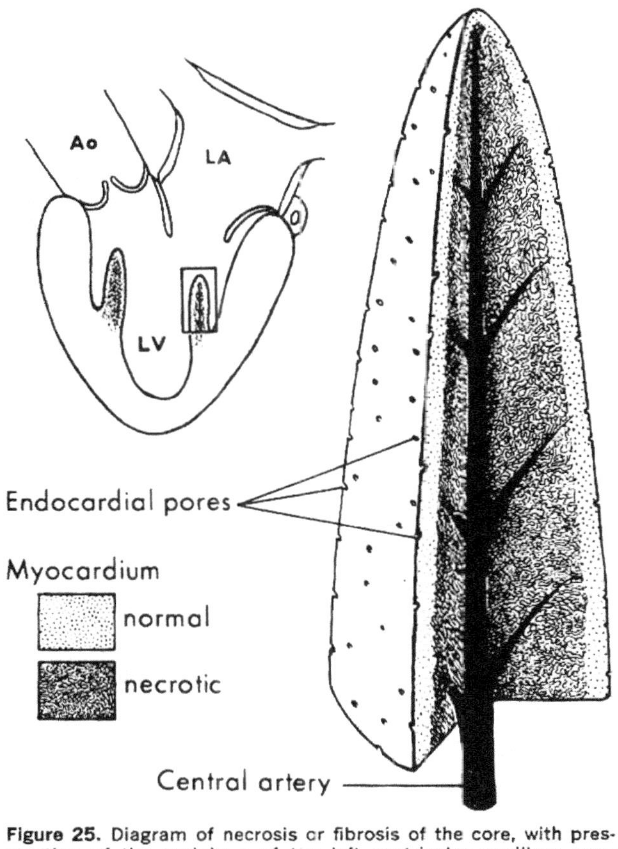

Figure 25. Diagram of necrosis or fibrosis of the core, with preservation of the periphery of the left ventricular papillary muscles. The exact mechanism whereby the periphery of these structures is preserved is uncertain, but it is presumed that blood from the left ventricular (LV) cavity diffuses, possibly via endocardial pores, into their outer portions. The central artery appears to supply only the inner portion of the papillary muscle with arterial blood. Ao = aorta; LA = left artery.

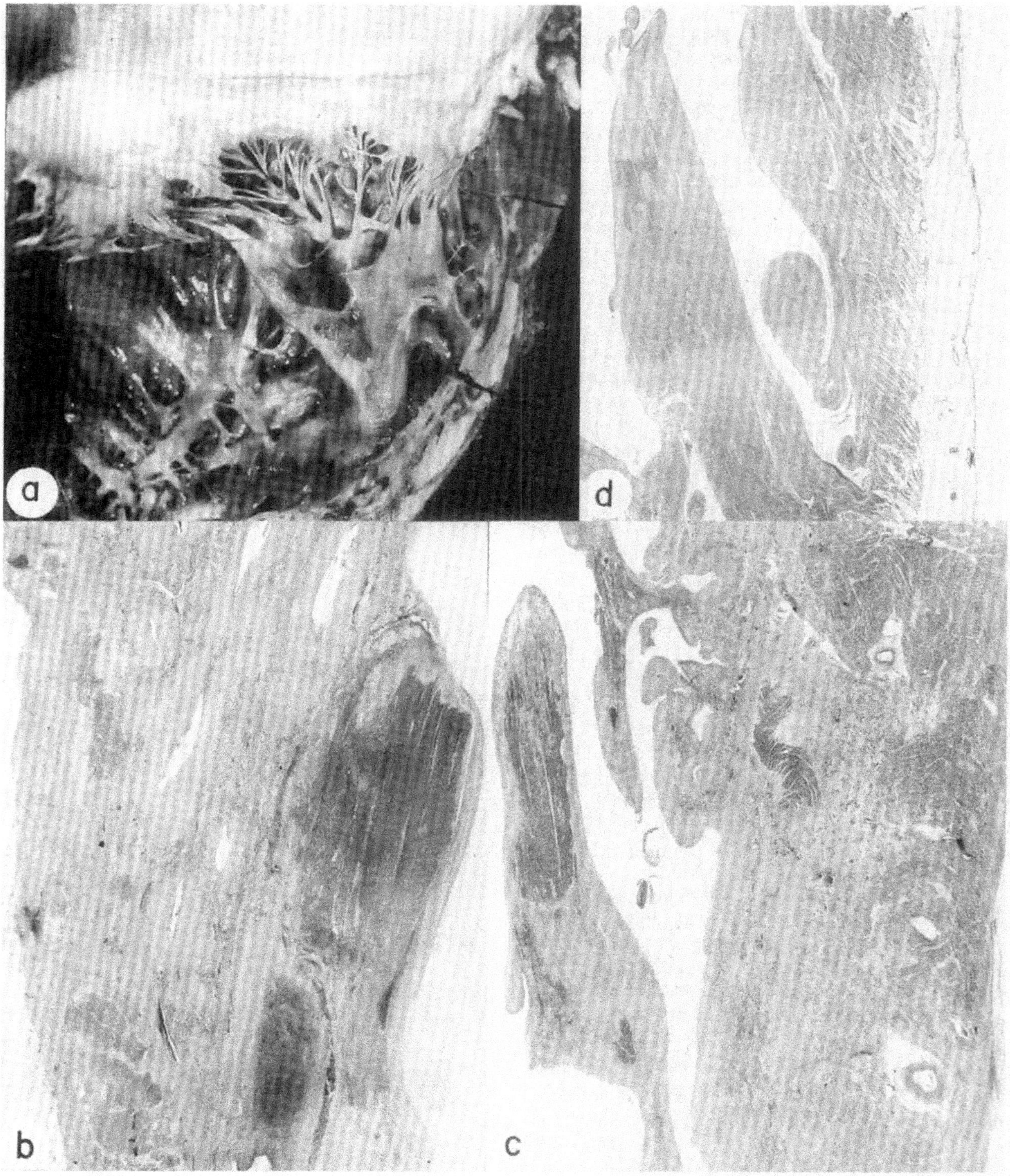

Figure 26. Papillary muscle necrosis without rupture during silent acute myocardial infarction in a 71-year-old man who developed congestive cardiac failure 2 months before death and a grade 4/6 systolic murmur of mitral regurgitation 2 weeks before death. Electrocardiograms did show an evolving acute myocardial infarction. **a.** Opened left ventricle, showing extensive necrosis of the posteromedial papillary muscle and of the left ventricular free wall beneath it. **b.** Histologic section, showing diffuse necrosis of the entire posteromedial papillary muscle and extensive fibrosis with patchy necrosis of the free wall beneath it. **c.** Anterolateral papillary muscle that is also necrotic and fibrotic. **d.** Anterior papillary muscle of right ventricle showing focal necrosis in its apical third. (Hematoxylin and eosin. Original magnification: **b** and **c**, × 6; **d**, × 3.)

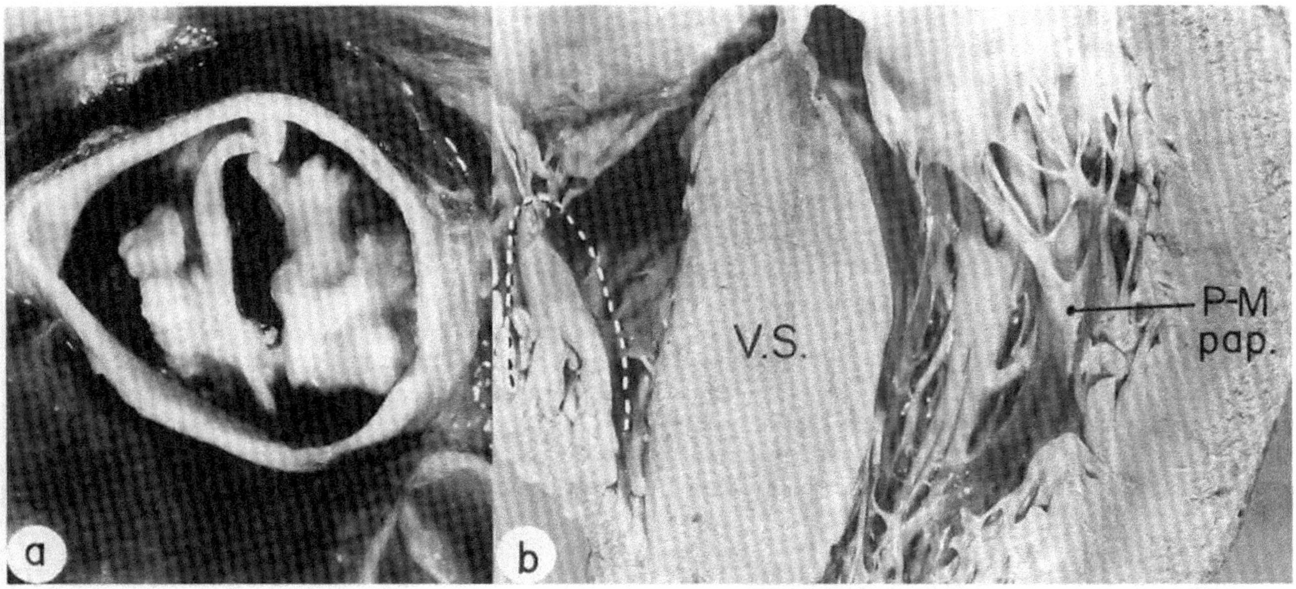

Figure 27. Papillary muscle fibrosis and atrophy associated with aortic stenosis involving a congenitally bicuspid aortic valve and unassociated with coronary arterial luminal narrowing. This 52-year-old woman had symptoms of cardiac dysfunction for 3 years and a precordial murmur typical of mitral regurgitation in addition to murmurs of aortic stenosis and regurgitation. The peak systolic gradient across the valve was 130 mm Hg. **a.** Stenotic aortic valve from above. **b.** Longitudinal section, showing portions of all four chambers. The posteromedial papillary muscle (*P-M pap.*) is severely atrophied (it hardly protrudes into the left ventricular cavity) and scarred. The apical portion of the anterior papillary muscle of the right ventricle is also scarred (*dots*). The reason for papillary muscle scarring and atrophy in patients with aortic stenosis superimposed on congenitally malformed valves is unknown. VS = ventricular septum.

Fibrosis with atrophy of the papillary muscles is to be expected in patients with primary endocardial fibroelastosis of the left ventricle (82). Histologically, the thickened endocardium in this condition is similar to the media of the aorta, being characterized by elastic fibrils running parallel to one another and to the surface. Primary left ventricular endocardial fibroelastosis may be an anatomic expression of chronically inadequate coronary arterial perfusion of the left ventricle; since the posteromedial papillary muscle is the least well perfused portion of the heart, this structure is affected the most. In the congenital anomaly, origin of the left (69) or both (83) coronary arteries from the pulmonary trunk, diffuse endocardial fibroelastosis of the left ventricle is nearly always an associated lesion. Fibrosis and atrophy of the left ventricular papillary muscles are to be expected in this anomaly, and these patients may present clinically with features of pure mitral regurgitation (84) (Figure 28).

Foci of fibrosis or necrosis in the left ventricular papillary muscles are infrequent in patients with the congestive or dilated type of cardiomyopathy (85) (Figure 29). Severe scarring of one papillary muscle and of the free wall beneath it was responsible for severe mitral regurgitation in a patient with primary myocardial disease studied by Marcus and coworkers (86). Generally, however, left ventricular cavity dilation alone is the cause of mitral regurgitation in these patients. Rarely, myocarditis may be localized to papillary muscle and adjacent left ventricular free wall (39). Patients with the neurogenic heart diseases (Friedreich's ataxia, progressive musculary dystrophy, and myotonic muscular dystrophy) (87) generally have scarred left ventricular papillary muscles, especially posteromedial ones. The African cardiomyopathy, endomyocardial fibrosis, may be associated with extensive scarring of the papillary muscles (2). In this condition the posteromedial muscle is usually covered by a thrombus or by dense fibrous tissue that may be organization of thrombus. Likewise, Löffler's fibroplastic parietal endocarditis (Figure 30), which may be one stage of endomyocardial fibrosis (88), is usually associated with extensive scarring of one or both papillary muscles (89).

The papillary muscles are subject to various infiltrative processes, just like any other portion of myocardium. Pyogenic abscesses, Aschoff bodies (Figure 31), granulomas (85), neoplasms, amyloid (90), and iron (91) have all been observed in these structures. Congestive heart failure from severe mitral regurgitation may be the initial symptom of sarcoidosis (2).

The most frequent congenital malformation of papillary muscles is the occurrence of only one such muscle in the left ventricle (22) (Figure 9). In this condition, described as the parachute mitral valve, all mitral chordae tendineae are attached to the one left ventricular papillary muscle. The resulting mitral valve is usually stenotic (22), but it may be purely incompetent (23), or it may function normally (23). The single papillary muscle is usually associated with other malformations, including a supramitral valve ring, diffuse subaortic stenosis, and coarctation of the aorta. Other malformations, including valvular aortic stenosis, ventricular septal defect, and valvular pulmonic stenosis may also occur.

There may be not only one too few papillary muscles but also one too many. An accessory papillary muscle is usually of no functional significance, but it has been seen in association with congenital mitral regurgitation (58). When two papillary muscles are present, one or both may still be congenitally malformed. Each of the papillary muscles may be abnormally large and malpositioned, so that the primary orifice of the valve is narrowed (24, 25). Both papillary muscles also may be poorly developed and small. This finding is particularly characteristic with origin of the left coronary artery from the pulmonary trunk. In the latter anomaly the papillary muscles also arise high on the left ventricular wall (24), in contrast to the normal heart, in which the papillary muscles arise at the junction of the middle and lower thirds of the left ventricle. Minor, functionally insignificant, abnormalities of the papillary muscles may occur. A not uncommon one consists of insertion of one papillary muscle directly into one or both mitral leaflets. In acquired rheumatic mitral stenosis,

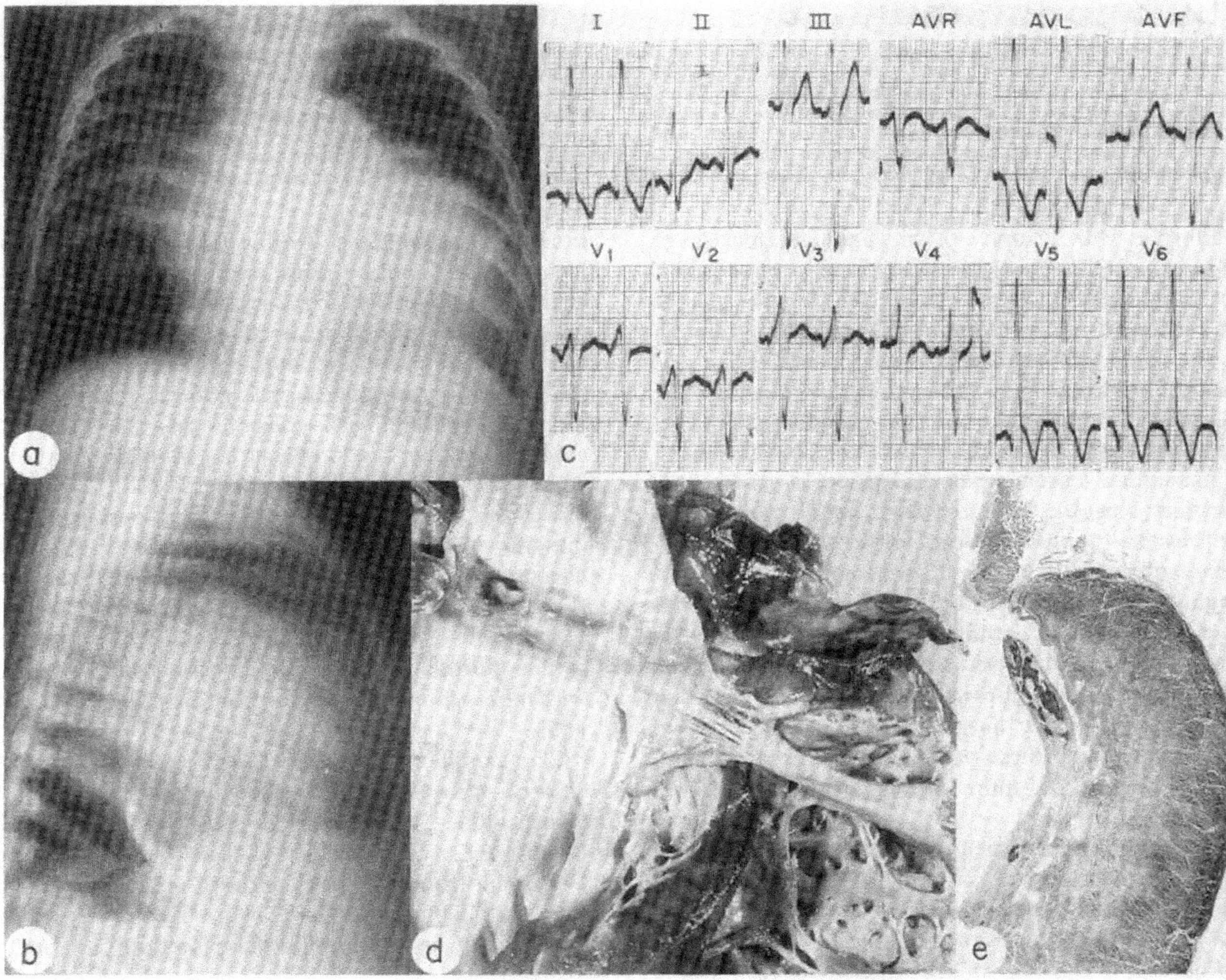

Figure 28. Severe fibrosis and calcification of the anterolateral left ventricular papillary muscle in a 9-month-old girl in whom the left coronary artery arose from the pulmonary trunk. She had had evidence of congestive cardiac failure since age 3 weeks. Examination at age 8 months showed a grade 3/6 systolic precordial murmur, consistent with mitral regurgitation. The heart was large (*a* and *b*), and an electrocardiogram (*c*) showed evidence of left ventricular hypertrophy and ischemia. She died during cardiac operation. At necropsy the left ventricle was considerably dilated, and its endocardium showed diffuse fibroelastosis (*d*). The anterolateral papillary muscle was severely thinned, scarred, and calcified (*e*). (Hematoxylin and eosin; original magnification, × 4.)

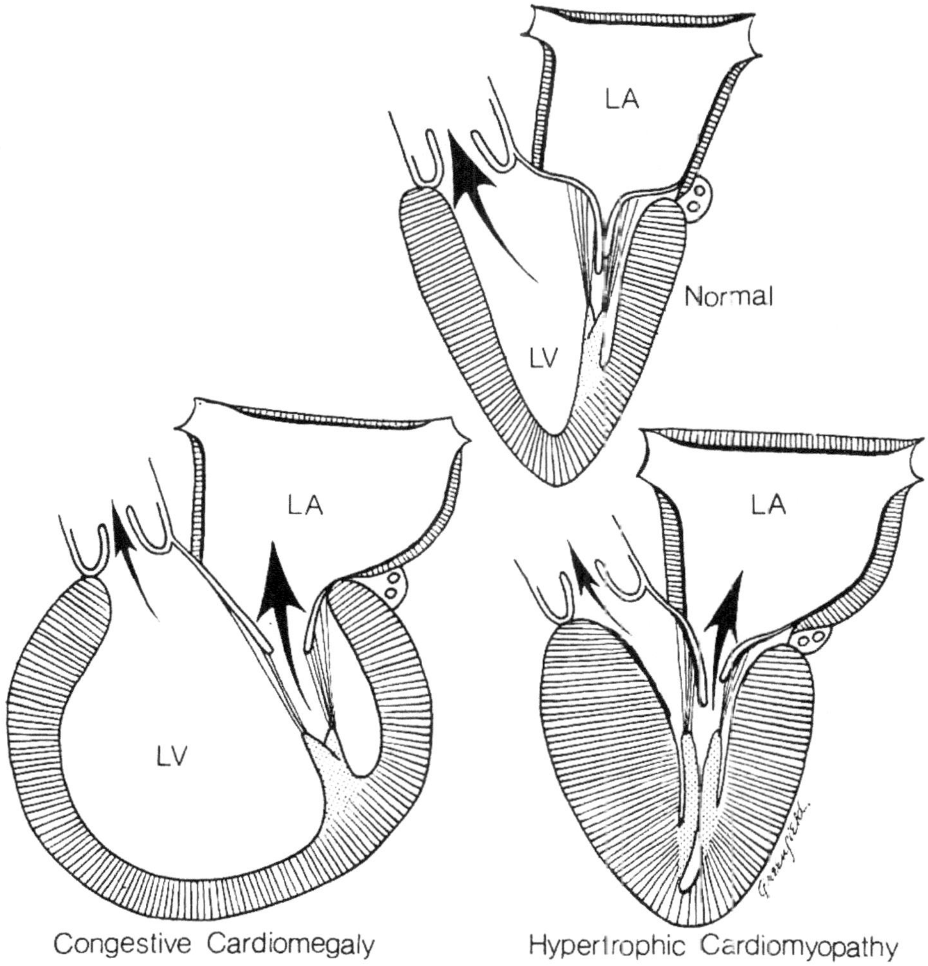

Figure 29. Diagram of how a dilated left ventricle (*LV*) (congestive cardiomyopathy) may lead to mitral regurgitation by pulling the papillary muscles laterally and caudally, and how a small left ventricular cavity, produced mainly by severe disproportional hypertrophy of the ventricular septum (hypertrophic [asymmetric] cardiomyopathy) may lead to mitral regurgitation by distorting or bending the papillary muscles and thus preventing their proper contraction during ventricular systole. The normal left ventricle is shown for comparison. Normally, the axes of the papillary muscles are more or less parallel to the major axes of the left ventricular walls. LA = left artery.

fusion and shortening of the chordae tendineae may be so extensive that both papillary muscles appear to insert directly into the mitral leaflets.

Both left ventricular papillary muscles are excised by most surgeons at the time of mitral valve replacement. The myocardium of the free wall at the sites of excision of these muscles is always infiltrated by inflammatory cells when this area is examined in the early postoperative period (19). With time these areas are covered by dense fibroelastic tissue simulating the composition of the media of the aorta (19). If the papillary muscles are not excised when the mitral leaflets and chordae tendineae are excised during mitral valve replacement, the papillary muscles atrophy and are focally replaced by fibrous tissue (92). When the papillary muscles are excised at operation, each is grasped by a clamp extending through the mitral orifice from the left atrium. If the papillary muscles are pulled too vigorously by the clamp when the muscle is excised, a portion of left ventricular papillary muscle also may be excised. This may result in perforation of the left ventricular wall or in severe thinning of the wall, with formation of a functioning or anatomic aneurysm, or both.

LEFT VENTRICULAR WALL AND MITRAL ANULUS

Dr. Perloff: I shall complete this discussion by commenting on the left ventricular wall and mitral anulus as important components of the mitral apparatus.

Regurgitation may have no other effect on a normal mitral apparatus except for changing the shape of the left ventricle. Such is the case in patients with ordinary heart failure, left ventricular dilation, and mitral regurgitation. It has often been assumed that under these circumstances the mitral anulus dilates, thus accounting for the incompetence. This explanation is an oversimplification (8). Left ventricular dilation—an undoubted cause of mitral regurgitation—may exert its effects independently of dilation of the mitral anulus. Nevertheless, the size of the anulus does play a role in preserving competence of the mitral orifice—albeit a role that relates less to dilation than to failure to decrease its circumference dur-

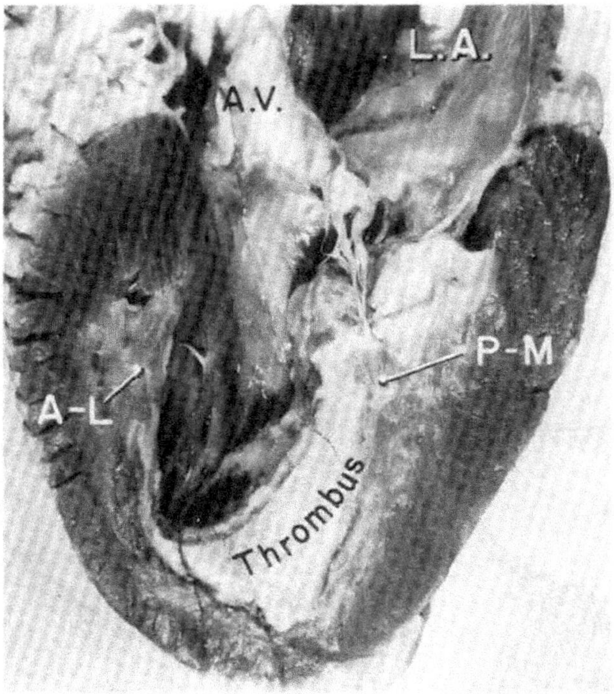

Figure 30. Opened left ventricle, aortic valve (*A.V.*) and left atrium (*L.A.*) in a 47-year-old man with Löffler's fibroplastic parietal endocarditis. This patient had been well until 13 months before death, when congestive cardiac failure associated with leukocytosis (62 000 leukocytes/mm^3) and eosinophilia (33%) appeared. He died of heart failure. At necropsy a large thrombus filled the inflow portion of the left ventricle, completely encasing the posteromedial (*P-M*) papillary muscle. In addition, both papillary muscles and portions of the left ventricular free wall subendocardium were fibrotic. No precordial murmur had been present during life. A-L = anterolateral papillary muscle.

ing systole. In the presence of ventricular dilation there are many stresses on the mitral apparatus that precede dilation of the anulus. Normally, the contracting papillary muscles exert vertical tension on the mitral leaflets, pulling them into apposition. As the left ventricle becomes globular, there is lateral migration of the papillary muscles, so that the normal vertical axis of tension is replaced by lateral tension, which tends to keep the leaflets apart (58). Accordingly, the average person with heart failure and a dilated globular left ventricle has lateral migration of the papillary muscles, lateral pull of these muscles on the chordae tendineae and leaflets, and mitral regurgitation because of that mechanism. In other patients, for example those with aortic regurgitation, the left ventricle becomes principally elongated rather than globular. Under these circumstances the papillary muscles elongate with the ventricle, and the interval between apex and anulus is too long for closure of the leaflets. The anulus still may not dilate significantly.

One final comment on the shape of the left ventricle as a cause of mitral regurgitation in idiopathic hypertrophic subaortic stenosis. In this disorder the following mechanism has been proposed for mitral regurgitation, based on a change in the shape of the left ventricle at the site of attachment of the anterolateral papillary muscle (93, 94). Early in systole there is rapid ejection. Then, as obstruction to outflow develops, the anterior mitral leaflet is pulled away from its closed position as the septum angulates at the site of origin of the anterolateral papillary muscle. The anterior mitral leaflet is pulled across the left ventricular outflow tract as late systolic mitral regurgitation develops.

Dr. Roberts: Although it may accompany left ventricular dilation, mitral anular dilation is probably a rare cause of mitral regurgitation, and in the past most patients with mitral regurgitation that was believed to be the result of mitral anular dilation probably had papillary muscle dysfunction. Mitral anular dilation to a degree capable of causing mitral regurgitation probably does not occur, because the surface area of the mitral leaflets is more than twice the area of the mitral orifice (1), and the anulus contracts during ventricular systole (9, 10). Indeed, as Dr. Perloff has pointed out, the mitral ring has a sphincter-like action, since the mitral orifice is smaller during systole than during diastole. In patients with dilated left ventricles the widest diameter does not occur at the left ventricular base, the area that includes the mitral anulus, but in the midportion of the chamber between apex and base. In fact, the base of the left ventricle is prevented from dilating freely because the "fibrous skeleton" is attached to it, whereas the midportion of the left ventricle is not so restricted. Severe left ventricular dilation may occur without any dilation of the mitral anulus.

Although it is now well known that mitral regurgitation may occur in patients with dilated left ventricles from any cause without associated left ventricular necrosis or fibrosis, it is less well recognized that necrosis or fibrosis of the left ventricular free wall, unassociated with left ventricular dilation or papillary muscle or mitral tissue lesions, also may be associated with mitral regurgitation (2). Generally, the scarring or necrosis of the myocardium adjacent to the papillary muscles fails to move or moves paradoxically during ventricular systole, and the abnormal ventricular contraction may lead to abnormal papillary muscle anchoring, resulting in mitral regurgitation. Anatomic left ventricular aneurysms unassociated with papillary muscle necrosis or fibrosis may cause mitral regurgitation by the same mechanism.

Abnormal pulling on the papillary muscles unassociated with left ventricular necrosis or fibrosis or

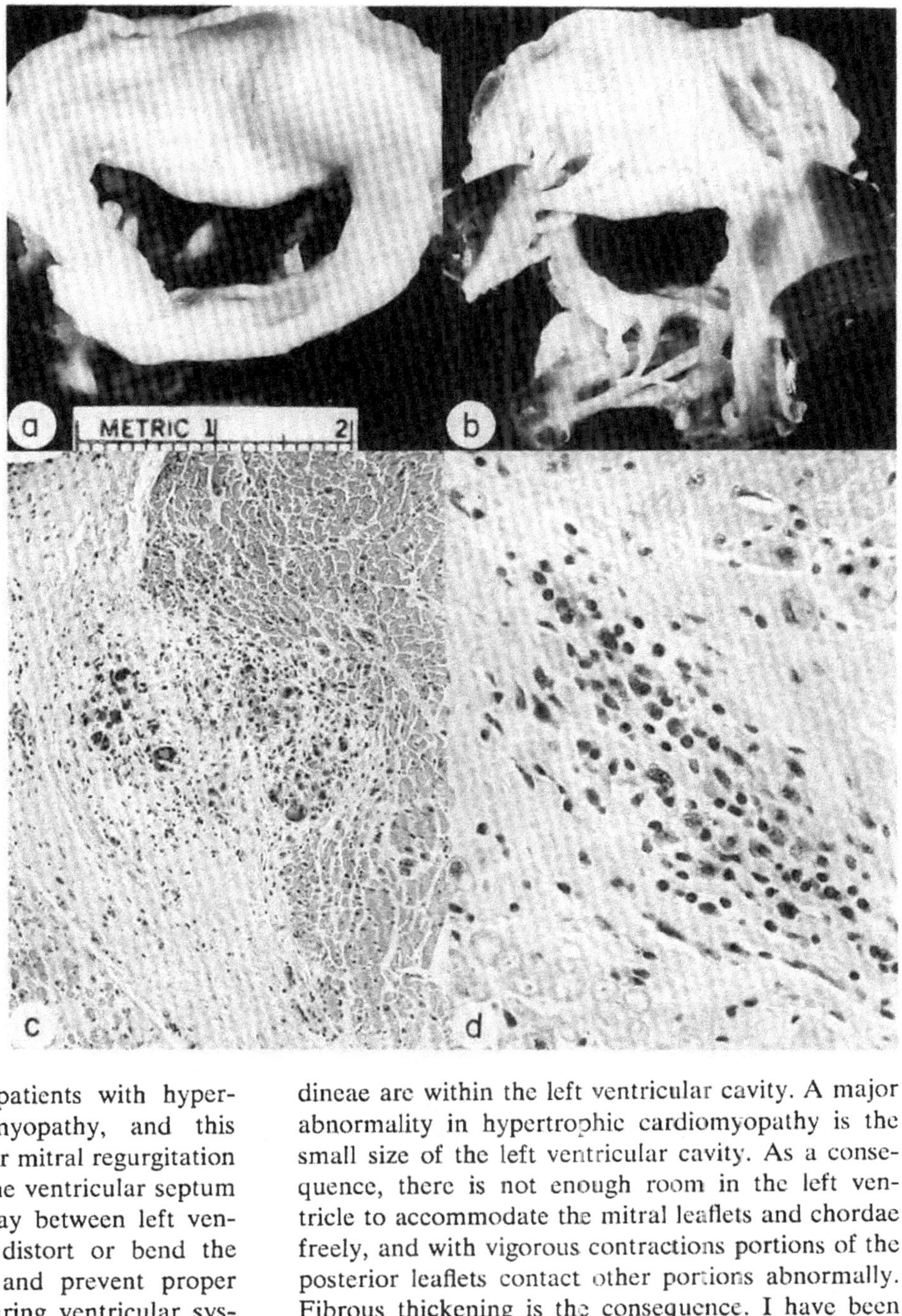

Figure 31. Excised mitral valve in a 23-year-old Indian woman with mitral stenosis (13 mm Hg mean diastolic pressure gradient between pulmonary artery wedge and left ventricle) and regurgitation. This patient had had acute rheumatic fever initially at age 7 and recurrence of migratory polyarthritis at age 22 years (14 months before operation). During the early postoperative period after mitral replacement she had swelling and pain in one knee and one ankle and erythema about two joints. When heard from 9 months postoperatively, she was much improved, although a murmur of tricuspid regurgitation was heard, and the liver pulsated. At operation earlier, mild (1+/4+) tricuspid regurgitation had been palpated, but the tricuspid leaflets and chordae were normal by palpation. Shown are the excised valve viewed from the left atrium (a) and from left ventricle (*b*) and Aschoff bodies (c and *d*), which were numerous in both excised left ventricular papillary muscles. (Hematoxylin and eosin. Original magnification: **c**, × 110; **d**, × 400.)

cavity dilation may occur in patients with hypertrophic (asymmetric) cardiomyopathy, and this mechanism may account for their mitral regurgitation (80). The huge thickening of the ventricular septum —the thickest portion is midway between left ventricular base and apex—may distort or bend the anterolateral papillary muscle and prevent proper contraction of this structure during ventricular systole. In addition to actual bending of the anterolateral left ventricular papillary muscle, however, the mitral leaflets in adults with hypertrophic cardiomyopathy are always thickened (80). It is easy to explain the thickening of the anterior mitral leaflet as being caused by its contraction of the mural endocardium in the left ventricular outflow tract during ventricular systole. But the posterior mitral leaflet also is thickened, probably as a result of its contacting itself abnormally during ventricular systole. It must be remembered that the mitral leaflets and chordae tendineae are within the left ventricular cavity. A major abnormality in hypertrophic cardiomyopathy is the small size of the left ventricular cavity. As a consequence, there is not enough room in the left ventricle to accommodate the mitral leaflets and chordae freely, and with vigorous contractions portions of the posterior leaflets contact other portions abnormally. Fibrous thickening is the consequence. I have been shown a mitral valve, excised because of incompetence, with the question, "Is the thickening rheumatic in origin?" The leaflets and chordae were focally thickened, and other features in retrospect clearly showed that the patient had had hypertrophic (asymmetric) cardiomyopathy presenting as mitral regurgitation. Of the 32 patients with hypertrophic cardiomyopathy studied by me at necropsy, 1 presented initially with pure mitral regurgitation associated with aneurysmal dilation of the pulmonary trunk (Figure 32). The mitral regurgitation in hypertrophic cardiomyopathy usually disappears after operative excision or incision of myocardium in the left ventricular outflow tract (95).

Calcification of the Mitral Anulus

Dr. Perloff: Now to the sixth element in the mitral apparatus, the anulus. As indicated, the anulus provides systolic sphincteric action, decreasing the area that the leaflets must seal. We have all seen calcified mitral anuli on roentgenograms. The J- or U-shaped appearance of a calcified anulus in an elderly person is typical. The calcific deposits assume J or U shapes because they are located nearly always only behind the posterior leaflet; they are rarely circumferential because the anulus is not circumferential. The anterior leaflet has no anulus because it is continuous with the aorta. A thick calcified anulus cannot act as a sphincter, cannot decrease the size of the mitral orifice during systole, and, accordingly, may be responsible for mitral regurgitation, generally only mild to moderate. Mitral anular calcification may occur in Marfan's syndrome and is an additional cause of mitral regurgitation in that disorder (96).

Dr. Roberts: Calcification of the mitral anulus is one of the more frequent abnormalities of the heart. Mitral anular calcification is generally considered to be a disease of elderly women. Indeed, of 14 patients with "massive" mitral anular calcification reported by Korn, DeSanctis, and Sell (97) in 1962, all were women and all were over 65 years of age. It is incorrect, however, to believe that this entity is reserved for a particular sex at a particular time in life. During

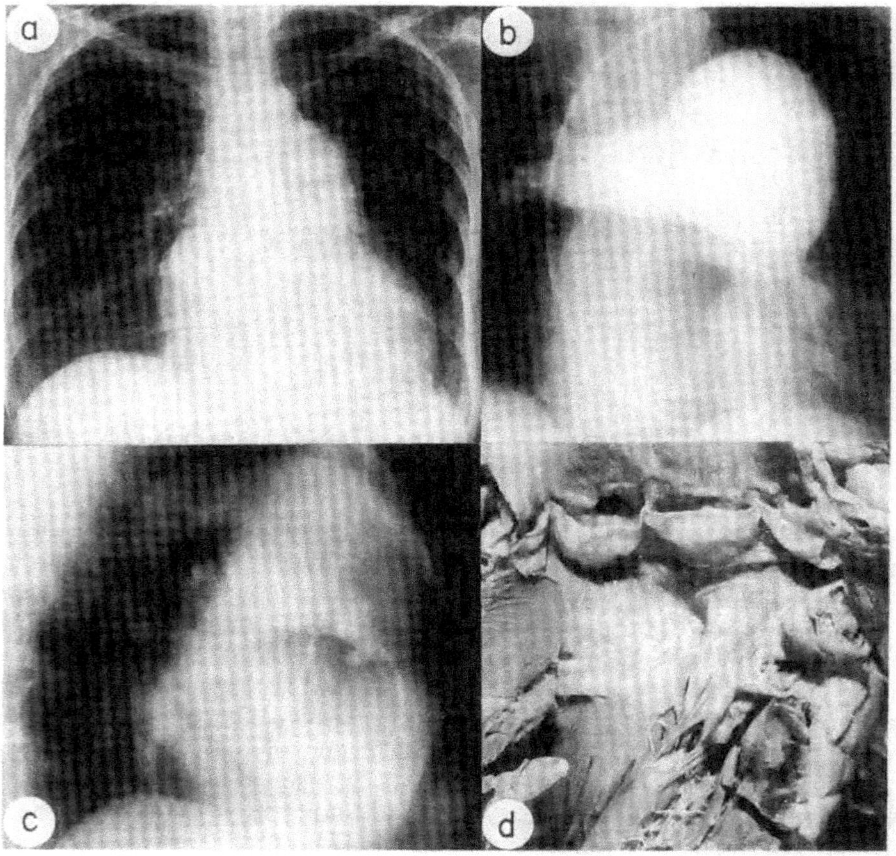

Figure 32. Hypertrophic (asymmetric) cardiomyopathy (idiopathic hypertrophic subaortic stenosis) presenting as pure mitral regurgitation. This 41-year-old woman had a precordial murmur and cardiomegaly on insurance examination at age 33 years, and overt right- and left-sided congestive cardiac failure, which progressed, appeared at age 38 years. When examined a month before death, she was severely ill, functionally class IV. A grade 4/6 blowing pansystolic precordial murmur, loudest along the lower left sternal border, was audible. Electrocardiogram showed atrial fibrillation and a marked clockwise rotation. By X ray (*a, b, c*) the heart was enlarged, and the pulmonary trunk was aneurysmally dilated. The total serum protein level was 5.3 g/100 ml, with an albumin level of 1.9 g/100 ml, and 2.2 g of protein were measured in the urine in a 24-hour period. The total serum cholesterol was 318 mg/100 ml. At catheterization the pressures (in mm Hg) were as follows: pulmonary artery, 34/7; right ventricle, 34/5; right atrial mean, 4; pulmonary arterial wedge—mean, 11 and V wave, 14; left ventricle, 112/11; and femoral artery, 122/65. The cardiac output (Fick method) was 1.6 litre/min·m^2 body surface area. Left ventricular cineangiogram showed 4+/4+ mitral regurgitation. (Retrospective examination showed this angiogram to be strongly suggestive of hypertrophic cardiomyopathy.) Aortic root injection of contrast material showed no aortic regurgitation. A day before death cardiotomy was performed, to replace the severely incompetent mitral valve. At operation, however, no systolic thrill was palpable over the left atrium, which expanded hardly at all during ventricular systole. Examination of the mitral valve after cardiopulmonary bypass had been instituted showed that the mitral leaflets and chordae were "normal" and that the left ventricular cavity was not dilated. Therefore, valve replacement was not carried out. The patient died the next day because of inadequate cardiac output. Necropsy showed a large transmural acute myocardial infarct involving the posterior left ventricular free wall. Histologic study indicated that the infarct was about 14 days old. The mitral leaflets and chordae were focally thickened, but the anulus was not dilated, and the left ventricular cavity was of normal size. In the outflow tract of the left ventricle a mural endocardial plaque was in direct apposition to the anterior mitral leaflet (*d*). Since the aortic valve cusps were normal, it was clear that this endocardial plaque indicated that hypertrophic cardiomyopathy was the proper diagnosis. The ventricular septum was nearly twice as thick as was the left ventricular free wall. Thus, this patient shows how idiopathic hypertrophic subaortic stenosis may present as pure mitral regurgitation. The cause of the aneurysmal dilation of the pulmonary trunk is uncertain. (At operation, a diastolic thrill had been palpated over this artery, indicating the presence of pulmonic regurgitation.)

the past 4 years I have examined at necropsy the hearts of 87 patients in whom various amounts of calcium involved the mitral anulus. Of the 87 patients, 44 were male and 43 were female. Sixty-one patients (26 male, 35 female) were age 65 years or greater, and 26 patients (18 male, 8 female) were less than 65 years of age. Of the latter 26 patients, 8 were less than 40 years of age: 3 of them had Marfan's syndrome, 2 had Hurler's syndrome, and 3 had metabolic disturbances with hypercalcemia.

The extent of mitral anular calcification was graded 1+ to 4+ (Figure 33); 45 patients (28 male, 17 female) had 1+ or 2+ deposits, and 42 (16 male, 26 female) had 3+ or 4+ deposits. Thus, this condition is slightly more frequent in the male, but the larger deposits (those likely to be seen on chest roentgenogram) are more frequent in the female. The smaller deposits (grades 1+ and 2+) almost surely have no functional importance. The larger deposits (grades 3+ and 4+), in contrast, may produce mitral regurgitation by the mechanism discussed by Dr. Perloff. Although stenosis has been mentioned as a possible complication of "massive" mitral anular calcification, obstruction has never been shown either anatomically or functionally to be caused by this mechanism. Wide-open severe mitral regurgitation, likewise, is probably never caused by mitral anular calcification.

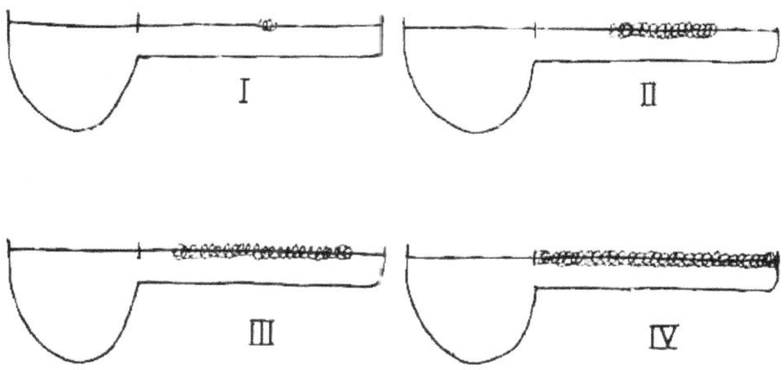

Figure 33. Method of grading mitral anular calcification. Grade I indicates only a single small deposit; grade II, a large single, or more than one small, deposit. Grade III and IV represent extensive deposits. The entire anulus behind the posterior leaflet is involved in grade IV, and, on rare occasion, calcific deposits also may extend across the anterior leaflet.

In patients with calcific deposits in the mitral

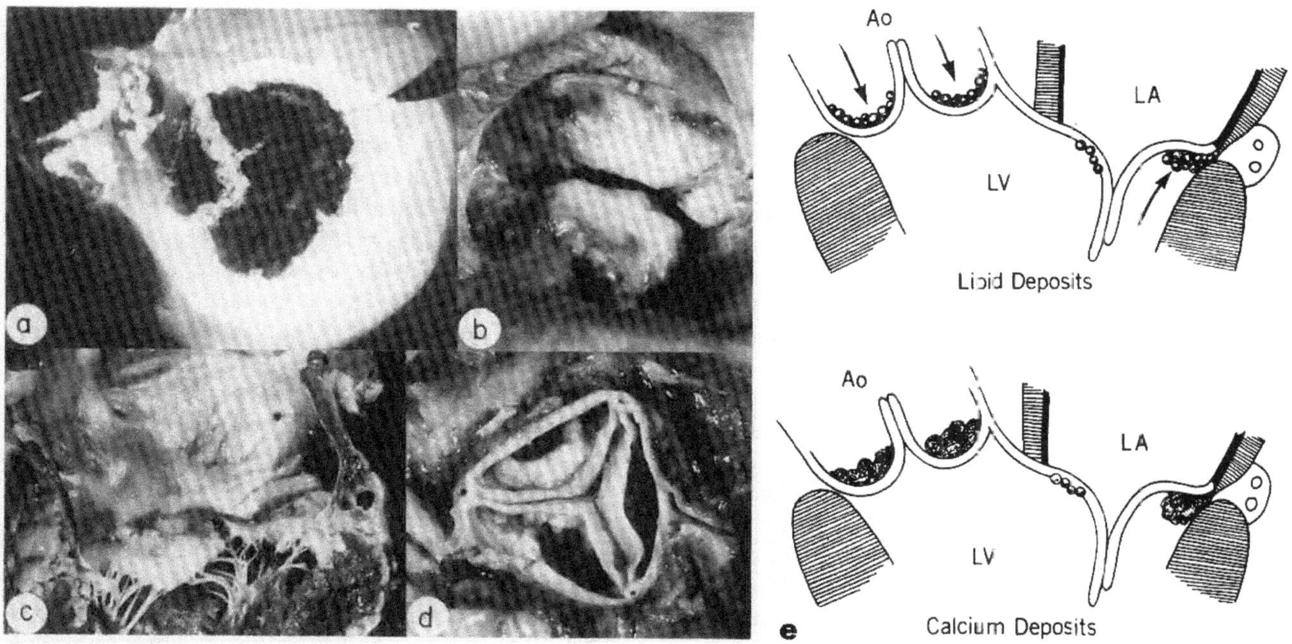

Figure 34 A-D. Massive mitral anular calcification associated with aortic valvular and coronary arterial calcification in an 82-year-old woman who died of volvulus of the caecum. She never had symptoms of cardiac dysfunction. **a.** Radiograph of heart at necropsy, showing circumferential mitral anular calcification. Most of the calcium is located behind the posterior mitral leaflet. Calcific deposits are also present in the aortic valve, root of aorta, and coronary arteries. **b.** Mitral valve as viewed from left atrium. The valve orifice appears to be only slightly incompetent. **c.** Opened dilated left atrium, mitral valve, and left ventricle. Calcium is apparent beneath the posterior leaflet. **d.** Aortic valve from above. Calcific deposits are present on the aortic aspects of each cusp, and none of the three commissures are fused. This valve is stenotic, as evidenced by left ventricular hypertrophy and by decreased mobility of the cusps. The heart weighed 440 g. **e.** The cause of calcification of the mitral anulus is uncertain. Since most patients with mitral anular calcific deposits also have calcific deposits in the aortic valve cusps and coronary arteries, it seems reasonable to believe that the cause of the calcification in each of these sites is similar. In young adults, yellow deposits are nearly always seen on the ventricular surface of both mitral leaflets and on the aortic surface of the aortic valve cusps. The lipid may be both intra- and extra-cellular in location. Degeneration of the lipid appears to lead to the calcification. The latter occurs behind the posterior mitral leaflet and on the aortic aspects of the cusps, since these are sites of high pressure, and there is nowhere else for the blood to go—it is, in effect, pushed into the valve leaflets. In contrast, the high pressure on the anterior leaflets is reflected off into the aorta. In other words, the impact of pressure contacts the posterior mitral leaflet and aortic valve cusps at right angles to the cusps, whereas the angle of contact with the anterior leaflet approaches a 180-deg angle.

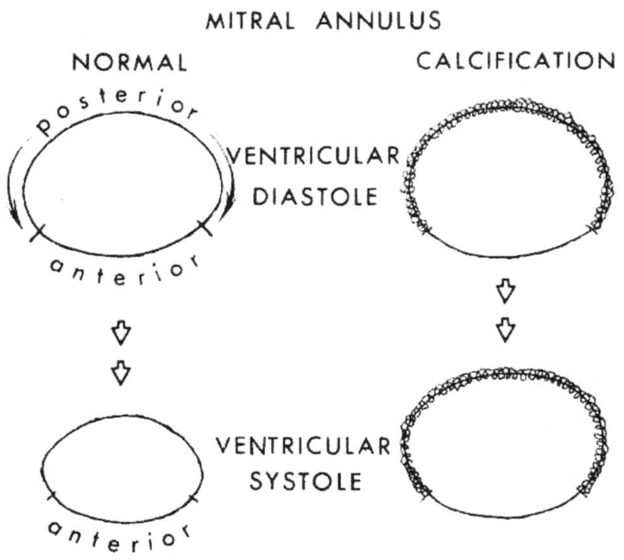

Figure 35. The mechanism of mitral regurgitation in patients with calcification of the mitral anulus. During ventricular systole the base of the left ventricle contracts like a sphincter. Included in the base of the left ventricle is the anulus behind the posterior mitral leaflet. Thus, this circumference decreases during systole. If, however, the anulus behind the posterior mitral leaflet is calcified, the sphincter-like contraction of the left ventricular base no longer occurs. The area of the mitral orifice thus is not decreased, and mild degrees of mitral regurgitation may result.

anulus, similar calcific deposits are often also observed in the aortic valve cusps and in the extramural or epicardial coronary arteries (Figure 34 *A-D*). Of the 87 patients with mitral anular calcification, 64 (74%) also had calcific deposits in the aortic valve, and in 35 of them the deposits were so extensive that the aortic valve orifice appeared stenotic. In several of them large peak systolic pressure gradients were recorded across the aortic valve (78). In this situation the aortic valve usually contains calcific deposits only on its aortic surfaces, the commissures are not fused, and there is no associated incompetence (78). Calcific deposits were observed grossly in the coronary arteries in 76 (87%) of the 87 patients. Of the 11 patients without deposits, 8 were less than age 53 years, and only 3 were more than age 65 years. Thus, of the 61 patients with mitral anular calcification aged 65 years or more, 58 (85%) had calcific deposits in the coronary arteries, and 47 (77%) had calcific deposits in the aortic valve cusps. Calcification in these three locations—mitral anulus, aortic valve, and coronary arteries—therefore is extremely common in the elderly population and suggests that the cause of the deposits in each location is similar. The deposits occur on the undersurface, that is, the ventricular surface, of the posterior mitral leaflet at or below the anulus and on the aortic surfaces of the aortic valve cusps. Foam cells are common in these locations in younger adults. Breakdown of these lipid deposits is probably responsible for the calcification at these sites (Figure 34*E*).

Calcification in the mitral anular area appears to be accelerated by conditions that elevate left ventricular pressure—namely, systemic hypertension, aortic valvular stenosis, and hypertrophic cardiomyopathy—and by conditions that accelerate atherosclerosis—for example, diabetes mellitus. The former conditions increase the mitral closing pressure, and the latter conditions increase the supply of lipids. An intrinsic defect of the fibrous skeleton of the heart appears to be the explanation for early mitral anular calcification in Marfan's and Hurler's syndromes. The mechanism by which mitral regurgitation is produced in patients with calcified mitral anuli is illustrated in Figure 35.

Conclusion

In closing, I refer you to Figure 36. Until the last 20 years or so, valvular cardiac disease in adults was considered rheumatic in origin. A major purpose of this review has been to call attention to many conditions other than rheumatic heart disease that may cause the mitral valve to function abnormally. One of the major contributions to cardiology in the 1960s was the realization that the left ventricular papillary muscles played an important role in closing the mitral orifice during ventricular systole and that ischemia, necrosis, or fibrosis of these structures could be the cause of severe mitral regurgitation even when the leaflets and chordae were normal. With the introduction of the concept of papillary muscle dysfunction, the role played by the mitral anulus in causing regurgitation has been deemphasized. With few exceptions it no longer seems reasonable to attribute mitral regurgitation to anular dilation. Papillary muscle dysfunction usually is a better explanation. Although numerous conditions can affect the mitral leaflets and cause regurgitation (far fewer conditions produce stenosis), myocardial disease with or without coronary arterial luminal narrowing now is recognized as the commonest cause of mitral regurgitation, even though the conditions that affect primarily the leaflets and chordae lead to the more severe degrees of regurgitation.

ACKNOWLEDGMENTS: Received 14 September 1972; accepted 2 October 1972.

► Requests for reprints should be addressed to William C. Roberts, M.D., Chief, Section of Pathology, National Heart and Lung Institute, Bldg. 10A, Room 3E-30, National Institutes of Health, Bethesda, Md. 20014.

References

1. Brock RC: The surgical and pathological anatomy of the

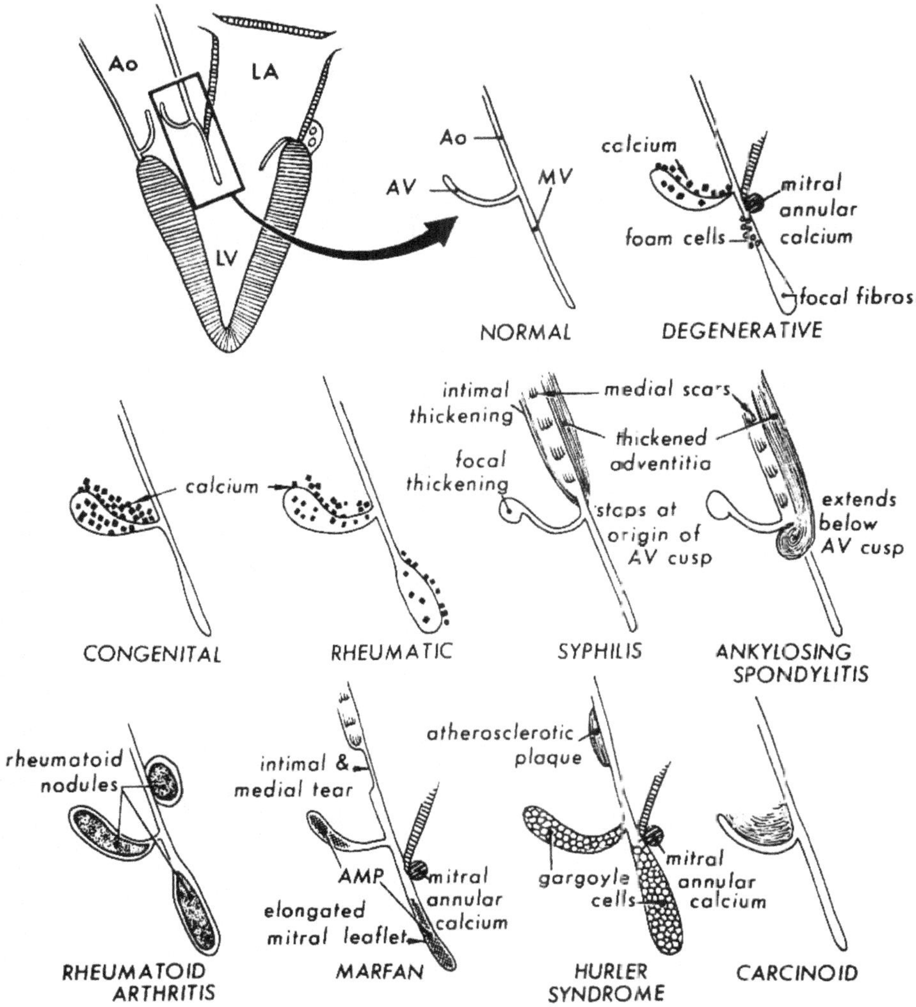

Figure 36. Diagram of some of the conditions affecting the mitral leaflets, most of which also affect the aortic valve. Degenerative, congenital, and rheumatic conditions frequently are associated with some degree of valvular stenosis. Syphilis never affects the mitral leaflets, but ankylosing spondylitis extends below the aortic valve and may lead to some degree of mitral regurgitation. Rheumatoid arthritis, floppy valves with or without Marfan's syndrome, and the Hurler syndrome produce purely incompetent lesions. Carcinoid usually affects, or more severely affects, the right-sided cardiac valves, but carcinoid plaques also have been observed on the mitral and aortic leaflets. Ao = aorta; LV = left ventricle; LA = left atrium; AV = aortic valve; MV = mitral valve; AMP = acid mucopolysaccharide material.

mitral valve. *Br Heart J* 14:489-513, 1952
2. Roberts WC, Cohen LS: Left ventricular papillary muscles. Description of the normal and a survey of conditions causing them to be abnormal. *Circulation* 46:138-154, 1972
3. Estes EH Jr, Dalton FM, Entman ML, et al: The anatomy and blood supply of the papillary muscles of the left ventricle. *Am Heart J* 71:356-362, 1966
4. Sell S, Scully RE: Aging changes in the aortic and mitral valves. Histologic and histochemical studies, with observations on the pathogenesis of calcific aortic stenosis and calcification of the mitral annulus. *Am J Pathol* 46:345-365, 1965
5. Perloff JK, Roberts WC: The mitral apparatus. Functional anatomy of mitral regurgitation. *Circulation* 46:227-239, 1972
6. Cheng TO: Some new observations on the syndrome of papillary muscle dysfunction. *Am J Med* 47:924-945, 1969
7. Rushmer RF, Finlayson BL, Nash AA: Movements of the mitral valve. *Circ Res* 4:337-342, 1956
8. Levy MJ, Edwards JE: Anatomy of mitral insufficiency. *Prog Cardiovasc Dis* 5:119-144, 1962
9. Davis PKB, Kinmonth JB: The movements of the annulus of the mitral valve. *J Cardiovasc Surg (Torino)* 4:427-431, 1963
10. Brolin I: The mitral orifice. *Acta Radiol [Diagn] (Stockh)* 6:273-295, 1967
11. Selzer A, Cohn KE: Natural history of mitral stenosis. A review. *Circulation* 45:878-890, 1972
12. Blackmon JR, Murray JA: Valvular heart disease, in *Cardiovascular Hemodynamics*, edited by Rushmer RF. Philadelphia, W. B. Saunders Co., 1970, p. 469
13. Perloff JK: *The Clinical Recognition of Congenital Heart Disease*. Philadelphia, W. B. Saunders Co., 1970, pp. 116-120
14. Short DS: Radiology of the lung in severe mitral stenosis. *Br Heart J* 17:33-40, 1955
15. Roberts WC: Anatomically isolated aortic valvular disease. The case against its being of rheumatic etiology. *Am J Med* 49:151-159, 1970
16. Roberts WC: Pathologic aspects of valvular and subvalvular (discrete and diffuse) aortic stenosis, in *The Natural History and Progress in Treatment of Congenital Heart Disease*, edited by Kidd BSL, Keith JD. Springfield, Ill., Charles C Thomas, Publisher, 1971, pp. 221-244
17. Roberts WC, Sjoerdsma A: The cardiac disease associated with the carcinoid syndrome (carcinoid heart disease). *Am J Med* 36:5-34, 1964
18. Roberts WC, Morrow AG: Mechanisms of acute left atrial thrombosis after mitral valve replacement. Pathologic findings indicating obstruction to left atrial emptying. *Am J Cardiol* 18:497-503, 1966
19. Roberts WC, Morrow AG: Causes of death and other anatomic observations after cardiac valve replacement. *Adv Cardiol* 7:226-247, 1972
20. Perloff JK: Auscultatory and phonocardiographic manifestations of pulmonary hypertension. *Prog Cardiovasc Dis* 9:303-340, 1967
21. Wood P: An appreciation of mitral stenosis. *Br Med J* 1: 1051-1063, 1113-1124, 1954
22. Shone JD, Sellers RD, Anderson RC, et al: The development complex of "parachute mitral valve," supravalvular ring of left atrium, subaortic stenosis, and coarctation of aorta. *Am J Cardiol* 11:714-725, 1963
23. Glancy DL, Chang MY, Dorney ER, et al: Parachute

mitral valve. Further observations and associated lesions. *Am J Cardiol* 27:309-313, 1971

24. Castaneda AR, Anderson RC, Edwards JE: Congenital mitral stenosis resulting from anomalous arcade and obstructing papillary muscles. Report of correction by use of ball valve prosthesis. *Am J Cardiol* 24:237-240, 1969
25. Davachi F, Moller JH, Edwards JE: Diseases of the mitral valve in infancy. An anatomic analysis of 55 cases. *Circulation* 43:565-579, 1971
26. Nasser WK, Davis RH, Dillon JC, et al: Atrial myxoma. I. Clinical and pathologic features in nine cases. *Am Heart J* 83:694-704, 1972
27. Ferrans VJ, Roberts WC: Structural features of cardiac myxomas. Histology, histochemistry and electronmicroscopy. *Hum Pathol.* In press
28. MacClowery JD, Roberts WC: Metastatic choriocarcinoma of the lung. Invasion of pulmonary veins with extension into left atrium and mitral orifice. *Am J Cardiol* 18:938-941, 1966
29. Sterns LP, Eliot RS, Varco RL, et al: Intracavitary cardiac neoplasms. A review of fifteen cases. *Br Heart J* 28:75-83, 1966
30. Buchbinder NA, Roberts WC: Active infective endocarditis confined to mural endocardium. A study of six necropsy patients. *Arch Pathol* 93:435-440, 1972
31. Zvaifler N: Chronic postrheumatic-fever (Jaccoud's) arthritis. *N Engl J Med* 267:10-14, 1962
32. Braunwald E, Awe WC: The syndrome of severe mitral regurgitation with normal left atrial pressure. *Circulation* 27:29-35, 1963
33. Perloff JK, Harvey WP: Auscultatory and phonocardiographic manifestations of pure mitral regurgitation. *Prog Cardiovasc Dis* 5:172-194, 1962
34. Edwards JE, Burchell HB: Endocardial and intimal lesions (jet impact) as possible sites of origin of murmurs. *Circulation* 18:946-960, 1958
35. Roberts WC, Braunwald E, Morrow AG: Acute severe mitral regurgitation secondary to ruptured chordae tendineae. Clinical, hemodynamic, and pathologic considerations. *Circulation* 33:58-70, 1966
36. Ronan JA Jr, Steelman RB, DeLeon AC, et al: The clinical diagnosis of acute severe mitral insufficiency. *Am J Cardiol* 27:284-290, 1971
37. Cohen LS, Mason DT, Braunwald E: Significance of an atrial gallop sound in mitral regurgitation. A clue to the diagnosis of ruptured chordae tendineae. *Circulation* 35:112-118, 1967
38. Gross L: Lesions of the left auricle in rheumatic fever. *Am J Pathol* 11:711-735, 1935
39. Roberts WC, Ross RS, Eggleston JC, et al: Chronic mitral regurgitation of unresolved etiology in the elderly. A clinico-pathologic study of two patients. *Johns Hopkins Med J* 122:26-36, 1968
40. Buchbinder NA, Roberts WC, Morrow AG: The pathology of healed infective endocarditis. Unpublished
41. Buchbinder NA, Roberts WC: Left-sided valvular active infective endocarditis. A study of forty-five necropsy patients. *Am J Med* 53:20-35, 1972
42. Haller JA Jr, Morrow AG: Experimental mitral insufficiency. An operative method of chronic survival. *Ann Surg* 142:37-51, 1955
43. Rockoff SD, Ross J Jr, Oldham NN Jr, et al: Ventriculoatrial regurgitation following prosthetic replacement of the mitral valve. Angiocardiographic and hemodynamic findings. *Am J Cardiol* 17:817-824, 1966
44. Edwards JE: Mitral insufficiency resulting from overshooting of leaflets. *Circulation* 43:606-612, 1971
45. Barlow JB, Bosman CK, Pocock WA, et al: Late systolic murmurs and non-ejection ("mid-late") systolic clicks. An analysis of 90 patients. *Br Heart J* 30:203-218, 1968
46. Bittar N, Sosa JA: The billowing mitral valve leaflet. *Circulation* 38:763-770, 1968
47. Dillon JC, Haine CL, Chang S, et al: Use of echocardiography in patients with prolapse mitral valve. *Circulation* 43:503-507, 1971
48. Ronan JA, Perloff JK, Harvey WP: Systolic clicks and the late systolic murmur. Intercardiac phonocardiographic evidence of their mitral valve origin. *Am Heart J* 70:319-325, 1965
49. Jeresaty RM: The syndrome associated with mid-systolic click and/or late systolic murmur. Analysis of 32 cases. *Chest* 59:643-647, 1971
50. Ehlers KH, Engle MA, Levin AR, et al: Left ventricular abnormality with late mitral insufficiency and abnormal electrocardiogram. *Am J Cardiol* 26:333-340, 1970
51. Osler W: On a remarkable heart murmur heard at a distance from the chest wall. *Med Times Gazette* 2:432, 1880
52. Rizzon P, Biasco G, Maselli-Campagna G: The precordial honk. *Br Heart J* 33:707-715, 1971
53. Leon DF, Leonard JJ, Kroetz FW, et al: Late systolic murmurs, clicks, and whoops arising from the mitral valve. A transseptal intracardiac phonocardiographic analysis. *Am Heart J* 72:325-336, 1966
54. Gooch AS, Vicencio F, Maranhao V, et al: Arrhythmias and left ventricular asynergy in the prolapsing mitral leaflet syndrome. *Am J Cardiol* 29:611-620, 1972
55. Baron MG: Abnormalities of the mitral valve in endocardial cushion defects. *Circulation* 45:672-680, 1972
56. Berry WB, Roberts WC, Morrow AG, et al: Corrected transposition of the aorta and pulmonary trunk. Clinical, hemodynamic and pathologic findings. *Am J Med* 36:35-53, 1964
57. Roberts WC, Ross RS, Davis FW Jr: Congenital corrected transposition of the great vessels in adulthood simulating rheumatic valvular disease. *Bull Johns Hopkins Hosp* 144:157-172, 1964
58. Carney EK, Braunwald E, Roberts WC, et al: Congenital mitral regurgitation. Clinical, hemodynamic and angiographic findings in nine patients. *Am J Med* 33:223-235, 1962
59. Cohn LH, Morrow AG, Braunwald E: Operative treatment of atrial septal defect: clinical and haemodynamic assessments in 175 patients. *Br Heart J* 29:725-734, 1967
60. Braunwald E, Ross RS, Morrow AG, et al: Differential diagnosis of mitral regurgitation in childhood: clinical pathological conference at the National Institutes of Health. *Ann Intern Med* 54:1223-1242, 1961
61. Brockenbrough EC, Braunwald E, Roberts WC, et al: Partial persistent atrioventricular canal simulating pure mitral regurgitation. *Am Heart J* 63:9-17, 1962
62. Rosenberg J, Roberts WC: Double orifice mitral valve. Study of the anomaly in two calves and a summary of the literature in humans. *Arch Pathol* 86:77-80, 1968
63. Morrow AG, Cohen LS, Roberts WC, et al: Severe mitral regurgitation following acute myocardial infarction and ruptured papillary muscle. Hemodynamic findings and results of operative treatment in four patients. *Circulation* 37 and 38 (suppl II):124-132, 1968
64. Burch GE, DePasquale NP, Phillips JH: Clinical manifestations of papillary muscle dysfunction. *Arch Intern Med* 112:112-117, 1963
65. Phillips JH, Burch GE, DePasquale NP: The syndrome of papillary muscle dysfunction. Its clinical recognition. *Ann Intern Med* 59:508-520, 1963
66. Burch GE, DePasquale NP, Phillips JH: The syndrome of papillary muscle dysfunction. *Am Heart J* 75:399-415, 1968
67. Shelburne JC, Rubinstein D, Gorlin R: A reappraisal of papillary muscle dysfunction. Correlative clinical and angiographic study. *Am J Med* 46:862-871, 1969
68. Brody W, Criley JM: Intermittent severe mitral regurgitation. Hemodynamic studies in a patient with recurrent acute left-sided heart failure. *N Engl J Med* 283:673-676, 1970
69. Noren GR, Raghib G, Moller JH, et al: Anomalous origin of the left coronary artery from the pulmonary trunk with special reference to the occurrence of mitral insufficiency. *Circulation* 30:171-179, 1964
70. Miller GE Jr, Cohn KE, Kerth WJ, et al: Experimental papillary muscle infarction. *J Thorac Cardiovasc Surg* 56:611-616, 1968
71. Tsakiris AG, Rastelli GC, Amorim D deS, et al: Effect of experimental papillary muscle damage on mitral valve closure in intact anesthetized dogs. *Mayo Clin Proc* 45:275-285, 1970
72. Mittal AK, Langston M Jr, Cohn KE, et al: Combined papillary muscle and left ventricular wall dysfunction as a cause of mitral regurgitation. An experimental study. *Circulation* 44:174-180, 1971
73. Estes EH Jr, Entman ML, Dixon HB II, et al: The vascular supply of the left ventricular wall. Anatomic observations, plus a hypothesis regarding acute events in coronary artery disease. *Am Heart J* 71:58-67, 1966
74. Heikkilä J: Mitral incompetence as a complication of acute myocardial infarction. *Acta Med Scand* 182 (suppl 475):1-

149, 1967
75. Moller JH, Nakib A, Edwards JE: Infarction of papillary muscles and mitral insufficiency associated with congenital aortic stenosis. *Circulation* 34:87-91, 1966
76. Arosemena E, Moller JH, Edwards JE: Scarring of the papillary muscles in left ventricular hypertrophy. *Am Heart J* 74:446-452, 1967
77. Roberts WC: The congenitally bicuspid aortic valve. A study of 85 autopsy cases. *Am J Cardiol* 26:72-83, 1970
78. Roberts WC, Perloff JK, Costantino T: Severe valvular aortic stenosis in patients over 65 years of age. A clinicopathologic study. *Am J Cardiol* 27:497-506, 1971
79. Falcone MW, Roberts WC, Morrow AG, et al: Congenital aortic stenosis resulting from a unicommissural valve. Clinical and anatomic features in twenty-one adult patients. *Circulation* 44:272-280, 1971
80. Roberts WC: Valvular, subvalvular, and supravalvular aortic stenosis. Morphologic features. *Cardiovasc Clin.* In press
81. Roberts WC, Buchbinder NA: Papillary muscle necrosis in active valvular infective endocarditis (abstract). *Am J Cardiol* 29:287, 1972
82. Moller JH, Lucas RV Jr, Adams P Jr, et al: Endocardial fibroelastosis. A clinical and anatomic study of 47 patients with emphasis on its relationship to mitral insufficiency. *Circulation* 30:759-782, 1964
83. Roberts WC: Anomalous origin of both coronary arteries from the pulmonary artery. *Am J Cardiol* 10:595-600, 1962
84. Burchell HB, Brown AL Jr: Anomalous origin of coronary artery from pulmonary artery masquerading as mitral insufficiency. *Am Heart J* 63:388-393, 1962
85. Roberts WC, Ferrans VJ: Morphologic observations in the cardiomyopathies, in *The Cardiomyopathies*, edited by Fowler NO. New York, Grune & Stratton. In press, 1973
86. Marcus FI, Gomez L, Glancy DL, et al: Papillary muscle fibrosis in primary myocardial disease. *Am Heart J* 77:681-685, 1969
87. Perloff JK, Roberts WC, deLeon AC, et al: The distinctive electrocardiogram of Duchenne's progressive muscular dystrophy. An electrocardiographic-pathologic correlative study. *Am J Med* 42:179-188, 1967
88. Roberts WC, Buja LM, Ferrans VJ: Löffler's fibroplastic parietal endocarditis, eosinophilic leukemia, and Davies' endomyocardial fibrosis: the same disease at different stages? *Pathol Microbiol (Basel)* 35:90-95, 1970
89. Roberts WC, Liegler DG, Carbone PP: Endomyocardial disease and eosinophilia. A clinical and pathologic spectrum. *Am J Med* 46:28-42, 1969
90. Buja LM, Khoi NB, Roberts WC: Clinically significant cardiac amyloidosis. Clinicopathologic findings in 15 patients. *Am J Cardiol* 26:394-405, 1970
91. Buja LM, Roberts WC: Iron in the heart. Etiology and clinical significance. *Am J Med* 51:209-221, 1971
92. Rastelli GC, Kirklin JW, Titus JL: Fate of papillary muscles after prosthetic replacement of mitral valve. *Mayo Clin Proc* 42:210-217, 1967
93. Adelman AG, McLoughlin MJ, Marquis Y, et al: Left ventricular cineangiographic observations in muscular subaortic stenosis. *Am J Cardiol* 24:689-697, 1969
94. Oakley CM: Hypertrophic obstructive cardiomyopathy—patterns of progression, in *Hypertrophic Obstructive Cardiomyopathy*, edited by Wolstenholme GEW, O'Connor M. London, J. & A. Churchill, Ltd., 1971, p. 9
95. Morrow AG: Hypertrophic subaortic stenosis. Some physiologic concepts and the role of operative treatment. *Arch Surg* 99:677-683, 1969
96. Grossman M, Knott AP Jr, Jacoby WJ Jr: Calcified annulus fibrosis with mitral insufficiency with Marfan's syndrome. *Arch Intern Med* 121:561-563, 1968
97. Korn D, DeSanctis RW, Sell S: Massive calcification of the mitral annulus. A clinicopathological study of fourteen cases. *N Engl J Med* 267:900-909, 1962
98. Brawley RK, Roberts WC, Morrow AG: Intestinal infarction resulting from nonobstructive mesenteric arterial insufficiency. With a note on hepatic hypoglycemia as a possible aid in diagnosis. *Arch Surg* 92:374-378, 1966

Results of Valve Replacement for Severe Mitral Regurgitation Due to Papillary Muscle Rupture or Fibrosis

D. LUKE GLANCY, MD, FACC
EDWARD B. STINSON, MD
RICHARD L. SHEPHERD, MD
SAMUEL B. ITSCOITZ, MD
WILLIAM C. ROBERTS, MD, FACC
STEPHEN E. EPSTEIN, MD
ANDREW G. MORROW, MD, FACC

Bethesda, Maryland

Late results of mitral valve replacement for papillary muscle rupture (four patients) or fibrosis without rupture (five patients) are described for the first time. Patients underwent operation 3 months to more than 13 years (median 14 months) after the onset of severe mitral regurgitation. Preoperatively all had holosystolic murmurs, atrial and ventricular gallops, cardiomegaly and cardiac failure. Three had class III and six had class IV functional capacity (New York Heart Association Classification). Atrial fibrillation developed ir the three patients who had mitral regurgitation for more than 3 years. Left atrial mean pressure (average 27 mm Hg) and *V* waves (average 46 mm Hg) were greatly increased in all but one patient and cardiac index (average 2.0 liters/min per m^2) was reduced i all but one. No finding distinguished patients with rupture from thos without rupture. The left ventricular angiogram was the best preoperative guide to postoperative results. Of five patients with poor le ventricular contractions, four died (one suddenly 2 days postopera tively and three with cardiac failure, two 6 months and one 6 months postoperatively); 4 months after operation one is limited b the residua of a cerebral embolus. None of the three studied postop eratively showed hemodynamic improvement. In contrast, of fou patients with fair or good left ventricular contractions preoperatively three have class I or II functional capacity 23, 60, 64 months, re spectively, after operation, and one died suddenly 41 months afte operation. All three studied postoperatively showed marked hemody namic improvement.

The early results of operation for mitral regurgitation due to papilla ry muscle rupture or dysfunction without rupture have been de scribed,[1-22] but the late results have not. Four patients we[1] hav previously described were followed up for 5 years after mitral valv replacement for papillary muscle rupture. During this interval w studied and operated upon an additional five patients who had se vere mitral regurgitation due to papillary muscle fibrosis and dy function without rupture. This report describes the clinical, hemod namic and anatomic features in the nine patients, compares the features in patients with and without papillary muscle rupture an assesses the effects of operation and the factors influencing the la postoperative results.

From the Cardiology Branch, Section of Pathology, and Clinic of Surgery, National Heart and Lung Institute, Bethesda, Md. 20014. Accepted February 28, 1973.

Address for reprints: D. Luke Glancy, MD, Section of Cardiology, Department of Medicine, Louisiana State University Medical Center, 1542 Tulane Ave., New Orleans, La. 70112.

Results

Preoperative Clinical Features

All nine patients were men aged 49 to 69 years (average 57 year at the time of operation (Table I). Seven had been hospitalized wi clinical features of acute myocardial infarction 3 to 65 months

Preoperative Clinical Features, Operative Findings, Postoperative Follow-Up

Case no.	Age at Operation (yr)	Months from Infarct to Operation (mo)	AP	Edema	NYHA Functional Class	Cardiac Rhythm	ECG	Chest X-ray C/T	Chest X-ray LA Enlargement	Involved Papillary Muscle	Prosthesis Model	Prosthesis Size	Follow-up (mo)	Current Status
								Papillary Muscle Rupture						
1	59	15	0	+	IV	Sinus	AMI	0.56	2+/4+	Anterior	S-E6120	2M	62	Died of CHF
2	51	3	0	+	IV	Sinus	IMI	0.54	1+/4+	Posterior	S-E6120	2M	41	Died suddenly
3	69	13	0	+	IV	Sinus	IMI	0.62	2+/4+	Posterior	S-E6120	2M	64	Early class II
4	59	14	+	0	IV	Sinus	SEI	0.50	0	Anterior	S-E6120	2M	60	Class II (PAF → III)
								Papillary Muscle Fibrosis Without Rupture						
5	49	6	0	0	III	Sinus	AMI	0.55	1+/4+	Posterior	S-E6120	2M	6	Died of CHF
6	57	?	0	+	III	AF	IMI	0.65	3+/4+	Both	S-E6300	3M	6	CHF, died suddenly
7	51	42	+	+	IV	AF	IMI	0.75	3+/4+	Both	S-E6310	3M	0	Died postop day 2
8	65	8	+	+	III	Sinus	SEI	0.56	1+/4+	Posterior	Kay-Shiley	#4	23	Class I
9	53	65	0	+	IV	AF	IMI	0.63	3+/4+	Posterior	S-E6520	3M	4	Limited by stroke

AF = atrial fibrillation; AMI = anterior myocardial infarct; AP = angina pectoris; CHF = congestive heart failure; C/T = cardiothoracic ratio; ECG = electrocardiogram; IMI = inferior myocardial infarct; LA = left atrial; NYHA = New York Heart Association; PAF = paroxysmal atrial fibrillation; postop = postoperative; S-E = Starr-Edwards; SEI = subendocardial ischemia or infarct.

fore operation, and in each a cardiac murmur had been noted before discharge. Two patients had not been hospitalized for myocardial infarction. One of the two patients (Case 7) experienced pain in the right jaw during exertion 42 months before operation, but the pain had been replaced by dyspnea when he presented to a hospital several months later with congestive failure and the electrocardiographic findings of remote inferior wall infarction. The second patient (Case 6) had never had precordial pain. He was known to have had a cardiac murmur for 13 years; 4 years before operation atrial fibrillation and heart failure developed. His electrocardiogram suggested old inferior wall infarction. All patients experienced severe dyspnea, fatigue and orthopnea before operation, and seven also had right-sided failure with marked peripheral edema. Only three of the nine patients had angina pectoris, and in one (Case 8) it appeared for the first time after myocardial infarction. In no patient was angina the limiting symptom. Three patients had class III functional capacity (New York Heart Association classification) at the time of operation, and the other six, including all four with papillary muscle rupture, had class IV functional capacity.

At the time of operation, six patients had sinus rhythm and three, each with papillary muscle dysfunction and mitral regurgitation for at least 3 years, had atrial fibrillation. Seven patients were examined during sinus rhythm, and each had an atrial (S_4) gallop. All nine patients had a ventricular (S_3) gallop and a holosystolic apical murmur (Fig. 1).

The electrocardiogram showed inferior wall infarction in five patients, and anterior wall infarction in two. The electrocardiogram was of no help in determining whether a papillary muscle was ruptured and was only partially accurate in predicting which muscle was involved. All five whose electrocardiogram showed an inferior wall infarction had involvement of the posterior papillary muscle, but two also had involvement of the anterior muscle. The electrocardiographic patterns of anterior wall infarction and of subendocardial ischemia were each associated with involvement of the anterior muscle in one patient and of the posterior muscle in another.

All patients had generalized cardiomegaly with a cardiothoracic ratio of 0.5 or more on the posteroanterior chest roentgenogram (Table I); in four patients this ratio exceeded 0.6. In one patient left atrial size appeared to be normal on roentgenograms taken in the four standard views after barium swallow. The other eight patients had various degrees of left atrial enlargement. Cardiothoracic ratio and left atrial size were greatest in the three patients who had papillary muscle fibrosis without rupture, long-standing mitral regurgitation and atrial fibrillation. No patient had a giant left atrium.

Preoperative Hemodynamic Findings

All patients underwent preoperative cardiac catheterization (Table II, Fig. 2). Despite digitalis and diuretic therapy, pulmonary arterial pressure was in-

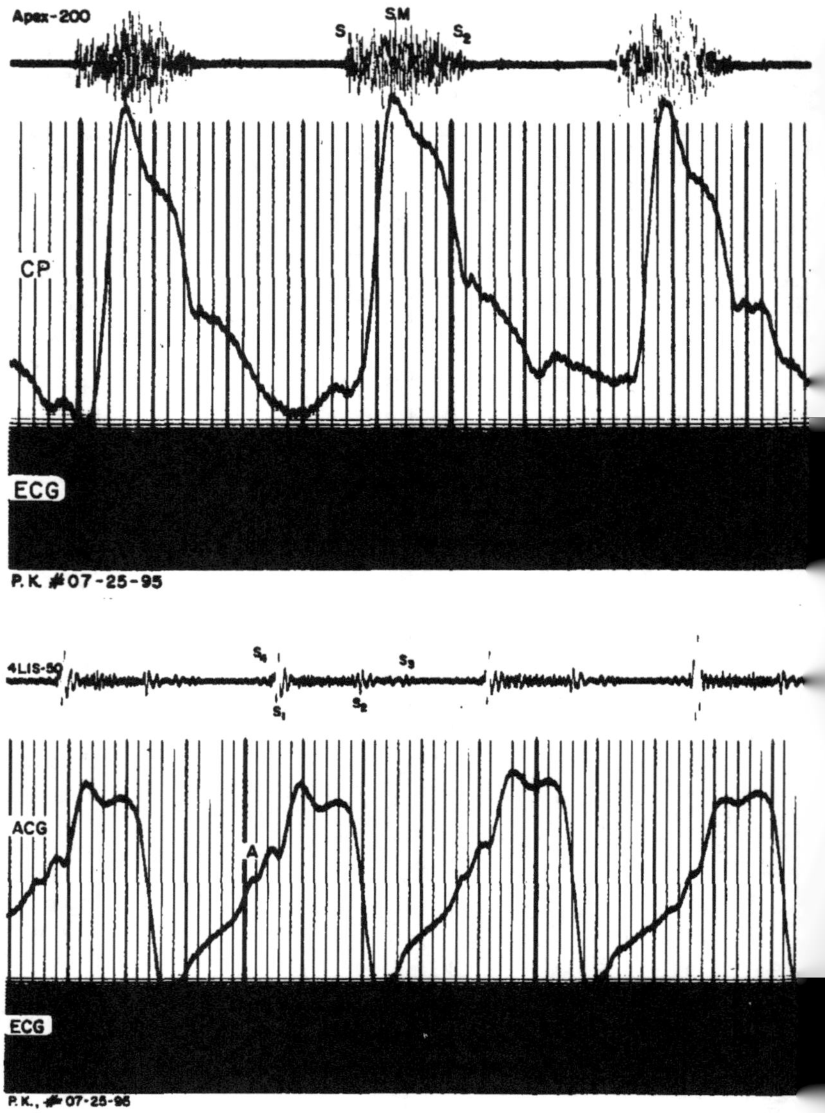

FIGURE 1. Case 4. Phonocardiograms. The systolic murmur (SM) begins with the first heart sound (S_2) and extends to the second sound (S_2). Third (S_3) and fourth (S_4) heart sounds are present, and a large *A* wave is seen on the apex cardiogram (ACG). CP = carotid pulse tracing; 4 LIS = fourth left intercostal space.

creased in all patients, and the levels of right ventricular end-diastolic and right atrial mean pressure were above the upper limits of normal in six. Eight patients had increased left atrial or pulmonary arterial wedge mean pressure and unusually large *V* waves (40 to 62 mm Hg) (Fig. 3). In one patient (Case 4), left atrial *V* wave and mean pressures were at the upper limits of normal. The left ventricular end-diastolic pressure level was abnormally high in eight of the nine patients, and the cardiac index was low in six of the seven patients in whom it was measured.

Mitral regurgitation was judged by selective left ventricular angiogram to be severe in all nine patients. Regurgitant volume was not quantified, but appeared to be equally large in patients with and without papillary muscle rupture. Prolapse of a mitral valve leaflet into the left atrium was seen only in Patient 7, who had papillary muscle fibrosis without rupture and a prolapsing posterior leaflet. Generalized or focal abnormalities, or both, of left ventricul contraction were recognized in all but one patie (Case 8). Contractions were judged to be fair or goc in four patients (Fig. 4), three of whom had rupture papillary muscles, and poor in five patients, four whom had papillary muscle dysfunction witho rupture. Coronary arteriograms were not obtained.

Operative Findings and Early Results

Rupture involved a single head of the anterior p pillary muscle in two patients and a single head of t posterior muscle in the other two (Table I). In t patient (Case 2) with the shortest interval (3 month between infarction and operation, necrotic my cardial fibers were observed in the ruptured pap lary muscle head. In the other three patients, the ru tured papillary muscle head was composed of fibro tissue with only a few viable subendocardial fibers. three of the five patients without rupture, the post rior papillary muscle was fibrotic (Fig. 5), and in t

TABLE II

Hemodynamic Data

Case no.	Pressures (mm Hg) RA mean Pre	RA mean Post	RV S/ED Pre	RV S/ED Post	PA S/ED (mean) Pre	PA S/ED (mean) Post	PAW or LA V wave (mean) Pre	PAW or LA V wave (mean) Post	LV S/ED Pre	LV S/ED Post	Carciac Index (liters/min/per m²) Pre	Carciac Index Post	Quality of LV Contractions on Angiogram
					Papillary Muscle Rupture								
1	4	7	60/6	62/10	60/30(37)	62/31(42)	49(29)	44(32)	75/19	93/28	1.9	2.0	Poor
2	14	1	60/13	28/3	60/28(40)	28/8(16)	42(28)	14(7)	74/17	...	1.7	1.5	Fair
3	10	2	80/16	42/3	80/33(52)	42/17(27)	42(28)	17(11)	110/10	...	1.2	2.9	Good
4	0	...	37/5	...	37/13(27)	...	17(12)	...	97/13	...	2.3	...	Fair
					Papillary Muscle Fibrosis Without Rupture								
5	13	15	72/15	73/15	72/42(53)	73/35(47)	..(27)	42(29)	90/30	90/36	1.7	2.4	Poor
6	2	...	32/3	...	32/12(22)	...	40(20)	...	85/16	...	3.2	...	Poor
7	21	...	112/20	62/10	112/50(80)	62/35(45)	52(33)	44(36)	120/19	74/24	...	...	Poor
8	15	8	95/19	67/11	95/40(60)	67/32(47)	60(35)	37(22)	125/20	225/14	...	3.0	Good
9	10	...	88/16	...	88/35(54)	...	62(30)	...	120/18	...	2.2	...	Poor

LA = left atrial; LV = left ventricular; PA = pulmonary arterial; PAW = pulmonary arterial wedge; Pre = preoperative; Post = postoperative; RA = right atrial; RV = right ventricular; S/ED = systolic/end-diastolic.
Figures in parentheses indicate mean pressures.

other two, both papillary muscles were scarred. The excised mitral valve was replaced by a Starr-Edwards caged-ball prosthesis in seven cases, and by a disc-type prosthesis in Cases 8 and 9 (Table I).

Patient 7 had signs of low cardiac output and died on the second postoperative day of intractable ventricular arrhythmias. Autopsy revealed severe triple vessel coronary artery disease, marked cardiomegaly (heart weight 750 g) and left ventricular dilatation, an extensive old posteroinferior infarct, thrombi in the right atrial appendage and recent pulmonary emboli with infarcts.

Patient 9 had had atrial fibrillation for 4 months before operation, but reversion to sinus rhythm occurred at the end of the procedure. Two weeks after operation he had a cerebral embolus, despite continued anticoagulation with warfarin, and was found to have atrial fibrillation again. His condition has steadily improved, but he remains limited by right hemiparesis and expressive aphasia. The condition of the other seven patients improved dramatically in the early postoperative period.

Postoperative Hemodynamic Findings

Six patients underwent postoperative cardiac catheterization (Table II, Fig. 2). The studies were usually performed 6 months after operation, but in Case 7 the data shown were obtained on the operat-

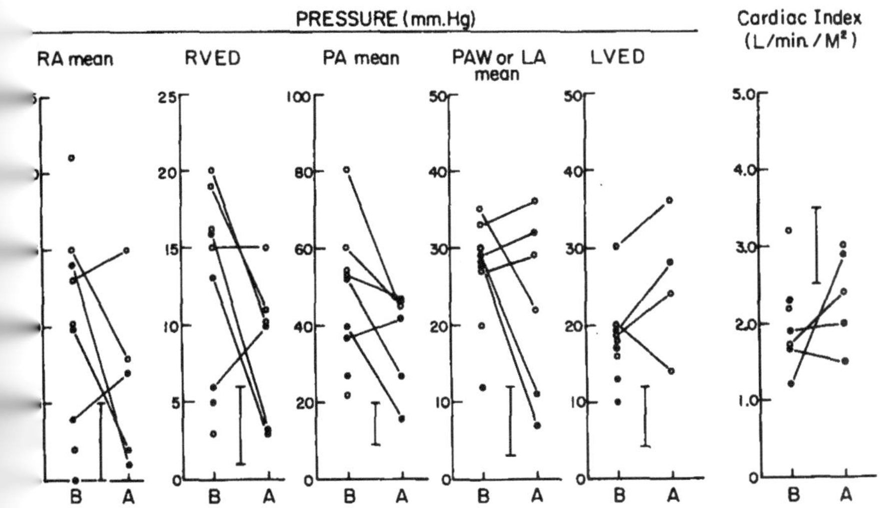

FIGURE 2. Intracardiac pressures and cardiac index before (B) and after (A) mitral valve replacement in patients with papillary muscle rupture **(solid circles)** and papillary muscle fibrosis without rupture **(open circles)**. Each **vertical bar** indicates the range of normal values. LA = left atrial; LVED = left ventricular end-diastolic; PA = pulmonary arterial; PAW = pulmonary arterial wedge; RA = right atrial; RVED = right ventricular end-diastolic.

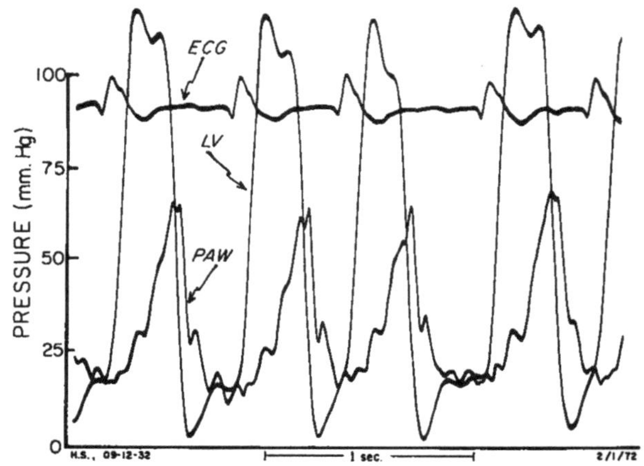

FIGURE 3. Case 9. Pulmonary arterial wedge (PAW) and left ventricular (LV) pressure tracings. The pulmonary arterial wedge *V* waves are huge, and left ventricular end-diastolic pressure is increased.

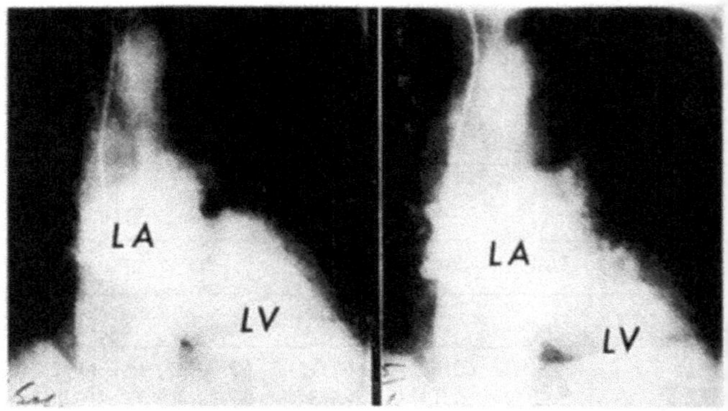

FIGURE 4. Case 3. Left ventricular angiograms exposed in dias- tole **(left)** and systole **(right)**. There is marked regurgitation contrast material from left ventricle (LV) to left atrium (LA) Overall left ventricular contraction was judged to be good de spite poor motion of the inferior wall.

ing table after valve replacement. Of the three patients with ruptured papillary muscles, the two whose preoperative angiograms revealed fair or good left ventricular contractions (Cases 2 and 3) showed striking hemodynamic improvement postoperatively; the patient with poor contractions had essentially unchanged hemodynamics postoperatively (Case 1). Of the three patients with papillary muscle dysfunction, two had a poorly contracting left ventricle preoperatively, and their hemodynamic status was not improved by operation. Patient 8 had good contractions before operation, and his postoperative hemodynamic status was improved although the left atrial pressure remained increased, because of a large (11 mm Hg) mean diastolic gradient across a small Kay-Shiley prosthesis. He also has had systemic arterial hypertension since operation.

Late Results of Operation

Of the eight patients who survived the early postoperative period, four have subsequently died. Patient 5 died of progressive congestive failure 6 months after operation. Patient 6 also continued to have signs and symptoms of cardiac failure, but his death, 6 months after operation, was sudden and presumably due to an arrhythmia. The condition of Patient 2 was greatly improved after operation both symptomatically and hemodynamically. Aside from several episodes of atrial fibrillation, he did well until 39 months after operation when he was hospitalized for a prolonged episode of chest pain and paroxysmal atrial tachycardia with heart block. He died suddenly 2 months after leaving the hospital and 41 months after operation. Again, death presumably was due to an arrhythmia. Necropsy revealed old complete occlusion of the right coronary artery, an old aneurysm of the inferior wall of the left ventricle and a normal mitral valve prosthesis. After operation Patient 1 had a marked decrease in symptoms but showed no hemodynamic improvement. Symptoms of congestive failure gradually recurred, but with use of digitalis and diuretic agents and with careful attention to sodium intake for 5 years his functional capacity remained in late class II or early class III and he had no angina pectoris although he had symptoms of dyspnea and fatigue. For several months before death his failure grew worse, and weeks before death he had a cerebral embolus. Although he gradually recovered from the stroke, his cardiac status steadily deteriorated and he died with shock 62 months after operation.

Four patients are alive 64, 60, 23 and 4 months respectively, after operation (Table I). Patient 3 is now 74 years old and has early class II functional capacity. He can walk a mile slowly, but experiences dyspnea if he walks rapidly. Patient 4 usually has late class II functional capacity, but has paroxysms of atrial fibrillation that cause his symptoms of dyspnea and fatigue to increase to class III severity. Patient 8 was completely asymptomatic, but 20 months after operation therapy with warfarin was temporarily discontinued in anticipation of dental extractions. Five days later he presented with pulmonary edem with faint prosthetic valve sounds and an apic grade 2/6 blowing holosystolic murmur. He underwent emergency operation. The disc of his Kay-Shiley mitral prosthesis was virtually immobilized b old and new thrombi. The prosthesis was replace with a porcine aortic valve mounted on a flexibl stent,[23] and 3 months after operation the patient i again asymptomatic. Four months postoperativel Patient 9 remains limited by hemiparesis, as described earlier.

Neither the intracardiac pressure measurement nor the cardiac output determinations could be use preoperatively to predict postoperative survival hemodynamic results. Patients who had papillar muscle fibrosis without rupture, especially thos with long-standing mitral regurgitation, an enlarge heart and atrial fibrillation, seemed to have a less fa vorable course after valve replacement than the pa tients with papillary muscle rupture. However, th

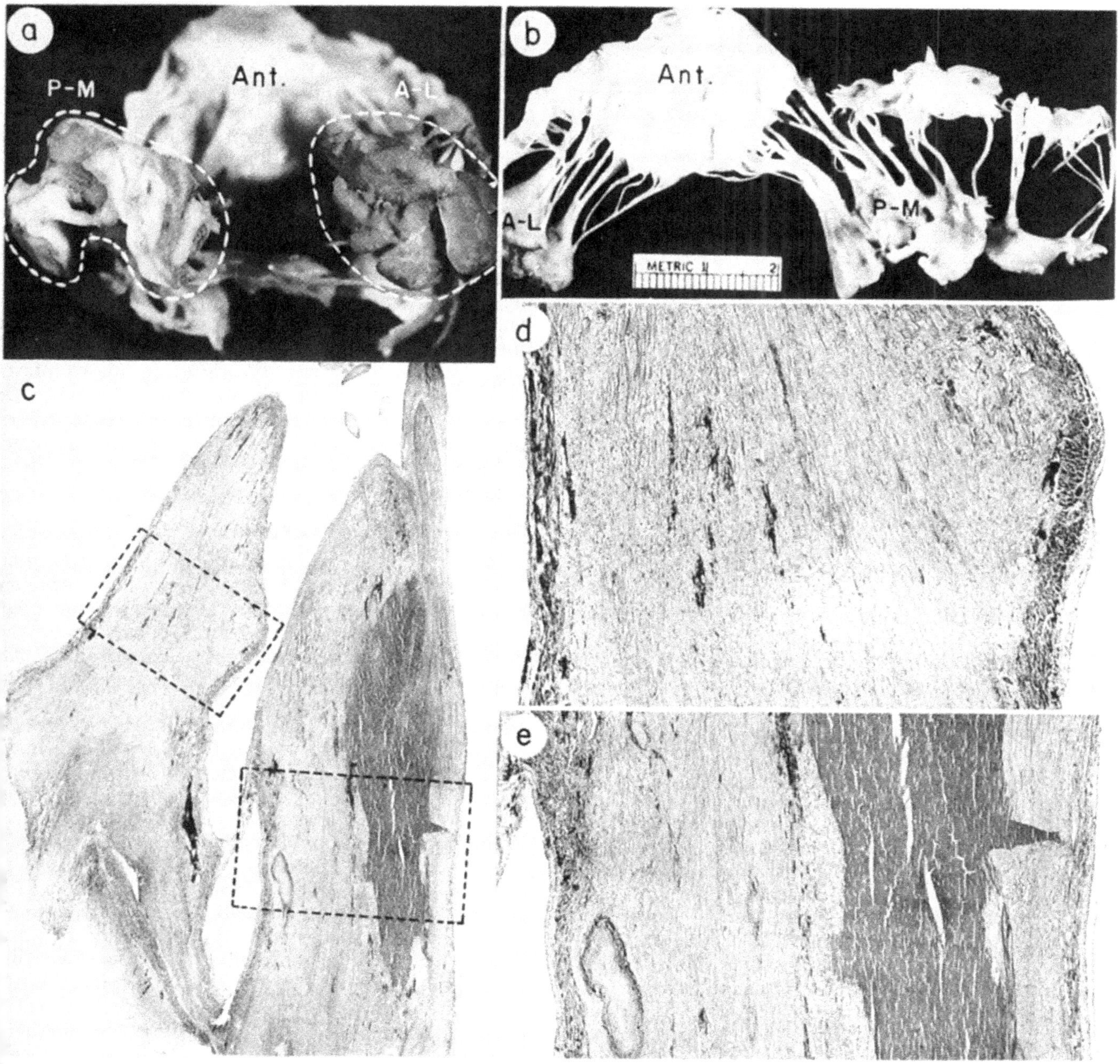

IGURE 5. Case 5. Excised mitral valve **(a,b)** and photomicrographs **(c,d,e)** of portions of posteromedial (P-M) left ventricular papilla- muscle in a patient who had papillary muscle necrosis *without* rupture during acute myocardial infarction 6 months before valve re- acement. This patient was the only one among the five without rupture who had myocardial necrosis in the excised papillary muscle. intact mitral valve showing extensive necrosis and fibrosis of the posteromedial papillary muscle. The anterolateral muscle (A-L) is ormal. **b** opened valve showing atrial aspects of the leaflets. **c** section of each of two trunks of the posteromedial muscle showing ly fibrous scarring in one (close-up in **d**) and both fibrosis and necrosis in the other (close-up in **e**). Only the myocardial fibers in e most peripheral portions of the muscles are preserved. (These peripheral fibers probably are oxygenated directly by blood from the ft ventricular cavity and not by blood from the coronary arteries, which supply the remainder of the papillary muscle.) Hematoxylin- osin ×8.5 **(c)**, ×25 **(d)**, and ×20 **(e)** all reduced by 10 percent. Ant. = anterior mitral leaflet.

eoperative left ventriculogram was clearly the best edictor of operative results (Table III). Patients ith poor left ventricular contractions had no emodynamic improvement and had a low rate of ng-term survival, whereas the opposite was true for tients with fair or good left ventricular contrac- ons.

Discussion

Clinical Features

Mitral regurgitation and coronary artery disease frequently coexist. Although the two conditions are often unrelated, as in patients with both coronary

TABLE III

Quality of Left Ventricular Contractions as Determined by Angiogram vs. Postoperative Results

LV Contractions	Total Patients (no.)	Patients Who Died (no.)	Patients Who Survived (no.)
Poor	5	4* (2 days, 6 mo, 6 mo, 62 mo)	1 (4 mo)
Fair–good	4	1† (41 mo)	3† (23 mo, 60 mo, 64 mo)

* In the three patients in this group who underwent postoperative catheterization studies, the findings demonstrated unimproved hemodynamic status.

† The patient who died and two of the three survivors underwent postoperative catheterization studies. The findings in all three cases demonstrated improved hemodynamic status.

Figures in parentheses indicate time after operation.

atherosclerosis and rheumatic mitral valve disease, mitral regurgitation is commonly caused by coronary disease and papillary muscle infarction. When one or more heads of an infarcted papillary muscle rupture, severe mitral regurgitation invariably results and is often rapidly fatal.[16] If the remainder of the left ventricular myocardium has not been too severely damaged, the patient may survive the acute infarction to be left with chronic severe mitral regurgitation. This was the case in our first four patients.

Burch et al.[24] have drawn attention to mitral regurgitation occurring as the result of papillary muscle dysfunction without actual rupture. Mild mitral regurgitation due to papillary muscle dysfunction appears to be a common disorder, occurring in up to 55 percent of patients with acute myocardial infarction[25] and in 15 to 25 percent of patients with severe chronic ischemic heart disease.[26-28] Severe regurgitation is unusual but, when it occurs, the findings are similar to those in patients with papillary muscle rupture. The murmur is usually first heard during hospitalization for acute infarction. If the patient survives, he subsequently presents with chronic mitral regurgitation and symptoms of congestive failure rather than with angina pectoris. The cardiac rhythm is sinus during the first few years of mitral regurgitation, but atrial fibrillation eventually supervenes. A ventricular gallop is invariably heard, and an atrial gallop also is heard when the patient has sinus rhythm.

In patients with mild mitral regurgitation due to papillary muscle dysfunction, holosystolic,[25] ejection[24,25] and late[25,29,30] systolic murmurs have been described, but when mitral regurgitation is severe, the murmur is always holosystolic. It often is harsher than the blowing murmur of rheumatic mitral regurgitation and may be crescendo-decrescendo in character (Fig. 1). The electrocardiographic pattern is most often that of old inferior wall infarction, but patterns of anterior wall infarction or subendocardial ischemia also are seen. If severe mitral regurgitation has been present for 3 months or more, generalized cardiomegaly with left atrial enlargement is the rule and, in patients surviving several years, the heart is as large as in many patients with rheumatic mitral regurgitation. The longer duration of mitral regurgitation probably accounts for the larger size of the heart in our patients without papillary muscle rupture than in those with rupture. With occasional exceptions, as in Case 4, and regardless of left atrial size, cardiac catheterization reveals marked left atrial hypertension with large *V* waves. Angiocardiograms demonstrate severe mitral regurgitation with focal or generalized impairment, or both, of left ventricular contraction, but prolapse of a mitral leaflet into the left atrium can be recognized only occasionally. Thus, severe mitral regurgitation due to infarction of a papillary muscle usually has characteristic features that distinguish it from mitral regurgitation due to other causes, but we know of no way to determine preoperatively whether the papillary muscle is ruptured.

Operative Findings and Results

Repair of the mitral apparatus has been attempted in patients with mitral regurgitation due to papillary muscle infarction,[2,3] but the results have not been encouraging. Valve replacement appears to be the operation of choice under most circumstances. Although eight of our nine patients survived the first postoperative month (a survival rate approximatin[g] that of all patients undergoing isolated mitral valv[e] replacement at the National Heart and Lung Insti[tu]te[23,31,32]), only 23 (61 percent) of 38 patients pre[]viously reported on[4-22] survived the early postopera[]tive period. Thus, operative mortality rates for valv[e] replacement are probably higher in patients with mi[]tral regurgitation due to coronary disease than i[n] those with other types of mitral regurgitation. Al[]though the number of patients in our study is sma[ll] our results also suggest that the long-term prognosi[s] after mitral valve replacement is less favorabl[e] in patients with papillary muscle infarction than i[n] patients with other types of isolated mitral valv[e] disease. As assessed by the life-table metho[d] 50 percent of the first 100 patients undergoing mitr[al] valve replacement at the National Heart and Lun[g] Institute were alive 8 1/2 years postoperatively, and results were better in patients with pre[]dominant regurgitation than in those with predomi[]nant stenosis. In our study, 50 percent of patien[ts] were dead within 5 years. Patients in our stud[y] were older and more severely ill than most patien[ts] undergoing valve replacement for rheumatic mitr[al] regurgitation. In addition, they had various degre[es] of left ventricular impairment due to coronary arte[ry] disease and myocardial infarction. These factors u[n]doubtedly are responsible for the less favorable lon[g] term results in our study. Nevertheless, the resul[ts] are at least as good as the results in patients unde[r]going double valve replacement for mitral and aort[ic] disease, for in this group 50 percent of patients we[re] dead in slightly less than 3 years.[34]

Both in our series and in that reported from the Massachusetts General Hospital,[20] operative results were somewhat better in patients with papillary muscle rupture than in those with dysfunction without rupture, but in our series we were unable to determine preoperatively whether the papillary muscle was ruptured. This is not a serious disadvantage because the preoperative left ventricular cineangiogram appears to be an even better predictor of operative results. Thus, patients with fair or good left ventricular contractions and gross mitral regurgitation usually show clinical and hemodynamic improvement, but patients with poor left ventricular contractions, especially those with only moderate mitral regurgitation, usually do not.

Operative indications: None of our patients and few of those reported on by others[15,17,19,22] were operated upon within a month of myocardial infarction and the onset of mitral regurgitation. Although some patients are alive who might not have survived without operation, valve replacement under these circumstances seems to carry a high risk. Moreover, the onset of left ventricular failure in a patient with acute infarction and severe mitral regurgitation is not necessarily indicative of progressive deterioration and death. For example, in one patient referred to us for valve replacement because of severe mitral regurgitation and several episodes of pulmonary edema, cardiac failure began to decrease 3 weeks after infarction. Five years later this patient is receiving no cardiac medications, experiences no symptoms, has a normal-sized heart and a soft, short apical systolic murmur. Thus, we believe that the indications for valve replacement in patients with chronic severe mitral regurgitation are the same whether or not the cause is papillary muscle infarction, but the indications for valve replacement during acute infarction need to be defined further.

Role of aortocoronary bypass: The role of concomitant aortocoronary bypass in patients undergoing mitral valve operations for chronic regurgitation due to papillary muscle infarction also needs to be established. Both enthusiastic[35] and discouraging[36] reports of combined operations have appeared. Although the operation might prevent or delay arrhythmic deaths or future infarction, our experience[37] suggests that left ventricular performance is more often adversely affected than improved by bypass operation, a finding of particular relevance in a group of patients whose major problem after mitral valve replacement often is chronic left ventricular failure.

Acknowledgment

We thank Dr. James Bacos, Washington Hospital Center, who performed the preoperative cardiac catheterizations in Cases 8 and 9 and generously allowed us to use the data.

References

1. **Morrow AG, Cohen LS, Roberts WC, et al:** Severe mitral regurgitation following acute myocardial infarction and ruptured papillary muscle. Hemodynamic findings and results of operative treatment in four patients. Circulation 37: suppl II:124–132, 1968
2. **Adicoff A, Alexander CS, Ferguson JN, et al:** Surgical repair of ruptured papillary muscle complicating posterior myocardial infarction. Amer J Cardiol 11:246–252, 1963
3. **Horlick L, Merriman JE, Robinson CLN:** Case of mitral insufficiency following myocardial infarction with rupture of a papillary muscle: improvement following re-attachment of the papillary muscle and plication of the mitral valve. Canad Med Ass J 94:192–195, 1966
4. **Holloway DH Jr, Whalen RE, McIntosh HD:** Systolic murmur developing after myocardial ischemia or infarction. JAMA 191:888–892, 1965
5. **De La Torre A, Linhart JW, Bartley TD:** Mitral valve replacement in a patient with mitral regurgitation secondary to rupture of a papillary muscle. Ann Intern Med 67:387–392, 1967
6. **Shelburne JC, Rubinstein D, Gorlin R:** A re-appraisal of papillary muscle dysfunction. Correlative clinical and angiographic study. Amer J Med 46:862–871, 1969
7. **Bartle SH, Hermann HJ:** Acute mitral regurgitation in man: hemodynamic evidence and observations indicating an early role for the pericardium. Circulation 36:839–851, 1967
8. **Spencer FC, Reppert EH, Stertzer SH:** Surgical treatment of mitral insufficiency secondary to coronary artery disease. Arch Surg (Chicago) 95:853–861, 1967
9. **Bashour RA:** Mitral regurgitation following myocardial infarction: the syndrome of papillary mitral regurgitation. Dis Chest 48:113–122, 1965
10. **Fluck DC, Taubman JO, Cleland WP, et al:** Acute mitral incompetence after acute myocardial infarction, with successful early treatment by mitral valve prosthesis. Lancet 2:1052–1054, 1966
11. **Klughaupt M, Flamm MD, Hancock EW, et al:** Nonrheumatic mitral insufficiency. Determination of operability and prognosis. Circulation 39:307–316, 1969
12. **Berman DA, Grismer JT:** Postmyocardial infarction syndrome followed by left ventricular aneurysm with papillary muscle dysfunction. Amer J Cardiol 25:349–352, 1970
13. **Ronan JA Jr, Steelman RB, De Leon AC Jr, et al:** The clinical diagnosis of acute severe mitral insufficiency. Amer J Cardiol 27:284–290, 1971
14. **Lee KS, Johnson T, Karnegis JN, et al:** Clinical pathologic conference. Amer Heart J 79:258–264, 1970
15. **Schimert G, Lajos TZ, Greene DG, et al:** Surgery for postinfarction complications (abstr). Circulation 38: suppl VI:VI-174, 1968
16. **De Busk RF, Harrison DC:** The clinical spectrum of papillary muscle disease. New Eng J Med 281:1458–1467, 1969
17. **De Busk RF, Kleiger RE, Ebnother CL, et al:** Successful early operation for papillary muscle rupture. Chest 58:175–178, 1970
18. **Austen WG, Sanders CA, Averill JH, et al:** Ruptured papillary muscle: report of a case with successful mitral valve replacement. Circulation 32:597–601, 1965
19. **Austen WG, Sokol DM, De Sanctis RW, et al:** Surgical treatment of papillary muscle rupture complicating myocardial infarction. New Eng J Med 278:1137–1141, 1968
20. Case records of the Massachusetts General Hospital. Case 22–1969. New Eng J Med 280:1228–1236, 1969
21. Case records of the Massachusetts General Hospital. Case 6–1970. New Eng J Med 282:327–335, 1970
22. Case records of the Massachusetts General Hospital. Case 26–1970. New Eng J Med 282:1421–1429, 1970
23. **Reis RL, Hancock WD, Yarbrough JW, et al:** The flexible stent: a new concept in the fabrication of tissue heart valve prostheses. J Thorac Cardiovasc Surg 62:683–689, 1971

24. **Burch GE, De Pasquale NP, Phillips JH:** The syndrome of papillary muscle dysfunction. Amer Heart J 75:399–415, 1968
25. **Heikkila J:** Mitral incompetence complicating acute myocardial infarction. Brit Heart J 29:162–169, 1967
26. **Hamilton GW, Murray JA, Kennedy JW:** Quantitative angiocardiography in ischemic heart disease. The spectrum of abnormal left ventricular function and the role of abnormally contracting segments. Circulation 45:1065–1080, 1972
27. **Rackley CE, Dear HD, Baxley WA, et al:** Left ventricular chamber volume, mass and function in severe coronary artery disease. Circulation 41:605–613, 1970
28. **Glancy DL:** Unpublished data
29. **Steelman RB, White RS, Hill JC, et al:** Midsystolic clicks in arteriosclerotic heart disease: a new facet in the clinical syndrome of papillary muscle dysfunction. Circulation 44:503–515, 1971
30. **Cheng TO:** Late systolic murmur in coronary artery disease. Chest 61:346–356, 1972
31. **Morrow AG, Oldham NH, Elkins RC, et al:** Prosthetic replacement of the mitral valve: preoperative and postoperative clinical and hemodynamic assessments in 100 patients. Circulation 35:962–979, 1967
32. **Winter TQ, Reis RL, Glancy DL, et al:** Current status of the Starr-Edwards cloth-covered prosthetic cardiac valves. Circulation 45: suppl I: 14–24, 1972
33. **Levine FH, Copeland JC, Morrow AG:** Prosthetic replacement of the mitral valve. Continuing assessments in the 100 patients operated upon during 1961–1965. Submitted for publication
34. **Melvin DB, Tecklenberg PL, Hollingsworth JF, et al:** Computer-based analysis of preoperative and postoperative prognostic factors in 100 patients with combined aortic and mitral valve replacement. Circulation; in press
35. **Cheng TO, Bashour T, Adkins, PC:** Acute severe mitral regurgitation from papillary muscle dysfunction in acute myocardial infarction. Successful early surgical treatment by combined mitral valve replacement and aortocoronary saphenous vein bypass graft. Circulation 46:491–497, 1972
36. **Spencer FC, Green GE, Tice DA, et al:** Coronary artery bypass graft for congestive heart failure: a report of experiences with 40 patients. J Thorac Cardiovasc Surg 62:529–542, 1971
37. **Itscoitz SB, Shepherd RL, Glancy DL, et al:** Deterioration o myocardial function following aortocoronary bypass opera tion (abstr). Clin Res 21:427, 1973

Dilatation of the Mitral Anulus

A Rare Cause of Mitral Regurgitation

BERNADINE H. BULKLEY, M.D.*
WILLIAM C. ROBERTS, M.D.
Baltimore, Maryland

To confirm or deny the thesis that mitral anular dilatation is a cause of mitral regurgitation, this anulus was measured in 102 patients, 24 of whom had normal hearts and 78 of whom had dilated left ventricles, some associated with mitral regurgitation, others not. The circumference of the mitral anulus in the 24 patients with normal hearts averaged 9 cm (range 7 to 11 cm); in 24 patients with idiopathic cardiomyopathy of the ventricular dilated type, both with (12 patients) and without (12 patients) mild to moderate regurgitation, 11 cm (range 10 to 14 cm); and in 31 patients with severe mitral regurgitation, 12 cm (range 8 to 18 cm). Among the latter 31 patients with severe mitral regurgitation, the anulus was only mildly dilated in the 15 with rheumatic disease (average 11 cm) and in the six with ruptured chordae tendineae on previously normal valves (average 10 cm); in contrast, in the 10 patients with floppy mitral valves with or without the Marfan syndrome the mitral anulus was greatly dilated (average 15.5 cm). Thus, only in patients with floppy valves with or without the Marfan syndrome or both does anular dilatation by itself appear great enough to cause mitral regurgitation. It appears, therefore, that dilatation of the mitral anulus is a rare cause of mitral regurgitation and that abnormality of the fibrous skeleton of the heart is necessary for the mitral anulus to dilate enough to cause mitral regurgitation.

Although believed for many years to be an important cause of mitral regurgitation, anular dilatation today is considered an infrequent cause. Surprisingly, supportive anatomic evidence for or against this view is lacking. To reexamine this concept, the mitral anulus and other left ventricular dimensions were measured in 102 human hearts, including some with and some without mitral regurgitation.

METHODS AND DESCRIPTION OF PATIENTS STUDIED

From among approximately 2,500 hearts with various cardiovascular conditions on file in the Pathology Laboratory of the National Heart and Lung Institute, 78 recently accessioned hearts (all in patients greater than 14 years of age) with dilated left ventricles were selected for study. Only well

From the Section of Pathology, National Heart & Lung Institute, National Institutes of Health, Bethesda, Maryland 20014. Requests for reprints should be addressed to Dr. William C. Roberts, Bldg. 10A, Rm. 3E30, National Institutes of Health, Bethesda, Maryland 20014. Manuscript accepted January 22, 1975.

* Present address: Department of Medicine, Division of Cardiology, The Johns Hopkins Hospital, Baltimore, Maryland.

preserved hearts in which few histologic sections had been taken, or extraneous cuts made, were utilized. The measurements in each of the 102 hearts were performed separately by each of us.

In addition to measuring the circumferences of the mitral anuli, several other left ventricular dimensions were measured (Figure 1): left ventricular length; the distance from the base of right anterior aortic valve cusp to the apex or the distance from the anulus behind the posterior mitral leaflet to the apex; and left ventricular circumference interiorly, at its base and midway between its base and apex.

The 24 patients with normal hearts ranged in age from 19 to 69 years (average 43 years), and the 78 patients with abnormal hearts, from 15 to 78 years (average 41 years) (Table I). The latter 78 patients were divided into three major groups depending on the presence or absence of mitral regurgitation (Tables II and III): 23 patients without mitral regurgitation; 24 patients with idiopathic cardiomyopathy of the ventricular dilated type [1] who may or may not have had mitral regurgitation; and 31 patients with mitral regurgitation of varying etiology. Cardiac catheterization, including measurement of left ventricular pressures, and left ventricular angiographic studies were performed in 48 of the 78 patients: in 16 of 23 without mitral regurgitation, in three of 24 with cardiomyopathy and in 29 of 31 with mitral regurgitation. None of the 78 patients had stenotic valvular lesions. Aortic regurgitation was present in 14 of the 23 patients without mitral regurgitation, in none of the 24 with cardiomyopathy and in three of the 21 with mitral regurgitation (Table I).

Of the 23 patients without mitral regurgitation, 10 had pure aortic regurgitation of non-Marfan etiology [2] (Figure 2), seven had floppy mitral valves (all incidental necropsy findings because none had had precordial murmurs) [2],

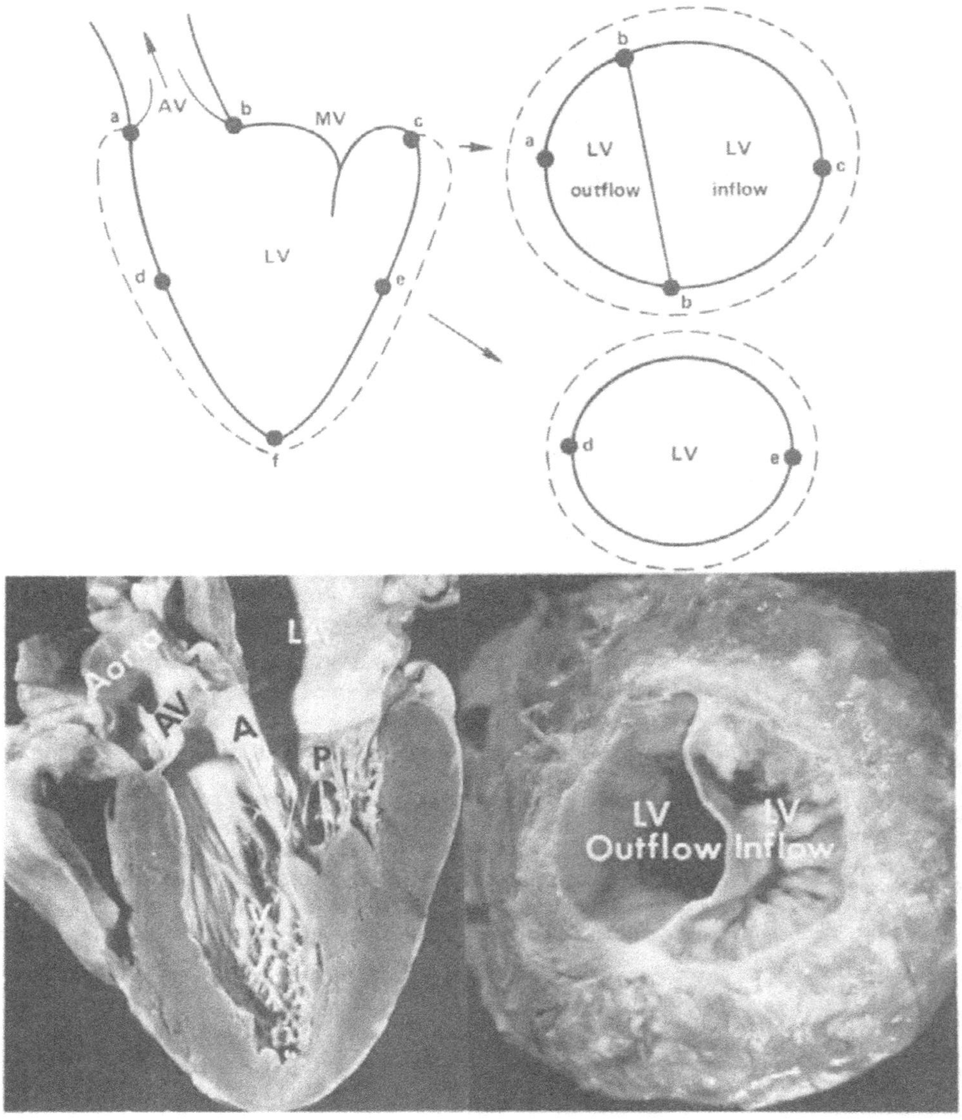

***Figure 1.** Left ventricular dimensions. The upper left diagram is a longitudinal view of the left ventricle, and the specimen itself is shown in the lower left. The upper right diagram is a view of left ventricle (LV) at its base, and the specimen itself after removal of the atria and right ventricle is shown in the lower right. The anterior mitral leaflet (A) divides the left ventricular cavity into inflow and outflow tracts. Measurements were made of the circumferences of the mitral anulus (b to c [upper left]; b to b via c [upper right]). The LV base (a to c through b [upper left]; a back to a via b, c and b [upper right]); the mid-portion of the LV (d to e [upper left]) and the length of LV from base to apex (a to f via d or c to f via e [upper left]).*

and six had the Marfan syndrome [2], five of whom had aortic regurgitation also.

Of the 24 patients with idiopathic cardiomyopathy of the ventricular dilated type (Figure 3), 12 had had precordial murmurs strongly suggestive of mitral regurgitation, and in three of them the mitral regurgitation was confirmed by left ventricular angiography. A precordial murmur was not described in any of the other 12 patients.

The 31 patients with mitral regurgitation included 15 whose mitral regurgitation was of rheumatic etiology (Figure 4), six whose mitral regurgitation was secondary to ruptured chordae tendineae on previously normal valves [3], six whose mitral regurgitation was secondary to floppy or prolapsing mitral leaflets unassociated with the Marfan syndrome (Figure 5) and four whose mitral regurgitation was secondary to floppy mitral leaflets associated with the Marfan syndrome [2]. Mitral regurgitation appears to have been present over many years in the 25 patients with rheumatic, floppy and Marfan etiologies, but for only a

TABLE I Clinical Data on Patients Studied

Patients Studied	No.	Ages (yr) Range	Ages (yr) Average	Male (no.)	Female (no.)	No. with AR	No. with MR
Normal hearts	24	19–69	43	11	13	0	0
Abnormal hearts	78	15–78	41	48	30	17	43
Pure AR	10	39–56	47	9	1	10	0
Floppy	7	18–67	54	3	4	0	0
Marfan	6	21–48	36	5	1	4	0
CM	24	21–66	45	17	7	0	12
Rheumatic	15	16–40	25	3	12	0	15
Ruptured CT	6	20–62	44	2	4	0	6
Floppy	6	41–78	54	5	1	0	6
Marfan	4	15–31	24	4	0	3	4

NOTE: AR = aortic regurg tation; f oppy = floppy mitral valves; CM = cardiomyopathy; CT = chordae tendineae; MR = mitral regurgitation.

TABLE II Left Ventricular Dimensions (cm) and Heart Weights (g) of Patients with and without Mitral Regurgitation

Dimensions	Patients without MR: Normal Hearts (24)	Pure AR (10)	Floppy (7)	Marfan (6)	±MR: CM (24)	Patients with MR: Rheumatic (15)	Ruptured Chordae (6)	Floppy (6)	Marfan (4)
Mitral anulus circ	7–11 (9)*	11–13 (11)	7–13 (12)	9–13 (11)	10–14 (11)	9–13 (11)	8–13 (10)	13–18 (15)	14–17 (16)
LV circ, base	10–12 (11)	12–17 (14)	9–12 (12)	9–14 (12)	12–18 (14)	11–14 (13)	9–16 (12)	13–18 (15)	15–18 (17)
LV circ, mid	9–10 (10)	14–17 (15)	9–10 (11)	12–14 (9)	14–22 (16)	12–15 (14)	11–13 (13)	11–16 (13)	13–20 (16)
LV length	6–10 (7)	9–14 (12)	7–9 (8)	10–11 (11)	9–13 (10)	8–10 (9)	9–10 (9)	7–9 (8)	8–11 (10)
Heart weight (g)	250–350 (300)	680–1,250 (930)	300–650 (505)	520–920 (645)	440–830 (600)	360–675 (500)	400–650 (550)	370–880 (575)	750–850 (800)

NOTE: AR = aortic regurgitation; circ = circumference; Floppy = floppy mitral valve leaflets; CM = idiopathic cardiomyopathy of the ventricular dilated type; LV = left ventricle; MR = mitral regurgation.
* Figures in parentheses in body of table represent the average.

TABLE III Per Cent Changes in Mean Left Ventricular Dimensions and Heart Weights with Dilatation

Dimension	Patients without MR: Normal Hearts (24)	Pure AR (10)	Floppy (7)	Marfan (6)	±MR: CM (24)	Patients with MR: Rheumatic (15)	Fuptured Chordae (6)	Floppy (6)	Marfan (4)
Mitral anulus (% ↑ >9 cm)	0	22	28	22	22	22	11	66	77
LV circ, base (% ↑ >11 cm)	0	27	9	9	27	18	9	36	54
LV circ, mid (% ↑ >10 cm)	0	50	0	10	60	40	30	30	60
LV length (% ↑ >7)	0	64	14	36	43	21	29	14	43
Heart weight (% ↑ 300 g)	0	210	68	115	100	66	83	92	166

NOTE: AR = aortic regurgitation ; circ = circumference; CM = idiopathic cardiomyopathy of the ventricular dilated type; LV = left ventricle; MR = mitral regurgitation.

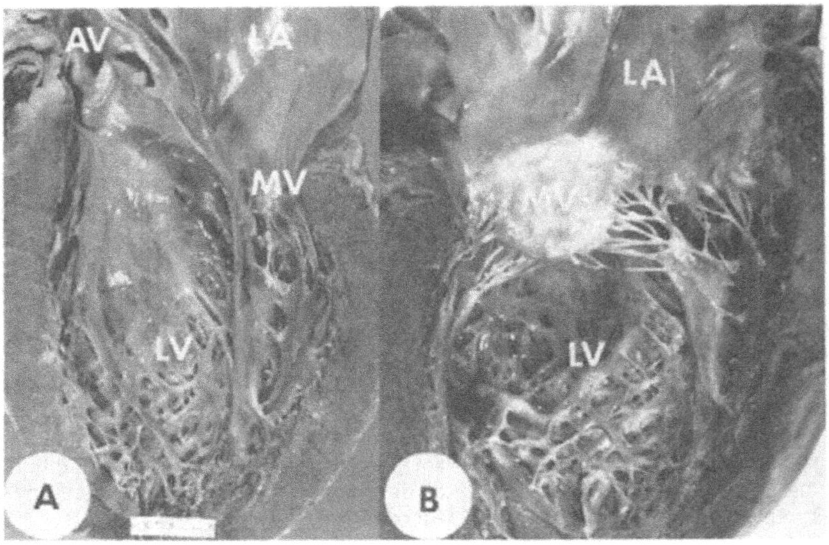

Figure 2. *Heart of a 54 year old man (A68-300) with severe aortic regurgitation associated with ankylosing spondylitis.* ***a,*** *longitudinal view exposing left atrium (LA), mitral valve (MV), left ventricle (LV) and aortic valve (AV). The dilatation is primarily in length rather than in width.* ***b,*** *opened mitral valve; the leaflets and its chordae are normal and the anulus is only mildly dilated.*

few months in the patients with ruptured chordae tendineae.

RESULTS

The mean circumferences of the mitral anuli in all 78 patients with dilated left ventricles were increased: in the 23 patients without mitral regurgitation, in the 24 patients with cardiomyopathy with or without mitral regurgitation and in the 21 patients with mitral regurgitation secondary to rheumatic or ruptured chordal origin the mean mitral anular circumferences ranged from 10 to 12 cm or from 11 to 28 per cent above the normal mean mitral anular circumference of 9 cm (Tables II and III). In the 10 patients with mitral regurgitation secondary to floppy mitral valves (unassociated with the Marfan syndrome in six and with the Marfan syndrome in four), however, the circumferences of the mitral anuli were greatly dilated, averaging 15 and 16 cm, respectively, each more than 65 per cent above the normal circumference of 9 cm. The differences between the anuli less than 30 per cent dilated and those more than 65 per cent dilated, and the differences between the normal and dilated mitral anuli are significant ($p < 0.001$).

The per cent increase in the left ventricular dimensions in the various conditions over the normal also are summarized in Table III. All left ventricular dimensions increased with cavity dilatation. The mid-cir-

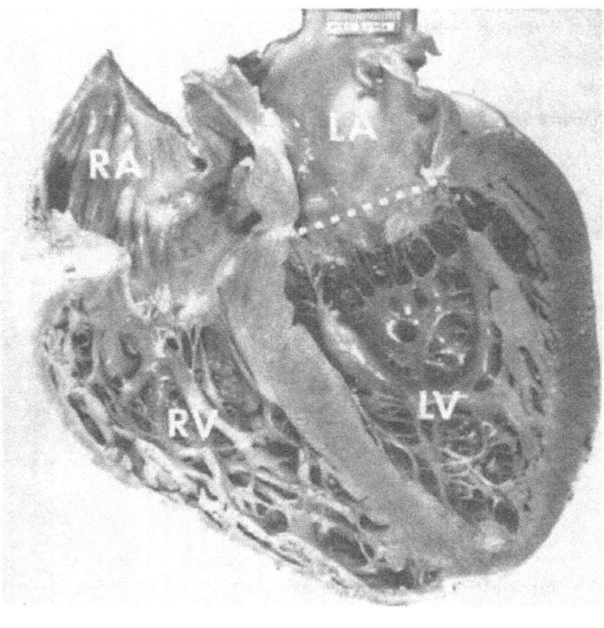

Figure 3. *Longitudinal section of heart of a 22 year old woman (DCGH No. 73A-2) with fatal idiopathic cardiomyopathy of the ventricular dilated type. The mid-left ventricular (LV) circumference is considerably larger than its basal circumference which includes the mitral anulus (dashed line). A precordial murmur suggestive of mitral regurgitation had been audible. RA = right atrium; LA = left atrium; RV = right ventricle.*

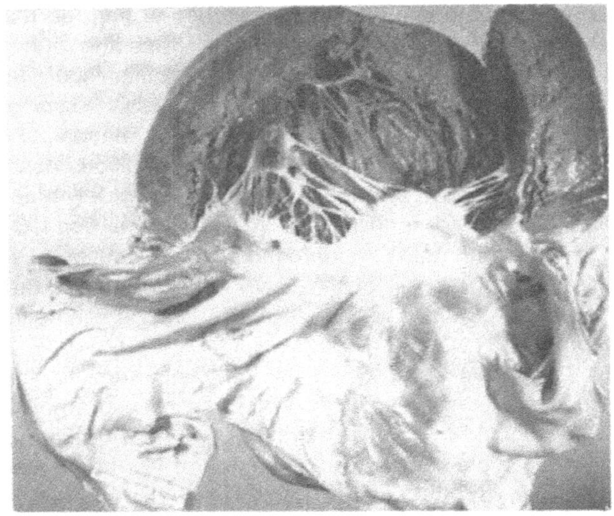

Figure 4. Opened left side of heart in a 43 year old man (A67-178) with severe mitral regurgitation of presumed rheumatic etiology. Both left atrium and left ventricle are dilated. A jet lesion is present in the left atrial wall posteriorly. The mitral anulus measured only 12.0 cm in circumference despite severe regurgitation of long duration.

cumference increased the most, and next, the length. With the exception of the patients with ventricular dilatation associated with floppy mitral valves (with or without the Marfan syndrome), the circumference of the mitral anulus was the least affected. In these patients, the dilatation of the mitral anulus was proportionately greater than the enlargement of the other left ventricular dimensions.

The left ventricular base usually dilated in proportion to the mitral anulus. Exceptions to this were the patients with floppy mitral valves (with or without the Marfan syndrome); in them, the mitral anuli were proportionately more dilated than their ventricular bases, irrespective of whether or not mitral regurgitation was present.

The weights of the hearts (Tables II and III) did not correlate with the degree of mitral anular dilatation. Patients with aortic regurgitation had the largest hearts, and they had only a mild (less than 30 per cent) increase in the circumference of the mitral anulus unless the aortic regurgitation was associated with the Marfan syndrome.

COMMENTS

The measurements delineated clearly indicate that mitral anular dilatation is an uncommon cause of mitral regurgitation. How the belief that anular dilatation was a common cause of mitral regurgitation originated is unclear. In 1870, Flint [4] wrote: "mitral insufficiency may also be due to enlargement of the mitral orifice in connection with dilatation of the left ventricle." This view was supported by Osler [5]. In 1908, Mackenzie [6] described "functional" mitral regurgitation due to "dilatation of the orifice from depression of the tonicity of the muscle supporting the valves." Levine [7] described "relative" mitral regurgitation due to ventricular cavity dilatation in all five editions of his book from 1936 to 1958. In his last edition, he stated that the "left ventricular cavity is enlarged or dilated, and in this process of dilatation

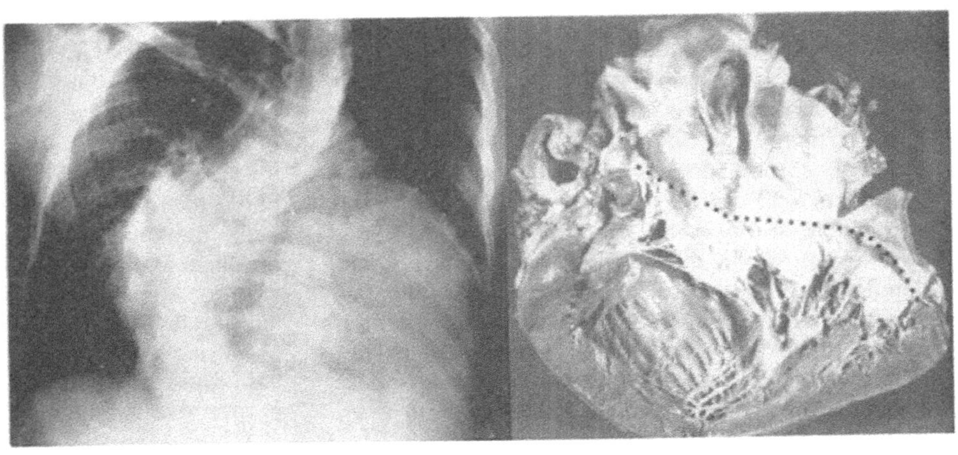

*Figure 5. Shown here is the chest roentgenogram **(left)** and opened left side of the heart **(right)** of a 28 year old man (A63-25) with the Marfan syndrome associated with kyphoscoliosis and pectus excavatum. He died of severe congestive cardiac failure due to mitral regurgitation; he did not have aortic regurgitation. The mitral valve is floppy and its anulus is enormously dilated (17 cm in circumference).*

the mitral ring is sufficiently stretched so that normal leaflets can no longer completely close the orifice during ventricular systole and there results regurgitation of blood" [7]. In the New York Heart Association's 1964 nomenclature and criteria manual, the occurrence of mitral regurgitation in conditions associated with left ventricular hypertrophy or dilatation was attributed to dilatation of the mitral ring [8]. Other recent texts of cardiology have continued to describe stretching of the valve ring as an important cause of "functional" or "relative" mitral regurgitation [9–13].

There were, however, some dissenters to this concept. On the basis of necropsy measurements, Cabot in 1926 [14] deemed the concept of anular dilatation's causing mitral regurgitation as unprovable because many patients had dilated mitral anuli at necropsy but no signs of mitral regurgitation during life, and conversely, patients with murmurs of mitral regurgitation during life had normal sized mitral anuli at necropsy. In 1931, White [15] suggested that "displacement downwards of the papillary muscles as a result of the ventricular dilatation is a more important factor in causing mitral regurgitation than is dilatation of the . . . valve ring." During the past decade the importance of papillary muscle dysfunction as a cause of mitral regurgitation has been stressed in many reports [16–21]; these reports, mainly by implication, have tended to deemphasize dilatation of the anulus as a possible cause of mitral regurgitation. Nevertheless, dimensional studies of the mitral anulus and left ventricular cavity have been lacking.

Our study demonstrates that the mitral anulus dilates whenever the left ventricle dilates (from any cause), but that anular dilatation, with few exceptions, is not sufficient by itself to cause mitral regurgitation. The circumference of the mitral anulus in our patients was increased up to 30 per cent above normal by cavity dilatation alone, irrespective of the etiology of the dilatation, irrespective of whether or not mitral regurgitation was present and irrespective of the increase in muscle mass (heart weight). Anular dilatation of mild degree (less than 30 per cent above normal) was related solely to the occurrence of left ventricular dilatation and not to the occurence of mitral regurgitation. The degree of anular dilatation was mild (11 to 28 per cent above normal) and similar in the patients with dilated left ventricles without mitral regurgitation, in those with dilated left ventricles and either absent or only mild to moderate mitral regurgitation and in the patients with severe mitral regurgitation secondary to rheumatic disease or to ruptured chordae tendineae on previously normal valves. The only patients with severely dilated anuli were those with mitral regurgitation secondary to floppy or prolapsing mitral valves with or without the Marfan syndrome. In them, the mean mitral anular dilatation was more than 65 per cent above normal. In the patients with floppy mitral valves but without mitral regurgitation, however, anular dilatation was less than 30 per cent above normal.

Examination of other left ventricular dimensions after dilatation indicates that the greatest enlargement occurs not at its base, which includes the mitral anulus, but at its mid-portion, between the apex and base. The base of the left ventricle is prevented from dilating freely because of its attached fibrous skeleton; its mid-portion, in contrast, is not restricted by any fibrous structure. The mid-left ventricle in our patients with idiopathic cardiomegaly of the ventricular dilated type was three times more dilated than the mitral anulus, and proportionately more enlarged than the length of the left ventricle. In this cardiomyopathy, the spatial relationships between the papillary muscles and the mitral leaflets consequently are distorted, primarily by lateral movement of the left ventricular wall, and the latter probably accounts for the mitral regurgitation in these patients [19–21].

In our patients with dilated left ventricles due to aortic regurgitation alone, both the mid-circumference and the basal-to-apex length of the left ventricle were equally enlarged, and the papillary muscles were displaced both caudally and laterally. In the patients with mitral regurgitation due to floppy valves with or without the Marfan syndrome, the fibrous skeleton of the heart did not restrict the base of the left ventricle, including the mitral anulus, from dilating even more than the mid-portion. In patients with the Marfan syndrome, an underlying connective tissue defect may account for the lax fibrous skeleton. A similar defect may be present in the mitral anulus of patients with floppy valves unassociated with other signs of the Marfan syndrome.

A frequent examination at necropsy is measurement of the circumferences of cardiac valve anuli. This practice appears to have been recommended initially in 1897 by Mallory and Wright [22], who believed that "inspection and measurement of the valve after the heart had been opened will usually enable one to judge fairly accurately concerning the degree of competence." So great was their authority that the convenient method they recommended soon came to be standard [23]. Our present study, however, demonstrates that measuring circumferences of mitral anuli is rarely helpful in predicting the presence or absence of mitral competence. The "unrolling" technic at necropsy which includes the incising of valve rings is not ideal because it distorts the spatial relations of intracardiac structures and prevents proper examination of the intact three-dimensional valve. Thus, at necropsy, emphasis should be placed on study of the intact valve, and not on study of the opened valve, a procedure most often done solely for the purpose of measuring valve anuli [24].

REFERENCES

1. Roberts WC, Ferrans VJ: Pathological aspects of certain cardiomyopathies. Circ Res 34, 35 (suppl): II-128, 1974.
2. Roberts WC, Dangel JC, Bulkley BH: Nonrheumatic valvular cardiac disease: clinicopathologic survey of 27 different conditions causing valvular dysfunction. Cardiovasc Clin 5: 333, 1973.
3. Roberts WC, Braunwald E, Morrow AG: Acute severe mitral regurgitation secondary to ruptured chordae tendineae. Clinical, hemodynamic, and pathologic considerations. Circulation 33: 58, 1966.
4. Flint A: A Practical Treatise on the Diagnosis, Pathogenesis and Treatment of Diseases of the Heart, Philadelphia, Henry C. Lea, 1870, p 134.
5. Osler W: The Principles and Practice of Medicine, New York, D. Appelton & Co., 1895, p 645.
6. Mackenzie J: Diseases of the Heart, London, Oxford University Press, 1914, p 334.
7. Levine SA: Clinical Heart Disease, Philadelphia, W. B. Saunders, 1958, p 317.
8. Kossmann CE, Chasis H, Connor Car, De La Chapelle CE, Foley WT, Harvey RM, Maynard EP Jr, Schwedel JB: Diseases of the Heart and Blood Vessels, Nomenclature and Criteria for Diagnosis, 6th ed., Boston, 1964, p 103.
9. Evans W: Diseases of the Heart and Arteries, Baltimore, Williams & Wilkins Co., 1964, p. 370.
10. Friedberg CK: Diseases of the Heart, 3rd ed., Philadelphia, W. B. Saunders, 1966, p 1030.
11. Leonard JC, Galea EG: A Guide to Cardiology, Edinburgh and London, E. & S. Livingstone,1966, p 200.
12. Somerville W, et al: Paul Wood's Diseases of the Heart and Circulation, 3rd ed., Philadelphia, J. B. Lippincott Co., 1968, p 602.
13. Oram S: Clinical Heart Disease, London, William Heinemann Medical Books Ltd., 1971, p 343.
14. Cabot RC: Facts on the Heart, Philadelphia, W. B. Saunders, 1926, p 291.
15. White PD: Heart Disease, New York, MacMillan Co., 1931, p 485.
16. Mc Kusick VA: Cardiovascular Sounds in Health and Disease, Baltimore, Williams & Wilkins Co., 1958, p 314.
17. Burch GE, De Pasquale ND, Phillips JH: Clinical manifestations of papillary muscle dysfunction. Arch Intern Med 112: 112, 1963.
18. Phillips JH, Burch GE, De Pasquale NP: The syndrome of papillary muscle dysfunction. Its clinical recognition. Ann Intern Med 59: 508, 1963.
19. Roberts WC, Perloff JK: Mitral valvular disease. A clinicopathologic survey of the conditions causing the mitral valve to function abnormally. Ann Intern Med 77: 939, 1972.
20. Roberts WC, Cohen LS: Left ventricular papillary muscles. Description of the normal and a survey of conditions causing them to be abnormal. Circulation 46: 138, 1972.
21. Perloff JK, Roberts WC: The mitral apparatus. Functional anatomy of mitral regurgitation. Circulation 46: 227, 1972.
22. Mallory FB, Wright JH: Pathological Technique: A Practical Histology and Bacteriology, Including Directions for the Performance of Autopsies and for Clinical Diagnosis by Laboratory Methods, Philadelphia, W. B. Saunders, 1897.
23. Chapman CB: On the study of the heart. A comment on autopsy techniques. Arch Intern Med 113: 318, 1964.
24. Roberts WC: Examining the precordium and the heart. Chest 57: 567, 1970.

THE MALFUNCTIONING MITRAL VALVE: MORPHOLOGIC FEATURES

WILLIAM C. ROBERTS, M.D.

From the Section of Pathology, National Heart and Lung Institute, National Institutes of Health, Bethesda, Maryland 20014.

This presentation will describe the structure of the normal and the malfunctioning mitral valve. The leaflets of the normal mitral valve during ventricular systole contact one another over a broad area and not just at their margins. During ventricular diastole blood enters the left ventricle not only through the valve's primary orifice but also it flows between the various chordae tendineae. Thus, fusion of chordae eliminates interchordal space through which blood can flow. The anterior mitral leaflet is continuous with the aortic valve cusps and the wall of ascending aorta. Each of the 2 left ventricular papillary muscles receives half their chordae from the anterior leaflet and the other half from the posterior leaflet. The posterior mitral leaflet is simply an extension of the mural endocardium of left atrium. The anterior leaflet, however, is not an extension of the endocardium of the atrial septum. The basal to margin distance of the anterior mitral leaflet is considerably greater than that of the posterior leaflet; the actual surface area of the posterior and anterior leaflets, however, is similar. There are about 60 chordae tendineae, from each papillary muscle, which actually contact the valve leaflets, and they arise from about 12 chordae that insert onto a papillary muscle. There are about 6 "heads" on each papillary muscle, and from each head an average of 2 chordae arise.

Of the various fatal valvular lesions, excluding papillary muscle dysfunction, the most frequent is stenosis, followed by pure regurgitation, followed by the mixed valvular lesions, i.e., more than one valve functions abnormal and one malfunctioning valve is stenotic and another is purely incompetent. The most common stenotic lesion is aortic stenosis, followed by mitral stenosis, and then comes combined aortic and mitral stenosis. The most common purely incompetent valve lesion observed at necropsy is aortic regurgitation followed by mitral regurgitation.

Now to *mitral stenosis.* This lesion is more often isolated than associated with another valvular lesion. Most stenotic mitral valves also have elements of regurgitation. There are, for practical purposes, only 2 etiologies of mitral stenosis, namely, rheumatic and congenital. The evidence that mitral stenosis is usually (>99%) rheumatic in origin is indirect because Aschoff bodies, the only direct evidence of rheumatic heart disease, is found in only about 5% of necropsy patients with mitral stenosis. The degree of obstruction in rheumatic mitral stenosis is determined primarily by the degree of shortening and fusion of the chordae tendineae: the shorter the chordae and the greater the fusion of the chordae, the tighter the stenosis. All chordae may be fused together in the most obstructed mitral valve. The stenotic mitral valves in men tend to contain more calcific deposits than do stenotic mitral valves in women. Thrombi may occur in the left atrial appendage in any patient with poor cardiac output (increased residual intracardiac blood and therefore increased stasis) but thrombi occur in the *body* of left atrium only in patients with mitral stenosis, nearly always of severe severity.

Now to *mitral regurgitation,* the fifth most common of the nine major combinations of valve dysfunction or 10% of all fatal valve disease (excluding papillary muscle dysfunction). In contrast to mitral stenosis which has only 2 causes, pure mitral regurgitation has many causes. Its most common cause in the absence of ischemic heart disease and idiopathic cardiomyopathy of the ventricular dilated type is the *prolapsing mitral valve syndrome.* The process probably starts only with a systolic click(s) followed later by a late systolic murmur. As the prolapse worsens, combined with progressive dilatation of the mitral anulus, the click disappears and the murmur becomes pansystolic rather than just late systolic in time. The click and/or late systolic murmur is a benign condition (with extremely rare exception) and consequently little anatomic information is available on the status of the mitral valve in this situation. I have studied at necropsy 3 patients with a click and/or click plus late systolic murmur and none during life had symptoms of cardiac dysfunction. Each, a girl, aged 9, 13 and 17 years, respectively, died of cancer. The child with 3 clicks and no murmur had 3 areas of leaflet overlap involving the posterior leaflet but no space between the 2 leaflets during simulated ventricular systole. The 13-year-old girl had multiple "scallops" involving both leaflets and small openings for regurgitation between the scallops. The 17-year-old girl had a similar valve but the margins were thickened, and the chordae focally shortened and fused. The scallops represent excessive leaflet tissue simulating an accor dion partially compressed. The prolapsing mitral (and tricuspid valve also) may occur in patients with the Marfan syndrome or forme fruste varieties of it. The prolapsing valve may be present at birth or acquired later in life. It may well be one of the natural consequences of aging, the result of the old-age contracture of the left ventricle without similar contracture of the mitral leaflets which are pushed back toward the left atrium by the small "senile" left ventricle. The mitral valve, as do all valves, consists of 2 major components: the fibrosa and the spongiosa. The fibrosa element is the one that proliferates in most valvular diseases. In patients with floppy valves the fibrosa element does not appear to proliferate; it is the spongiosa element and this component contains a great deal of acid mucopolysaccharide (AMP) material in it. The result, therefore, is excessive AMP material in these valves but there is no evidence that the AMP which is present is degenerated. "AMP degeneration," however, has been one of the morphologic terms to describe the floppy valve.

Certain complications of the prolapsing mitral valve are well known. Probably most prolapsing mitral valves observed at necropsy had been competent during life. Thus, regurgitation is a complication of "floppiness" and not an integral part of this condition. Other definite complications of this condition include infective endocarditis and calcification of the mitral anulus. Other less well appreciated complications include rupture of chordae tendineae unassociated with infection ("spontaneous"), and rupture or perforation of a cusp. The morphology of the sudden death, electrocardiographic changes, arrhythmias, and chest pain in this condition is unknown.

Now to another cause of mitral regurgitation, *infective endocarditis*, which usually causes sudden rupture of chordae tendineae and acute mitral regurgitation. It is the previously normal chorda that tends to rupture, not the thick short one of mitral stenosis. When the normal chorda suddenly ruptures, massive mitral regurgitation is the usual result and because the left atrium cannot distend acutely, the left ventricular pressure is not "absorbed" by the left atrium but reflected into the pulmonary vessels with rapid development of severe pulmonary hypertension. The syndrome of small left atrium and high left atrial pressure due to sudden development of mitral regurgitation may be contrasted to the extreme of the chronic form of mitral regurgitation characterized by a giant-sized left atrial cavity and normal left atrial pressures. Here the left atrial "bag" is capable of absorbing the left ventricular pressure and consequently pulmonary hypertension does not develop. The latter situation occurs predominantly in the patient with rheumatic heart disease. These giant atria are devoid of thrombi in their bodies.

Now to rheumatic mitral regurgitation. It is infrequent, in my experience, to observe in adults at necropsy pure mitral regurgitation, i.e., no element whatsoever of stenosis, on a rheumatic basis. This is not the case in children. The valve with thick chordae and diffusely thickened mitral leaflets, the one considered to be of rheumatic type, is rarely purely incompetent. It usually has some element of obstruction across it.

There has been much discussion through the years of so-called functional mitral regurgitation, that is, the left ventricular cavity dilates and the mitral anulus dilates resulting in regurgitation. The concept of anular dilatation as a cause of mitral regurgitation, however, is not supported by facts. Indeed, anular dilation of up to 30% may occur in nearly any condition associated with left ventricular dilatation but this much anular dilatation does not produce mitral regurgitation. The latter occurs as a result of anular dilatation only when the anulus is greater than 60% dilated, and in my experience, that has occurred only in patients with floppy mitral valves. On the other hand, the tricuspid valve dilates preferentially when the right ventricular cavity dilates, and consequently tricuspid anular dilatation is the most common cause of tricuspid valve regurgitation.

Now to *calcification of the mitral anulus*. The study by Korn and associates at the Massachusetts General Hospital about 15 years ago disclosed that all of their 14 patients with "massive" mitral anular calcification were old women. If all degrees of mitral anular calcification are lumped together, however, the sex ratio is similar ,but those with the largest amounts of anular calcium do indeed tend to be women. About 75% of patients with mitral anular calcification also have calcific deposits in the aortic valve cusps and 100% of them have calcific deposits at necropsy in the coronary arteries. Certain conditions clearly predispose to mitral anular calcification: these include any condition which raises the left ventricular systolic pressure, namely, systemic hypertension, valvular aortic stenosis, and hypertrophic obstructive cardiomyopathy. Diabetes mellitus, floppy mitral valves, and hpyercalcemia also predispose to mitral anular calcification. The mechanism of development of mitral regurgitation in patients with mitral anular calcification is uncertain, but the amount or regurgitation from this mechanism is never more than mild.

Mitral valve "anular" calcium forming a complete circle or "O" configuration: Clinical and necropsy observations

Attention is called to the occurrence of a complete circle or "O"-shaped ring of calcium at the mitral anular region in each of two women, aged 67 and 82 years. Extension of mitral anular calcium from behind the posterior mitral leaflet across the ventricular aspect of the anterior mitral leaflet to form a complete circle has not been reported previously. (Am Heart J 101:619, 1981.)

William C. Roberts, M.D., and Bruce F. Waller, M.D. *Bethesda, Md.*

Calcification of the mitral anulus is a common occurrence in hearts of older persons in the Western World. The anular calcific deposits on radiographs generally are "J," "C," or "U"-shaped because they are located nearly always entirely in or below the anulus of the posterior mitral leaflet. Recently, we encountered two patients in whom calcific deposits not only were located in and beneath the anulus of the *posterior* mitral leaflet, but they extended across the ventricular aspect of the *anterior* leaflet to form a complete calcific circle or "O." Because we have not encountered this "O" configuration in over 200 other patients with mitral anular calcium studied at necropsy in our laboratory[1] and because we have found no reports by others describing a complete circumferential calcific ring at the site of the mitral "anulus," a brief description of the clinical and morphologic findings in our two patients appeared warranted.

From the Pathology Branch, National Heart, Lung and Blood Institute, National Institutes of Health.

Received for publication Jan. 7, 1981; accepted Jan. 29, 1981.

Reprint requests: Dr. William C. Roberts, Bldg. 10A, Room 3E30, National Institutes of Health, Bethesda, MD 20205.

METHODS AND RESULTS

Pertinent clinical and morphologic features in the two patients are summarized in Table I. Both were older women who died of noncardiovascular conditions. Both had precordial murmurs consistent with mitral regurgitation and one had a murmur of aortic stenosis. Neither patient had chest pain consistent with myocardial ischemia and neither had evidence of congestive cardiac failure. One had systemic hypertension, diabetes mellitus (adult onset), and chronic atrial fibrillation. Chest radiographs (Fig. 1) in each disclosed heavy mitral anular calcific deposits.

At necropsy, the hearts of both were mildly increased in weight. Neither had dilated cardiac ventricles, but both had dilated atria. One had severe (> 75% in cross-sectional area) narrowing of all three major epicardial coronary arteries by atherosclerotic plaques. The mitral "anular" circular calcium in each is shown in Figs. 2 and 3. Patient No. 2 also had calcific deposits in the aortic valve cusps to an extent to produce aortic valve stenosis. Both also had relatively heavy calcific deposits in the aorta, arch and abdominal portions. Patient No. 1 had a small transmural left ventricular scar.

DISCUSSION

Extension of calcium from the anulus of the posterior mitral leaflet across the ventricular aspect

Table I. Clinical and morphologic findings in patients with circle "O" mitral anular calcium

Pt.	*Age (yrs)*	*Associated disease*	*Murmurs* *MR*	*AS*	*SH*	*DM*	*AF*	*Cause of death*	*Heart wt. (gm)*	*Calcium (0-4+)* *AV*	*CA*	*Ao*	*AS*	*CA > 75%*
1	67	Habitual alcoholism	3/6	0	+	+	+	Werniche's encephalopathy	390	0	2+	3+	0	+
2	82	Paget's, bone	3/6	2/6	0	0	0	Caecal volvulus	400	3+	2+	2+	+	0

Abbreviations: AF = atrial fibrillation; Ao = aorta; AS = aortic valve stenosis; AV = aortic valve; CA = coronary arteries; DM = diabetes mellitus; MR = mitral regurgitation; SH = systemic hypertension.

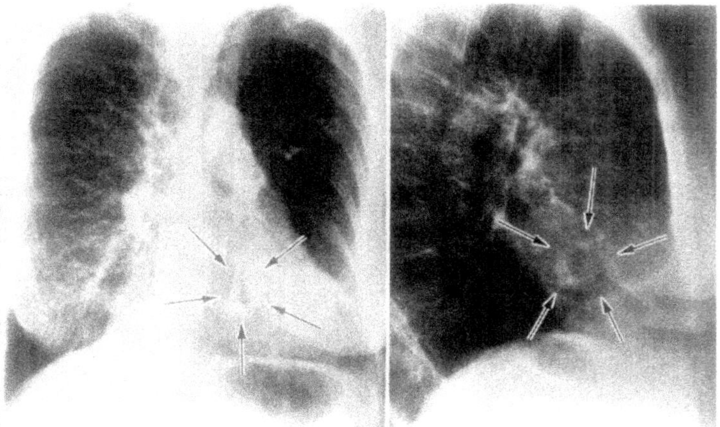

Fig. 1. Patient No. 1. Posteroanterior *(left)* and lateral *(right)* radiographs showing mitral anular calcium forming a complete circle *(arrows)*.

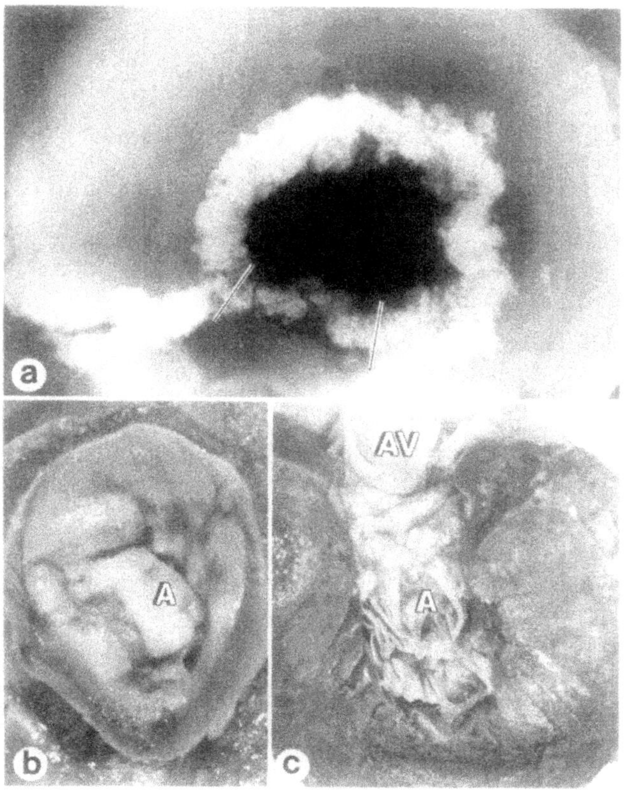

Fig. 2. Patient No. 1. Heart at necropsy. *a,* Radiograph of the heart specimen showing complete circle of "anular" calcium. The short distance between the lines designates the width of the anterior mitral leaflet. *b,* View of mitral valve from left atrium. *A* = anterior mitral leaflet. *c,* Opened left ventricular outflow tract and aortic valve *(AV)* showing calcium extending across the anterior *(A)* mitral leaflet.

of the *anterior* mitral leaflet to form a complete circle of calcium has not been reported previously to our knowledge. The stimulus to its extension across the anterior leaflet is unknown. It should be recalled that the anterior mitral leaflet does not have a true anulus because its ventricular aspect is continuous with the wall of the aorta and the aortic valve cusps and its atrial aspect is continuous with the mural endocardium of the atrial septum. The posterior mitral leaflet, in contrast, represents in effect the caudal extension of the mural endocardium of the entire free wall of left atrium. The site where the posterior mitral leaflet meets mural endocardium of left atrial free wall is the mitral anulus.

Calcium rarely is limited, however, to just the anulus, or if it were it would not be visible by radiography during life. Radiographically visible anular calcium in actuality is located primarily beneath the anulus, in the angle between posterior mitral leaflet and mural endocardium of left ventricle. The linear bar of calcium which extended across the anterior mitral leaflet in our two patients was located only on the ventricular aspect of the leaflet and at a level caudal to the anulus behind the posterior mitral leaflet. Thus because the anterior leaflet lacks a true anulus and because the calcium attached to it was located caudal to that behind posterior mitral leaflet, it is actually improper to designate the bar of calcium extending across anterior leaflet as "anular," although for convenience and to prevent confusion with leaflet calcium observed in patients with rheumatic mitral stenosis, calcium extending across the anterior leaflet and

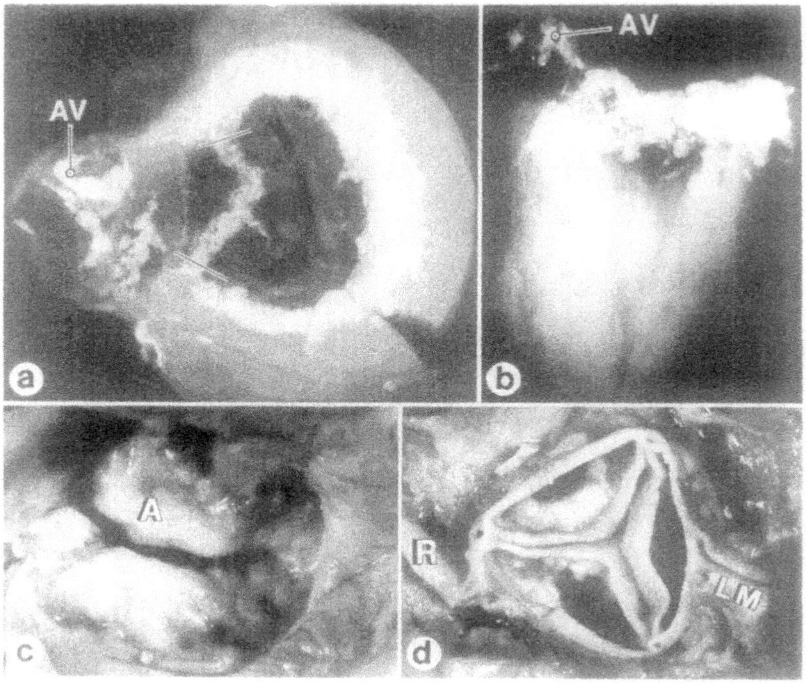

Fig. 3. Patient No. 2. Heart at necropsy. *a,* Radiograph of heart specimen. The short bar of calcium *between the lines* is that extending across the anterior mitral leaflet. Calcific deposits also are present in the aortic valve *(A V)* cusps and in coronary arterial atherosclerotic plaques. *b,* Radiograph of heart, lateral view, showing massive mitral anular calcific deposits. *c,* Mitral valve from left atrium. *A* = anterior mitral leaflet. *d,* Aortic valve from above showing calcific deposits on the aortic aspects of each of the three cusps. *R* = right and *LM* = left main coronary artery.

continuous with that in the angle behind posterior mitral leaflet might, nevertheless, be considered "anular."

Despite the circumferential nature of the mitral calcific deposits in our two patients, neither had functional (diastolic apical murmur or evidence of pulmonary venous or arterial hypertension) or anatomic evidence of mitral stenosis.

REFERENCE

1. Roberts WC, Perloff JK: Mitral valvular disease. A clinicopathologic survey of the conditions causing the mitral valve to function abnormally. Ann Intern Med **77**:939, 1972.

Etiology of clinically isolated, severe, chronic, pure mitral regurgitation: Analysis of 97 patients over 30 years of age having mitral valve replacement

Bruce F. Waller, M.D.,* Andrew G. Morrow, M.D., Barry J. Maron, M.D.,
Albert A. Del Negro, M.D., Kenneth M. Kent, M.D., Francis J. McGrath, M.D.,
Robert B. Wallace, M.D., Charles L. McIntosh, M.D., and William C. Roberts, M.D.
Bethesda, Md., and Washington, D.C.

For many years rheumatic heart disease was considered the major cause of mitral regurgitation (MR) severe enough to necessitate mitral valve replacement (MVR). In most past studies of patients with mitral valvular disease, patients were subdivided on the basis of predominant mitral stenosis (MS) or predominant MR. This type of subdivision, however, does not provide as much information about etiology as can be obtained by dividing patients with mitral valve dysfunction into two groups based on the presence or absence of mitral valve obstruction. MS of any degree is recognized as usually having a rheumatic etiology. Likewise, most patients who have combined dysfunction of both mitral and aortic valves usually have a rheumatic etiology of their valvular lesions. The present study examines the etiology of the valvular disease in 97 patients over the age of 30 years in whom MVR was carried out for severe, chronic, pure MR unassociated with MS or aortic valve dysfunction.

PATIENTS STUDIED AND METHODOLOGY

Operatively excised mitral valves accessioned in the Pathology Branch, National Heart, Lung, and Blood Institute from July, 1968, through December, 1981, were reexamined and those which on anatomic grounds were purely regurgitant or possibly purely regurgitant were selected. The medical records including results of cardiac catheterization and angiographic procedures were then reviewed and the anatomic diagnosis of a purely regurgitant valve was substantiated by preoperative studies or the case was excluded. In addition to excluding patients with associated MS or aortic valve dysfunction, patients with intracardiac shunts or hypertrophic cardiomyopathy also were excluded.

After the exclusions noted, the study group comprised 97 patients (Table I). All fulfilled the following criteria: (1) severe (3+ or 4+/4+) MR by left ventricular (LV) angiography; (2) mean diastolic pressure gradient between left atrium (LA) (or pulmonary arterial wedge position) and LV of 2 mm Hg or less and no gradient at end-diastole between LA and LV; (3) no dysfunction (either stenosis or regurgitation or both) of the aortic valve; (4) age greater than 15 years (all patients were older than 30 years); and (5) clinical evidence of congestive heart failure (CHF) for 2 months or longer. Hereafter, the patients included in this study will be referred to as having *pure* MR, a word to signify the absence of associated MS, and *isolated* MR, a word to signify the absence of associated aortic valve stenosis or regurgitation.

The *circumference* (in centimeters) and *area* (in centimeters squared) of each excised mitral valve were determined in all 97 patients: the circumference, by measuring the length of the anulus of the excised mitral leaflets, and the area, by outlining the basal and distal margins of the leaflets on paper after opening the valve and then measuring the resulting area by videoplanimetry[1] (Fig. 1).

Criteria for etiologic subgrouping— Rheumatic. Both

From the Pathology, Surgery, and Cardiology Branches, National Heart, Lung and Blood Institute, National Institutes of Health; and the Departments of Medicine (Cardiology) and Surgery, Georgetown University Medical Center.

Received for publication Feb. 23, 1982; accepted March 2, 1982.

Reprint requests: William C. Roberts, M.D., Pathology Branch, NIH-NHLBI, Bldg. 10A, Room 3E-30, Bethesda, MD 20205.

*Present address: Department of Pathology, Indiana University Medical Center, Indianapolis, IN 46223.

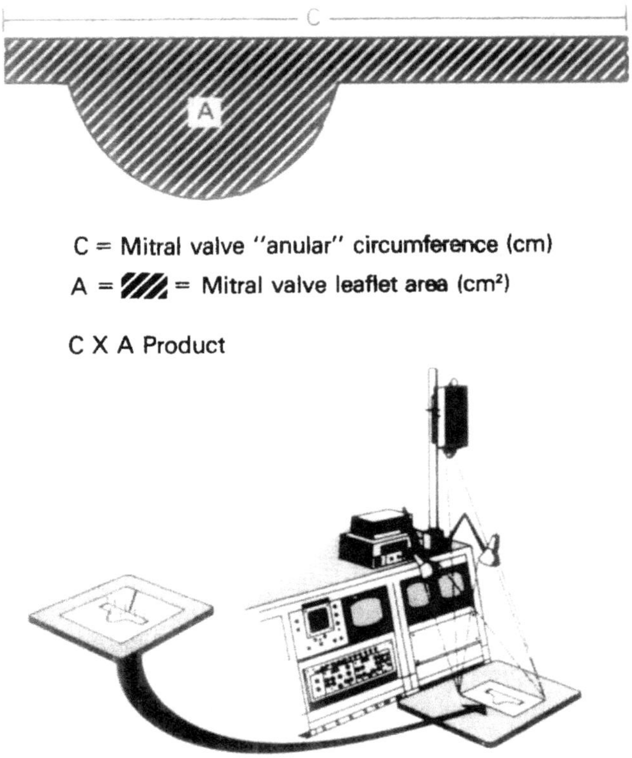

Fig. 1. Schematic drawing of opened operatively excised mitral valve showing methods of measuring the circumference and area. The videoplanimetry method of measuring leaflet area is shown in the lower drawing.

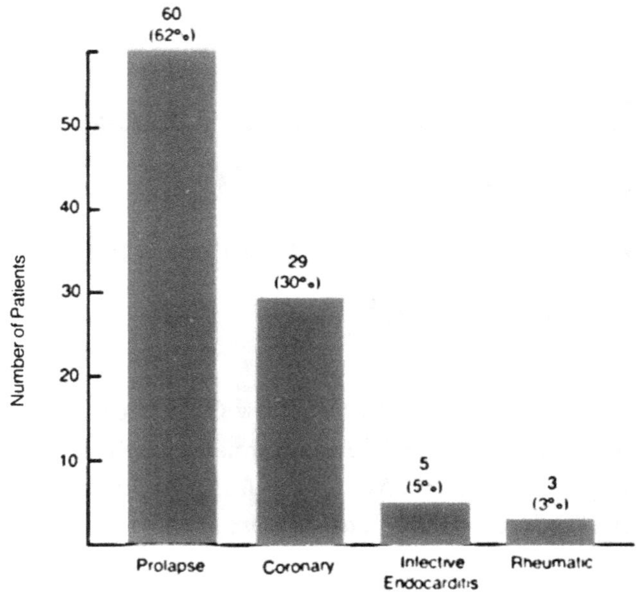

Fig. 2. Bar graph showing the four conditions causing chronic, isolated, pure, mitral regurgitation in the 97 patients with operatively excised valves.

mitral leaflets were diffusely thickened by fibrous tissue. The chordae tendineae may or may not have been abnormal.[2] Although the papillary muscles may have been focally scarred, neither was transmurally scarred. The mitral leaflet area was less than 12 cm^2 and the anular circumference was equal to or less than 11 cm.

Healed infective endocarditis on previously normal values. The major portion of leaflet and most chordae were normal. Several chordae, however, attached to one or both leaflets were absent or ruptured and the adjacent leaflet was thickened by fibrous tissue and a portion was either missing (indentation) or one or more perforations were present in one leaflet. The mitral leaflet area was less than 12 cm^2 and the mitral anular circumference was equal to or less than 11 cm.

Coronary heart disease with papillary muscle dysfunction. The mitral leaflets and chordae tendineae were either normal or only slightly and focally thickened. No leaflet indentation or perforations or ruptured or absent chordae tendineae were present. The mitral leaflet area was less than 12 cm^2 and the mitral circumference less than or equal to 11.5 cm. One or both papillary muscles were extensively scarred and usually atrophied.

Mitral valve prolapse with intact chordae tendineae. These valves had leaflet areas greater than 11 cm^2 and anular circumferences greater than 11 cm. The distance from basal attachment to distal margin in the posterior leaflet was not uniform in that one or more segments were elongated compared to other segments. No leaflet perforations or indentations were present and all chordae tendineae were intact.

Mitral valve prolapse with ruptured (or absent) chordae tendineae. These valves had focal thickening of one or both leaflets at sites of rupture of several chordae tendineae. Additionally, leaflet indentations or perforations were present. These values differed from those classified as "ruptured chordae tendineae on previously normal valves" by the presence of one or more elongated posterior leaflet segments as observed in the patients with mitral valve prolapse with intact chordae tendineae. Usually also the leaflet area and anular circumference were increased but neither was essential for classification in this subgroup.

OBSERVATIONS

Anatomic findings. Gross examinations of the 97 mitral valves revealed that the etiology of regurgita-

Table I. Certain clinical observations in 97 patients undergoing mitral valve replacement for isolated, severe, pure mitral regurgitation from various conditions

	Mitral valve prolapse (MVP)			
Item	*With RCT (n = 13)*	*Without RCT (n = 47)*	*Subtotal (n = 60)*	*Coronary (n = 29)*[d]
1. Age (yr) at MVR	46-71 (57)	36-73 (55)	36-73 (55)	39-78 (56)
2. Men: Women	7(54%):6(46%)	22(47%):25(53%)	29(48%):31(52%)*	23(73%):6(27%)*
3. History of ARF	0	5 (11%)	5 (8%)	0
4. History of IE	4[a]	0	4 (7%)	0
5. History of AMI	0	2 (4%)	2 (3%)*	24 (83%)*
6. Angina pectoris	0	0	0[b]	19 (66%)
7. Systolic click(s)	0[c]	0	0	0
8. Duration (yr) MR, m	2-20 (8)	2-22 (9.5)	2-22 (9)	1-6 (4)
9. Duration (mo) CHF	6-24 (16)*	4-60 (31)*	4-60 (25)	10-36 (20)
10. Atrial fibrillation	0	4 (8%)	4 (7%)*	7 (24%)*
11. Abnormal Q waves on ECG	0	4 (8%)	4 (7%)*	29*
12. Total cholesterol (mg/dl) No. patients	4	25	25	13
Values (range [mean])	195-243 (221)	177-263 (234)	177-263 (228)*	242-305 (277)*
13. MVP by E only/total No. E	3/11	16/32 (50%)	19/43 (44%)	2/22 (9%)
14. MVP by A only/total No. A	0/13	3/47 (6%)	3/60 (5%)	0/29
15. MVP by both E and A/total No. with both E + A	3/11	10/32 (31%)	13/43 (30%)	0/22
16. Pressures (mm Hg)				
PAW: range (avg)				
a	10-18 (15)	9-20 (14)	9-20 (14)	10-16 (15)
v	18-48 (35)	16-42 (32)	16-48 (33)	13-34 (26)
mean	16-24 (19)	12-24 (18)	12-24 (18)	14-24 (19)
LV: range (avg)				
systolic	115-168 (149)	120-165 (131)	115-168 (137)	120-165 (146)
diastolic	16-24 (25)	12-24 (18)	12-24 (18)	14-24 (19)
SA: range (avg)				
systolic	115-168 (149)	120-165 (131)	115-168 (137)	120-165 (146)
diastolic	70-88 (81)	84-90 (83)	70-90 (82)	70-90 (86)
17. Direct systolic SAP > 140 or diastolic SAP > 90 mm Hg	11 (85%)*	11 (23%)*	22 (37%)	9 (31%)
18. One or more major CA narrowed > 50% in D by A/total No. A	0/1	3[g]/22 (14%)	3[g]/23 (13%)	29/29 (100%)

—*(horizontal only) = $p < 0.05$.
The four patients with MVP and RCT with a history of active IE were included in the prolapse group rather than in the IE group because MV function was bnormal before the active IE.
Three patients had chest pain not judged to be angina pectoris unassociated with AMI.
One patient had a systolic click and a late systolic murmur about 4 months before developing active IE murmur but the precordial murmur became olosystolic and the click disappeared.
Of 29 patients, 28 (97%) had MVR with aortocoronary bypass grafting and one (3%) had MVR with LV aneurysmectomy. Only 1 of the 29 had neither ngina pectoris nor past evidence of AMI.
Iealed in all.
One patient with opiate abuse was treated for active IE 15 months before MVR. Both anterior and posterior MV leaflets were diffusely thickened by fibrous ssue, indicating underlying rheumatic mitral disease.
Only the right coronary artery was narrowed in each patient, only one of whom had chest pain which was nonanginal in type.
bbreviations: A = angiogram; ARF = acute rheumatic fever; AMI = acute myocardial infarction; CA = coronary arteries; CHF = congestive heart failure; = diameter; E = echocardiogram; ECG = electrocardiogram; IE = infective endocarditis; LV = left ventricular; m = precordial murmur; mo = months; IR = mitral regurgitation; MVR = mitral valve replacement; PAW = pulmonary arterial wedge; RCT = ruptured chordae tendineae; SA = systemic artery; AP = systemic artery pressure; yr = years.

on was leaflet prolapse in 60 patients (62%); 13 of nese 60 valves had ruptured chordae tendineae Fig. 2) while in the other 47 the chordae were intact Figs. 3, 4, and 5). In 29 patients (30%), the MR esulted from papillary muscle dysfunction secondary to coronary heart disease; neither the chordae nor papillary muscles were ruptured (Figs. 2 and 6). In five patients (5%) the regurgitation occurred after infective endocarditis involving an apparently normal mitral valve, and in all five patients the

Infective endocarditis (n = 5)[c]	*Rheumatic (n = 3)*	*Totals (n = 97)*
33-56 (42)	32,35,52, (40)	32-78 (54)
3:2	2:1	57(59%):40(41%)
0	2	7 (7%)
4	1[f]	9 (9%)
0	0	26 (27%)
0	0	19 (20%)
0	0	0
0.8-1.8(1.3)	1.3,14,20(12)	1-22 (10)
3-5 (3.8)	1.3,4,5(3.4)	2-60 (23)
1	1	13 (13%)
0	0	33 (34%)
4	3	49 (51%)
224-226 (241)	226,232,243(234)	177-305(248)
0/5	0/2	21/72 (29%)
0/5	0/3	3/97 (3%)
0/5	0/2	13/72 (18%)
10-14 (12)	-,10,27 (19)	9-27 (14)
18-36 (32)	21,24,40 (28)	16-48 (31)
16-18 (17)	10,18,27 (18)	12-27 (18)
140-155 (147)	130,145,160(145)	115-168 (143)
16-18 (17)	10,18,27 (18)	12-27 (18)
140-155 (147)	130,145,160(145)	115-168 (143)
75-90 (79)	70,78,85 (78)	70-90 (83)
4	2	37 (38%)
0/1	-/0	32/53 (60%)

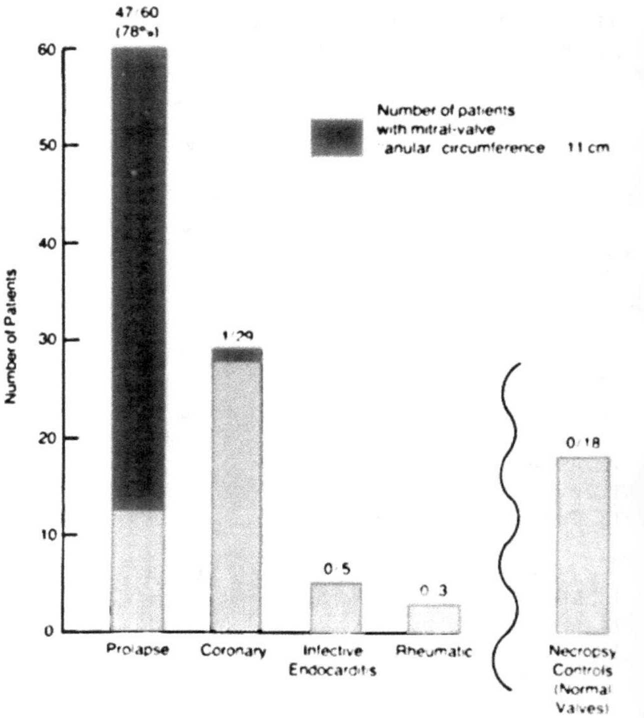

Fig. 3. Bar graph showing the frequency of mitral valve "anular" circumference of greater than 11 cm in the four conditions causing chronic, isolated, pure, mitral regurgitation in the 97 patients with operatively excised valves. The normal mitral valves used as controls were excised from hearts of 18 necropsy patients who had no cardiac abnormalities. The frequency of men and women and age range was similar in the control and study patients.

chordae were ruptured (Figs. 2 and 7). The remaining three patients had MR as the result of rheumatic heart disease (Figs. 2 and 8).

Anular circumference. The circumferences of the mitral anuli measured in the 18 control patients without heart disease ranged from 8.0 to 10.5 cm (average 9.4) (Table II, Fig. 9). Anular circumferences were not significantly different in the valves rendered regurgitant by coronary heart disease, infective endocarditis, rheumatic fever, or in prolapsed valves with ruptured chordae (Figs. 10 and 11). The anular circumferences of the prolapsed valves without chordae rupture were significantly larger than those of all other groups.

Leaflet area. In the 18 control patients, the areas of the excised leaflets ranged from 7.0 to 12.5 cm^2 (average 9.5) (Table II, Fig. 12). In 59 of the 60 patients with mitral valve prolapse, the leaflet area was greater than 11.0 cm^2; in the remaining patient the area was 10.6 cm^2. In the patients with prolapse and ruptured chordae the leaflet areas were 10.6 to 18.4 cm^2 and averaged 14.3 cm^2. In those with prolapse and intact chordae, the leaflet areas ranged from 11.7 to 27.5 cm^2 (average 18.3). The leaflet areas of both groups of prolapsed valves were significantly larger than the valves rendered incompetent by coronary heart disease, infective endocarditis, or rheumatic heart disease (Fig. 12).

Product of valve circumference and area. The product of the circumference (in centimeters) times the area (in centimeters squared) calculated for the normal valves ranged from 45 to 140 cm^3 (average 91) (Fig. 13). The average product was 150 cm^3 in the prolapsed valves with ruptured chordae, and much larger, 273 cm^3, in the prolapsed valves with intact chordae (Table II). The products were 87, 93, and 106 cm^3, respectively, in the valves regurgitant because of papillary muscle dysfunction, infective endocarditis, or rheumatic disease, and these proc

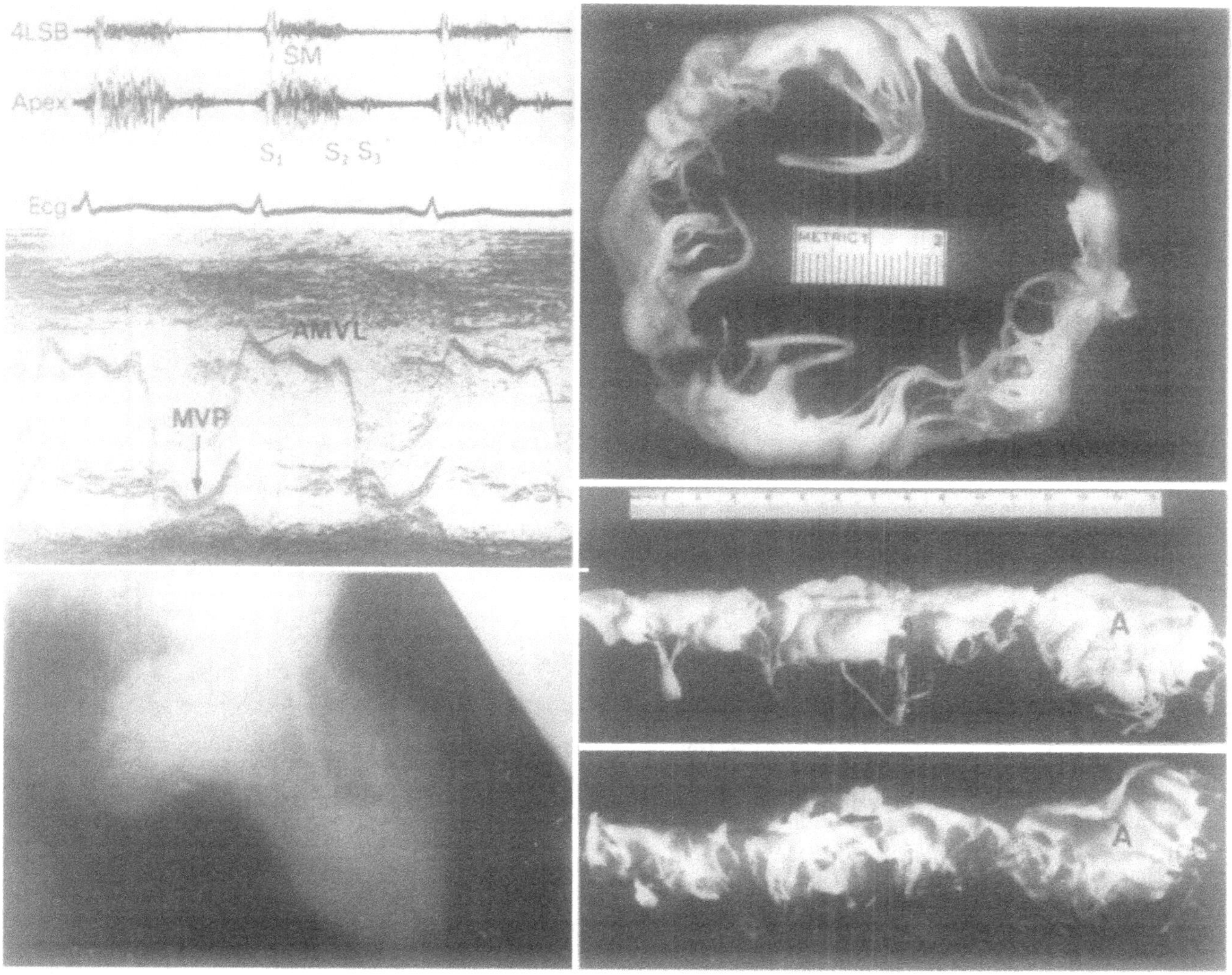

Fig. 4. Preoperative data and operatively excised mitral valve from a 51-year-old woman (S80-33) with *mitral valve prolapse* causing severe, isolated, pure mitral regurgitation. *Left upper,* Phonocardiogram recorded at the fourth left sternal border *(LSB)* and apex showing a holosystolic murmur *(SM)* and third heart sound *(S_3)*. *Ecg* = electrocardiogram; S_1 and S_2 = *first and second heart sounds. Left middle,* Echocardiogram of anterior *(A)* and posterior mitral valve leaflets *(MVL)* showing prolapse *(MVP)* during ventricular systole. *Left lower,* Frame from left ventricular angiogram showing mitral valve prolapse. *Right upper,* Operatively excised mitral valve with an "anular" circumference of 17 cm. *Right middle,* Opened mitral valve showing areas of focal fibrous thickening and an elongated posterior leaflet. *A* = anterior leaflet. *Right lower,* Postmortem radiogram showing focal and minimal calcific deposits *(between arrows)*.

ucts did not differ from those of the normal valves (Fig. 13).

COMMENTS

The cause of the pure MR in these 97 patients was determined by examination of the operatively excised mitral valves, but the correct etiology of the MR was usually predictable from the *history alone.* Of the 29 patients with papillary muscle dysfunction from atherosclerotic coronary heart disease, all have clinical evidence of myocardial ischemia: history of acute myocardial infarction which had healed in 24, a LV aneurysm from a silent infarction in one, and angina pectoris in four. Of the five patients found to have MR secondary to infective endocarditis, four had well-documented episodes of infection, which had been cured by antibiotic therapy, and none had evidence of valvular dysfunction before the episode of infective endocarditis. Of the three patients with MR secondary to a clinical rheumatic etiology, two

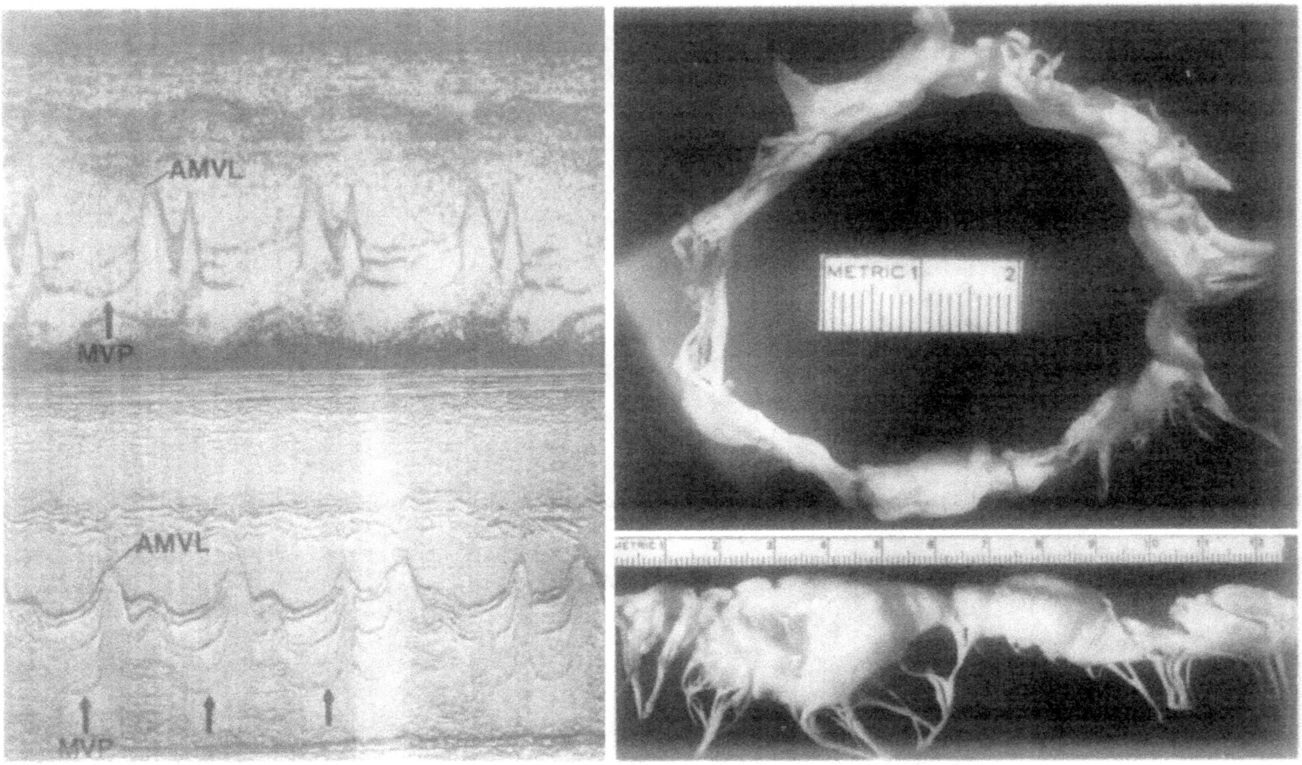

Fig. 5. Operatively excised mitral valve from a 52-year-old man (S80-17) with *mitral valve prolapse* causing chronic, severe, isolated, pure mitral regurgitation. *Left upper,* Echocardiogram of the anterior *(A)* and posterior mitral valve leaflets *(MVL)* obtained 7 years before operation showing prolapse *(MVP)*. *Left lower,* Echocardiogram obtained 2 months before operation showing more severe mitral valve prolapse *(arrows)*. *Right upper,* Operatively excised mitral valve showing a dilated "anular" circumference measuring 12.5 cm. *Right lower,* Opened mitral valve showing areas of focal fibrous thickening.

had a history of acute rheumatic fever, whereas this item was positive in only five of the other 94 patients. Clinical diagnosis of mitral valve prolapse was by a process of exclusion. Only two (3%) of these 60 patients had historical evidence of previous acute myocardial infarction; five (11%) had histories of acute rheumatic fever, and four (7%) had histories of active infective endocarditis. Compared to the five patients classified as having ruptured chordae tendineae on previously normal valves (four of whom had histories of infective endocarditis), the four patients with healed infective endocarditis and mitral prolapse were older (mean age 61 years vs 42 years), had previous systolic murmurs of MR before the episode of infective endocarditis (four of four vs none of five), and had a longer mean duration of CHF (11 months vs 4 months). Thus, of the 60 patients with prolapse, 51 (85%) had no historical evidence of myocardial ischemia, acute rheumatic fever, or infective endocarditis.

The etiology of the MR also was suggested preoperatively by more objective means. The *electrocardiogram* was most useful in delineating the patients with MR secondary to coronary heart disease. Of these 29 patients, all had abnormal Q waves whereas abnormal Q waves were present in only 4 of the 60 patients with mitral valve prolapse, and in none of the eight patients in whom the regurgitation resulted from either infective endocarditis or rheumatic disease. Atrial fibrillation was significantly ($P < 0.05$) more frequent in the patients in whom the MR resulted from coronary heart disease. It was present in seven (24%) of these 29 patients whereas it occurred in only four (7%) of the 60 patients with mitral valve prolapse and in two of the eight patients with either infective endocarditis or a rheumatic etiology.

The *M-mode echocardiogram* was helpful in delineating the patients in whom the MR resulted from mitral valve prolapse. Of the 60 patients with mitral valve prolapse, 43 had an M-mode echocardiogram performed and in 32 (74%) of them it

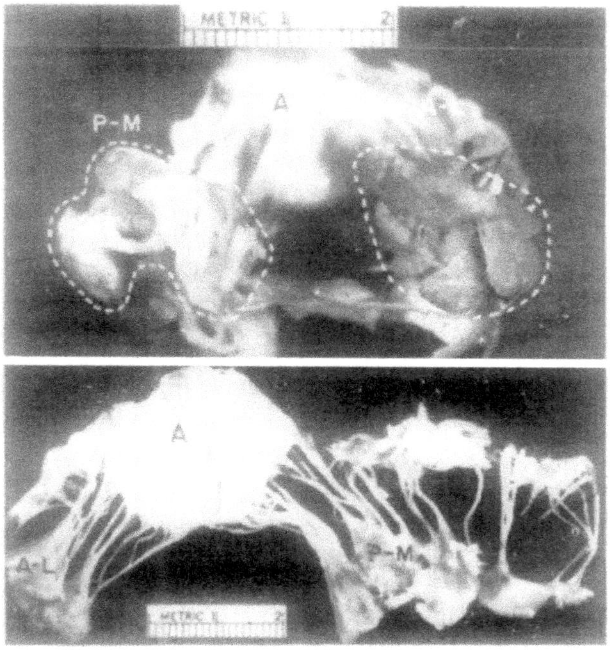

Fig. 6. Operatively excised mitral valve from a 53-year-old man who had chronic, pure mitral regurgitation from *papillary muscle dysfunction secondary to coronary heart disease. Upper,* Photography of cut surfaces of portions of the anterolateral *(A-L)* and posteromedial *(P-M)* papillary muscle showing extensive scarring of the P-M papillary muscle. *A* = anterior leaflet. *Lower,* Opened mitral valve showing anatomically normal leaflets and "anular" circumference of 7 cm.

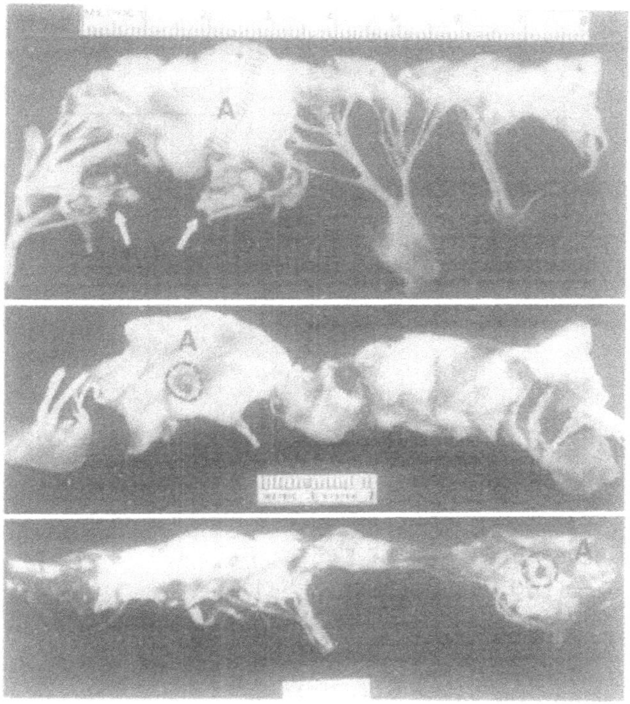

Fig. 7. Operatively excised mitral valves from three patients with chronic, isolated, pure mitral regurgitation from *healed infective endocarditis* occurring on previously anatomically and functionallly normal valves. *Upper,* Valve from a 32-year-old man (S80-131) showing a focally thickened anterior *(A)* leaflet with ruptured chordae tendineae *(arrows). Middle,* Valve from a 48-year-old man (S74-54) showing a perforation *(dashed circle)* in the anterior leaflet. *Lower,* Valve from a 42-year-old man (S79-38) showing a perforation *(dashed circle)* in the anterior leaflet.

indicated the presence of mitral prolapse. In contrast, of the 29 patients with MR secondary to coronary heart disease, M-mode echocardiograms were done in 22 and only two (9%) indicated the presence of mitral prolapse. M-mode echocardiograms were performed in seven of the eight patients with infective endocarditis and rheumatic etiologies and in none of them was mitral prolapse present by this procedure.

Left ventriculograms were performed in all 97 patients. Mitral prolapse was present by this procedure in 16 (27%) of the 60 patients in whom the MR was caused by mitral valve prolapse and in none of the other 37 patients with coronary or infective endocarditis or rheumatic etiologies.

Selective coronary angiograms were performed in 53 (55%) patients. All 29 with MR secondary to coronary heart disease had significant (> 50% diameter reduction) coronary narrowing demonstrated angiographically and 24 of them had evidence of past acute myocardial infarction and the others had other clinical evidences of myocardial ischemia. In 23 (38%) of the 60 patients with mitral valve prolapse coronary angiograms were performed and three (13%) had significant coronary narrowing, limited in each to one (right) coronary artery. In contrast, all 29 patients with MR from papillary muscle dysfunction had two or three of the three major coronary systems with significant narrowing.

Auscultation and hemodynamics at *cardiac catheterization* were not helpful in delineating the etiology of the MR. None of the 97 patients—including the 60 classified as mitral valve prolapse—had systolic clicks on precordial examination, and the systolic precordial murmurs in all 97 patients were holosystolic immediately before MVR. The average pulmonary arterial, LA (or pulmonary arterial wedge), and LV pressures were similar in all four etiologic groups. The systolic systemic arterial pressures, however, were significantly higher in the patients with mitral valve prolapse and ruptured chordae tendineae than in those with mitral valve prolapse with intact chordae tendineae.

Table II. Morphologic observations of operatively excised mitral valves in 97 patients with isolated, pure mitral regurgitation and in 18 normal necropsy valves

	Mitral valve prolapse						
Mitral valve observation	*With RCT (n = 13)*	*Without RCT (n = 47)*	*Subtotals (n = 60)*	*Coronary (n = 29)*	*Infective endocarditis (n = 5)*	*Rheumatic (n = 3)*	*Necropsy controls (n = 18)*
Circumference (C)(cm)	9.5-11.0 (10.5)†	11.5-19.5 (14.8)‡	9.5-19.5 (13.4)‡	8.0-11.5 (9.7)†	9.0-10.5 (9.7)†	9.5,10.5,11.0 (10.5)†	8.0-10.5 (9.4)†
Leaflet area (A) (cm^2)	10.6-18.4 (14.3)†	11.7-27.5 (18.3)‡	10.6-27.5 (16.8)‡	5.5-11.1 (8.9)*	9.2-10.6 (9.7)*	9.5,10.2,10.6 (10.1)*	7.0-12.5 (9.5)*
C x A product (cm^3)	111-225 (150)†	128-536 (273)§	111-536 (268)§	45-112 (87)*	87-111 (93)*	90,112,116 (106)*	45-140 (91)*
No. with C > 11 cm	0	13	47	1	0	0	0
No. with ruptured chordae tendineae (RCT)	13	0	13	0	5	0	0
No. with calcific deposits	0	3[a]	3[a]	0	0	1	0

[a]Primarily in the mitral valve anulus.
—, †—†,§—§(horizontal) = p = ns.
‡—‡(horizontal) = $p < 0.05$.
*—†, *—‡, †—‡, †—§ (horizontal) = $p < 0.01$.

Table III. Summary of causes of mitral regurgitation in 230 patients reported by Selzer and Katayama (Medicine 51:337, 1972)

Etiology	*No. (%) pts.*	*Ages (yr) range (mean)*	*MV op*	*No. without or only mild symptoms of CD*	*Probable no. with MS*	*AF*	*M:F*
1. Rheumatic	88[a] (38)	< 10-> 60 (43)	61	22	42[b]	50 (57%)[c]	26:62 (29%):(71%)
2. Rupture chordae tendineae[d]	44 (19)	21-> 60 (~ 55)	31	11	0	10 (23%)	36:8 (82%):(18%)
3. Late systolic murmur with or without click	28[e] (12)	17-72 (~ 40)	0	28	0	0	10:18 (35%):(65%)
4. Coronary (Post-myocardial infarct)	26 (11)	40-70 (~ 55)	11	2	0	2 (8%)	23:3 (88%):(12%)
5. Congenital[f]	23 (10)	1-56 (-)	11	0	0	4	11:12 (48%):(52%)
6. Infective endocarditis[g]	11 (5)	30-72 (-)	7	3	0	1	7:4
7. Miscellaneous	10[h] (5)	10-64 (45)	4[i]	4	0	1	0:10
Totals	230 (100)	1-72[j] (-)	125 (54%)	70 (30%)	0	68 (30%)	113:117 (49%):(51%)

[a]The MR in eight was attributed entirely to infective endocarditis. Probably several of them had previous mitral stenosis.
[b]Five patients had MR only after mitral valve commissurotomy for mitral stenosis. Of the 61 having mitral valve operations, 20 had calcific deposits on the valve observed at operation. Of the 27 patients not undergoing mitral valve operations, 13 appear to have had calcific deposits on the mitral valve observed radiographically. Probably at least four of the eight with infective endocarditis had previous mitral stenosis.
[c]Of the 61 patients having mitral valve operation, 46 (75%) had atrial fibrillation. Thus, only four (15%) of the 27 without mitral valve operations had atrial fibrillation.
[d]Defined by three characteristics: (1) sudden onset, (2) selective involvement of chordae supporting the posterior leaflet, and (3) a normal mitral valve except for the localized loss of chordal support. Ten of the 44 patients with isolated chordae rupture had mitral valve prolapse by LV angiogram.
[e]All were asymptomatic.
[f]Precordial murmur before age 3. At least two had associated atrial septal defect. Most had more than one congenital cardiovascular anomaly. Thirteen were under 18 years of age.
[g]None had previous evidence of cardiac disease.
[h]Of the 10, at least four had prolapsed mitral valves, two had left atrial myxomas, and in the other four clinical clues suggesting the proper cause were absent and operations were not performed.
[i]Two additional patients had left atrial myxomas excised.
[j]This is a minimal age, possibly older.
Abbreviations: AF = atrial fibrillation; CD = cardiac dysfunction; F = female; M = male; MS = mitral stenosis; MV = mitral valve; op = operation; pts = patients; yr = years.

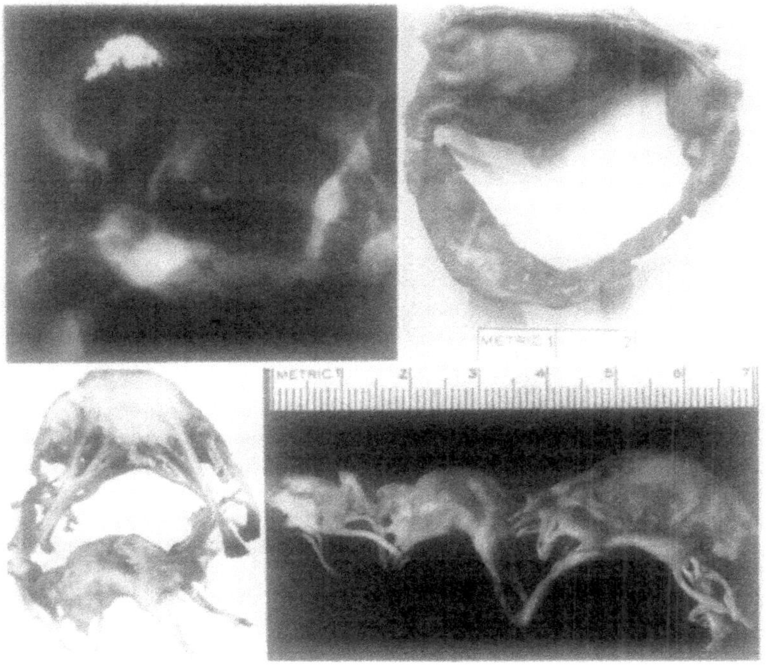

Fig. 8. Operatively excised mitral valves from two patients with chronic, isolated, pure mitral regurgitation from *rheumatic heart disease. Upper left,* Postmortem radiogram of the excised mitral valve from a 35-year-old man (S75-5148) showing focal and minimal calcific deposits. *Upper right,* Valve from the patient showing diffuse fibrous thickening of the anterior and posterior leaflets with an "anular" circumference of 11 cm. *Lower left,* Excised mitral valve from a 52-year-old woman (S78-8). *Lower right,* View of opened valve from the same patient showing diffuse fibrous thickening of both leaflets and a circumference of 7 cm.

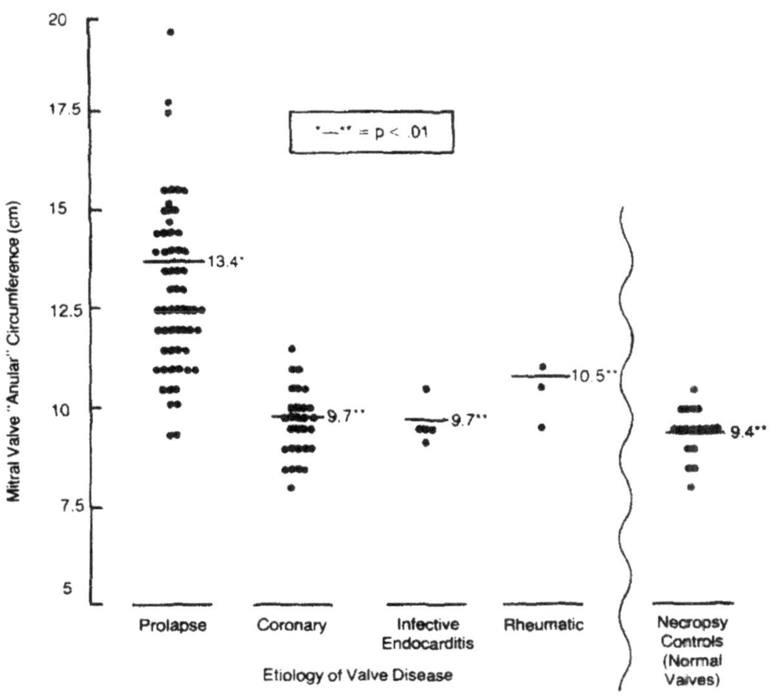

Fig. 9. Graph showing mitral valve "anular" circumference (in cm) in each of the 97 patients with operatively excised mitral valves in the four conditions causing chronic, isolated, pure mitral regurgitation, and in 18 necropsy control valves.

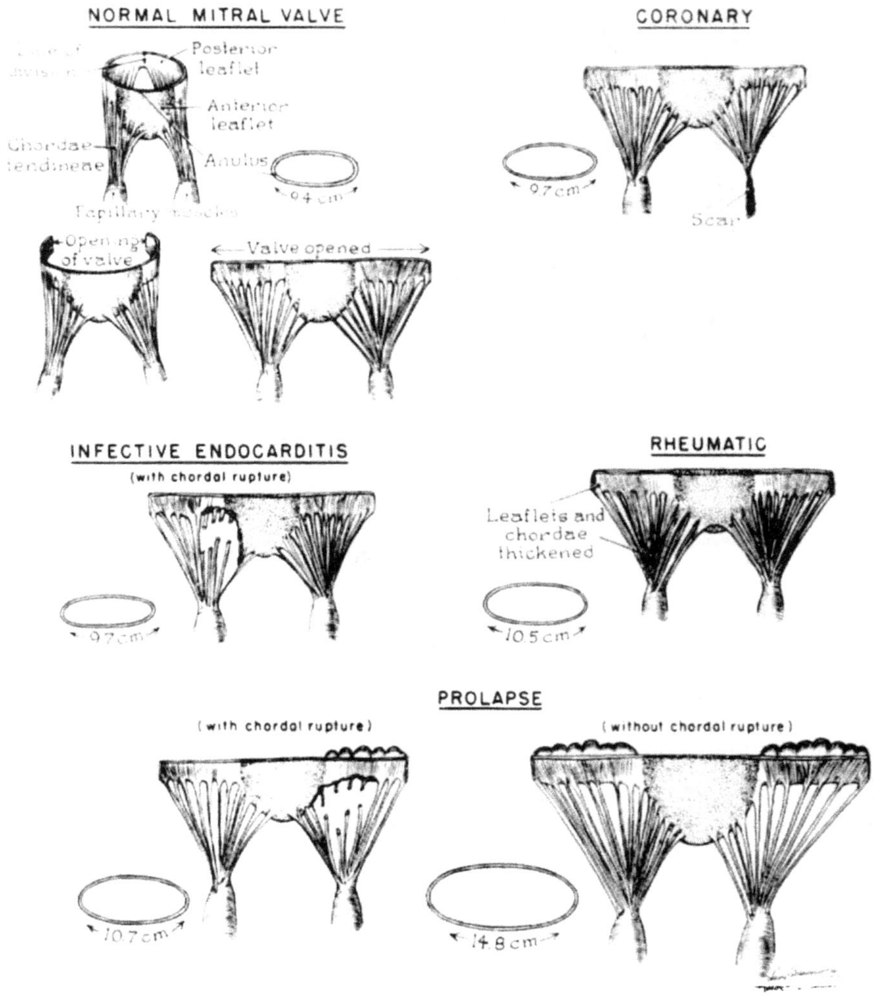

Fig. 10. Diagram showing morphologic variations in mitral valve "anular" circumference and leaflet area in four conditions causing isolated, pure mitral regurgitation.

Surprisingly few reports are available describing the various causes of MR in large numbers of patients. Furthermore, we were unable to find any reports concerning the etiology of pure MR in groups of patients in whom any associated MS or aortic valve dysfunction had been excluded by appropriate hemodynamic and angiographic studies.

The most frequently cited paper describing patients with MR appears to be that by Selzer and Katayama,[3] who summarized findings in 230 patients (Table III). Although 212 of their 230 patients had pure MR defined as the "absence of a late diastolic gradient across the valve . . . except in tachycardia . . . " at the time of cardiac catheterization, some of their patients had MS at other times. Of their 230 patients, 88 were classified as rheumatic in etiology, and we suspect that of them nearly half (42 patients) had MS at some time in their course:

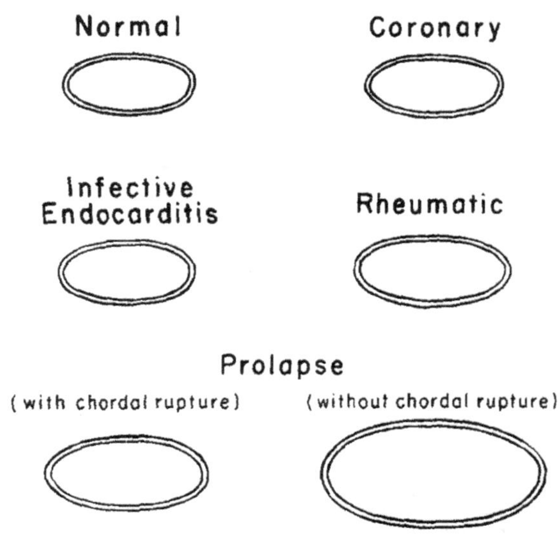

Fig. 11. Diagram showing variations in mitral valve anuli in conditions causing isolated, pure mitral regurgitation.

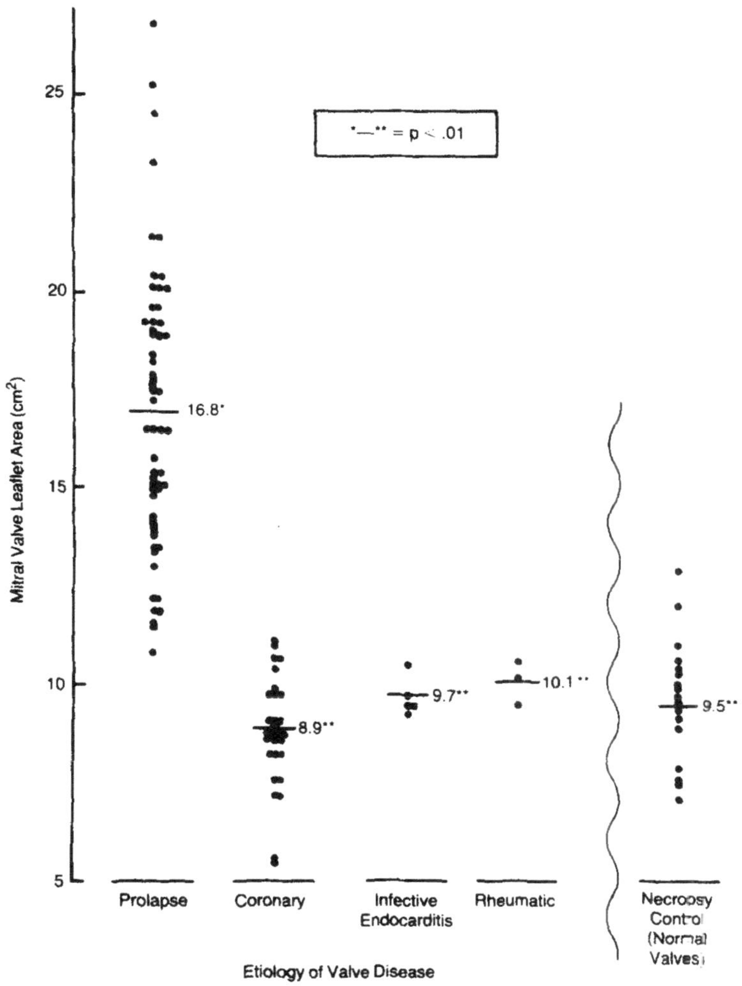

Fig. 12. Graph showing mitral valve leaflet area (in cm^2) in each of the 97 patients with operatively excised mitral valves in the four conditions causing chronic, isolated, pure mitral regurgitation and in 18 necropsy control valves.

five had had mitral commissurotomies for MS and severe MR developed subsequently; eight of their rheumatic patients had MR only after the development of infective endocarditis, and it is probable that one or more of them previously had had MS; 33 (38%) of their 88 rheumatic patients had sizable calcific deposits in their mitral valves, a finding quite unusual in patients without some degree of MS. (Only four of our 97 patients had grossly visible calcific deposits in their excised mitral valves.) It is also difficult to compare the observations in our patients to those reported by Selzer and Katayama because of differences in patient selection. We studied only patients who were in functional classes III and IV (New York Heart Association classification) because of CHF; all underwent MVR and all had their valves examined by the same observers (BFW and WCR). Seventy (30%) of the 230 patients reported by Selzer and Katayama were in functional classes I or II, and mitral valve operations were performed in just over half of the 230 patients. Additionally, they included children, which we did not. Finally, we excluded patients with any aortic valve dysfunction, which may or may not have been the case in the study by Selzer and Katayama.

In the past rheumatic heart disease has been considered the most common cause of severe MR, but it is likely that most or many patients so classified in older studies had some degree of MS. Because there has been such a strong tendency in the past to believe that severe MR was frequently the result of rheumatic heart disease, other etiologies commonly have not been sought and definitions of "rheumatic mitral regurgitation" have not been precisely stated. Before 1963, most prolapsing or floppy mitral valves almost certainly were called

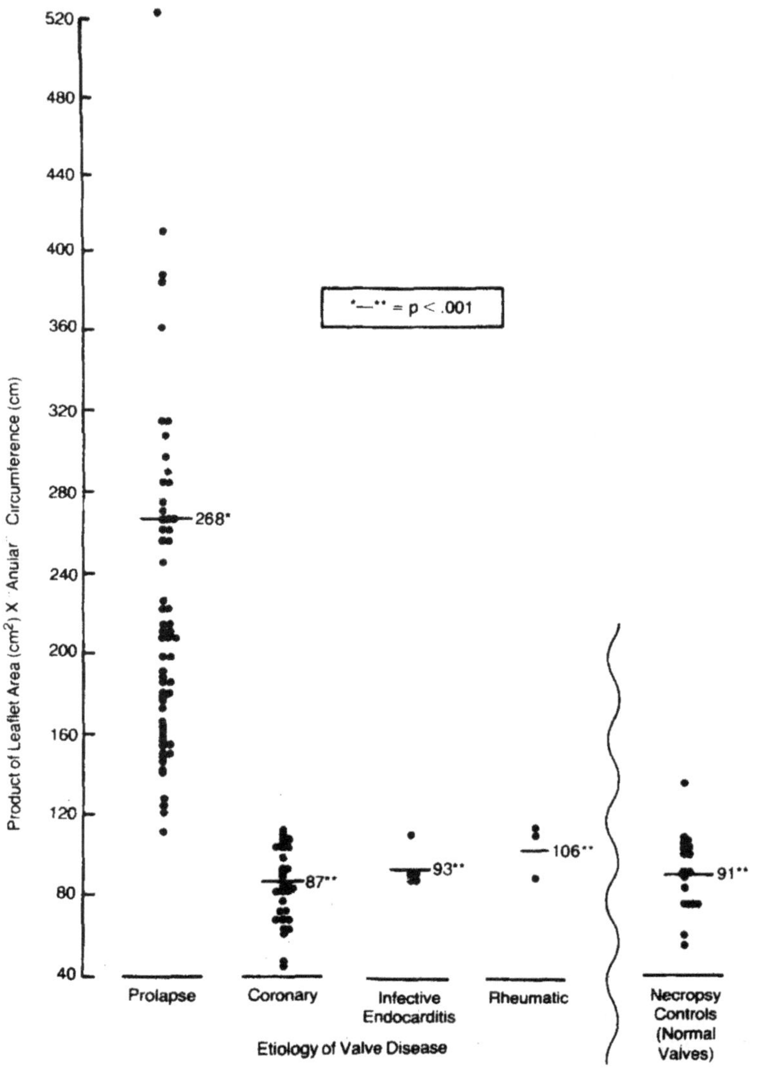

Fig. 13. Graph showing product of mitral valve leaflet area (in cm^2) times the "anular" circumference (in centimeters) in each of the 97 patients with operatively excised mitral valves in the four conditions causing chronic, isolated, pure mitral regurgitation, and in 18 necropsy control valves.

"rheumatic" in origin at necropsy or operation. The present report defines morphologically a prolapsed mitral valve which can cause severe MR: its anular circumference and leaflet area are clearly increased over that of other valves causing MR, except when the chordae tendineae of the prolapsing valve are ruptured. It is hoped that this definition will prevent indiscriminate labeling of mitral disease in the future as "rheumatic" when other evidences of previous rheumatic carditis are lacking.

CONCLUSIONS

The etiology of clinically isolated, severe, pure mitral regurgitation was determined in 97 patients over 30 years of age by examination of the operatively excised mitral valves. None had any degree of mitral stenosis or a dysfunctioning aortic valve as determined by preoperative catheterization. The etiology of the MR was leaflet *prolapse* in 60 patients (62%), *papillary muscle dysfunction* from coronary heart disease in 29 (30%), *infective endocarditis* on previously normally functioning valves in five (5%), and *rheumatic heart disease* in three (3%). Thus, nonrheumatic conditions caused the MR in 94 (97%) of the 97 patients. The history alone (previous acute myocardial infarction, rheumatic fever, active infective endocarditis) usually provided adequate information in the patients with coronary, infective endocarditis and rheumatic etiologies to predict accurately the cause of the MR preoperatively; conversely, the lack of a history of one of these other three conditions strongly suggested mitral valve prolapse as the cause of the MR preoperatively. All 60 patients with mitral valve prolapse had increased mitral valve circumferences, leaflet areas, and/or products of the circumference times the area. In contrast, only one of the 37 patients in whom the MR was due to another cause had increased mitral circumference, increased area, or the product of the two. A systolic click was not heard preoperatively in any of the 97 patients including the 60 with mitral valve prolapse.

REFERENCES

1. Dvorak JA, Schuette WH, Whitehouse WC: A simple video method for the quantification of microscopic objects. J Microsc **102**:71, 1974.
2. Roberts WC, Virmani R: Aschoff bodies at necropsy in valvular heart disease. Evidence from an analysis of 543 patients over 14 years of age that rheumatic heart disease, at least anatomically, is a disease of the mitral valve. Circulation **57**:803, 1978.
3. Selzer A, Katayama F: Mitral regurgitation: Clinical patterns, pathophysiology, natural history. Medicine **51**:337, 1972.

Morphologic Features of the Normal and Abnormal Mitral Valve

WILLIAM C. ROBERTS, MD

Anatomic and functional features of the normal and abnormal mitral valve are reviewed. Of 1,010 personally studied necropsy patients with severe (functional class III or IV, New York Heart Association) cardiac dysfunction from primary valvular heart disease, 434 (43%) had mitral stenosis (MS) with or without mitral regurgitation (MR): unassociated with aortic valve stenosis or regurgitation or with tricuspid valve stenosis in 189 (44%) patients, and associated with aortic stenosis in 152 (35%), with pure (no element of stenosis) aortic regurgitation in 65 (15%) patients, and with tricuspid valve stenosis with or without aortic valve stenosis in 28 (6%) patients. The origin of MS was rheumatic in all 434 patients. Of the 1,010 necropsy patients, 165 (16%) had pure MR (papillary muscle dysfunction excluded): unassociated with aortic valve stenosis or regurgitation or with tricuspid valve stenosis in 97 (59%) patients, and associated with pure aortic regurgitation in 45 (27%) and with aortic valve stenosis in 23 (14%) patients. When associated with dysfunction of the aortic valve, pure MR was usually rheumatic in origin, but when unassociated with aortic valve dysfunction it was usually nonrheumatic in origin. Review of operatively excised mitral valves in patients with pure MR unassociated with aortic valve dysfunction disclosed mitral valve prolapse (most likely an inherent congenital defect) as the most common cause of MR. Excluding the patients with MR from coronary heart disease (papillary muscle dysfunction), mitral prolapse was the cause of MR in 60 (88%) of the other 68 patients, and a rheumatic origin was responsible in only 3 of the 68 patients, all 68 of whom were >30 years of age.

Mitral anular calcification in persons aged >65 years is usually associated with calcific deposits in the aortic valve cusps and in the coronary arteries. Because calcium in each of these 3 sites is common in older individuals residing in the Western World, it is most reasonable to view mitral anular calcification in older individuals as a manifestation of atherosclerosis. Mitral anular calcium appears to be extremely uncommon in persons with total serum cholesterol levels <150 mg/dl. Mitral anular calcium may produce mild MR and, if the deposits are heavy enough, MS.

This report reviews anatomic findings in both the normally and abnormally functioning mitral valve. Major attention is directed to anatomic observations which have clinical usefulness. This review focuses primarily on studies carried out in my laboratory during the past 20 years.

From the Pathology Branch, National Heart, Lung, and Blood Institute, National Institutes of Health, Bethesda, Maryland. Manuscript received and accepted December 3, 1982.

Address for reprints: William C. Roberts, MD, Building 10A, Room 3E30, National Institutes of Health, Bethesda, Maryland 20205.

Normal Mitral Valve (Fig. 1)

The mitral valve, in comparison with the semiluna valves, is a complex structure consisting of 4 majo components: leaflets, chordae tendineae, papillar muscles, and anulus.[1,2] Unlike the other 3 cardiac valve each of which has 3 cusps, the mitral valve consists o only 2 *leaflets*. The anterior one has a much longe basal-to-margin length than does the posterior leafle but the length of the anular attachment of the posteric leaflet (about 6 cm) is about twice that of the anteric leaflet (about 3 cm) (Fig. 1). Although the basal-tc margin lengths and the lengths of the basal attachmen

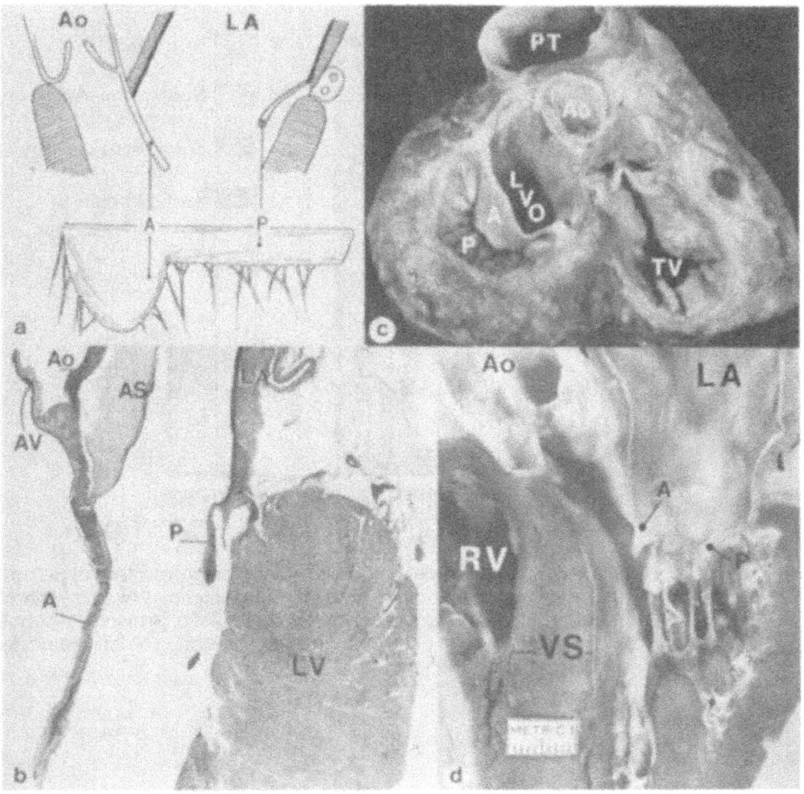

FIGURE 1. Normal mitral valve. **a,** diagram showing relation of anterior (A) and posterior (P) mitral leaflets to one another and to left atrium (LA), aortic valve (AV), and aorta (Ao). The inflow and outflow tracts of the left ventricle are divided by the anterior leaflet. The basal attachment of the posterior leaflet is twice as long as that of the anterior leaflet, although the basal-to-margin length of the anterior leaflet is twice that of the posterior leaflet. **b,** histologic sections of the mitral valve confirming the observations depicted in **a**. One section includes the anterior (A) mitral leaflet, the aortic valve cusp (AV), the wall of the aorta (Ao), and the atrial septal (AS) wall, and the other includes the left atrial and left ventricular free walls with intervening posterior mitral leaflet. (Elastic van Gieson stains; magnification ×4.5 and ×3, reduced 45%). **c,** view of the heart from above after excision of the atria. The anterior (A) mitral leaflet separates the left ventricular inflow from outflow (LVO). PT = pulmonary trunk; TV = tricuspid valve. **d,** longitudinal cut of the left ventricle, mitral valve, aorta, and left atrium, as would be seen by M-mode echocardiogram.

of each mitral leaflet are quite different, the surface area of each leaflet is virtually identical. The posterior leaflet has a true bundle of fibrous tissue (the anulus) separating the myocardium of left atrium from the myocardium of left ventricle. The posterior leaflet, in a large sense, is simply an extension of mural endocardium from the free walls of the left atrium. In contrast to the posterior mitral leaflet, the anterior leaflet does not have a true anulus but is continuous with the wall of the ascending aorta, aortic valve, membraneous ventricular septum, and atrial septum. The area of the leaflets is about 2.5 times that of the area of the mitral orifice at the level of the mitral anulus. In contrast to the semilunar cusps, which are independent or discontinuous of each other, the 2 mitral leaflets are continuous with each other, being connected at the commissures.

Chordae tendineae from both mitral leaflets insert into both papillary muscles. About 5 times as many

TABLE I Functional and Anatomic Classification of Valvular Heart Disease in 1,010 Necropsy Patients Aged ≥15 Years*

Functional Class	Patients (n [%])	Anatomic Class (n [%]) AV	MV	MV-AV	TV-MV	TV-MV-AV
1. Aortic stenosis (AS)	292 (29)	256 (87.5)	0	35 (12.1)	0	1 (0.3)
2. Mitral stenosis (MS)	189 (19)	0	117 (62)	40 (21)	13 (7)	19 (10)
3. MS + AS	152 (15)	0	0	120 (79)	0	32 (21)
4. Aortic regurgitation (AR)	119 (12)	107† (90)	0	10 (8)	0	2 (2)
5. Mitral regurgitation (MR)	97 (10)	0	85 (88)	8 (8)	1 (1)	3 (3)
6. MS + AR	65 (6)	0	52 (80)	0	0	13 (20)
7. MR + AR	45 (4)	0	0	39 (87)	0	6 (13)
8. AS + MR	23 (2)	0	0	21 (91)	0	2 (9)
9. Tricuspid stenosis + MS ± AS	28 (3)	0	0	0	4 (14)	24 (86)
Totals	1,010 (100)‡	363 (36)	254 (25)	273 (27)	18 (2)	102 (10)

AV = aortic valve; MV = mitral valve; TV = tricuspid valve.

* Excludes patients with mitral regurgitation secondary to coronary heart disease (papillary muscle dysfunction), carcinoid heart disease, and hypertrophic cardiomyopathy and those with infective endocarditis limited to 1 or both right-sided cardiac valves. Tricuspid valve regurgitation was present in many patients in most of the 9 functional groups. All patients were in functional class III or IV (New York Heart Association), and more than half had 1 or more cardiac operations.

† In many patients, the aortic valve cusps actually were normal and the regurgitation was the result of disease of the aorta (Marfan and Marfan-like syndromes, syphilis, systemic hypertension, healed aortic dissection).

‡ The hearts in all 1,010 patients were examined and classified by WCR.

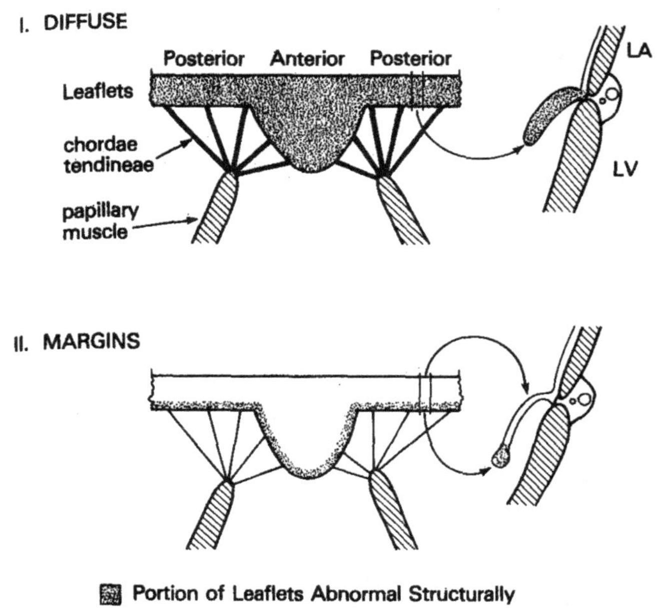

FIGURE 2. Diagram showing the 2 types of anatomic involvement of the mitral valve in rheumatic heart disease. Thickening of chordae are not required for diagnosis, only thickening of the leaflets, either diffusely or on all margins. LA = left atrium; LV = left ventricle. (Reprinted, by permission, from Roberts and Virmani.[11])

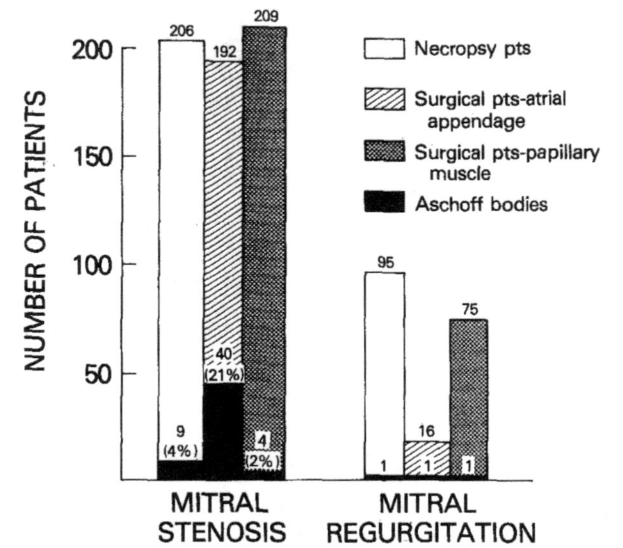

FIGURE 3. Bar graph demonstrating number and percentage of patients (pts) undergoing operations for either mitral stenosis (with or without mitral regurgitation) and pure mitral regurgitation in whom Aschoff bodies were found in either the left atrial appendage or left ventricular papillary muscle.

chordae are attached to leaflets as to papillary muscles. On an average, 24 chordae tendineae are attached to the papillary muscles (12 to each), and 120 chordae are attached to the leaflets.[3] The chordae insert onto the undersurfaces—that is, the ventricular surfaces—of both leaflets. The chordae subdivide as they progress from papillary muscle to leaflet. The subdivisions may be viewed as primary (first order), secondary (second order), and tertiary (third order) chordae. The spaces between the chordae serve as secondary orifices between left atrium and left ventricle. Obviously, the major orifice is the area between the leaflets, but much blood passes between the interchordal spaces. Therefore, fusion of chordae tendineae may narrow the mitral inlet.

The 2 *left ventricular papillary muscles* are preferably designated anterolateral and posteromedial.[3] There is considerable variation in the appearances of these 2 structures in the same person, and comparison of corresponding structures in different persons discloses considerable variation. The anterolateral papillary muscle is generally the more uniform of the 2. It usually consists of a single trunk that protrudes more into the cavity than does the posteromedial one. The posteromedial papillary muscle is generally smaller than the anterolateral structure and often consists of 2 or 3 smaller pillars rather than a single pillar. The posteromedial muscle usually has several connections to the left ventricular wall in addition to the base of the major trunk. Both papillary muscles are attached to the left ventricular free wall roughly at the junction of the caudal third and middle thirds.

With aging, the mitral valve, like other tissues, changes; this change consists mainly of focal fibrous thickening of both leaflets and chordae. The left ventricular cavity becomes smaller (presumably because the cardiac output decreases) as we grow older,[2,4] and consequently less area becomes available in the left ventricle to accommodate the mitral leaflets and chordae. The leaflets then contact one another abnormally during ventricular systole and focal fibrous thickening results. Since the left ventricular cavity diminishes with age, the mitral *anulus* does also. The latter change further increases the abnormal contact of the mitral leaflets with one other and furthers the leaflet scarring. This scarring from aging, however, is not enough to cause mitral dysfunction.

Abnormal Mitral Valve

Mitral Stenosis

The essential hemodynamic fault caused by mitra stenosis (MS) is the inability of the left atrium to empty normally.[2] In sinus rhythm, left atrial contraction serve to augment its emptying, but atrial contraction is los in atrial fibrillation. The obstruction, represented b a pressure gradient across the valve, results in pulmonary venous obstruction which may be apparent o chest roentgenography.

Of the 9 single or combined cardiac valve lesions severe enough to be fatal, MS, in my experience, rank second[5,6] (Table I). Of 1,010 patients >14 years of ag with functionally severe (class III or IV, New Yor Heart Association) valvular cardiac disease whom I ha studied at necropsy up to 1980, 434 (44%) had MS. Only aortic valve stenosis was more common.[7–9] Mitra

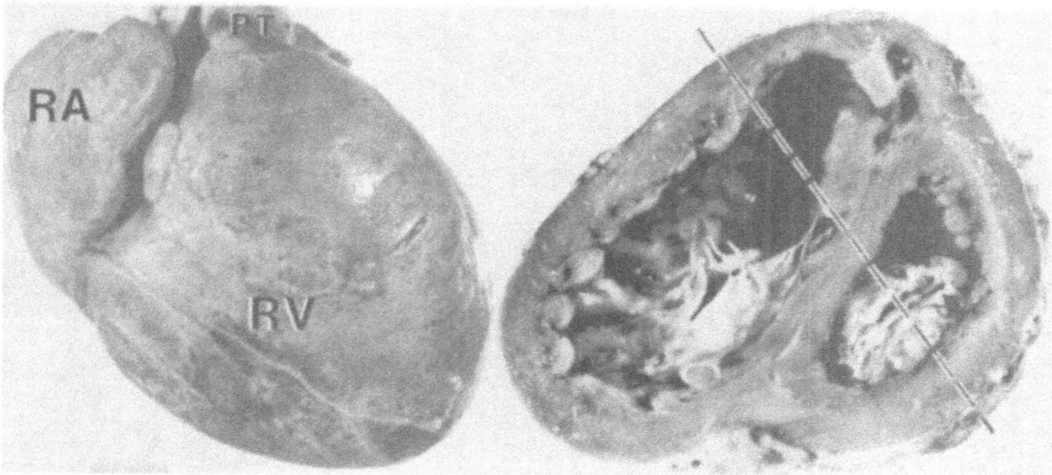

FIGURE 4. Heart in a 16-year-old boy (NIH #A77-232) who had acute rheumatic fever at age 6 years and chronic congestive heart failure beginning at age 10 years. By examination, the patient had evidence of severe mitral stenosis and tricuspid regurgitation. At cardiac catheterization 10 hours before death, the right ventricular pressure was 100/20 and the left ventricular pressure, 100/10 mm Hg. Neither pulmonary arterial wedge or left atrial pressures were obtained. Left ventriculogram disclosed no mitral regurgitation and a normal-sized left ventricular cavity. The patient had acute pulmonary edema after catheterization and underwent closed mitral commissurotomy as a terminal procedure on the ward. At necropsy, the heart weighed 450 g (the patient weighed 43 kg). The right atrium (RA) and ventricle (RV) were huge, and the thickness of the free walls of both ventricles were similar. Both mitral and tricuspid valve leaflets were diffusely thickened but free of calcific deposits. No Aschoff bodies were present. The **dashed straight line** is the line of the M-mode beam. PT = pulmonary trunk.

stenosis occurred alone in 189 (44%) patients and in combination with other functional valvular lesions in the other 245 (56%) patients. Mitral stenosis was rheumatic in origin in all 434 patients.[10,11]

Although a functional classification of valvular heart disease is most useful from physiologic and therapeutic standpoints, an anatomic classification is helpful from an etiologic standpoint. Five anatomic categories have proved useful: isolated mitral, isolated aortic, combined mitral and aortic, combined tricuspid and mitral with

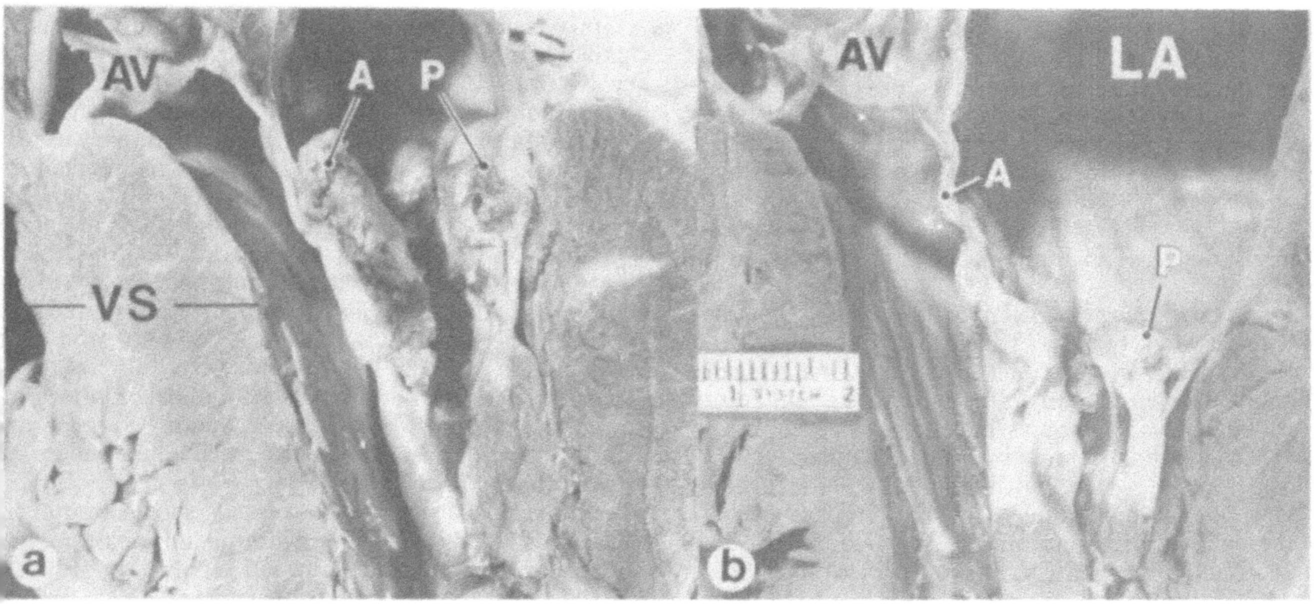

IGURE 5. Longitudinal views, as would be seen by M-mode echocardiogram, of 2 hearts of patients with severe mitral stenosis. **a,** in a 55-year-old ian (GT #74A-69) with equal peak systolic pressures in the right and left ventricles and no associated mitral regurgitation. The patient died from iassive bleeding during cannulation of the aorta for planned mitral valve replacement. Both anterior (A) and posterior (P) mitral leaflets are heavily alcified. AV = aortic valve; VS = ventricular septum. **b,** in a 64-year-old woman (GT #78A-129) with right and left ventricular peak systolic pressures f 100 and 135 mm Hg, respectively, and an 18 mm Hg mean diastolic gradient between pulmonary arterial wedge position and left ventricle just efore closed mitral commissurotomy 3 years before death. This patient died of progressive congestive cardiac failure. The heart weighed 410 The amount of calcium in the thickened mitral leaflets is relatively mild. LA = left atrium.

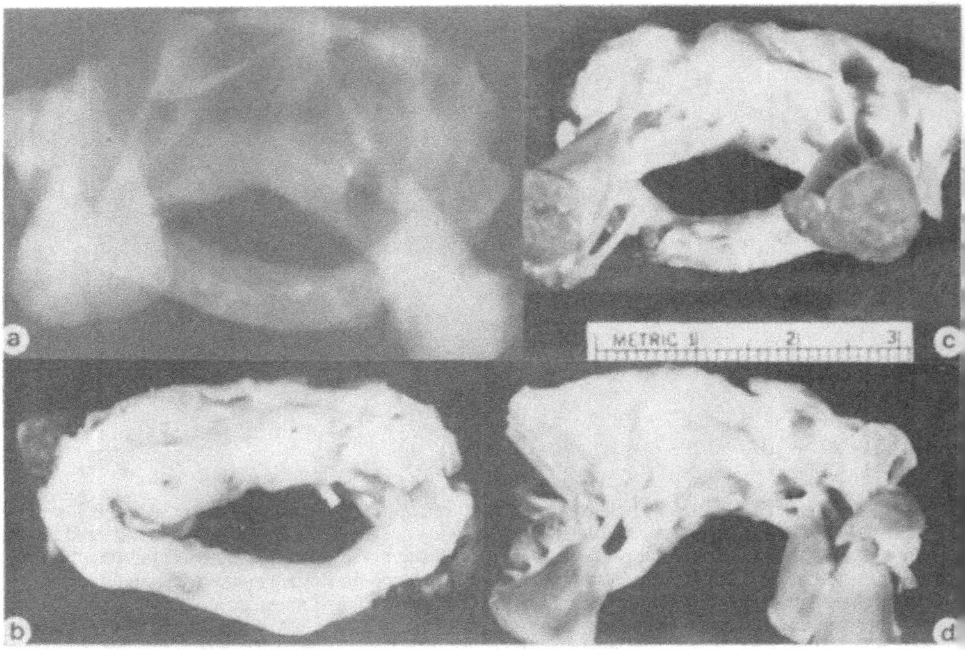

FIGURE 6. Operatively excised stenotic mitral valve in a 40-year-old woman with only a minute calcific deposit in the anterior leaflet. The mean diastolic gradient between the pulmonary arterial wedge position and the left ventricle was 13 mm Hg, the peak pulmonary arterial systolic pressure was 50 mm Hg, and 3+/4+ mitral regurgitation was present by left ventriculogram. **a,** radiogram of operatively excised valve. **b,** view from left atrial aspect. **c,** view from left ventricular aspect. **d,** view of anterior leaflet and papillary muscles. (Reprinted, by permission, from Lachman and Roberts.[18])

or without aortic, and both tricuspid and mitral (Table I). Anatomically isolated aortic valve disease is never rheumatic in origin.[5] Isolated mitral disease causing MS is, with rare exception, rheumatic in origin, but isolated mitral disease causing pure regurgitation is usually nonrheumatic in origin.[12] Anatomic valve disease involving more than 1 cardiac valve is usually rheumatic in origin. Isolated anatomic disease of the tricuspid or pulmonic valves, or both, is usually congenital or infectious in origin or is associated with the carcinoid syndrome.[13–17]

A valve may function normally and yet be anatomically abnormal. Only 62% of the 189 patients with isolated MS (with or without mitral regurgitation [MR]) had anatomic involvement limited to the mitral valve[6] (Table I). In contrast, 88% of the 292 patients with clinically isolated aortic valve stenosis (with or without regurgitation) had anatomic disease limited to the aortic valve only.

Rheumatic heart disease may be viewed as a disease of the mitral valve; other valves also may be involved both anatomically and functionally, but anatomically the mitral valve is always involved[11] (Fig. 2). To my knowledge, *Aschoff bodies* have never been found in hearts without anatomic disease of the mitral valve.[11] Of the first 543 patients with severe valvular heart disease whom I studied at necropsy, 11 (27%) had Aschoff bodies, and all had anatomic mitral valve disease. The ages of the 11 patients with Aschoff bodies ranged from 18 to 68 years (mean 38) and 9 had a history of acute rheumatic fever earlier in life. Clinical study revealed that 9 of the 11 patients had MS with or without dysfunction of 1 or more other cardiac valves, 1 had isolated pure aortic regurgitation, and 1 had both mitral and aortic regurgitation. All 11 patients had diffuse fibrous thickening of the mitral valve leaflets and all but 1 had diffuse anatomic lesions of at least 2 other cardiac valves. No patient with anatomic lesions limited to the aortic valve had Aschoff bodies. Thus, among patients with chronic valvular heart disease, Aschoff bodies, the only anatomic lesion pathognomonic of rheumatic heart disease, usually indicate diffuse anatomic lesions of 2 or more other cardiac valves. The functional mitral lesion is usually stenosis.

Although they are rare at necropsy in patients with fatal chronic valvular heart disease, Aschoff bodies are fairly common in the heart in patients having mitral valve commissurotomy for MS.[10] Among 481 patients undergoing various mitral valve operations, Aschof bodies were found in 40 (21%) of 191 operatively excise left atrial appendages, in 4 (2%) of 273 operatively excised left ventricular papillary muscles (1 per patient) and in 1 (6%) of 17 patients with both left atrial appendage and papillary muscle operatively excised (Fig 3). Of the 45 patients with Aschoff bodies, 44 had MS preoperatively, and only 1, a 10-year-old boy, had pur MR. Sinus rhythm was present in 38 (84%), and atria fibrillation in 7 (16%). Perioperatively, only 1 of the 4 patients with Aschoff bodies had clinical or laborator stigmata compatible with acute rheumatic fever, an 58% had an illness compatible with acute rheumati fever at any time.

Rheumatic heart disease not only is a disorder of th cardiac valves; it also affects mural endocardium, pe icardium, and myocardium. On histologic study, th atrial walls virtually always have increased amounts fibrous tissue in both myocardial interstitium and in th mural endocardium, atrophy of some and hypertroph of other myocardial cells, and hypertrophy of smoot muscle cells of the mural endocardium. In all patien with rheumatic MS, the leaflets are diffusely thicken either by fibrous tissue or calcific deposits or both; th

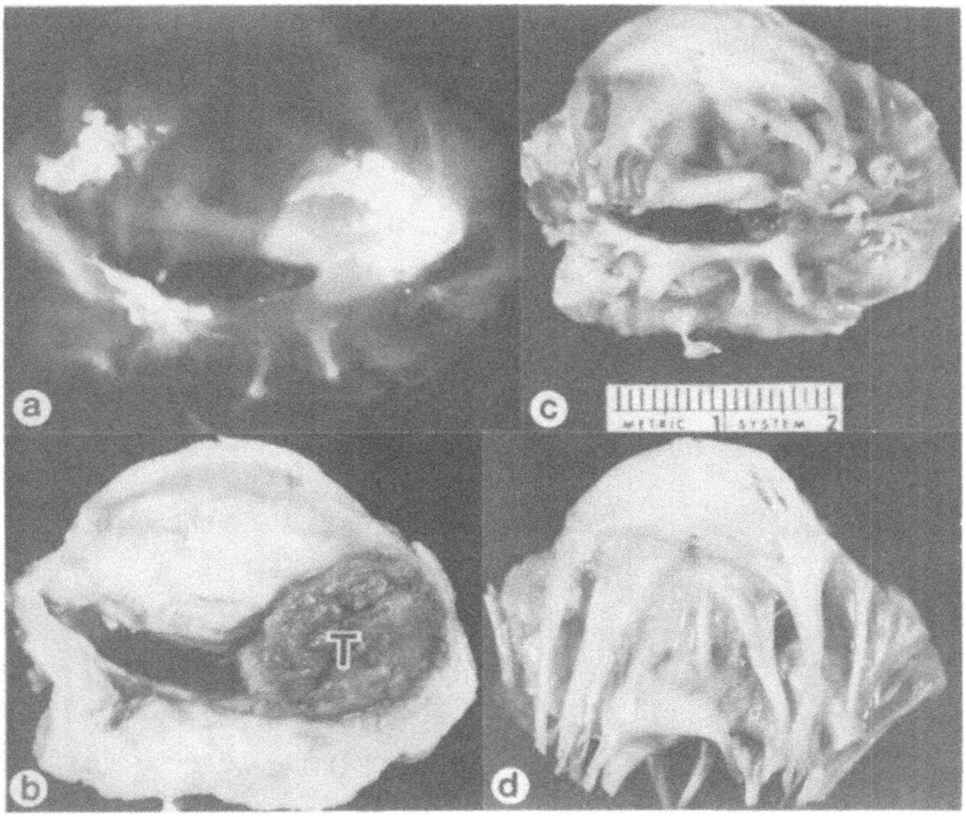

FIGURE 7. Operatively excised stenotic mitral valve in a 72-year-old woman (S76-76) who had had an embolus to a femoral artery 5 years earlier. **a,** radiogram of the operatively excised valve showing focal calcific deposits. **b,** view of the valve from the left atrial aspect showing an oval thrombus (T) over half of the orifice. No thrombus was present in the left atrial cavity. **c,** view of the valve from the left ventricular aspect. The orifice is eccentric. **d,** view of the anterior leaflet.

commissures are usually fused, and the chordae tendineae are shortened and usually fused to some degree (Fig. 4 to 8). The great obstruction to this funnel-shaped valve occurs at its apex, which is within the left ventricular cavity. The primary orifice, located at the level of the anulus, is far less narrowed. Fusion may involve 1 or both commissures. When only 1 is fused or 1 is fused more than the other, the stenotic orifice is eccentrically located. A centrally located orifice indicates symmetrical commissural fusion. In rheumatic MS, the chordae tendineae are occasionally so retracted that the leaflets appear to insert directly into the papillary muscles. When this occurs, the MS is always severe because the interchordal spaces are almost entirely obliterated. Sometimes chordae inserting into 1 papillary muscle are well preserved, whereas those inserting into the other papillary muscle are partially or completely fused. Mitral commissurotomy on a valve in which the leaflets insert almost directly into the papillary muscle(s) usually must include a splitting of the papillary muscle(s) as well as the commissure(s). If there are normally about 120 third-order chordae and about 24 first-order chordae, in MS these numbers are usually halved and, on occasion, even reduced to just 1.

The amount of *calcium* in the leaflets of stenotic mitral valves varies considerably[18] (Figs. 6 to 8). Generally, calcium is more frequent and in larger quantity in men than in women, in older than in younger patients, and in patients with higher compared with those with lower pressure gradients between left atrium and left ventricle[18] (Fig. 9). The rapidity with which calcium develops also varies considerably; it is present at a younger age in men than in women.[18] Lachman and I[18] determined the presence or absence and the extent of calcific deposits in operatively excised stenotic mitral valves by radiography of the excised valve in 164 patients aged 26 to 72 years. The extent of the mitral calcific deposits was determined by the percentage of the valvular circumference containing the deposits: grade 0 (14 patients); grade I = 1 to 25% (43 patients); grade II = 26 to 50% (34 patients); grade III = 51 to 75% (39 patients); and grade IV = 76 to 100% (34 patients). The amount of calcific deposits in the stenotic mitral valves correlated with *sex* and with the *mean diastolic pressure gradient across the mitral valve* ($p < 0.05$) (Fig. 9), but it did not correlate with the patient's age (after age 25 years), cardiac rhythm, pulmonary arterial or pulmonary arterial wedge pressure, previous mitral commissurotomy, presence of thrombus in the body of left atrium, or the presence of disease of 1 or more other cardiac valves.

Among the 164 patients with MS having mitral valve replacement and roentgenography of the excised mitral valve, 14 had no mitral calcium and 43 had only trace or minimal mitral calcific deposits. Thus, we[19] wondered why these 57 patients had mitral replacement rather than mitral commissurotomy. Of the 57 patients, 37 had moderate to severe MR and, therefore, clearly deserved mitral valve replacement. The remaining 20 had absent or minimal calcific deposits, but, nevertheless, they too

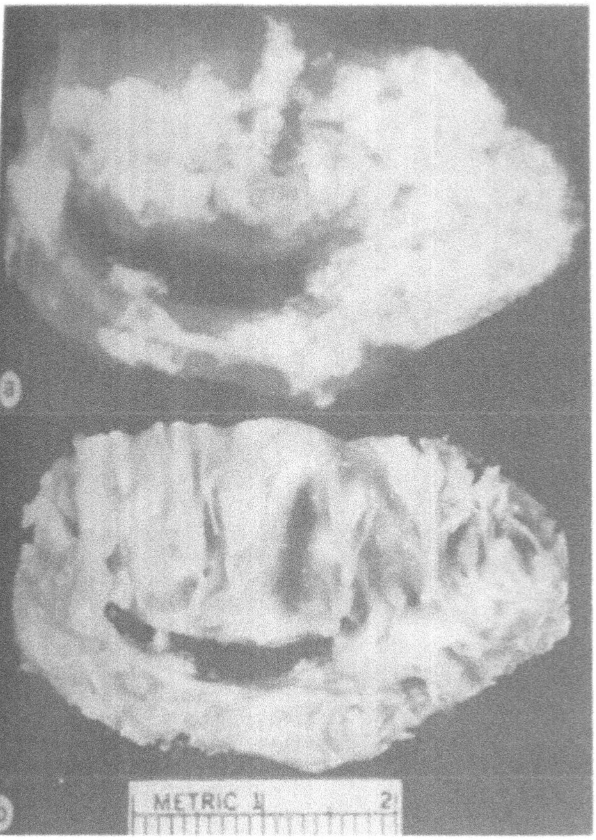

FIGURE 8. Operatively excised stenotic heavily calcified mitral valve in a 53-year-old woman (S67-867) in whom the mean diastolic gradient between the pulmonary arterial wedge position and the left ventricle was 26 mm Hg. She also had 1+/4+ mitral regurgitation by left ventriculogram; a thrombus was present in the body of left atrium. **a,** radiogram of the operatively excised valve. **b,** view of the valve from the left ventricle after excision of the papillary muscle. The orifice is eccentric. (Reprinted, by permission, from Lachman and Roberts.[18])

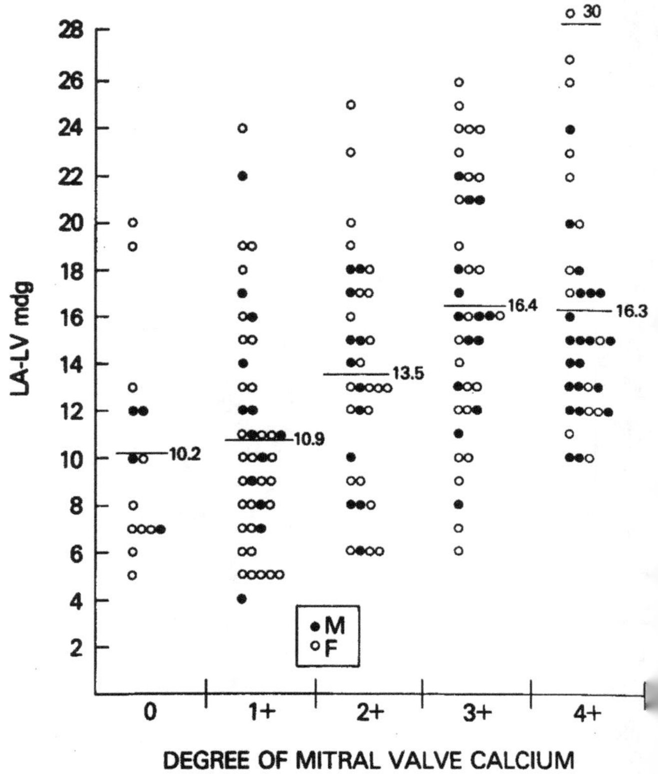

FIGURE 9. Relation between the left atrial (LA) left ventricular (LV) mear diastolic gradient (mdg) and degree of mitral valve calcium. (Reprinted by permission, from Lachman and Roberts.[18])

had mitral valve replacement. Although in the prevalve replacement era all 20 patients almost surely would have been considered good or ideal candidates for mitral commissurotomy, other factors swung the surgeon to valve replacement rather than commissurotomy. These factors included the need to replace 1 or more other cardiac valves (13 patients), the utilization of cardiopulmonary bypass allowing visual inspection rather than simple palpation of the diseased mitral valve (all 20 patients), relatively little experience with mitral commissurotomy in 4 of the 5 surgeons (17 patients), displeasure with attempted commissurotomy (3 patients), previous mitral commissurotomy (11 patients), and incorrect identification of mitral calcific deposits (2 patients). Even though mitral commissurotomy has been in use for 30 years, the mere alternative of valve replacement may have altered the definition of the stenotic mitral valve previously considered ideal for mitral commissurotomy.

A major complication of MS is *thrombus formation in the left atrial cavity.* The thrombus may be limited to atrial appendage (most common) or be located in both left atrial appendage and body (Fig. 10). The latte group hereafter will be referred to as "left atrial body thrombus." Left atrial body thrombus was observed in 5% of 1,010 personally studied necropsy patients with fatal valvular heart disease; all had severe MS (Table I). Left atrial body thrombus was not observed in any of the 165 patients with pure MR with or without aorti valve dysfunction. All patients with left atrial body thrombi had atrial fibrillation. Comparison of these necropsy patients with 46 patients with MS operated upon at the National Heart, Lung, and Blood Institute and in whom thrombus was found at operation in the left atrial body disclosed that 42 (91%) patients had atrial fibrillation. In contrast, of 40 living patient undergoing mitral valve replacement for pure MR and operated upon at the National Heart, Lung, and Blood Institute, none had thrombus in the body of the lef atrium, although 75% had atrial fibrillation. *Thrombu appears to occur in the body of the left atrium only i patients with MS, and atrial fibrillation without M is incapable of forming a thrombus in the left atria body.*

Calcific deposits on the mural endocardium of th left atrium are indicative of previous organization wit calcification of left atrial thrombi. Histologically, th "calcific thrombi" also contain cholesterol clefts and a identical to atherosclerotic plaques. The observatic that left atrial thrombi can organize into lesions ide

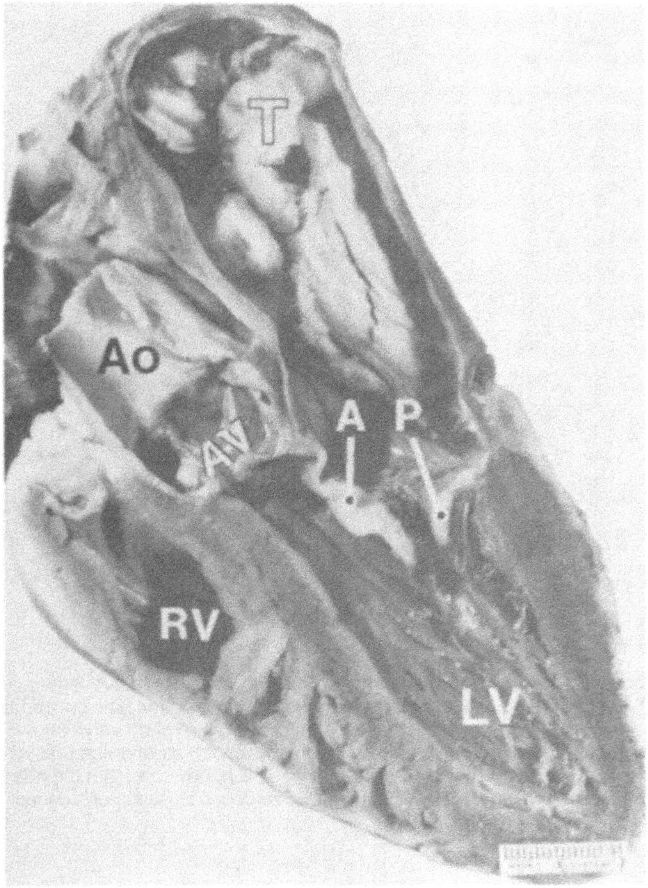

FIGURE 10. Long-axis view of the heart in a 53-year-old woman (GT#77A-190) in whom a huge thrombus (T) was found in the body of the left atrium at necropsy. The mitral valve is quite stenotic. The aortic valve (AV) is normal. A = anterior and P = posterior mitral leaflet; Ao = aorta; LV = left ventricle; RV = right ventricle. Mitral valve commissurotomy had been recommended when the patient was 40 years of age, but she declined. Her last 2 years were characterized by chronic progressive congestive cardiac failure complicated by anemia from multiple myeloma. The patient had chronic atrial fibrillation, but never had cardiac catheterization, a cardiac operation, or evidence of systemic emboli.

ical to atherosclerotic plaques supports the view that atherosclerotic plaques may be the result of organization of thrombi. If calcific deposits form on left atrial body endocardium before the left atrial cavity has had time to dilate, this cavity may be prevented thereafter from dilating. The elevated left atrial pressure may lead more rapidly to pulmonary venous, pulmonary arterial, and right ventricular dilatation with subsequent tricuspsid regurgitation and development of huge right atrial dilatation.[20]

Nonrheumatic causes of MS include *congenital anomalies*[21] (Fig. 11); *neoplasms* (Fig. 12) (particularly myxoma[22]) protruding through the mitral orifice from the left atrium (but malignant neoplasms primary or secondary in the lung may grow into the mitral orifice by way of the pulmonary veins[23]); *large vegetations from active infective endocarditis*[24,25]; and *massive mitral anular calcific deposits*, particularly when associated with small-sized left ventricular cavities and left ventricular outflow tract obstruction[26] (Fig. 13). A relatively new, acquired cause of MS is a *mechanical prosthetic or bioprosthetic cardiac valve.*[27–29] Since the native mitral valve is within the left ventricle, a prosthetic mitral valve also is located within this cavity. The prosthesis must be small enough for the contracting left ventricular wall not to interfere with movement of the prosthetic poppet or disk. When the prosthesis is too large for the cavity into which it was inserted, the poppet may be prevented from moving adequately and may therefore obstruct left atrial emptying. The latter state is far more common than obstruction to left ventricular emptying by the prosthesis. Thrombus formation on a mitral prosthesis also may obstruct left atrial emptying.

Pure Mitral Regurgitation

In contrast to MS, which has mainly 1 cause (rheumatic), pure MR has numerous causes.[2,3,12,16,17,23,30–60] Of the 1,010 patients with functionally severe valvular heart disease, excluding papillary muscle dysfunction, studied personally at necropsy, 165 (16%) had pure (no element of stenosis) MR[5] (Table I); the MR was isolated in 97 of these patients (59%) and associated with aortic valve dysfunction in 68 (41%) (aortic regurgitation in 45 and aortic stenosis in 23). In the 68 patients with associated aortic valve dysfunction, the origin of the valvular disease was rheumatic. Of the 97 patients with clinically isolated pure MR, the aortic valve or the tricuspid valve or both was anatomically abnormal (mild diffuse scarring) in 12 and therefore the cause of the mitral valve dysfunction in these patients was also rheumatic in origin (Table I). Of the remaining 85 patients, the origin of the pure MR was usually nonrheumatic, most commonly ruptured chordae tendineae from infection on a previously normal valve or spontaneous rupture with underlying prolapsing (or floppy) mitral leaflet(s).

Why the mitral valve affected by acute rheumatic fever becomes stenotic in some patients and purely regurgitant in others (mainly children) is unknown. Although the cause may be similar (rheumatic), the structural alterations in the purely regurgitant mitral valve are quite different from those in the stenotic valve. The purely regurgitant rheumatic valve infrequently contains calcific deposits, its commissures are virtually never fused, and its chordae tendineae are only mildly thickened, if at all; chordal fusion is infrequent (Fig. 14). It is often difficult to explain adequately the mechanism of MR in a valve made purely regurgitant by consequences of rheumatic fever. The mitral anuli in children with rheumatic MR usually are dilated but this mechanism is most often not applicable in adults with rheumatic MR.

Rheumatic disease is never limited to endocardium. Inflammatory cells are nearly always found in atrial walls of patients dying with acute rheumatic fever.[61] The inflammation appears to weaken the walls, and superimposed MR tends to dilate the chamber out of proportion to the dilation that would occur with similar degrees of MR into a left atrium with previously normal

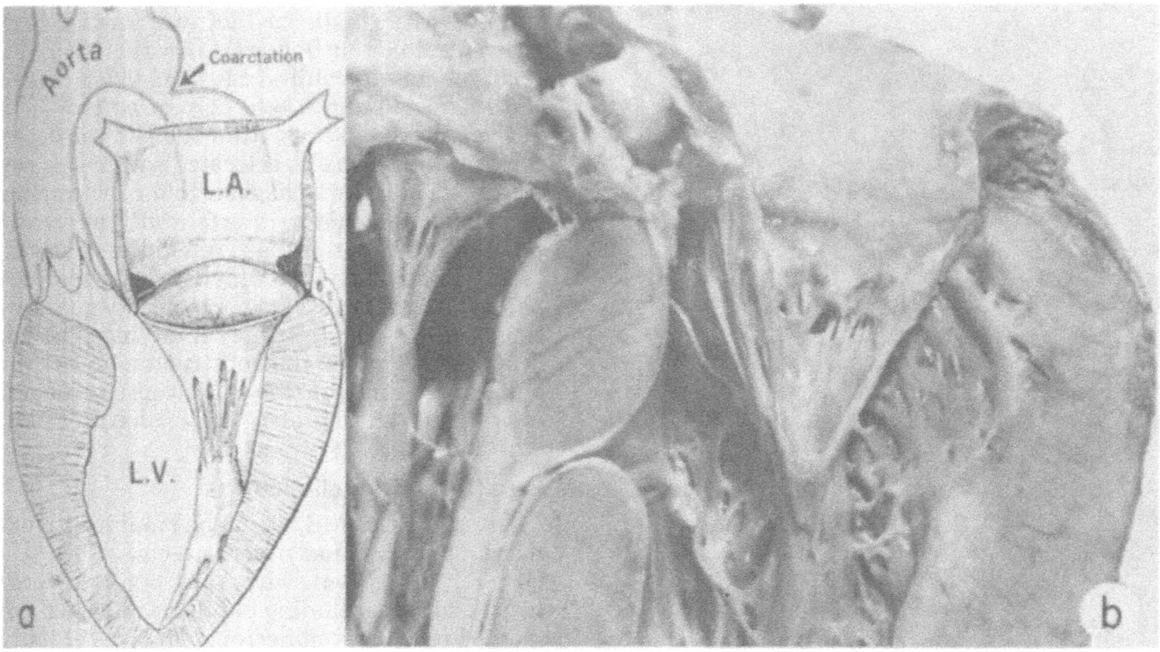

FIGURE 11. Parachute mitral valve causing mitral stenosis in a 14-year-old boy (GT #71A-215) who presented clinically with signs of left ventricular outflow obstruction. The peak systolic gradient between the left ventricle (L.V.) and a systemic artery was 80 mm Hg. Obstruction was caused by a small aortic "anulus" with a bicuspid aortic valve and by discrete obstruction just below the aortic valve. At necropsy, the mitral valve showed a parachute configuration, and all of its chordae inserted into a single left ventricular papillary muscle. Preoperatively, the left atrial mean pressure was 30 mm Hg, and the pulmonary arterial systolic pressure was 50 mm Hg. It was not realized while the patient was alive, however, that the mitral valve was stenotic. In addition, a functionally insignificant coarctation of the aorta was present. A ventricular septal defect had closed spontaneously. L.A. = left atrium. (Reprinted, by permission, from Roberts and Cohen.[3])

walls.[41] What causes the left atrium to dilate enormously in some patients with rheumatic MR is uncertain. Possibly, the patients with so-called giant atria have had more frequent or more severe attacks of acute rheumatic fever, with particularly severe destruction of atrial myocardial fibers. When the left atrium in pure MR is giant in size (Fig. 15), intimal proliferation is rarely found in the pulmonary veins or arteries, and the right ventricular walls are not hypertrophied.[41,47] The larger the left atrial cavity in pure MR, the lower it intracavity pressure. Since the right ventricular wall in these patients are usually not hypertrophied (becaus the right ventricular systolic pressures are normal o near normal), tricuspid regurgitation is infrequent. I contrast, patients with large left atria from MS or fron combined MS and MR have elevated left atrial, pul monary venous, pulmonary arterial, and right ventric ular pressures; the right ventricular walls therefore ar

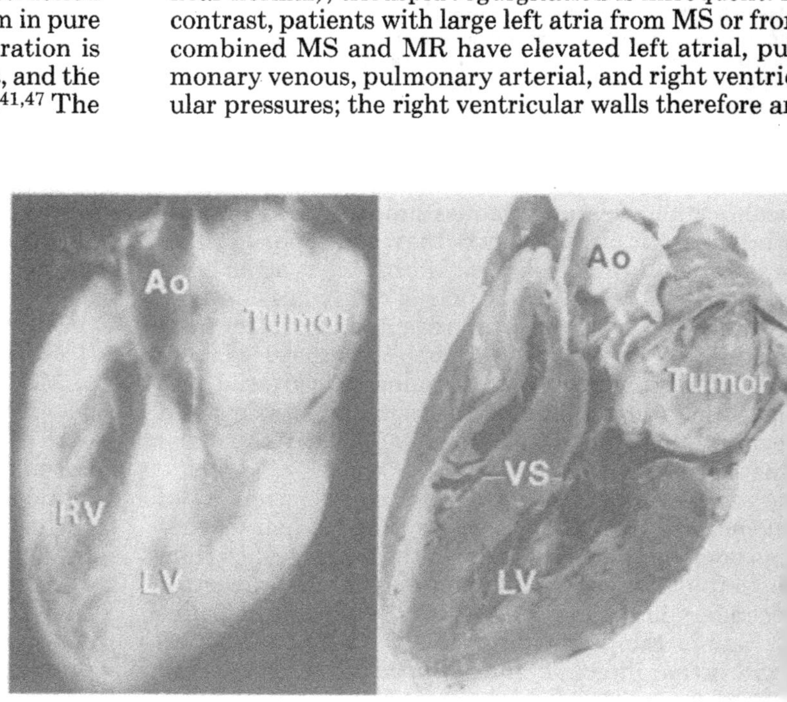

FIGURE 12. Metastatic ovarian carcinoma to the lung with extension into the pulmonary veins and from there into the left atrial body to partly obstruct the mitral orifice in a 44-year-old woman (NNMC #A76-150) who had been asymptomatic until 6 weeks before death, when evidence of congestive heart failure appeared. A precordial murmur was not recorded. **a,** radiogram of heart at necropsy showing a mass in the left atrium and **b,** a long-axis view of heart. Ao = aorta; LV = left ventricle; RV = right ventricle; VS = ventricular septum.

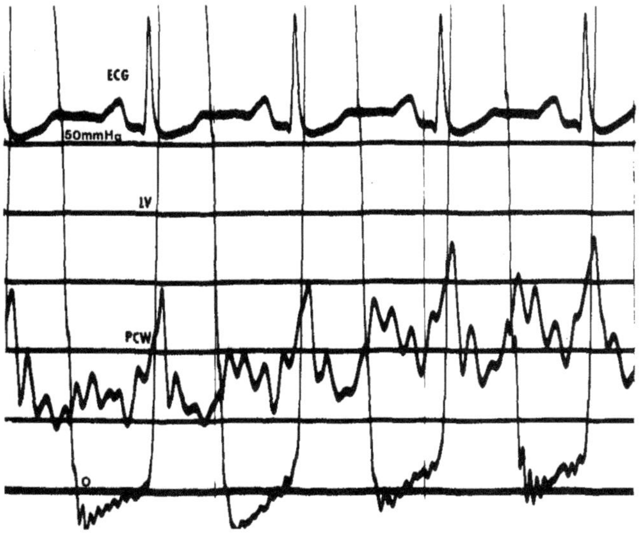

FIGURE 13. Simultaneous, equisensitive recording of pulmonary arterial wedge (PCW) and left ventricular (LV) pressures in a 70-year-old woman (GT #74A-287) with severe (153 mm Hg peak systolic gradient) aortic valve stenosis and massive (4+/4+) mitral anular calcium producing a 15 mm Hg mean diastolic pressure gradient at the level of the otherwise anatomically normal mitral valve. Thus, heavy mitral anular calcific deposits in the setting of left ventricular outflow obstruction can produce "mitral stenosis." ECG = electrocardiogram. (Reprinted, by permission, from Hammer et al.[26])

hypertrophied. Thus, tricuspid regurgitation is a common consequence.

Rupture of mitral chordae tendineae is another common cause of fatal or potentially fatal pure MR.[41,42] The normal chordae tendineae are the ones most likely to rupture, not the previously thickened ones. Thus, rupture of 1 or several thick chordae tendineae in patients with MS is extremely rare. The cause of the rupture varies. Infective endocarditis is the most common cause of acute rupture[41] (Fig. 16). Of 42 patients with healed ruptured mitral chordae tendineae studied by Buchbinder and me, however, only 14 had had infective endocarditis. Infective endocarditis causes acute severe MR by chordal rupture and rarely by leaflet perforation[16] (Fig. 17). The syndrome of acute severe MR associated with normal- or near-normal–sized left atria and severe elevations of left atrial, pulmonary venous, pulmonary arterial, and right ventricular pressures is usually the result of rupture of chordae tendineae by infective endocarditis involving previously normal valves[41] (Fig. 18). The left atrial myocardial fibers in these patients, as contrasted to those in patients with chronic rheumatic MR, have not been previously damaged by rheumatic fever, and, therefore, the left atrial wall is capable of responding to the sudden elevation of left atrial pressure by vigorous contractions, leading to myofiber hypertrophy. The ventricular sys-

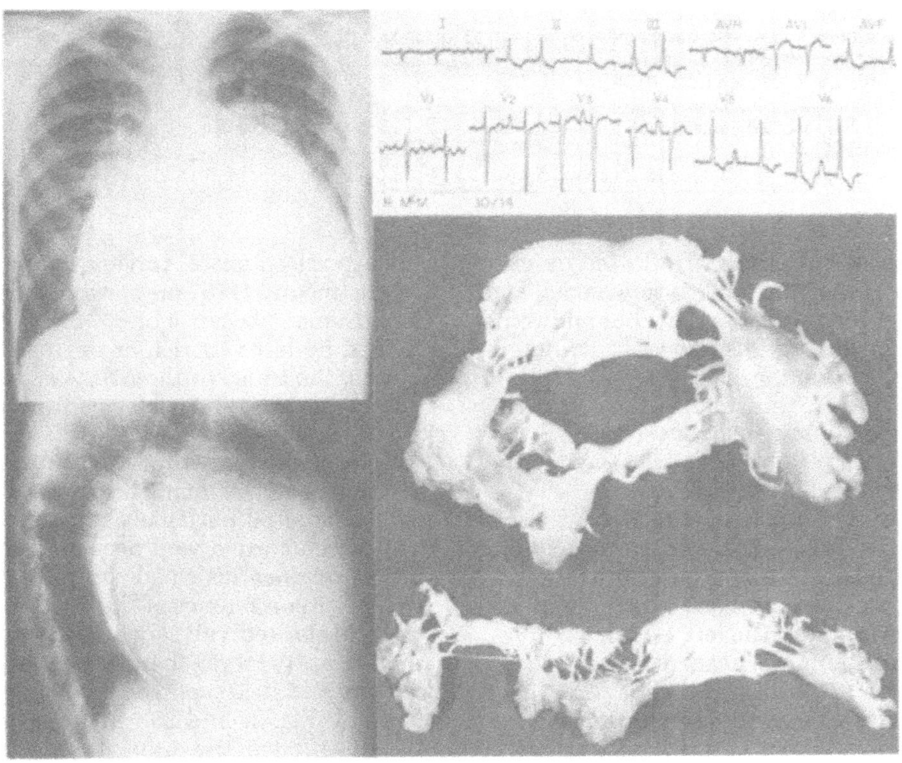

IGURE 14. Pure mitral and tricuspid valve regurgitation of rheumatic origin in a 15-year-old girl (A63-230) who died 2 days after mitral valve re-lacement. Shown are posteroanterior and lateral radiograms and an electrocardiogram immediately preoperatively and the intact and opened operatively excised mitral valve. The patient had acute rheumatic fever at ages 6 and 8 years and a prominent "malar flush." The right ventricular nd femoral arterial peak systolic pressures were 70 and 110 mm Hg, respectively, preoperatively. The mitral leaflets are diffusely thickened but nly mildly so. No Aschoff bodies were present.

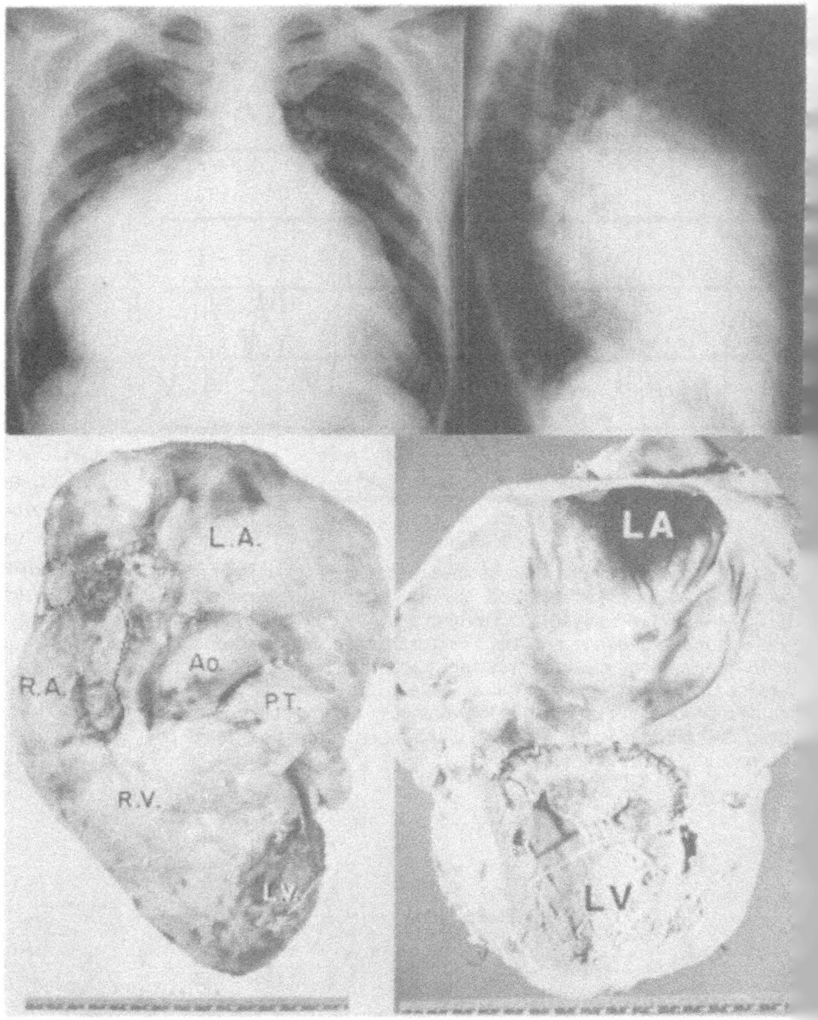

FIGURE 15. Giant-sized left atrium (LA) in a 49-year-old man (A61-84) with severe mitral regurgitation combined with mitral stenosis of rheumatic origin. The right and left ventricular peak systolic pressures were 30 and 100 mm Hg, respectively. The left atrium was entered by a needle inserted into the right mid-axillary line. The patient died 6 hours after mitral replacement. **Lower left,** the giant-sized left atrium is apparent. The **dotted line** outlines the right atrium (RA). Ao = aorta; LV = left ventricle; PT = pulmonary trunk; RV = right ventricle. **Lower right,** opened left atrium, mitral valve, and left ventricle (LV). The ruler units are in centimeters.

tolic pressures in these patients are reflected quickly into the vasculature of the lungs, and severe medial and intimal thickening of the pulmonary arteries and veins progress rapidly. The already diseased left atrium, in contrast, appears to respond to volume load by dilating, not by contracting. Thus, the smaller the left atrial cavity in pure MR, the thicker the right ventricular wall, and, conversely, the larger the left atrial cavity, the thinner the right ventricular wall[41] (Fig. 18).

A relatively new cause of acquired pure MR is *fistulas around the bases of prosthetic and bioprosthetic valves.*[29] Small peribasilar leaks around mitral prostheses are difficult to diagnose clinically without injecting contrast material into the left ventricle.

Although for years rheumatic heart disease has been considered the major cause of significant MR, most patients with rheumatic heart disease and MR also have some degree of MS as well. Of patients with *isolated* (aortic valve function normal), *pure* (no element of stenosis) MR severe enough to warrant mitral valve replacement, *mitral valve prolapse* is now recognized as the most common etiology (Fig. 19 to 22). My associates and I[12] recently reviewed the records and operatively excised mitral valves of 97 patients aged 32 to 7[illegible] years (mean 54) (57 men), who underwent mitral valv[illegible] replacement because of $3^+/4^+$ or $4^+/4^+$ MR as determined by left ventricular angiography. Of the 97 patients, the cause of the MR was leaflet prolapse in 6[illegible] (62%), papillary muscle dysfunction from coronar[illegible] heart disease in 29 (30%), infective endocarditis involving apparently previously normal mitral valve in [illegible] patients, and rheumatic heart disease in 3 patients (Fig 23). Of the 60 patients with mitral prolapse, 13 ha[illegible] ruptured chordae tendineae and all 5 patients with infective endocarditis had ruptured chordae.

The circumference of the mitral anuli in the patient[illegible] with prolapsed valves without ruptured chordae wa[illegible] significantly larger than those in the patients in othe[illegible] groups and in 18 control subjects, both of which wer[illegible] normal (Fig. 24 and 25). Likewise, the areas of the excised leaflets in the prolapsed valves were much large[illegible] than in the other groups and in the control subject[illegible] both of which were normal (Fig. 26). The product of th[illegible] circumference (in centimeters) multiplied by the are[illegible] (in centimeters squared) calculated for the norm[illegible] valves ranged from 45 to 140 cm^3 (average 91). The av[illegible] erage product was 150 cm^3 in the prolapsed valves with ruptured chordae, and 273 cm^3 in the prolapsed valves with intact chordae. The products were 87, 93, and 106 cm^3, respectively, in the valves regurgitant because of papillary muscle dysfunction, infective endocarditis, or rheumatic disease; these products did not differ from those of the normal valves.

The correct cause of the MR in the 97 patients was usually predictable from the history alone. Of the 29 patients with papillary muscle dysfunction from atherosclerotic coronary heart disease, all had clinical evidence of myocardial ischemia: history of acute myocardial infarction which had healed in 24, a left ventricular aneurysm from a silent infarction in 1, and angina pectoris in 4. Of the 5 patients with MR secondary to infective endocarditis, 4 had well-documented episodes of infection that had been cured by antibiotic therapy; none had evidence of valvular dysfunction before the episode of infective endocarditis. Of the 3 patients with MR secondary to a rheumatic origin, 2 had a history of acute rheumatic fever, whereas this item was positive in only 5 of the other 94 patients. Clinical diagnosis of mitral valve prolapse was by a process of exclusion. Only 2 (3%) of the 60 patients had historical evidence of previous acute myocardial infarction; 5 (8%) had a history of acute rheumatic fever and 4 (7%) had a history of active infective endocarditis. Compared with the 5 patients classified as having ruptured chordae tendineae on previously normal valves (4 of whom had a history of infective endocarditis), the 4 patients with healed infective endocarditis and mitral prolapse were older (mean age 61 years versus 42 years), had previous systolic murmurs of MR before the episode of infective endocarditis (4 of 4 versus 0 of 5), and had a longer mean duration of congestive heart failure (11 months versus 4 months). Thus, of the 60 patients with prolapse, 51 (85%) had no historical evidence of myocardial ischemia, acute rheumatic fever, or infective endocarditis.

The origin of the MR also was suggested preoperatively by more objective means. All 29 patients with MR secondary to coronary disease had abnormal Q waves by electrocardiogram, whereas abnormal Q waves were present in only 4 of the 60 patients with mitral prolapse and in none of the 8 patients with MR from either in-

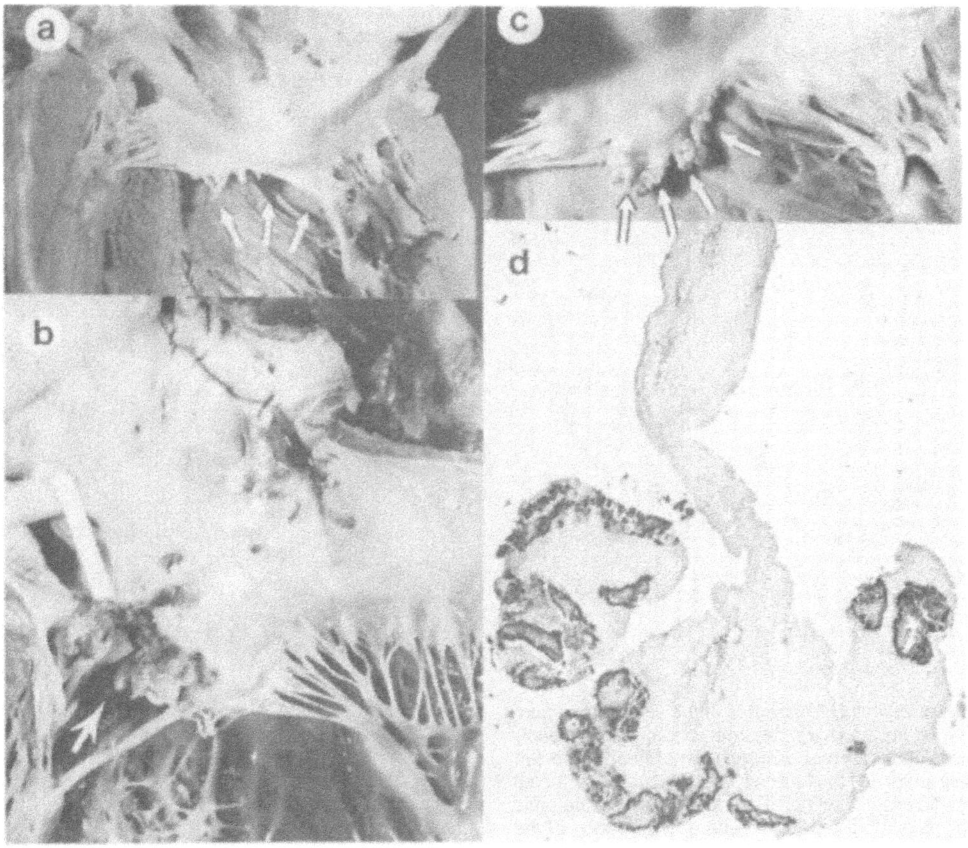

IGURE 16. Ruptured mitral chordae tendineae (**short arrows**) in 3 patients: **a,** in a 29-year-old woman (A63-97) who had had Staphylococcus epi-ermidis endocarditis 5 years earlier on what appears to have been a previously anatomically normal valve. The peak systolic pulmonary arterial ressure was 105 mm Hg and the left atrial V wave, 35 mm Hg. **b,** in a 19-year-old girl (A61-221) who had had Streptococcus group D endocarditis 6 months earlier. The peak systolic pulmonary arterial pressure was 70 mm Hg and the left atrial V wave, 36 mm Hg. **c** and **d,** in a 24-year-old oman (A62-19) who had had enterococcus endocarditis 5 months earlier. The peak systolic pulmonary arterial pressure was 72 mm Hg and the ft atrial V wave, 66 mm Hg. **d,** histologic section of mitral leaflet at site of chordal rupture showing calcific deposits. Hematoxylin and eosin stain. Reprinted, by permission, from Roberts et al.[41])

fective endocarditis or rheumatic disease. Atrial fibrillation was significantly ($p < 0.05$) more common in the patients in whom the MR resulted from coronary disease: in 7 (24%) of these 29 patients, in only 4 (7%) of the 60 patients with mitral prolapse, and in 2 of the 8 patients with either infective endocarditis or a rheumatic origin. Of the 60 patients with prolapse, 43 had M-mode echocardiograms; in 32 (74%) prolapse was demonstrated. Of the 29 patients with coronary heart disease, M-mode echocardiograms were done in 22; only 2 (9%) demonstrated prolapse. Of the 8 patients with MR from infective endocarditis or rheumatic etiologies, 7 had

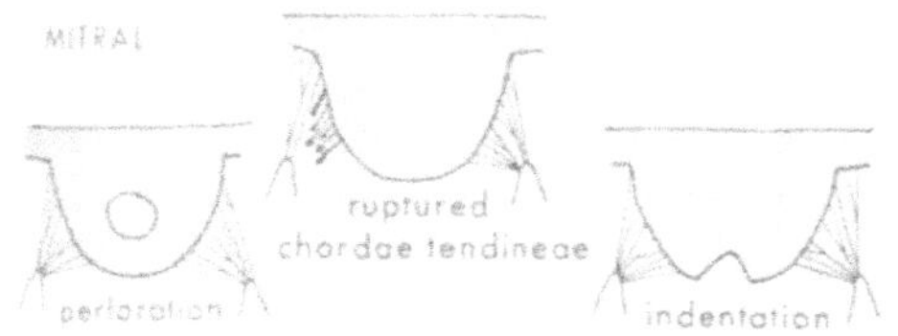

FIGURE 17. Types of mitral valve damage resulting from infective endocarditis.

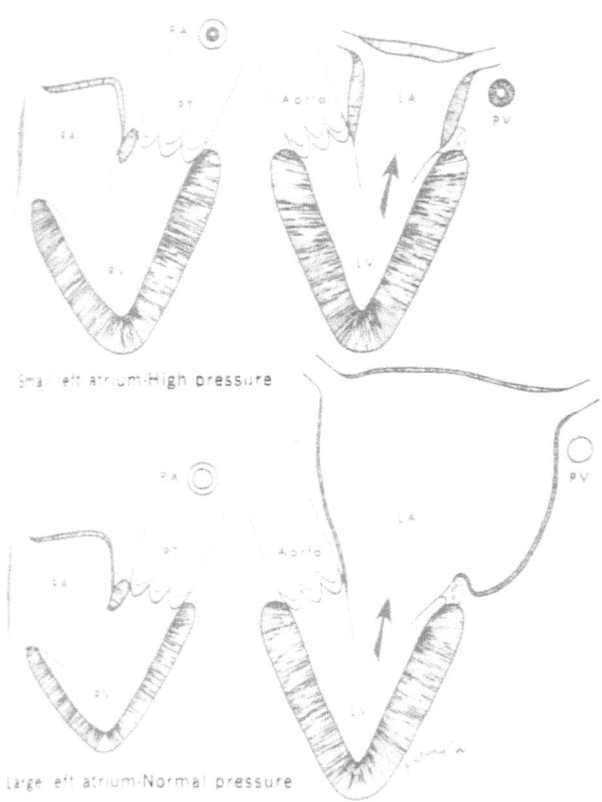

FIGURE 18. Diagram depicting the 2 extremes of the spectrum of pure mitral regurgitation. When severe mitral regurgitation appears suddenly in individuals with previously normal or near-normal hearts, the left atrium (LA) is relatively small and the high pressure within it is reflected back into the pulmonary vessels and right ventricle (RV). The anatomic indicator of this latter physiologic event is severe hypertrophy of the left atrial and right ventricular walls and marked intimal and medial thickening of the pulmonary arteries (PA), arterioles, and veins (PV). In the other extreme, the left atrial cavity is of giant size and its wall is thin. It is thus able to "absorb" the left ventricular (LV) pressure without reflecting it back into the pulmonary vessels or right ventricle. As a consequence, the pulmonary vessels remain normal and the right ventricular wall does not thicken. PT = pulmonary trunk; RA = right atrium. (Reprinted, by permission, from Roberts et al.[47])

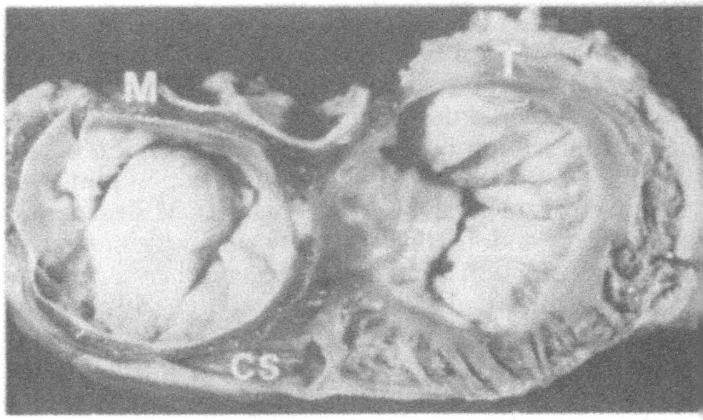

FIGURE 19. Prolapsing mitral (M) and tricuspid (T) valves from the atrial sides in a 55-year-old man (DCMEO #77-05-359) who died suddenly and unexpectedly while at a dance. The patient was known to have had a precordial systolic click and a late systolic murmur since age 36 years but had always been asymptomatic. The M-mode echocardiogram was typical of mitral prolapse. At necropsy, a huge prolapsing "scallop" of the posterior mitral leaflet was present and at least 1 chorda tendinea to this leaflet had ruptured. The leaflet area of the tricuspid valve also was considerably increased. CS = coronary sinus.

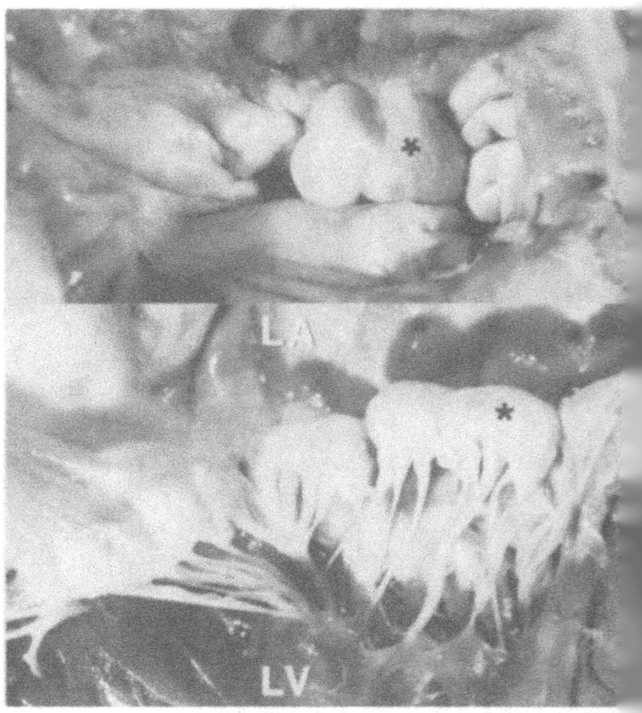

FIGURE 20. Prolapsed mitral valve from above (**top**) and after openir (**bottom**) in an 88-year-old woman who died when hit by an automobil The patient had had no symptoms of cardiac dysfunction. The **asteris** indicates the most prolapsed portion of posterior mitral leaflet. Th mural endocarium beneath the posterior leaflet is thickened by fibro tissue. LA = left atrium; LV = left ventricle.

echocardiograms; none demonstrated prolapse. Left ventriculograms, performed in all 97 patients, indicated prolapse in only 16 (27%) of the 60 prolapse patients and in none of the other 37 patients with other causes. Selective coronary angiograms were performed in 53 (55%) of the 97 patients. All 29 with MR secondary to coronary heart disease had significant (>50% diameter reduction) coronary narrowing demonstrated angiographically in at least 2 of the 3 major coronary arteries. Of the 60 patients with mitral prolapse, coronary angiograms were

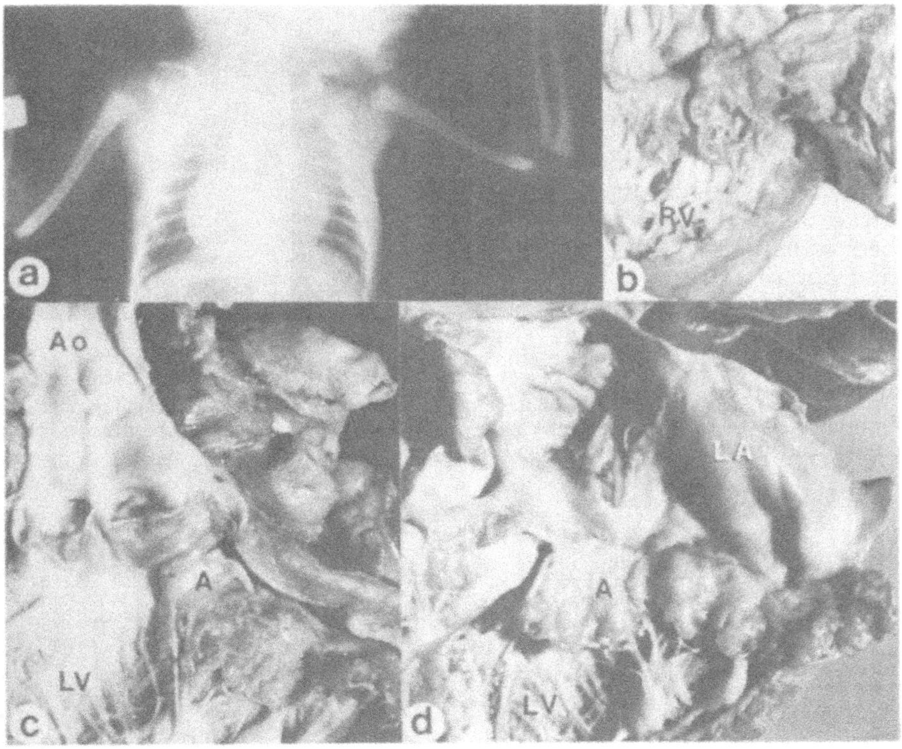

FIGURE 21. Congenital floppy mitral valve and floppy tricuspid valve in a 2-day-old boy (A67-236) who had long toes and fingers, a high-arched palate, and a grade 3/6 precordial systolic murmur typical of mitral regurgitation when examined. The heart was enlarged (**a**) and the infant died of congestive cardiac failure. At necropsy, the intima of the ascending aorta (Ao) was wrinkled (**c**), suggesting that the underlying media was abnormal at this early stage. Shown here are the opened aorta, aortic valve, and left ventricle (LV). A = anterior mitral leaflet. **d,** opened left atrium (LA), mitral valve, and left ventricle (LV). The mitral leaflets are considerably elongated in both longitudinal and transverse dimensions. The left atrium is dilated. **b,** the tricuspid valve leaflets also are elongated in both transverse and longitudinal dimensions. RA = right atrium; RV = right ventricle. (Reprinted, by permission, from Roberts and Honig.[40])

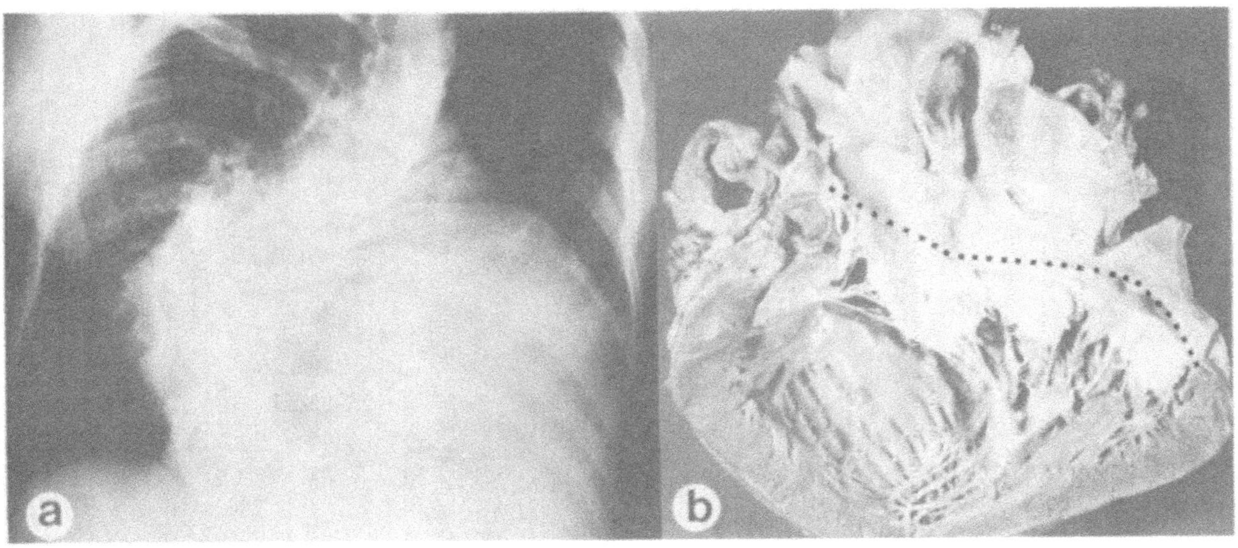

IGURE 22. Posteroanterior chest roentgenogram (**left**) and opened left atrium, mitral valve, and left ventricle (**right**) in a 28-year-old man (A63-25) who had the onset of exertional dyspnea 4 years before death and evidence of overt congestive heart failure for 1 year before death. He never had murmur of aortic regurgitation. At necropsy, the aorta was normal both grossly and histologically. The mitral valve anulus (**dotted line**) is greatly dilated (17 cm) and the length of the cusps from basal attachment to distal margin is elongated without elongation of the chordae tendineae. The vertebral column is greatly deformed (**left**). (Reprinted, by permission, from Roberts and Honig.[40])

performed in 23; only 3 (13%) had significant coronary narrowing, limited in each to 1 (right) coronary artery. Auscultation and hemodynamic data at cardiac catheterization were not helpful in delineating the origin of the MR. None of the 97 patients—including the 60 classified as having prolapse—had systolic clicks and the systolic precordial murmurs in all 97 patients were holosystolic. The average pulmonary arterial, left atrial (or pulmonary arterial wedge), and left ventricular pressures were similar in the 97 patients irrespective of the origin of the MR. The systolic systemic arterial pressures, however, were significantly higher in the patients with mitral prolapse and ruptured chordae tendineae than in those with mitral prolapse and intact chordae tendineae.

Surprisingly, few reports are available describing the various causes of MR in large numbers of patients. Furthermore, we[12] were unable to find any reports concerning the causes of pure MR in groups of patients in whom any associated MS or aortic valve dysfunction had been excluded by appropriate hemodynamic and angiographic studies. The most frequently cited report describing patients with MR appears to be that by Selzer and Katayama,[62] who summarized findings in

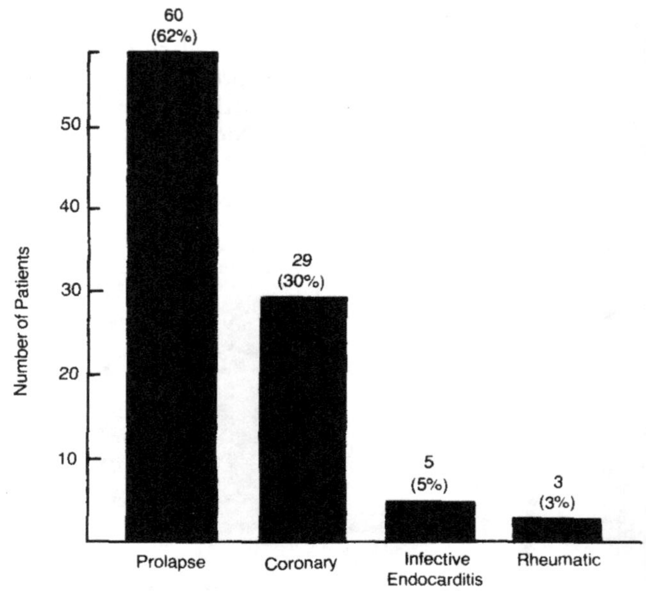

FIGURE 23. Bar graph showing the 4 conditions causing chronic, isolated, pure mitral regurgitation in 97 patients with operatively excised valves. (Reprinted, by permission, from Waller et al.[12])

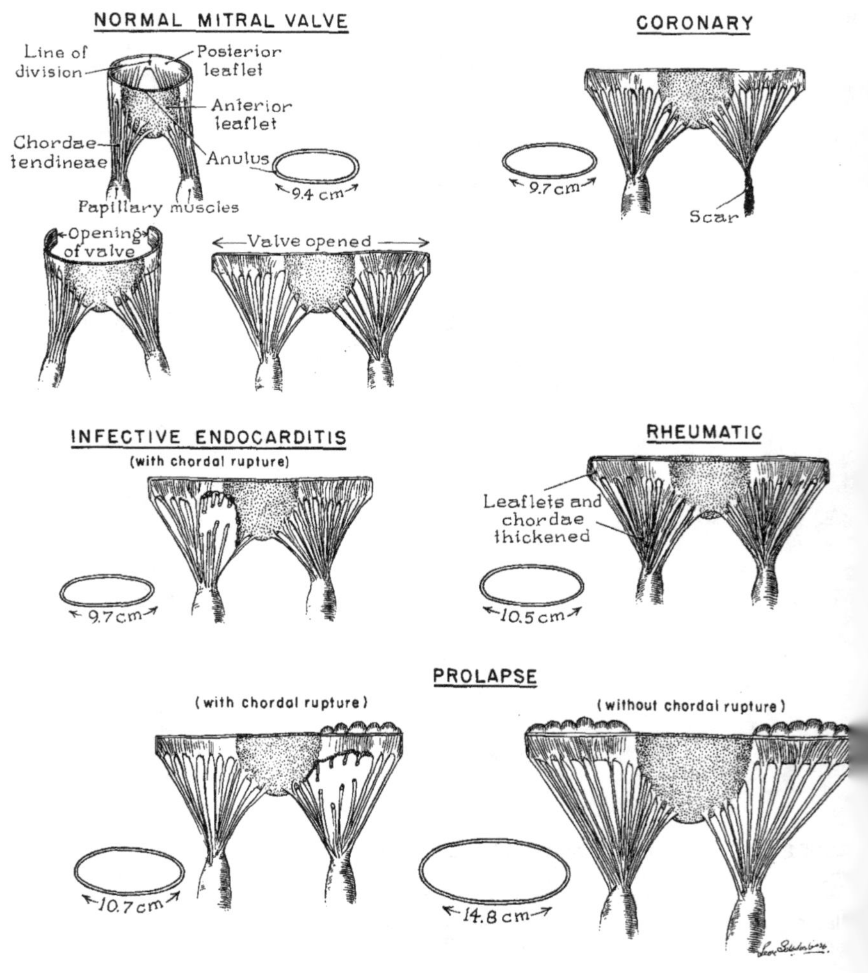

FIGURE 24. Diagram showing morphologic variations in mitral valve "anular" circumference and leaflet area in 4 conditions causing isolated, pure mitral regurgitation. (Reprinted, by permission, from Waller et al.[12])

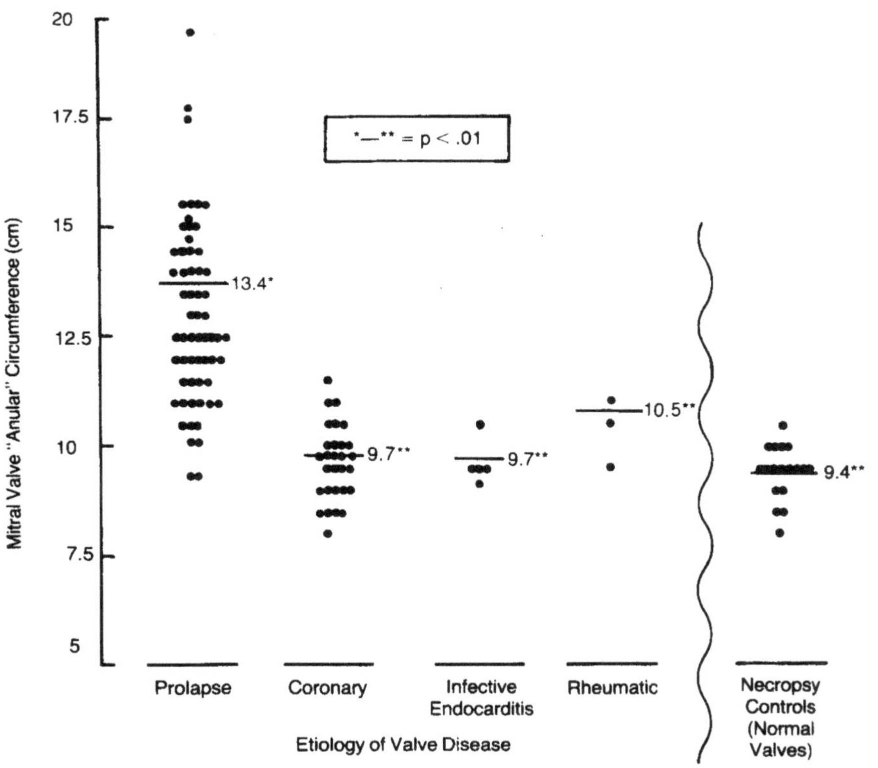

FIGURE 25. Graph showing mitral valve "anular" circumference (in centimeters) in each of the 97 patients with operatively excised mitral valves in the 4 conditions causing chronic, isolated, pure mitral regurgitation, and in 18 necropsy control valves. (Reprinted, by permission, from Waller et al.[12])

230 patients. Although 212 of their 230 patients had pure MR defined as the "absence of a late diastolic gradient across the valve . . . except in tachycardia" at the time of cardiac catheterization, some of their patients had MS at other times. Of their 230 patients, 88 were classified as having MR of rheumatic origin, and I suspect that nearly half (42 patients) had MS at some time in their course: 5 had had mitral commissurotomies for MS and severe MR developed subsequently; 8 of their rheumatic patients had MR only after the development of infective endocarditis, and it is probable that 1 or more previously had had MS; and 33 (38%) of their 88 rheumatic patients had sizeable calcific deposits in their mitral valves, a finding quite unusual in patients without some degree of MS. (Only 4 of our 97 patients had grossly visible calcific deposits in their excised mitral valves.) It is also difficult to compare the observations in our patients with those reported by Selzer and Katayama because of differences in patient selection. We[12] studied only patients who were in functional classes III and IV (New York Heart Association) because of congestive heart failure; all underwent mitral valve replacement and all had their valves examined by the same observer. Seventy (30%) of the 230 patients reported by Selzer and Katayama were in functional classes I or II, and mitral valve operations were performed in just over half of the 230 patients. Additionally, they included children, which we did not. Finally, we excluded patients with any aortic valve dysfunction, which may or may not have been the case in the study by Selzer and Katayama.

In the past, rheumatic heart disease has been considered the most common cause of severe MR, but it is likely that most or many patients so classified in older studies had some degree of MS. Because there has been such a strong tendency in the past to believe that severe MR was usually the result of rheumatic heart disease, other causes commonly have not been sought and definitions of "rheumatic" MR have not been precisely stated. Before 1963, most prolapsing or floppy mitral valves almost certainly were called "rheumatic" in origin at necropsy or operation. Our report[12] morphologically defined a prolapsed mitral valve which can cause severe MR; its anular circumference and leaflet area are clearly increased over that of other valves causing MR, except when the chordae tendineae of the prolapsing valve are ruptured. It is hoped that this definition will prevent indiscriminate labeling of mitral disease in the future as rheumatic when other evidences of previous rheumatic carditis are lacking.

Congenital MR is usually associated with other anomalities.[2,6,30–40] "*Isolated*" congenital MR is usually accompanied by *endocardial fibroelastosis of the left ventricle.* It is sometimes difficult, however, to determine what causes the mitral valve to be regurgitant in this circumstance. Neither is it always clear why the mitral valve is frequently regurgitant in patients with *partial atrioventricular canal* (endocardial cushion defect).[30,31,37] Nearly all patients with partial atrioventricular canal have a cleft, either partial or complete, in the anterior mitral leaflet. It would be easy to attribute the MR to the cleft, but the MR usually disap-

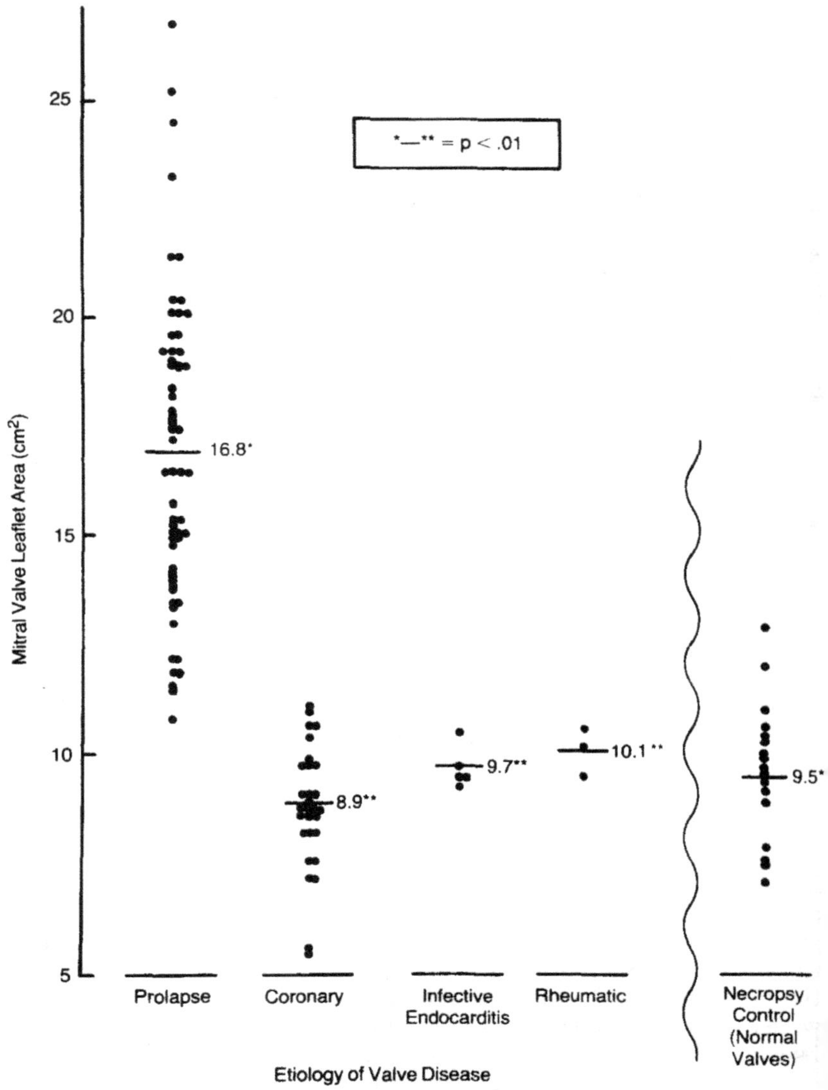

FIGURE 26. Graph showing mitral valve leaflet area (in centimeters squared) in each of the 97 patients with operatively excised mitral valves in the 4 conditions causing chronic, isolated, pure mitral regurgitation and in 18 necropsy control valves. (Reprinted, by permission, from Waller et al.[12])

pears after operative closure of the associated defect in the lowermost portion of the atrial septum (ostium primum defect), irrespective of whether the cleft in the anterior mitral leaflet is closed by suture. For the same reason, it is unlikely that the anomalous chordae tendineae that insert onto the crest of the ventricular septum play a significant role in the production of MR. It is helpful to think of partial atrioventricular canal as a syndrome consisting of 5 components: (1) defect in the lowermost portion of atrial septum; (2) cleft in the anterior mitral leaflet; (3) absence of tissue, either partial or complete, in the septal tricuspid valve leaflet; (4) anomalous chordae tendineae from the anterior mitral leaflet to the crest of ventricular septum; and (5) ventricular septal defect. The syndrome may include all 5 components or may have as few as 2; most commonly, the first 4 components are present. A cleft in the anterior mitral leaflet may occur, however, in the absence of a defect in the lowermost portion of the atrial septum.[63] These individuals usually present with evidence of isolated MR or with features of isolated ventricula[r] septal defect. Of 21 necropsy patients with a cleft in th[e] anterior mitral leaflet unassociated with a defect in th[e] lowermost portion of the atrial septum reported b[y] Segni and Edwards,[63] 11 had no defect in any portio[n] of the atrial or ventricular septa and the other 9 ha[d] associated defects, usually ventricular septal defect [o]r a fossa ovale type atrial septal defect or both. Occa[-]sionally, the ostium primum defect may be so small tha[t] the shunt through it is missed or is only trivial; thes[e] patients also may present with essentially pu[re] MR.[30,31]

Corrected transposition is an entity that has pr[o]duced much confusion. Corrected transposition an[d] complete transposition are quite different; the on[ly] thing they have in common is the word "transposition[."] Complete transposition is essentially 1 defect: the gre[at] arteries are transposed, so that the aorta arises from t[he] right ventricle and the pulmonary trunk from the le[ft] ventricle. In corrected transposition, the great arteri

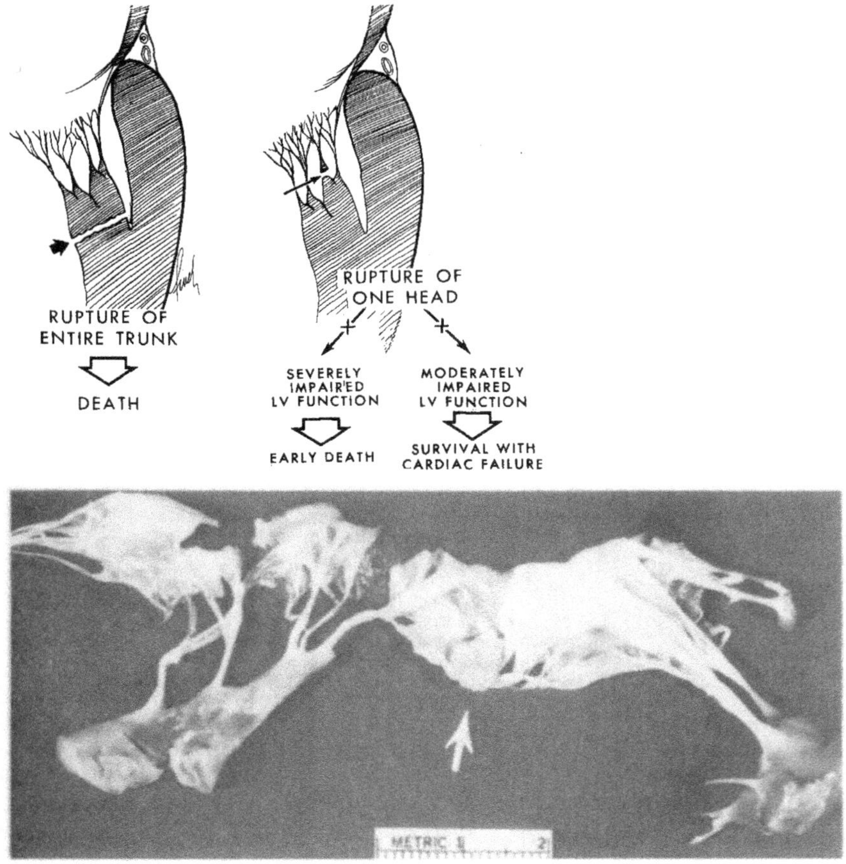

FIGURE 27. Top, diagram of the types of, and possible consequences of, papillary muscle rupture during acute myocardial infarction. It is likely that rupture of the entire trunk (**left**) is incompatible with survival in any patient since a major portion of the support to both valve leaflets is destroyed. With rupture of an apical head (**right**), survival would appear to depend on the extent to which the function of the left ventricle has been impaired by the infarct. With severely impaired ventricular function, the additional burden of even modest mitral regurgitation may be intolerable, and death will ensue. If the left ventricle is less severely compromised, survival is possible for weeks or months, but congestive cardiac failure will almost invariably develop. **Bottom,** rupture of a portion of 1 papillary muscle during acute myocardial infarction in a 51-year-old man (S67-813) who underwent mitral valve replacement 3 months after the onset of the infarction. Preoperatively, the pulmonary arterial pressure was 60/28 mm Hg; pulmonary arterial wedge pressure, mean 28, v42; left ventricular pressure 74/17 mm Hg; and cardiac index, 1.7 liters/min/m^2. The leaflets are normal but the posteromedial papillary muscle is necrotic and fibrotic and a portion of it (**arrow**) is entwined in chordae tendineae at the margin of the anterior mitral leaflet. This is a view of the ventricular aspects of the leaflets. LV = left ventricular. (Reprinted, by permission, from Roberts and Perloff.[2])

also are transposed, but, in addition, the ventricles, atrioventricular valves, coronary arteries, and conduction system are inverted. Patients with complete transposition die because they have inadequate communications between the 2 circuits. Patients with corrected transposition theoretically should be able to live a full lifespan, but usually this is not the case because associated defects—namely, ventricular septal defect or regurgitation of the left-sided atrioventricular valve, or both—cause the heart to function abnormally. Abnormalities of the left-sided atrioventricular valve, a systemic valve but anatomically a tricuspid valve, are the most common associated anomalies in corrected transposition.[64] Of the anomalies, the most frequent is the Ebstein-type malformation. These valves are intrinsically regurgitant because the chordae are short and the leaflets are closely adherent to the ventricular endocardium.

A mitral valve may be abnormal anatomically and yet function entirely normally. A congenital malformation illustrating this point is the *double-orifice mitral valve*, which looks like a double-barreled shotgun.[65] Generally, both orifices are totally competent and the patient should be asymptomatic.

Papillary Muscle Dysfunction

Rupture of a portion of a papillary muscle was not appreciated until 15 years ago.[48] The original concept of papillary muscle rupture was rupture of its entire trunk, caused either by myocardial infarction from coronary narrowing or by trauma (Fig. 27). Complete transsection of a left ventricular papillary muscle is incompatible with life because about 60 chordae tendineae are thus disrupted. More frequent is rupture of a portion of a papillary muscle. In this situation, the largest amount of MR is probably caused by the rupture, but all these patients have severe necrosis of the remaining portion of the papillary muscle and the latter probably contributes to the regurgitation. When 1 head of a papillary muscle is ruptured, about 10 third-order chordae tendineae are disrupted.

Necrosis or fibrosis of a papillary muscle without rupture is far more common than rupture. Table II lists conditions frequently associated with papillary muscle dysfunction, particularly necrosis or fibrosis.[3] Although coronary arterial luminal narrowing is the most frequent cause of papillary muscle necrosis or fibrosis, many other conditions may be accompanied by papillary muscle lesions. The papillary muscles are fibrotic or necrotic in so many conditions because they are the last structures in the heart to be perfused by arterial blood. Of the 2 left ventricular papillary muscles, the posteromedial one has the poorer blood supply, and, consequently, lesions are more frequent in it than in the anterolateral muscle. The posteromedial muscle receives its oxygen mainly from blood passing through the right coronary artery. The mouth of this artery may be >15 cm from the apex of the posteromedial muscle. To perfuse it, blood must pass through the entire thickness of left ventricular wall, turn uphill (so to speak), and ascend a distance equivalent to 2 more full thicknesses of left ventricular wall. Thus, the apices of the papillary muscles are the sites farthest from the coronary ostia, and they receive oxygen only after the other myocardium has had an opportunity to extract its oxygen needs. Although the surfaces of the papillary muscles are entirely bathed by intracavitary ventricular blood, only a small amount of oxygen diffuses into these structures from the intracavitary blood.

The most common cause of papillary muscle necrosis or fibrosis is *narrowing of the coronary arterial lumen by atherosclerotic plaques.* The posteromedial papillary muscle is usually involved in acute posterior myocardial infarction. In anterior wall infarction, however, the anterolateral papillary muscle may be spared, presumably because its blood supply is better than that of the posteromedial muscle. Since infarction limited to the ventricular septum or to the lateral portion of the left ventricular free wall (that is, the portions of the left ventricular wall unassociated with papillary muscles) is rare, the papillary muscles are usually involved when myocardial infarction occurs. It is, therefore, surprising that papillary muscle dysfunction is not more frequent during or after acute myocardial infarction.

In patients with *left ventricular outflow obstruction*, lesions often occur in the papillary muscles. Valvular aortic stenosis, whether in infants or in adults, when superimposed on a congenitally malformed valve, either unicuspid or bicuspid, is nearly always associated with fibrosis and atrophy of at least the posteromedial papillary muscle. Rheumatic valvular aortic stenosis combined with organic MS or MR, however, infrequently is associated with papillary muscle fibrosis or atrophy. Nearly all adult patients with discrete subaortic stenosis or hypertrophic cardiomyopathy with or without diffuse subaortic stenosis have small fibrous scars in both left ventricular papillary muscles, but atrophy of 1 or both muscles is uncommon.[39]

Foci of necrosis also are common in patients with fatal *severe valvular regurgitation of recent onset.* Among 47 patients dying of active valvular infective endocarditis and examined personally, 34 (72%) had necrotic lesions in 1 or both left ventricular papillary muscles; none had significant narrowing of the extramural coronary arteries. Most patients had pure aortic regurgitation, but some had pure MR secondary to the active infective endocarditis. Severely diminished cardiac output resulting in poor myocardial perfusion was believed the cause of the papillary muscle necrosis in these patients.

Small fibrous scars in the papillary muscles are common in patients with *systemic hypertension*, but atrophy of these muscles is infrequent in this condition, unless coronary heart disease also is present. In left ventricular hypertrophy of any cause, the hypertrophy of the papillary muscles should probably be proportional to that of the left ventricular free wall or ventricular septum. This proportional hypertrophy usually exists in patients with systemic hypertension but is infrequent in patients with left ventricular outflow obstruction.

Fibrosis with atrophy of the papillary muscles is to be expected in patients with primary *endocardial fibroelastosis* of the left ventricle. Histologically, the thickened endocardium in this condition is similar to the media of the aorta, being characterized by elastic fibrils running parallel to one another and to the surface. Primary left ventricular endocardial fibroelastosis may be an anatomic expression of chronically inadequate coronary arterial perfusion of the left ventricle; since the posteromedial papillary muscle is the least well-perfused portion of the heart, this structure is affected the most. In the congenital anomaly, origin of the left or both coronary arteries from the pulmonary trunk, diffuse endocardial fibroelastosis of the left ventricle is nearly always an associated lesion.[33] Fibrosis and atrophy of the left ventricular papillary muscles are to be expected in this anomaly, and these patients may present clinically with features of pure MR.

TABLE II Spectrum of Left Ventricular Papillary Muscle Dysfunction

- I. Rupture of papillary muscle
  - A. Total ("belly" or trunk)
    1. Rapid death
    2. Survival—not described
  - B. Partial ("head")
    1. Rapid death
    2. Survival but chronic congestive cardiac failure
- II. Fibrosis or necrosis of papillary muscle without rupture
  - A. With coronary arterial narrowing
    1. Acute myocardial infarct
    2. Healed myocardial infarct
  - B. Without coronary arterial narrowing
    1. Acute
    2. Chronic
       - a. Valvular, subvalvular (discrete and diffuse) and supravalvular aortic stenosis
       - b. Systemic hypertension
       - c. Origin of left coronary artery from pulmonary trunk
       - d. Primary endocardial fibroelastosis
       - e. Endomyocardial fibrosis
       - f. *Löffler's fibroplastic parietal endocarditis*
       - g. Diffuse (primary) myocardial disease
       - h. Focal myocardial disease
         1. Idiopathic
         2. "Neurogenic" heart disease
         3. Infectious
- III. Normal or near-normal papillary muscles but severe fibrosis or necrosis in adjacent left ventricular free wall with and without coronary arterial narrowing

Foci of fibrosis or necrosis in the left ventricular papillary muscles are infrequent in patients with dilated cardiomyopathy.[54,66] Rarely, *myocarditis* may be localized to papillary muscle and adjacent left ventricular free wall.[67] Patients with the *neurogenic heart disease* (Friedreich's ataxia, progressive muscular dystrophy and myotonic muscular dystrophy) generally have scarred left ventricular papillary muscles, especially the posteromedial ones.[68] The African cardiomyopathy, *endomyocardial fibrosis*, may be associated with extensive scarring of the papillary muscles.[54] In this condition the posteromedial muscle is usually covered by a thrombus or by dense fibrous tissue that probably represents organized thrombus. Likewise, *Löffler's fibroplastic parietal endocarditis*, which may be 1 stage of endomyocardial fibrosis,[53] is usually associated with extensive scarring of 1 or both papillary muscles.

The papillary muscles are subject to various infiltrative processes, just like any other portion of myo

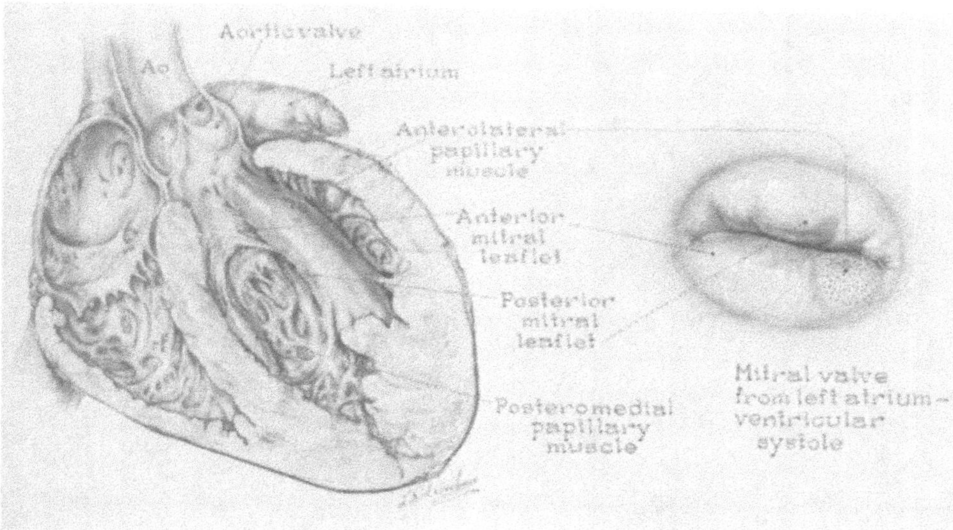

FIGURE 28. Drawing of heart in a 23-year-old man (DCMEO #80-02-134) who died from idiopathic dilated cardiomyopathy. An incidental finding at necropsy was the insertion of the anterolateral papillary muscle directly onto the anterior mitral leaflet. This congenital anomaly has been observed personally in about 5 cases at necropsy. It appears to have no functional significance. Ao = aorta.

cardium. *Pyogenic abscesses, Aschoff bodies, granulomas,*[67] *neoplasms,*[69–71] *amyloid,*[72] *iron,*[73] *and air*[74] have all been observed in these structures. Congestive heart failure from severe MR may be the initial symptom of cardiac *sarcoidosis.*[67]

The most frequent congenital malformation of papillary muscles is the occurrence of only 1 such muscle in the left ventricle. In this condition, described as the *parachute mitral valve*, all mitral chordae tendineae are attached to the 1 left ventricular papillary muscle (Fig. 11). The resulting mitral valve is usually stenotic, but it may be purely regurgitant or it may function normally.[35] The single papillary muscle is usually associated with other malformations, including a supramitral valve ring, diffuse subaortic stenosis, and coarctation of the aorta. Other malformations, including valvular aortic stenosis, ventricular septal defect, and valvular pulmonic stenosis, also may occur.

There may be not only 1 too few papillary muscles but also 1 too many. An *accessory papillary muscle* is usually of no functional significance, but it has been seen in association with congenital MR. When 2 papillary muscles are present, 1 or both may still be congenitally malformed. One or both papillary muscles may be abnormally large and malpositioned with attachment onto the anterior mitral leaflet, creating the potential at least for valvular stenosis or regurgitation (Fig. 28). Both papillary muscles also may be poorly developed and small. This finding is particularly characteristic with origin of the left coronary artery or both coronary arteries from the pulmonary trunk. In this situation, the papillary muscles arise more cephalad than normal from the left ventricular free wall.

Both left ventricular papillary muscles usually are excised either completely or incompletely at operations to replace the mitral valve. The myocardium of the free wall at the sites of excision of these muscles is always infiltrated by inflammatory cells when this area is examined in the early postoperative period. With time, these areas are covered by dense fibroelastic tissue simulating the composition of the media of the aorta. If the papillary muscles are not excised when the mitral leaflets and chordae tendineae are excised during mitral valve replacement, the papillary muscles atrophy and are focally replaced by fibrous tissue; the myocardial cells become disorganized.[75] When the papillary muscles are excised at operation, each is grasped by a clamp extending through the mitral orifice from the left atrium. If the papillary muscles are pulled too vigorously by the clamp during their excision, portions of left ventricular free wall also may be excised. The result may be perforation or severe thinning of the left ventricular wall. The latter may lead to the formation of a functioning or anatomic aneurysm or both.[76,77]

Mitral Anulus

Although it may accompany left ventricular dilation, mitral anular dilation, except in patients with prolapsing or floppy mitral valves,[12] is a rare cause of MR[59]; in the past, most patients with MR that was believed the result of mitral anular dilation probably had papillary muscle dysfunction. Mitral anular dilation to a degree capable of causing MR probably does not occur except in association with mitral valve prolapse because the surface area of the mitral leaflets is more than twice the area of the mitral orifice, and the anulus contracts during ventricular systole.[2] The mitral ring has a sphincter-like action because the mitral orifice is smaller during ventricular systole than during diastole. In patients with dilated left ventricles, the widest diameter does not occur at the left ventricular base, the area that includes the mitral anulus, but in the midportion of the chamber between apex and base (Fig. 29). In fact, the base of the left ventricle is prevented from dilating freely because the "fibrous skeleton" is attached to it, whereas the midportion of the left ventricle is not so restricted. Indeed, severe left ventricular dilation may occur without any dilation of the mitral anulus.

Although it is now well known that MR may occur in patients with dilated left ventricles from any cause

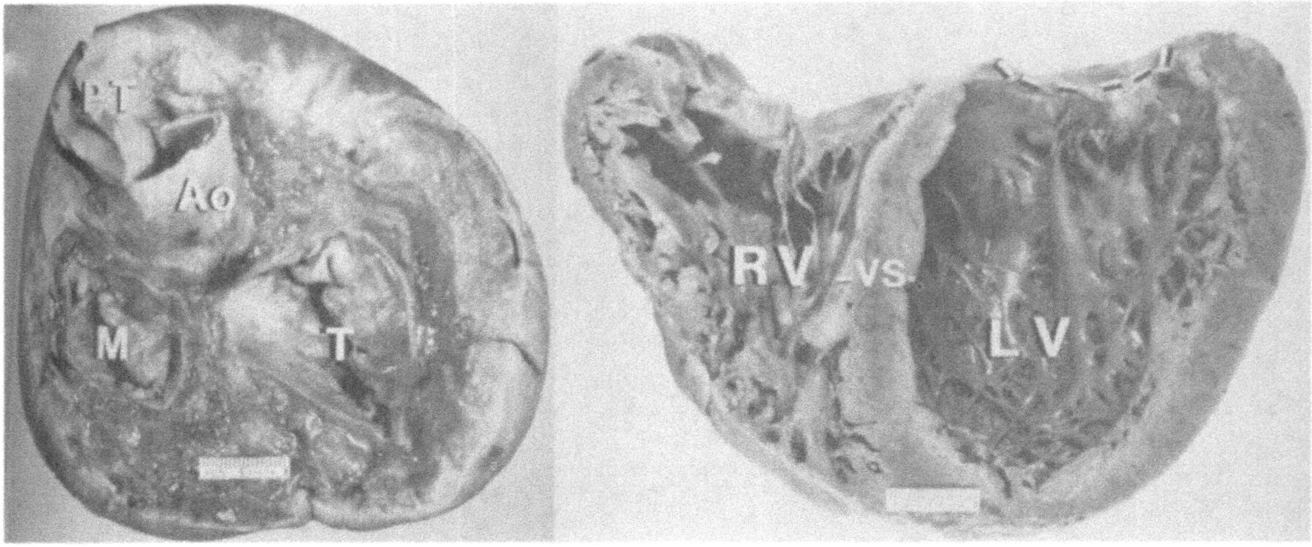

FIGURE 29. The heart of a 34-year-old man (DCGH #74A-65) with idiopathic dilated cardiomyopathy and clinical evidence of both tricuspid and mitral regurgitation of severe degree. Both ventricles are considerably dilated. The greatest increase in dimension of the right (RV) is in the area of the tricuspid valve anulus. The tricuspid valve orifice (T) admitted 4 fingers readily, indicating its proximal diameter to be about 8 cm. In contrast, the maximal diameter of the left ventricle (LV) was about midway between the apex and the mitral anulus. The mitral orifice (M) only admitted 2 fingers, indicating that its maximal diameter was about 4 cm. The mitral regurgitation resulted, therefore, not from anular dilatation, which was mild, but probably from altered angulation of the left ventricular papillary muscles. Ao = aorta.

without associated left ventricular necrosis or fibrosis, it is less well recognized that necrosis or fibrosis of the left ventricular free wall, unassociated with left ventricular dilation or papillary muscle or mitral tissue lesions, also may be associated with MR. Generally, the scarring or necrosis of the myocardium adjacent to the papillary muscles fails to move or moves paradoxically during ventricular systole, and the abnormal ventricular contraction may lead to abnormal papillary muscle anchoring, resulting in MR. Anatomic left ventricular aneurysms unassociated with papillary muscle necrosis or fibrosis may cause MR by the same mechanism.

Abnormal pulling on the papillary muscles unassociated with left ventricular necrosis or fibrosis or cavity

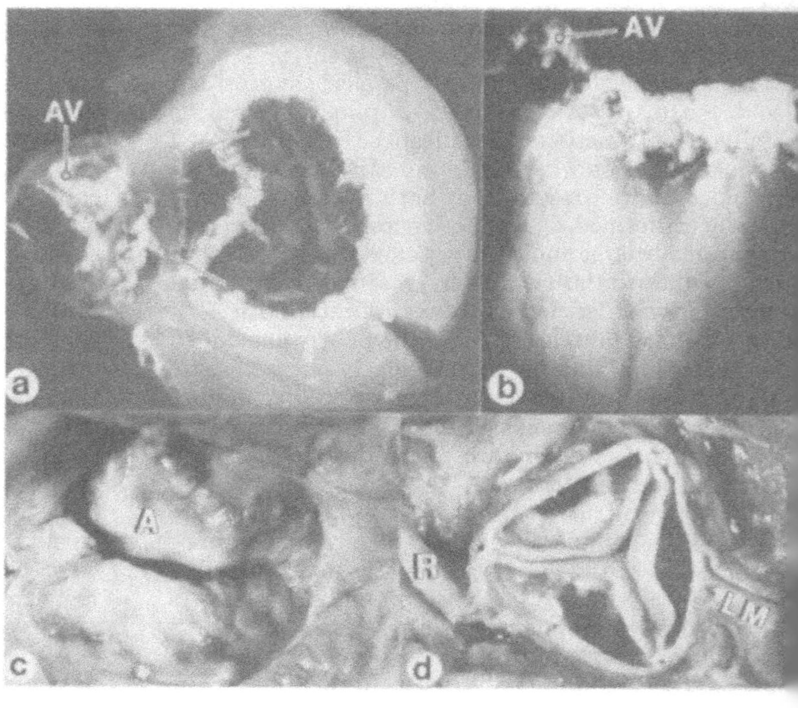

FIGURE 30. Massive calcific deposits in the mitral anulus (**a**, **b**, and **c**), aortic valve (AV) (**a**, **b**, and **d**), and coronary arteries (**a** and **b**) in an 82-year-old man (NNMC #A70-200) who had Paget's disease of bone. The short bar of calcium between the lines in **a** is that extending across the anterior (A) mitral leaflet. The radiogram in **a** is a cephalad-caudal orientation, and that in **b**, a lateral view. The mitral valve as observed from the left atrium is shown in **c**, and the aortic valve from the aorta in **d**. LM and R = left main and right coronary arteries. (Reprinted, by permission, from Roberts and Waller.[79])

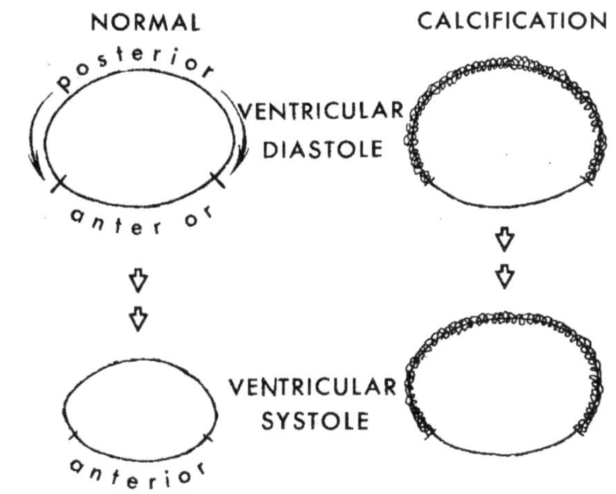

FIGURE 31. Mechanism of mitral regurgitation in patients with calcification of the mitral anulus. During ventricular systole, the base of the left ventricle contracts like a sphincter. Included in the base of the left ventricle is the anulus behind the posterior mitral leaflet. Thus, this circumference decreases during systole. If, however, the anulus behind the posterior mitral leaflet is calcified, the sphincter-like contraction of the left ventricular base may be prevented from occurring. The area of the mitral orifice thus is not decreased, and mild degrees of mitral regurgitation may result. (Reprinted, by permission, from Roberts and Perloff.[2])

dilation may occur in patients with *hypertrophic cardiomyopathy*; this mechanism may account for their MR.[51,54] The huge thickening of the ventricular septum may distort or bend the anterolateral papillary muscle and prevent proper contraction of this structure during ventricular systole. In addition to actual bending of the anterolateral left ventricular papillary muscle, however, the mitral leaflets in adults with hypertrophic cardiomyopathy are always thickened. The thickening of the anterior mitral leaflet appears to be the result of its contact with the mural endocardium in the left ventricular outflow tract during ventricular systole. But the posterior mitral leaflet also is thickened, probably a result of its contacting itself abnormally during ventricular systole. The mitral leaflets and chordae tendineae are within the left ventricular cavity, which in hypertrophic cardiomyopathy is relatively small; as a consequence, space within the left ventricle may be inadequate to easily accommodate the mitral leaflets and chordae, and with vigorous contractions portions of the posterior leaflet contact other portions of the same leaflet abnormally. Fibrous thickening is the consequence. The MR in hypertrophic cardiomyopathy usually disappears after operative excision or incision of myocardium in the left ventricular outflow tract.[51]

Calcification of the mitral anulus is one of the more frequent abnormalities of the heart. Mitral anular calcification is generally considered to be a disease of elderly women. Indeed, of 14 patients with "massive" mitral anular calcification reported by Korn et al[78] 21 years ago, all were women and all were over 65 years of age. It is incorrect, however, to believe that this entity is reserved for a particular sex at a particular time in life. During the past 14 years I have examined over 300 patients with mitral anular calcium at necropsy. Of the first 200 analyzed systematically, 47% were men and 53% were women. Of the 200 patients, 141 (70%) were over age 65 years and 17 (8%) were aged 45 years or less. The extent of the mitral anular calcium was graded 1^+ to 4^+: in 110 patients (55%) the deposits were graded 1^+ or 2^+ and in 90 patients (45%) grade 3^+ or 4^+. The calcium in 198 patients was limited to the anular region behind posterior mitral leaflet, usually forming a C-shaped configuration; in 2 patients, the calcium extended across the anterior mitral leaflet to form an O-shaped configuration[79] (Fig. 30). Of the 38 patients with 4^+ deposits, 76% were women. Thus, although mitral anular calcium of any degree appears to occur with similar frequency in men and women, the larger deposits (those likely to be seen on the chest roentgenogram) are more frequent in women. Calcium deposits also were present on the aortic aspects of the aortic valve cusps in 138 (69%) of the 200 patients (64 [32%] of whom had aortic valve stenosis) and in the coronary arteries in 168 (84%) patients.

Factors predisposing to mitral anular calcium were found in 80% of the 200 patients. These included elevation (>140 mm Hg) of left ventricular systolic pressure (142 patients), diabetes mellitus (39 patients), chronic hypercalcemia (9 patients),[30] prolapsing mitral valve (6 patients), the Marfan syndrome (5 patients),[40] left-to-right shunt (secundum type atrial septal defect) (3 patients), and the Hurler syndrome (2 patients).[46] Mitral anular calcium also may form late at sites of attachment of prosthetic mitral valves.[81]

The association of mitral anular calcium with calcific deposits in the coronary arteries and aortic valve cusps, the lack of mitral anular deposits in persons living in environments where the total serum cholesterol is ≤150 mg/dl, and the frequent occurrence of factors predisposing to atherosclerosis in patients with mitral anular calcium supports a common etiologic basis for both mitral anular calcium and atherosclerosis.

The functional consequences of mitral anular calcium are 2, namely MR or MS, and rarely, if ever, both. The presence of either MR or MS is a function of the amount of anular calcium present and also probably the size of the left ventricular cavity. The most common functional consequence, of course, is MR, which is nearly always of only mild degree and never of severe degree except in a patient with associated mitral anular dilatation in the setting of mitral valve prolapse.[12] The frequency of a murmur typical of MR is nearly always present in patients with $4^+/4^+$ anular deposits and is rarely the consequence of anular deposits if the extent of the latter is only $1^+/4^+$. The mechanism of MR in patients with mitral anular calcium is depicted graphically in Figure 31. Mitral stenosis as a consequence of mitral anular calcium has been observed only in the presence of huge ($4^+/4^+$) mitral anular deposits associated with severe left ventricular hypertrophy without dilatation, usually the consequence of associated left ventricular outflow obstruction.[25]

References

1. **Perloff JK, Roberts WC.** The mitral apparatus. Functional anatomy of mitral regurgitation. Circulation 1972;46:227–239.
2. **Roberts WC, Perloff JK.** Mitral valvular disease. A clinicopathologic survey of the conditions causing the mitral valve to function abnormally. Ann Intern Med 1972;77:939–975.
3. **Roberts WC, Cohen LS.** Left ventricular papillary muscles. Description of the normal and a survey of conditions causing them to be abnormal. Circulation 1972;46:138–154.
4. **Waller BF, Roberts WC.** Cardiovascular disease in the very elderly. An analysis of 40 necropsy patients aged 90 years or over. Am J Cardiol 1983;51:403–421.
5. **Roberts WC.** Anatomically isolated aortic valvular disease. The case against its being of rheumatic etiology. Am J Med 1970;49:151–159.
6. **Roberts WC, Dangel JC, Bulkley BH.** Non-rheumatic valvular cardiac disease: a clinicopathologic survery of 27 different conditions causing valvular dysfunction. Cardiovasc Clin 1973;5:333–446.
7. **Roberts WC.** The structure of the aortic valve in clinically-isolated aortic stenosis. An autopsy study of 162 patients over 15 years of age. Circulation 1970;42:91–97.
8. **Roberts WC.** The congenitally bicuspid aortic valve. A study of 85 autopsy cases. Am J Cardiol 1970;26:72–83.
9. **Roberts WC, Perloff JK, Costantino T.** Severe valvular aortic stenosis in patients over 65 years of age. A clinicopathologic study. Am J Cardiol 1971;27:497–506.
10. **Virmani R, Roberts WC.** Aschoff bodies in operatively excised atrial appendages and in papillary muscles. Frequency and clinical significance. Circulation 1977;55:559–563.
11. **Roberts WC, Virmani R.** Aschoff bodies at necropsy in valvular heart disease. Evidence from an analysis of 543 patients over 14 years of age that rheumatic heart disease, at least anatomically, is a disease of the mitral valve. Circulation 1978;57:803–807.
12. **Waller BF, Morrow AG, Maron BJ, Del Negro AA, Kent KM, McGrath FJ, Wallace RB, McIntosh CL, Roberts WC.** Etiology of clinically isolated, severe, chronic, pure mitral regurgitation: analysis of 97 patients over 30 years of age having mitral valve replacement. Am Heart J 1982;104: 276–288.
13. **Roberts WC, Sjoerdsma A.** The cardiac disease associated with the carcinoid syndrome (carcinoid heart disease). Am J Med 1964;36:5–34.
14. **Glancy DL, Marcus FI, Cuadra M, Ewy GA, Roberts WC.** Isolated organic tricuspid valvular regurgitation. Causes and consequences. Am J Med 1969;46:989–996.
15. **Andy JJ, Sheikh MU, Ali N, Barnes BO, Fox LM, Curry CL, Roberts WC.** Echocardiographic observations in opiate addicts with active infective endocarditis. Frequency of involvement of the various valves and comparison of echocardiographic features of right- and left-sided cardiac valve endocarditis. Am J Cardiol 1977;40:17–23.
16. **Arnett EN, Roberts WC.** Active infective endocarditis: a clinicopathologic analysis of 137 necropsy patients. Curr Probl Cardiol 1976;1:1–76.
17. **Roberts WC.** Characteristics and consequences of infective endocarditis (active or healed or both) learned from morphologic studies. In: Rahimtoola SH, ed. Infective Endocarditis. New York: Grune & Stratton, 1978:55–123.
18. **Lachman AS, Roberts WC.** Calcific deposits in stenotic mitral valves. Extent and relation to age, sex, degree of stenosis, cardiac rhythm, previous commissurotomy and left atrial body thrombus from study of 164 operatively-excised valves. Circulation 1978;57:808–815.
19. **Roberts WC, Lachman AS.** Mitral valve commissurotomy versus replacement. Considerations based on examination of operatively excised stenotic mitral valves. Am Heart J 1979;98:56–62.
20. **Roberts WC, Humphries JO, Morrow AG.** Giant right atrium in rheumatic mitral stenosis. Atrial enlargement restricted by mural calcification. Am Heart J 1970;79:28–35.
21. **Glancy DL, Roberts WC.** Congenital obstructive lesions involving the major pulmonary veins, left atrium, or mitral valve: a clinical, laboratory, and morphologic survey. Cathet Cardiovasc Diagn 1976;2:215–252.
22. **Ferrans VJ, Roberts WC.** Structural features of cardiac myxomas. Histology, histochemistry, and electron microscopy. Hum Pathol 1973;4:111–146.
23. **MacLowry JD, Roberts WC.** Metastatic choriocarcinoma of the lung. Invasion of pulmonary veins with extension into the left atrium and mitral orifice. Am J Cardiol 1966;18:939–941.
24. **Roberts WC, Ewy GA, Glancy DL, Marcus FI.** Valvular stenosis produced by active infective endocarditis. Circulation 1967;36:449–451.
25. **Waller BF, McManus BM, Roberts WC.** Mitral valve stenosis produced by or worsened by active bacterial endocarditis. Chest 1982;82:498–500.
26. **Hammer WJ, Roberts WC, de Leon AC Jr.** "Mitral stenosis" secondary to combined "massive" mitral anular calcific deposits and small, hypertrophied left ventricles. Am J Med 1978;64:371–376.
27. **Shepherd RL, Glancy DL, Stinson EB, Roberts WC.** Hemodynamic confirmation of obstruction to left ventricular inflow by a caged-ball prosthetic mitral valve. Case report. J Thorac Cardiovasc Surg 1973;65:252–254.
28. **Jones AA, Otis JB, Fletcher GF, Roberts WC.** A hitherto undescribed cause of prosthetic mitral valve obstruction. J Thorac Cardiovasc Surg 1977; 74:116–117.
29. **Roberts WC.** Complications of cardiac valve replacement: characteristic abnormalities of prostheses pertaining to any or specific site. Am Heart J 1982;103:113–122.
30. **Braunwald E, Ross RS, Morrow AG, Roberts WC.** Differential diagnosis of mitral regurgitation in childhood: clinical pathological conference at the National Institutes of Health. Ann Intern Med 1961;54:1223–1242.
31. **Brockenbrough EC, Braunwald E, Roberts WC, Morrow AG.** Partial persistent atrioventricular canal simulating pure mitral regurgitation. Am Heart J 1962;63:9–17.
32. **Carney EK, Braunwald E, Roberts WC, Aygen M, Morrow AG.** Congenital mitral regurgitation. Clinical, hemodynamic, and angiocardiographic findings in nine patients. Am J Med 1962;33:223–235.
33. **Roberts WC.** Anomalous origin of both coronary arteries from the pulmonary artery. Am J Cardiol 1962;10:595–600.
34. **Roberts WC, Ross RS, Davis FW Jr.** Congenital corrected transposition of the great vessels in adulthood simulating rheumatic valvular disease. Bull Johns Hopkins Hosp 1964;114:157–172.
35. **Glancy DL, Chang MY, Dorney ER, Roberts WC.** Parachute mitral valve. Further observations and associated lesions. Am J Cardiol 1971;27: 309–313.
36. **Roberts WC, Glancy DL, Seningen RP, Maron BJ, Epstein SE.** Prolapse of the mitral valve (floppy valve) associated with Ebstein's anomaly of the tricuspid valve. Am J Cardiol 1976;38:377–382.
37. **Waller BF, Sheikh MU, Roberts WC.** Prolapsing atrioventricular valve in partial atrioventricular defect. Am Heart J 1981;101:108–110.
38. **Cabin HS, Roberts WC.** Epstein's anomaly of the tricuspid valve and prolapse of the mitral valve. Am Heart J 1981;101:177–180.
39. **Roberts WC.** Congenital cardiovascular abnormalities usually "silent" until adulthood: morphologic features of the floppy mitral valve, valvular aortic stenosis, hypertrophic cardiomyopathy, sinus of Valsalva aneurysm, and the Marfan syndrome. In: Roberts WC, ed. Congenital Heart Disease in Adults. Philadelphia: FA Davis, 1979:407–453.
40. **Roberts WC, Honig HS.** The spectrum of cardiovascular disease in the Marfan syndrome: a clinico-morphologic study of 18 necropsy patients and comparison to 151 previously reported necropsy patients. Am Heart J 1982;104:115–135.
41. **Roberts WC, Braunwald E, Morrow AG.** Acute severe mitral regurgitation secondary to ruptured chordae tendineae. Clinical, hemodynamic, and pathologic considerations. Circulation 1966;33:58–70.
42. **Roberts WC, Buchbinder NA.** Healed left-sided infective endocarditis: a clinicopathologic study of 59 patients. Am J Cardiol 1977;40:876–888.
43. **Carpenter DF, Golden A, Roberts WC.** Quadrivalvular rheumatoid heart disease associated with left bundle branch block. Am J Med 1967;43: 922–929.
44. **Roberts WC, Kehoe JA, Carpenter DF, Golden A.** Cardiac valvular lesions in rheumatoid arthritis. Arch Intern Med 1968;122:141–146.
45. **Roberts WC, Hollingsworth JF, Bulkley BH, Jaffe RB, Epstein SE, Stinson EB.** Combined mitral and aortic regurgitation in ankylosing spondylitis. Angiographic and anatomic features. Am J Med 1974;56:237–243.
46. **Renteria VG, Ferrans VJ, Roberts WC.** The heart in the Hurler syndrome. Gross, histologic and ultrastructural observations in five necropsy cases. Am J Cardiol 1976;38:487–501.
47. **Roberts WC, Ross RS, Eggleston JC, Massumi RA.** Chronic mitral regurgitation of unresolved etiology in the elderly. A clinicopatholigic study of two patients. Johns Hopkins Med J 1968;122:26–36.
48. **Morrow AG, Cohen LS, Roberts WC, Braunwald NS, Braunwald E.** Severe mitral regurgitation following acute myocardial infarction and ruptured papillary muscle. Hemodynamic findings and results of operative treatment in four patients. Circulation 1968;37,38:Suppl II:II-124–II-132.
49. **Falcone MW, Ronan JA Jr, Roberts WC.** Silent mitral regurgitation complicating silent myocardial infarction: hemodynamic and morphologic documentation. Chest 1972;62:226–228.
50. **Glancy DL, Stinson EB, Shepherd RL, Itscoitz SB, Roberts WC, Epstein SE, Morrow AG.** Results of valve replacement for severe mitral regurgitation due to papillary muscle rupture or fibrosis. Am J Cardiol 1973;32:313–321.
51. **Roberts WC.** Operative treatment of hypertrophic obstructive cardiomyopathy. The case against mitral valve replacement. Am J Cardiol 1973 32:377–381.
52. **Roberts WC, Liegler DG, Carbone PP.** Endomyocardial disease and eosinophilia. A clinical and pathologic spectrum. Am J Med 1969;46:28–42.
53. **Roberts WC, Buja LM, Ferrans VJ.** Löffler's fibroplastic parietal endocarditis, eosinophilic leukemia, and Davies' endomyocardial fibrosis: the same disease at different stages? Pathol Microbiol 1970;35:90–96.
54. **Roberts WC, Ferrans VJ.** Pathologic anatomy of the cardiomyopathies Idiopathic dilated and hypertrophic types, infiltrative types, and endomyocardial disease with and without eosinophilia. Hum Pathol 1975;6:287–342.
55. **Harley JB, McIntosh CL, Kirklin JJW, Maron BJ, Gottdiener J, Roberts WC Fauci AS.** Atrioventricular valve replacement in the idiopathic hypereosinophilic syndrome. Am J Med 1982;73:77–81.
56. **Fauci AS, Harley JB, Roberts WC, Ferrans VJ, Gralnick HR, Bjornson BH** The idiopathic hypereosinophilic syndrome. Clinical, pathophysiologic, an therapeutic considerations. Ann Intern Med 1982;97:78–92.
57. **Bulkley BH, Roberts WC.** Systemic lupus erythematosus as a cause c severe mitral regurgitation. New problem in an old disease. Am J Cardi 1975;35:305–308.
58. **Bulkley BH, Roberts WC.** The heart in systemic lupus erythematosus ar the changes induced in it by corticosteroid therapy. A study of 36 necrops patients. Am J Med 1975;58:243–264.
59. **Bulkley BH, Roberts WC.** Dilatation of the mitral anulus. A rare cause mitral regurgitation. Am J Med 1975;59:457–463.
60. **Brosius FC III, Waller BF, Roberts WC,** Radiation heart disease. Analys of 16 young (aged 15 to 33 years) necropsy patients who received ov 3,500 rads to the heart. Am J Med 1981;70:519–530.
61. **Glancy DL, Massumi RA, Roberts WC.** Fatal acute rheumatic fever childhood despite corticosteroid therapy. A note on the spectrum of chil hood rheumatic fever. Am Heart J 1969;77:534–537.
62. **Selzer A, Katayama F.** Mitral regurgitation: clinical patterns, pathophys ology, natural history. Medicine 1972;51:337–350.
63. **di Segni E, Edwards JE.** Cleft anterior leaflet of mitral valve with intact sep A study of 20 cases. Am J Cardiol 1983;51:919–926.
64. **Berry WB, Roberts WC, Morrow AG, Braunwald E.** Corrected transpositi of the aorta and pulmonary trunk. Clinical, hemodynamic and patholog

findings. Am J Med 1964;36:35–53.
65. **Rosenberg J, Roberts WC.** Double orifice mitral valve. Study of the anomaly in two calves and a summary of the literature in humans. Arch Pathol 1968;86:77–80.
66. **Marcus FI, Gomez L, Glancy DL, Ewy GA, Roberts WC.** Papillary muscle fibrosis in primary myocardial disease. Am Heart J 1969;77;681–685.
67. **Roberts WC, McAllister HA Jr, Ferrans VJ.** Sarcoidosis of the heart. A clinicopathologic study of 35 necropsy patients (group I) and review of 78 previously described necropsy patients (group II). Am J Med 1977;63: 86–108.
68. **Perloff JK, Roberts WC, deLeon AC Jr, O'Doherty D.** The distinctive electrocardiogram of Duchenne's progressive muscular dystrophy. An electrocardiographic-pathologic correlative study. Am J Med 1967;42: 179–188.
69. **Roberts WC, Bodey GP, Wertlake PT.** The heart in acute leukemia. A study of 420 autopsy cases. Am J Cardiol 1968;21:388–412.
70. **Glancy DL, Roberts WC.** The heart in malignant melanoma. A study of 70 autopsy cases. Am J Cardiol 1968;21:555–571.
71. **Roberts WC, Glancy DL, DeVita VT Jr.** Heart in malignant lymphoma (Hodgkin's disease, lymphosarcoma, reticulum cell sarcoma and mycosis fungoides). A study of 196 autopsy cases. Am J Cardiol 1968;22:85–107.
72. **Buja LM, Khoi NB, Roberts WC.** Clinically significant cardiac amyloidosis. Clinicopathologic findings in 15 patients. Am J Cardiol 1970;26:394–405.
73. **Buja LM, Roberts WC.** Iron in the heart. Etiology and clinical significance. Am J Med 1971;51:209–221.
74. **Roberts WC, Berard CW.** Gas gangrene of the heart in clostridial septicemia. Am Heart J 1967;74:482–488.
75. **Pirolo JS, Hutchins GM, Moore GW, Weisfeldt ML.** Myocyte disarray develops in papillary muscles released from normal tension after mitral valve replacement. Circulation 1982;66:841–846.
76. **Roberts WC, Bulkley BH, Morrow AG.** Pathologic anatomy of cardiac valve replacement: a study of 224 necropsy patients. Progr Cardiovasc Dis 1973;15:539–587.
77. **Roberts WC, Isner JM, Virmani R.** Left ventricular incision midway between the mitral anulus and the stumps of the papillary muscles during mitral valve excision with or without rupture or aneurysmal formation. Analysis of 10 necropsy patients. Am Heart J 1982;104:1278–1287.
78. **Korn D, DeSanctis RW, Sell S.** Massive calcification of the mitral annulus. A clinicopathological study of fourteen cases. N Engl J Med 1962;267: 900–909.
79. **Roberts WC, Waller BF.** Mitral valve "anular" calcium forming a complete circle or "O" configuration: clinical and necropsy observations. Am Heart J 1981;101:619–621.
80. **Roberts WC, Waller BF.** Effect of chronic hypercalcemia on the heart. An analysis of 18 necropsy patients. Am J Med 1981;71:371–384.
81. **Bulkley BH, Morrow AG, Roberts WC.** Calcification of prosthetic valve anuli: a late complication of cardiac valve replacement. Am Heart J 1974;87: 129–133.

Frequency and Extent of Calcific Deposits in Purely Regurgitant Mitral Valves: Analysis of 108 Operatively Excised Valves

MARK T. BYRAM, BS,* and WILLIAM C. ROBERTS, MD

Operatively excised purely regurgitant mitral valves in 108 patients aged 21 to 73 years (mean 55) (63% men) undergoing isolated mitral valve replacement were examined for calcific deposits. Of the 108 patients, 19 (18%) had leaflet or chordal calcific deposits or both, but in each the deposits were small and did not appear to alter mitral function. Of the 19 patients with mitral calcium, 6 had had active infective endocarditis and the calcium likely represented healed vegetations; in 6 other patients, the leaflet calcium had extended from the mitral anulus in the setting of mitral valve prolapse. The average total serum cholesterol levels were higher in the patients with compared with those without mitral calcium. Thus, calcium deposits are relatively infrequent in adults with clinically isolated pure mitral regurgitation, and when they occur, the deposits are small and in themselves do not appear to contribute to mitral dysfunction.

(Am J Cardiol 1983;52:1059–1061)

Stenotic mitral and aortic valves in adults usually contain calcific deposits, which are often heavy.[1–4] A previous study of stenotic mitral valves from this laboratory indicated that the extent of the calcific deposits correlated with the patient's age and sex and the pressure gradient across the valve.[5] In contrast to the stenotic left-sided cardiac valves, purely regurgitant mitral or aortic valves usually do not contain calcific deposits and, if present, they are usually small. No studies, however, have described the precise frequency and extent of calcific deposits in purely regurgitant mitral or aortic valves. This report partially fills that void by analyzing 108 operatively excised purely regurgitant mitral valves for the presence and extent of calcific deposits.

Patients

Certain observations in the 108 patients are summarized in Table I. Criteria for inclusion in this study included the following: (1) presence of mitral regurgitation (MR) severe enough to warrent mitral valve replacement; (2) absence of mitral stenosis as determined by preoperative cardiac catheterization, i.e., the mean diastolic gradient between lef atrium (or pulmonary arterial wedge position) and left ventricle was ≤2 mm Hg; (3) absence of aortic valve dysfunction i.e., either aortic valve stenosis or regurgitation; (4) age >2 years at the time of mitral valve replacement; (5) absence o a defect in either the atrial or ventricular septum; (6) absenc of active infective endocarditis; and (7) availability of th operatively excised mitral valve for reexamination or presenc of photographs of the operatively excised valve.

From the several hundred operatively excised cardiac valve in our files, the mitral valves that appeared purely regurgitar by gross examination were analyzed. The medical records the patients in whom the mitral valve appeared to have bee purely regurgitant were then reviewed to be certain that th valves were classifiable according to our criteria for inclusior All 108 patients before mitral valve replacement were in Ne York Heart Association functional class III or IV. Other ir formation gathered from the medical records also is summa rized in Table I. The determination of calcium in the valv leaflets and chordae tendineae was made by gross inspectio Radiographs of the excised valve were performed in 40 of th 108 patients (Fig. 1 and 2).

The 108 patients ranged in age from 21 to 73 years (mea 55); 40 were women and 68 were men; 100 patients were whi and 8 were black. Total serum cholesterol values, available 63 patients, ranged from 116 to 366 mg/dl (mean 211); of th 63 values available, 6 (9%) were 101 to 150, 23 (37%) were 1 to 200, 24 (38%) were 201 to 250 and 10 (16%) were >2 mg/dl. Fasting serum triglyceride values, available in 41 p tients, ranged from 49 to 255 mg/dl (mean 141); in 25 patien

From the Pathology Branch, National Heart, Lung and Blood Institute, National Institutes of Health, Bethesda, Maryland. Manuscript received and accepted July 1, 1983.
Address for reprints: William C. Roberts, MD, Building 10A, Room 3E-30, National Institutes of Health, Bethesda, Maryland 20205.
* Freshman medical student, University of Tennessee.

(61%), they were ≤150, in 10 patients (24%), 151 to 200, 4 patients (10%), 201 to 250, and in 2 patients (5%), >250 mg/dl. Serum calcium levels, available in 60 patients, ranged from 3.6 to 5.2 mg/dl (mean 4.7).

Results

Of the 108 valves, 19 (18%) by gross inspection contained calcific deposits. The amount of calcium was trace or mild in all 19 patients, occupying <5% of the total leaflet area in 12 (63%). In none of the 19 patients did the leaflet calcific deposits appear to alter valvular function.

Table I is a list of the causes of the pure MR and certain comparisons in the patients with and without calcific deposits. Definitions of the various etiologic categories are described elsewhere.[6] The highest frequency (46%) (6 of 13) of calcific deposits occurred in the patients with ruptured chordae tendineae from infective endocarditis that had healed on previously anatomically normal valves (Group 3). The calcific deposits in these patients appeared to be the result of healing of vegetations of active infective endocarditis. In the patients with ruptured chordae tendineae complicating mitral valve prolapse (Group 1), the frequency of calcific deposits was 11% (4 of 36). Of the 30 patients with mitral prolapse without ruptured chordae (Group 2), 6 (20%) had calcific deposits. In each of them, the calcific deposits were located adjacent to the basal attachments of the posterior leaflets and therefore appear to have represented extension of anular calcium slightly onto the leaflet. Of the 7 patients with rheumatic MR (Group 4), 2 had calcific deposits. Each of the 4 patients with hypertrophic cardiomyopathy (Group 5) had had active infective endocarditis causing rupture of several mitral chordae; 1 had mitral calcific deposits. Of the 16 patients with MR secondary to papillary muscle dysfunction from coronary heart disease, only 1 had leaflet calcific deposits, and 1 had calcific deposits in a papillary muscle. (Calcium limited to papillary muscle was not considered "mitral calcium" for the purposes of this study.)

Of the 19 patients with mitral leaflet calcium, 6 (31%) had a history of active infective endocarditis that healed; of the 89 patients without leaflet calcium, 16 (18%) had a history of active infective endocarditis that healed.

The mean age, sex, serum triglyceride and serum calcium levels in the patients with and without mitral

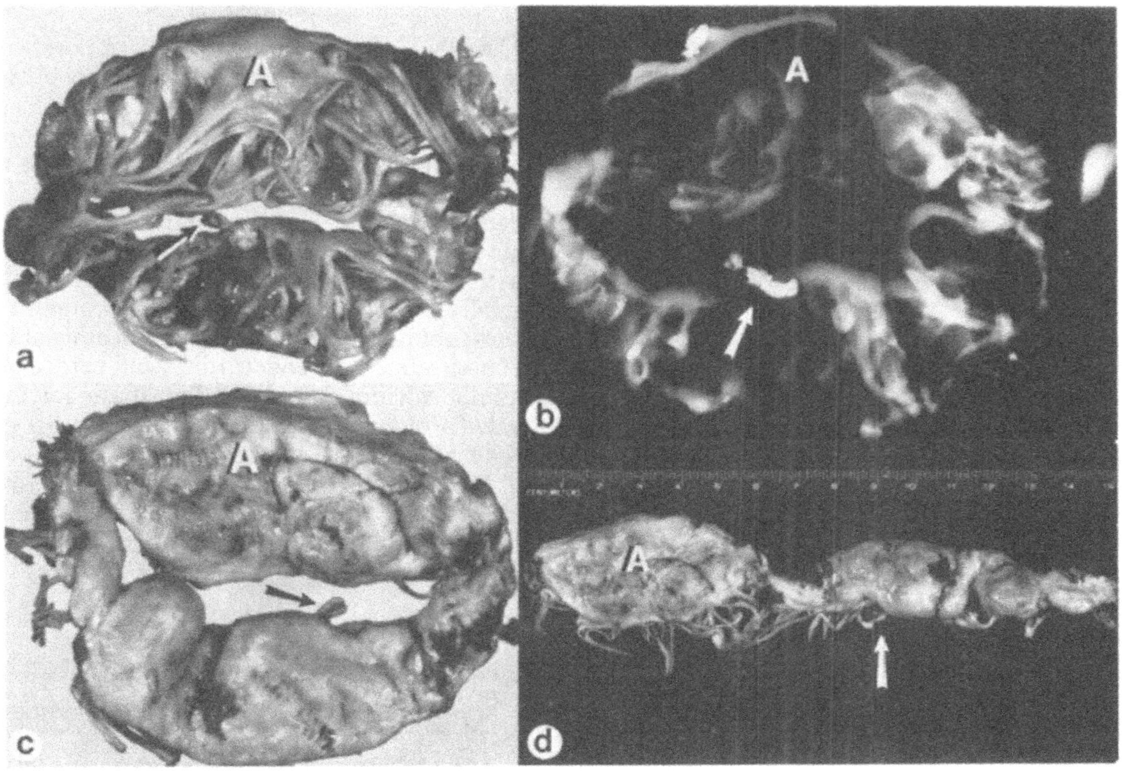

IGURE 1. Mitral valve prolapse with ruptured chordae tendineae in a 59-year-old man (S77-157) who was noted to have atrial fibrillation at age 3 years but was asymptomatic until age 49, when he had a stroke. At the time, atrial fibrillation was again noted and it was cardioverted to sinus ythm. At age 54, atrial fibrillation recurred and he was cardioverted on 5 additional occasions during the next 5 years. He was free of symptoms ntil age 59, when he had acute pulmonary edema while playing golf. Echocardiography then disclosed "hammocking" of the posterior mitral leaflet d probable rupture of several chordae tendineae. The pulmonary arterial wedge pressure was mean 30, v wave 50, and pulmonary arterial pressure)/25 mm Hg. Left ventricular angiography disclosed 4+/4+ mitral regurgitation. **a,** operatively excised mitral valve from its ventricular aspect. e **arrow** points to a ruptured chorda tendinea (also in **b, c** and **d**). A = anterior mitral leaflet. **b,** radiograph of the excised valve demonstrating e ruptured chorda to be calcified. An additional fragment of calcium is on the anterior (A) leaflet. **c,** valve from its atrial aspect. **d,** opened mitral lve. Both leaflets are redundant.

TABLE I Clinical Data in 108 Patients with Operatively Excised Purely Regurgitant Mitral Valves: 19 With Compared with 89 Patients Without Mitral Calcific Deposits

Group	Etiologic Group	MV Ca^{++}	No. of Patients	Ages (yr) Range (mean)	No. of Women	No. of Men	Hx IE	Total Serum Cholesterol (mg/dl)		
								No. Done	Range	(Mean)
1	Prolapse with ruptured chordae	+	4	55–66 (59)	2	2	1	4	208–314	(259)
		0	32	40–72 (56)	7	25	6	19	154–268	(211)
2	Prolapse without ruptured chordae	+	6	45–73 (60)	3	3	0	5	153–248	(205)
		0	24	26–71 (55)	11	13	4	13	150–272	(206)
3	Ruptured chordae without prolapse	+	6	24–65 (49)	2	4	4	2	180–260	(220)
		0	7	21–73 (54)	4	3	2	5	134–268	(185)
4	Rheumatic	+	2	35–52 (43)	1	1	0	1	230	(230)
		0	5	21–65 (34)	5	0	0	2	193–209	(201)
5	Hypertrophic cardiomyopathy	+	1	62 (62)	0	1	1	0	...	...
		0	3	28–46 (39)	1	2	2	0	...	...
6	Congenital	+	0	...	...	...	...	0	...	...
		0	1	23 (23)	1	0	0	1	194	(194)
7	Uncertain	+	0	...	...	...	...	0	...	...
		0	1	64 (64)	1	0	1	1	165	(165)
8	Coronary	+	0	...	0	0	...	...	...	...
		0	16	38–69 (59)	2	14	1	10	116–366	(215)
Totals		+	19	24–73 (55)	8	11	6	12	153–314	(228)
		0	89	21–73 (55)	32	57	16	51	116–366	(207)

Hx IE = history of infective endocarditis; MV = mitral valve.

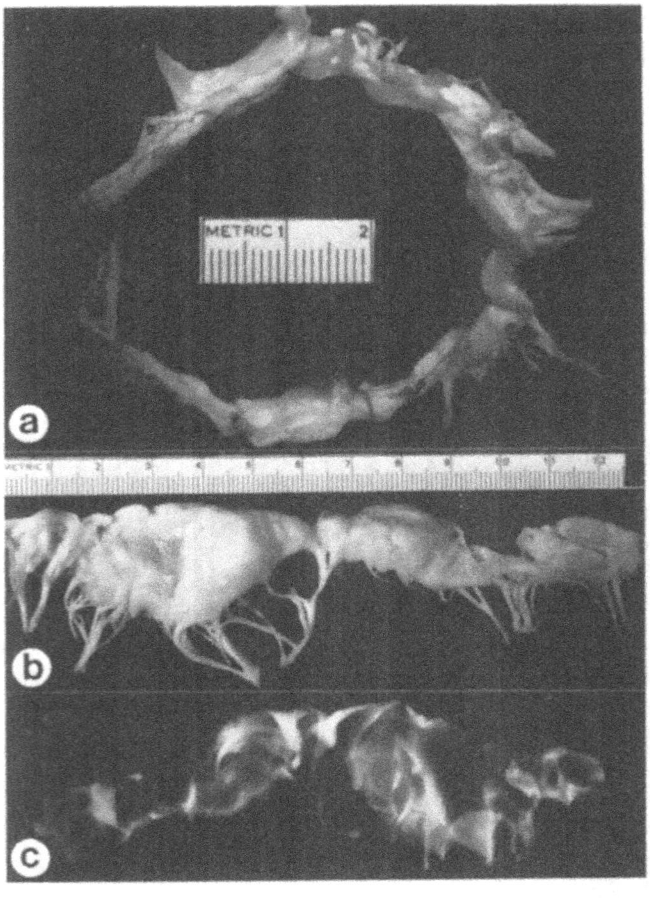

FIGURE 2. Mitral valve prolapse without ruptured chordae tendineae in a 62-year-old woman (S80-17) who was found to have a precordial murmur at age 37 years and the onset of exertional dyspnea at age 53 years. Just before mitral valve replacement, left ventricular angiography disclosed 4+/4+ mitral regurgitation; the cardiac index was 1.7 liters/min/m^2; the pulmonary arterial pressure was 44/16 mm Hg and the pulmonary capillary wedge pressure was mean 28, with v waves 40 mm Hg. **a,** excised mitral valve showing the anulus to be dilated. **b,** opened mitral valve showing its atrial aspect. **c,** radiograph of valve showing no calcific deposits.

leaflet calcific deposits were similar. The patients with calcific deposits had higher mean total serum cholesterol levels than those without (228 versus 207 mg/dl).

Discussion

Analysis of the operatively excised purely regurgitant mitral valves in 108 patients >20 years old at the time of isolated mitral valve replacement disclosed that 18% had calcific deposits in mitral leaflets, chordae tendineae or both, and that the calcific deposits were small and did not appear to alter mitral function. The calcific deposits were present in the mitral leaflets in only trace amounts (≤5% of leaflet area) in 12 of our 19 patients with pure MR; in the other 7 patients, the deposits were small (occupied 6 to 25% of the leaflet area). The 2 major causes of the leaflet calcium were healing of vegetations of active infective endocarditis and extension of mitral anular calcium onto the leaflets in the setting of mitral valve prolapse. If the latter 6 patients were eliminated the frequency of leaflet calcium would be only 12% (1 of 108). In contrast, calcific deposits were found in 91 (150 of 164) of operatively excised stenotic mitral valves in adults[5] and the deposits tended to be large.

References

1. **Roberts WC.** Morphologic features of the normal and abnormal mitral valv Am J Cardiol 1983;51:1005–1028.
2. **Roberts WC.** The structure of the aortic valve in clinically-isolated aor stenosis. An autopsy study of 162 patients over 15 years of age. Circulati 1970;42:91–97.
3. **Roberts WC.** The congenitally bicuspid aortic valve. A study of 85 autop cases. Am J Cardiol 1970;26:72–83.
4. **Roberts WC, Perloff JK, Costantino T.** Severe valvular aortic stenosis patients over 65 years of age. A clinicopathologic study. Am J Card 1971;27:497–506.
5. **Lachman AS, Roberts WC.** Calcific deposits in stenotic mitral valves. Exte and relation of age, sex, degree of stenosis, cardiac rhythm, previous co missurotomy and left atrial body thrombus from study of 164 operative excised valves. Circulation 1978;57:808–815.
6. **Waller BF, Morrow AG, Maron BJ, Del Negro AA, Kent KM, McGrath F Wallace RB, McIntosh CL, Roberts WC.** Etiology of clinically isolated, seve chronic, pure mitral regurgitation: analysis of 97 patients over 30 years age having mitral valve replacement. Am Heart J 1982;104:276–288.

Frequency and Significance of M-Mode Echocardiographic Evidence of Mitral Valve Prolapse In Clinically Isolated Pure Mitral Regurgitation: Analysis of 65 Patients Having Mitral Valve Replacement

BRUCE F. WALLER, MD, BARRY J. MARON, MD, ALBERT A. DEL NEGRO, MD, JOHN S. GOTTDIENER, MD, and WILLIAM C. ROBERTS, MD

To assess the reliability of M-mode echocardiographic patterns of mitral valve prolapse (MVP) (echo MVP) in detection of morphologic evidence of MVP (morphologic MVP), operatively excised mitral valves and corresponding M-mode echocardiograms from 65 patients with chronic, severe, isolated, pure mitral regurgitation (MR) were studied. Of the 65 patients, 45 (69%) had echo MVP (either holosystolic or mid-to-late systolic prolapse patterns on preoperative M-mode echograms) and 42 (93%) of them had morphologic MVP; of the 3 without morphologic MVP, 2 had ruptured chordae tendineae from infective endocarditis and 1 had papillary muscle dysfunction from atherosclerotic coronary heart disease. Of the 20 patients without echo MVP, 14 (70%) had no morphologic MVP (9 had papillary muscle dysfunction from coronary heart disease, 4 had infective endocarditis on previous normal valves and 1 had rheumatic heart disease). Of the 48 patients with morphologic MVP, 42 (88%) had echo MVP and most had considerably dilated mitral anulae; the other 6 had ruptured chordae tendineae with less degrees of anular dilatation. Of the 17 patients without morphologic MVP, 3 had echo MVP (coronary artery disease in 1 and infective endocarditis on a previous normal valve in 2); of the 14 with neither echo nor morphologic MVP, 9 had papillary muscle dysfunction from coronary artery disease, 4 had infective endocarditis on previously normal valves and 1 had rheumatic heart disease. The patients with very dilated mitral anuli and leaflet areas generally had holosystolic (hammocking) patterns on echo; the patients with small anuli and leaflet areas usually had mid-to-late systolic (buckling) prolapse patterns. **(Am J Cardiol 1984;53:139–147)**

Numerous clinical, echocardiographic (echo) and angiographic studies have attempted to establish criteria for the diagnosis of mitral valve prolapse (MVP). The echo signs of MVP have usually been established by auscultatory or angiographic signs, or both, considered diagnostic of MVP, and the echo signs of MVP infrequently have been compared to valves that possess characteristic morphologic features of MVP.[1–4] To assess the reliability of M-mode echo patterns of MVP (echo MVP) in detecting morphologic evidence of MVP (morphologic MVP), preoperative M-mode echocardiograms and operatively excised mitral valves were analyzed from 65 patients undergoing mitral valve replacement for isolated, pure mitral regurgitation (MR) associated with normally functioning aortic valves.

Methods

Patients studied: Operatively excised purely regurgitant mitral valves accessioned in the Pathology Branch of the National Heart, Lung, and Blood Institute from December 1973 through August 1982 were examined. Preoperative precordial auscultatory, cardiac catheterization pressure and angiographic observations substantiated the anatomic diagnosis of a purely regurgitant valve. Patients with associated mitral stenosis, aortic valve dysfunction, intracardiac shunts or hypertrophic cardiomyopathy were excluded. After these exclusions, 97 patients had clinically *isolated*, *severe*, *chronic* and *pure* MR and each met the following criteria[5]: (1) severe (3+ or 4+/4+) MR by left ventricular angiography; (2) mean diastolic pressure gradient between the left atrium or pulmonary arterial wedge position and left ventricle of ≤2 mm

[Fr]om the Pathology and Cardiology Branches, National Heart, Lung, and [Bl]ood Institute, National Institutes of Health, Bethesda, Maryland, and [th]e Department of Medicine (Cardiology), Georgetown University [M]edical Center, Washington, D.C. Manuscript received and accepted [Au]gust 22, 1983.
Address for reprints: Bruce F. Waller, MD, Department of Pathology, [In]diana University School of Medicine, University Hospital, N-340, In[di]anapolis, Indiana 46223.

Hg, and no gradient at end-diastole between the left atrium and left ventricle; (3) no stenosis or regurgitation of the aortic valve; and (4) clinical evidence of congestive heart failure for ≥2 months. Of the 97 patients (described earlier[5]), 65 had preoperative echocardiograms available for review, and they constitute the study group.

Morphologic criteria for etiologic subgrouping: The circumference (in cm), by measuring the length of the anulus of the excised mitral valve, and the leaflet area, by outlining the basal and distal margins of the opened leaflets and measuring the area by videoplanimetry, were determined in all patients.[5] The patients were divided into 4 groups based upon "anular" circumference, leaflet area, status of the chordae tendineae and attached portions of papillary muscles (Tables I, II and III).

Morphologic mitral valve prolapse: These valves had leaflet areas >11 cm^2 and the distance from basal attachment to leaflet free margin of the posterior leaflet was focally increased in that ≥1 segment was elongated compared to other segments. Valves with intact chordae tendineae had circumferences of >11 cm, while the valves with absent or ruptured chordae tendineae had circumferences of >10 cm. The valves with ruptured chordae had focal thickening of 1 or both leaflets at sites of the ruptured chordae. Additionally, a portion of leaflet was missing (indented) or perforated.

Healed infective endocarditis on previously normal valves: The major portion of leaflet and most chordae tendineae in these valves were normal. The valve leaflet area was <11 cm^2 and the "anular" circumference was <11 cm. Several chordae attached to 1 or both leaflets were ruptured (or absent), and the adjacent leaflet was thickened by fibrous tissue and a portion was either indented or perforated. These valves differed from those classified as "prolapsed mitral valves with ruptured chordae tendineae" by the *absence* of ≥1 elongated posterior leaflet segment and smaller total leaflet areas.

Atherosclerotic coronary heart disease with papillary muscle dysfunction: The mitral leaflets and chordae tendineae were either normal or only slightly and focally thickened, the leaflet areas were <11 cm^2, the "anular" circumferences ≤10 cm, and no leaflet indentations, perforations or ruptured chordae were present and 1 or both papillary muscles was extensively scarred and usually atrophied.

Rheumatic: Both mitral leaflets were diffusely thickened by fibrous tissue and the chordae tendineae may or may not have been abnormal.[6] The mitral leaflet areas and "anular" circumferences were <11 cm^2 and <11 cm, respectively.

Echocardiographic techniques: Preoperative M-mode echocardiograms from the 65 patients were retrospectively and independently reviewed by 2 echocardiographers (BJM, AADN) who had no knowledge of the morphologic classification. M-mode echocardiograms were performed using a 2.25-MHz, 1.25-cm-diameter transducer and either a Hoffrel 201, Smith-Kline Ekoline or Irex ultrasound receiver interfaced with a Honeywell or Irex strip-chart recorder. Mitral valve echocardiograms were recorded using an ultrasound window at the left sternal border with the transducer perpendicular to the anterior chest wall. Each M-mode echocardiogram was analyzed for the presence or absence of the following 4 mitral valve echo signs or patterns: prolapse (mid-to-late systolic ["buckling"], holosystolic ["hammocking"]), ruptured chordae tendineae and vegetations.

Characterization of prolapse: Two echo patterns of MVP were observed: mid-to-late systolic and holosystolic. Mid-to-late systolic prolapse ("buckling") was defined as posterior motion of 1 or both mitral leaflets beginning at or during the latter half of ventricular systole. Holosystolic ("hammocking")

TABLE I Clinical Observations in 65 Patients with Mitral Valve Replacement for Isolated, Pure Mitral Regurgitation

Observation	Floppy: With RCT (n = 13)	Floppy: Without RCT (n = 35)	Floppy: Total (n = 48)	Coronary (n = 10)‡	Infective Endocarditis (n = 6)‖	Rheumatic (n = 1)
1. Age (yr) at MVR (range, mean)	48–69 (58)	26–74 (56)	24–74 (57)	47–78 (61)	32–56 (41)	53
2. Men (%)/Women (%)	9 (69):4 (31)	17 (49):18 (51)	26 (54):22 (46)	8:2	5:1	0:1
3. History of IE	4	0	4 (6%)	0	5	0
4. Systolic clicks	0*	0	0	0	0	0
5. Duration (yr) MR mur	2–20 (8)	2–22 (9)	2–22 (8.5)	1–5 (4)	0.8–1.8 (1.2)	12
6. Direct SAP (mm Hg) (range, mean)	115–160 (140) 70–85 (82)	110–168 (136) 62–90 (76)	110–168 (138) 62–90 (79)	100–160 (129) 75–88 (81)	138–155 (146) 65–88 (80)	160 90
7. Direct systolic SAP >140 or diastolic >90 mm Hg	6 (46%)	9 (28%)	15 (31%)	2	4	1
8. MVP by E/total no. E	7/13	35/35	42/48 (88%)	1/10	2/6	0
9. E pattern of MVP						
Holosystolic	6/7	20/35 (57%)	26/42 (62%)	1/1	1/2	0
Mid-to-late systolic	1/7	15/35 (43%)	16/42 (38%)	0	1/2	0
10. E pattern of RCT	10/13	5/35 (14%)	15/48 (31%)	0	4/6	0
(No. with both RCT + MVP patterns)	(4/10)	(5/5)	(9/15 [60%])		2/4	
11. E pattern of vegetation	5	6 (17%)	11 (23%)	0	2	0
12. Interval (days) from E to MVR (range, avg)	3–406 (47)	6–377 (94)	3–406 (82)	8–26 (18)	13–156 (43)	83
13. One or more major CA narrowed >50% in D by angio/total no. angio	0/1	3/22 (14%)†	3–23 (13%)†	10/10§	0/1	—

* One patient had a systolic click and late systolic murmur 4 months before active IE developed but the precordial murmur became holosysto[lic] and the click disappeared.

† Only the right coronary artery was narrowed in each patient and only 1 had anginal pain.

‡ Of 10 patients, 9 had MVR with aortocoronary bypass grafting and 1 had MVR with left ventricular aneurysmectomy. All 10 patients had angi[na] pectoris and evidence of past myocardial infarction.

§ All 3 major coronary arteries (left anterior descending, left circumflex and right) were narrowed in each patient and each patient had at lea[st] one and most 2 artery systems bypassed.

‖ Healed in all.

Angio = angiogram; CA = coronary arteries; D = diameter; Da = days; E = M-mode echocardiogram; IE = infective endocarditis; MR = mi[tral] regurgitation; Mur = precordial murmur; MVP = mitral valve prolapse; MVR = mitral valve replacement; RCT = ruptured (or absent) chordae tendine[ae]; SAP = systemic arterial pressure.

TABLE II Morphologic Criteria for Etiologic Subgrouping or Purely Regurgitant Mitral Valves

	Floppy				
	+RCT	−RCT	Coronary	Infective Endocarditis	Rheumatic
1. Leaflets					
A. Elongated (distance from basal attachment to distal margin of closure)	+	+	0	0	0
B. Increased area (anterior plus posterior >11 cm²)	+	+	0	0	0
C. Indented or perforated	+	0	0	+	0
D. Diffuse fibrous thickening	0	0	0	0	+
2. Anular circumference >11 cm	0*	+	0	0	0
3. Chordae tendineae ruptured	+	0	0	+	0
4. Papillary muscles scarred	0	0	+	0	0

* Anular circumference ≥10.5 cm but ≤11.0 cm.
+ = present; 0 = absent.

prolapse was defined as posterior motion of 1 or both leaflets beginning at the onset of and continuing throughout ventricular systole with posterior excursion from the CD line of ≥3 mm. The echo prolapse pattern was observed on multiple recordings. Three patients had both late systolic and holosystolic patterns of MVP on the same recording, but the holosystolic pattern was the predominant one, and thus, each patient was classified under the holosystolic subgroup.

Characterization of ruptured chordae tendineae: Rupture of mitral chordae tendineae was diagnosed echocardiographically if ≥1 of the following patterns was observed: (1) abnormal echoes in the left atrium during ventricular systole; (2) coarse, irregular, erratic diastolic fluttering of the anterior or posterior leaflets; (3) systolic fluttering of 1 or both leaflets; and (4) early and sustained diastolic, anterior ("paradoxical") motion of the posterior leaflet.

Characterization of leaflet vegetations: The M-mode echo diagnosis of mitral valve leaflet "vegetation" was based on the presence of thick, irregularly bordered ("shaggy") echoes that involved the anterior or posterior leaflet, or both, in ventricular systole or diastole, or both, without significant impairment of leaflet movement.

TABLE III Morphologic Observations and M-Mode Echocardiographic Patterns of Operatively Excised Mitral Valves in 65 Patients with Isolated Pure Mitral Regurgitation and in 18 Necropsy Valves

Mitral Valve (MV) Observation	Floppy: With RCT (n = 13)	Floppy: Without RCT (n = 35)	Floppy: Total (n = 48)	Coronary (n = 10)	Infective Endocarditis (n = 6)	Rheumatic (n = 1)	Necropsy Controls (n = 18)
1. Circumference (C) (cm)	10.5–11.0 (10.9)*	11.5–16.0 (13.4)**	10.5–16.0 (12.8)**	8.5–10.0 (9.4)*	9.5–10.5 (9.7)*	10.5 ...	8.0–10.5 (9.4)*
2. Leaflet area (A) (cm²)	11.6–16.0 (14.0)*	11.9–25.2 (17.5)**	11.6–25.2 (16.6)**	8.8–10.9 (9.9)***	9.2–10.6 (9.7)***	10.6 ...	7.0–12.5 (9.5)***
3. C X A product (cm³)	128–178 (152)*	149–391 (240)**	128–391 (216)**	81–107 (94)***	87–113 (95)***	111 ...	45–140 (91)***
4. No. with C >11 cm	0	35	35 (73%)	0	0	0	0
5. No. with ruptured chordae tendineae (RCT)	13	0	13 (27%)	0	6	0	0
6. No. with vegetations	0‡	0§	0	0	0‖	0	0
7. Echo(E) pattern of mitral valve prolapse (MVP) *only*	3/13	30/35 (86%)	33/48 (69%)	1	0	0	...
C	11.0 (11.0*)	11.5–16.0 (13.4**)	11.0–16.0 (14.1**)†	9.5***			
A	15.4–16.2 (15.9)*	11.9–23.2 (17.2*)†	11.9–23.2 (17.1)*	9.7***			
C X A Product	165–178 (171)*	149–360 (235)**†	149–360 (229)**	92***			
8. E pattern of RTC *only*	6/13	0/35	6/48	0	2	0	...
C	10.5–11.0 (10.8)		10.5–11.0 (10.8)		9.5 (9.5)		
A	11.6–13.4 (12.6)		11.6–13.4 (12.6)		9.2,9.8 (9.5)		
C X A product	128–147 (136)		128–147 (136)		87,93 (90)		
9. E pattern of *both* MVP + RCT	4/13	5/35	9/48	0	2	0	...
C	10.5–11.0 (11.0)	12.5–15.5 (13.9)	10.5–15.5 (12.5)†		9.5,10.5 (10.0)		
A	14.6–15.3 (15.0)	13.4–25.2 (19.1)†	13.4–25.2 (17.1)		10.6,9.5 (10.1)		
C X A product	161–176 (165)	161–391 (266)†	161–391 (216)		90,113 (102)		

*-** (Horizontal only) = $p < .01$.
*-***,**-*** (Horizontal only) = $p < 0.001$.
†-† (vertical only) = $p < .05$.
‡ Five patients had echocardiographic patterns of leaflet vegetations. All 5 valves were free of vegetations but had focal areas of leaflet fibrous ickening and indentation at sites of ruptured chords.
§ Six patients had echocardiographic patterns of leaflet vegetations. All 6 valves were free of vegetations but had large leaflet areas ("redundant") ith focal sites of fibrous thickening.
‖ Two patients had echocardiographic patterns of vegetations but both operatively excised valves were free of vegetations and each had focal eas of fibrous thickening and leaflet indentation at sites of ruptured chords.

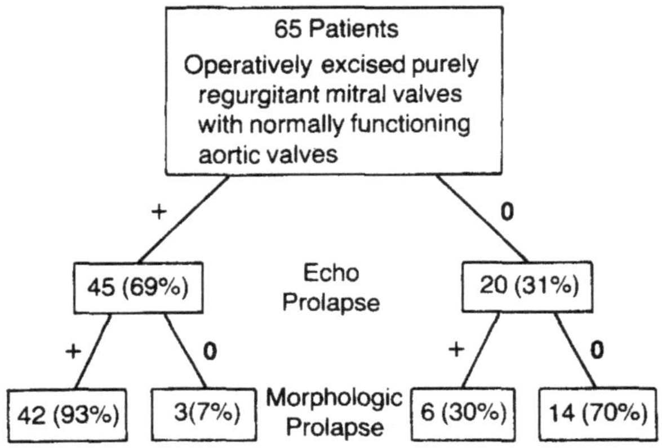

FIGURE 1. The frequency of echocardiographic (Echo) and morphologic mitral valve prolapse in the 65 patients with clinically isolated pure mitral regurgitation.

Temporal relation of echocardiogram to mitral valve replacement: The echocardiograms were recorded 3 to 406 days (mean 82) before MVR. Of 48 patients with morphologic MVP, the echocardiogram was performed within 30 days (mean 15) of operation in 26 patients, within 31 to 60 days (mean 43) in 6, 61 to 180 days (mean 104) in 7, and 6 to 12 months (mean 9) before operation in 8 patients. Two patients had echocardiograms done 377 and 406 days, respectively, before valve replacement; neither had ruptured chordae tendineae echocardiographically or morphologically. Patients with infective endocarditis on previously normal valves had echocardiograms recorded 13 to 156 days (mean 43) before valve replacement; patients with papillary muscle dysfunction had echograms 8 to 26 days (mean 18) preoperatively, and the only patient with rheumatic heart disease had an echocardiogram 83 days before valve replacement.

Statistical analysis: Data were compared using the chi-square test or unpaired t test, with statistical significance achieved if p was <0.05. The extent of agreement between the 2 independent echocardiographers was evaluated for each of the echo signs or patterns analyzed. Of 48 interpretations for the presence or absence of each of 3 patterns, 11 interobserver differences occurred, as follows: echo MVP, 5 patients (10%); ruptured chordae tendineae, 4 (8%); and leaflet vegetation, 2 (4%). These differences were then resolved by the third echocardiographer (JSG), who was unaware of the morphologic classification of the valve disease.

Results

Morphologic observations: Gross examination of the 65 mitral valves (Fig. 1) disclosed 48 with (Fig. 2) and 17 without (Fig. 3) morphologic MVP. In 10 patients (15%), the MR resulted from papillary muscle dysfunction secondary to atherosclerotic coronary heart disease (neither the chordae nor papillary muscles were ruptured); in 6 patients (9%), the cause was infective endocarditis that involved an apparently normal mitral valve (in all 6 valves the chordae were ruptured and the leaflets perforated or indented), and 1 patient had MR from rheumatic heart disease (Fig. 4). Results of morphologic measurements of anular circumference, leaflet area and circumference-area product for each subgroup are summarized in Table III. None of the 65 valves had vegetations of active infective endocarditis, but 19 valves (13 with morphologic MVP) with ruptured chordae tendineae had focal fibrous thickening of 1 or both leaflets at sites of ruptured chordae, and leaflet indentations or perforations indicative of healed infective endocarditis.[7]

Echocardiographic observations: Of the 65 patients, 45 (69%) had echo MVP, 42 (93%) of whom had morphologic MVP (Fig. 1); of the other 3 patients, 2 had healed infective endocarditis on previously normal valves and 1 had papillary muscle dysfunction from atherosclerotic coronary heart disease. Of the 20 patients without echo MVP, 6 (30%), nevertheless, had morphologic MVP and 14 (70%) did not (Fig. 1). Of the 48 patients with morphologic MVP (Fig. 2), 42 patients (88%) had echo MVP, and 7 of them had ruptured chordae; of the 6 patients with morphologic MVP without echo MVP, each had ruptured chordae tendineae. Of the 17 patients without morphologic MVP, 14 (82%) had no echo MVP; of the other 3 patients, 1 had papillary muscle dysfunction and 2 had healed infective endocarditis on previously normal valves (Fig. 3).

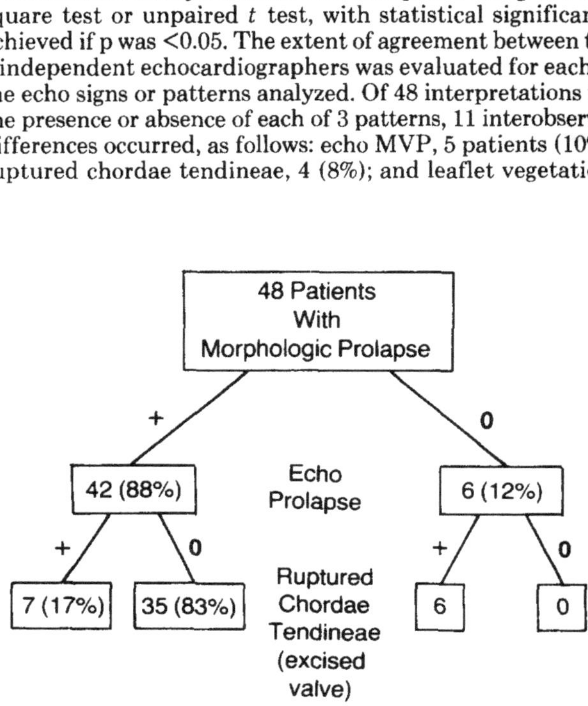

FIGURE 2. The frequency of echocardiographic (Echo) mitral valve prolapse (MVP) and ruptured chordae tendineae in the patients with morphologic MVP.

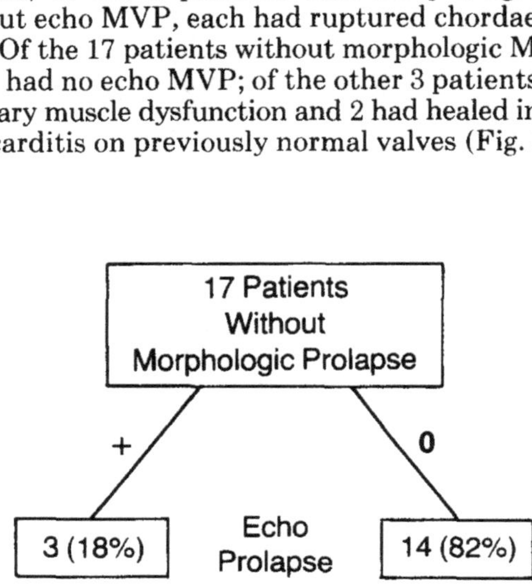

FIGURE 3. The frequency of echocardiographic (Echo) mitral valve prolapse (MVP) among the patients without morphologic MVP. Of the 3 patients with echo MVP, 1 had papillary muscle dysfunction from coronary heart disease and 2 had healed infective endocarditis on previously normal mitral valve. Of the 14 patients without echo MVP, 9 had MR from coronary heart disease, 9 had healed infective endocarditis on previously normal valves, and 1 patient had rheumatic heart disease.

The 48 patients with morphologic MVP were divided into 3 groups: those with holosystolic echo MVP (26 patients) (Fig. 5 to 9), those with mid-to-late systolic echo MVP (16 patients) (Fig. 5–7 and 10) and those without echo MVP (6 patients) (Fig. 5, 6, 7 and 11). The mean mitral anular circumferences (Fig. 5), leaflet areas (Fig. 6) and the products of the leaflet areas (in cm^2) times the anular circumferences (in cm) (Fig. 7) were significantly different in each of the 3 groups of morphologic MVP. The 13 patients with morphologic MVP with ruptured chordae tendineae (7 with and 6 without echo MVP) are displayed in the dashed boxes in Figures 5 to 7. Of the 7 valves with echo MVP, 6 had holosystolic patterns. The 7 patients with ruptured chordae and combined echo and morphologic MVP had similar average "anular" circumferences (Fig. 5), but significantly different mean leaflet areas (Fig. 6) and circumference-area products (Fig. 7) than did the 6 patients with ruptured chordae and morphologic MVP without echo MVP.

M-mode echo patterns of ruptured chordae tendineae were observed in 19 patients (29%); 15 (79%) had morphologic MVP (Fig. 11) and 4 (21%) had infective endocarditis without morphologic MVP (Fig. 12). Of 15 patients with morphologic MVP and echo patterns of ruptured chordae (Table I), 10 had morphologically confirmed ruptured chordae and 5 had intact chordae

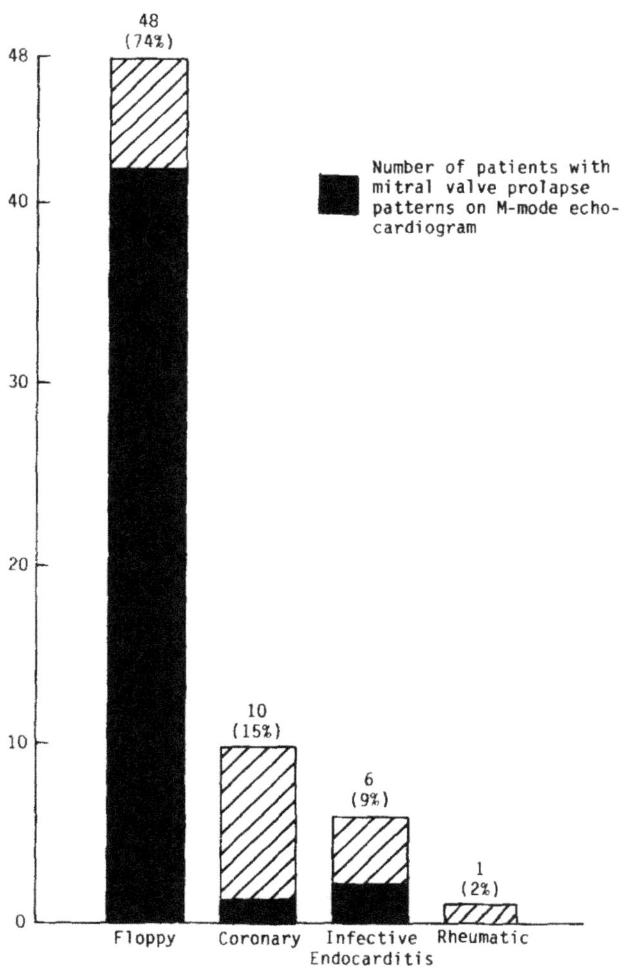

...URE 4. The etiology of isolated pure mitral regurgitation and number ...patients and frequency of echocardiographic mitral valve prolapse ...the 65 patients.

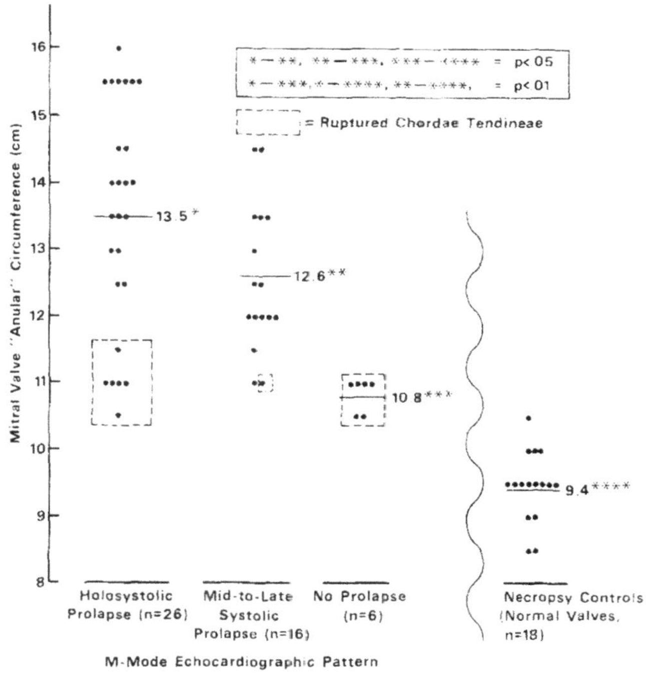

FIGURE 5. The relation of mitral valve anular circumference to M-mode mitral valve prolapse (MVP) patterns in the 48 patients with morphologic MVP and in 18 necropsy control valves.

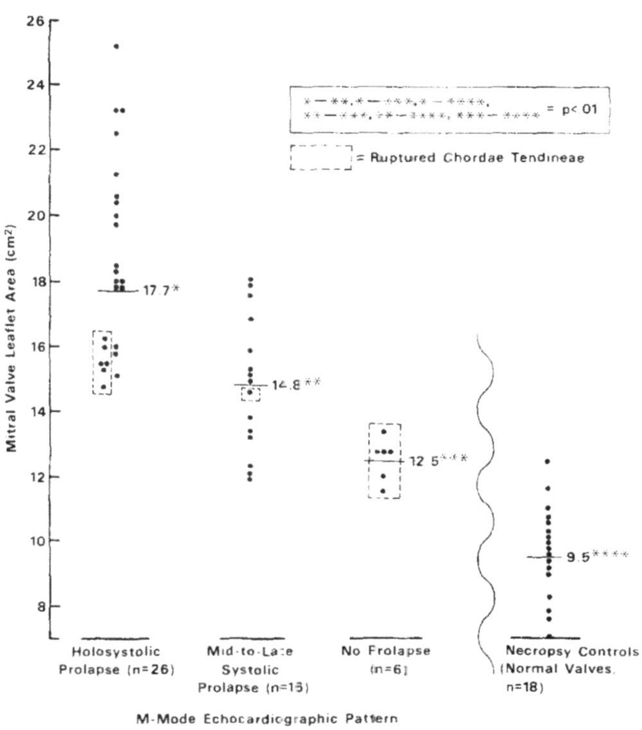

FIGURE 6. The relation of mitral valve leaflet area (in cm^2) to M-mode echocardiographic mitral valve prolapse (MVP) pattern in the 48 patients with morphologic MVP and in 18 necropsy control valves.

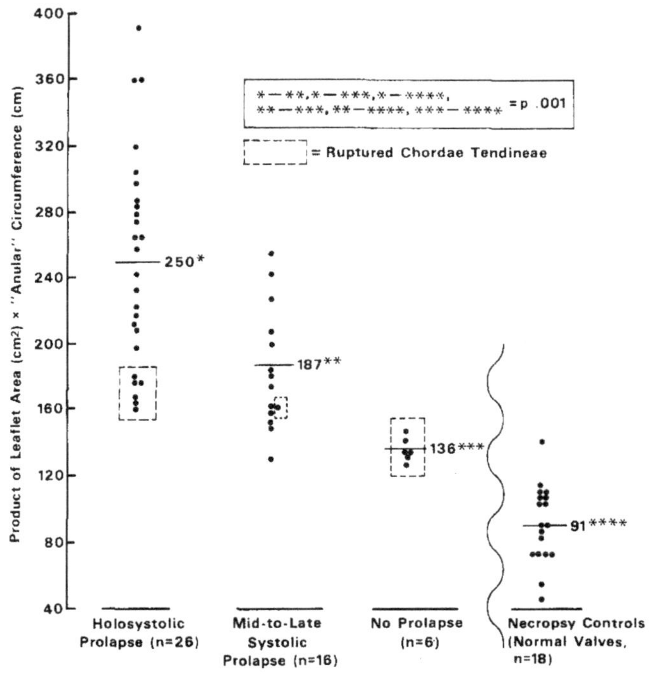

FIGURE 7. The relation of product of mitral valve leaflet area (in cm²) times "anular" circumference (in cm) to M-mode echocardiographic mitral valve prolapse (MVP) pattern in the 48 patients with morphologic MVP and in 18 necropsy control valves.

tendineae. Of 13 patients with morphologic MVP with ruptured chordae, 10 had echo patterns of ruptured chordae (Table I). Of 6 patients without morphologic MVP but with ruptured chordae, 4 had echo patterns of ruptured chordae. The 5 false-positive echograms were from patients with morphologic MVP with large anuli (14.0 to 15.5 cm) (Fig. 1) and leaflet areas (20 to

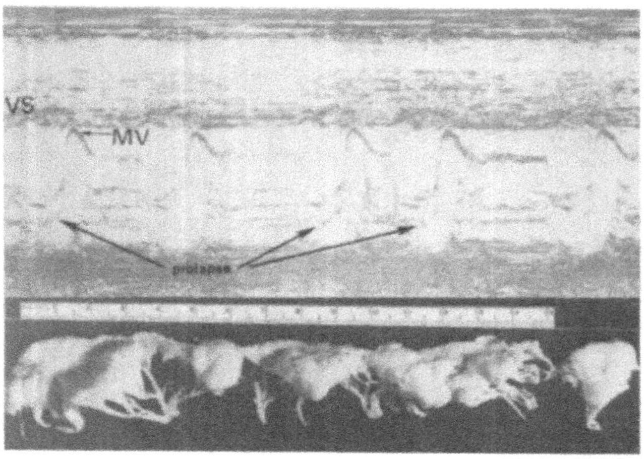

FIGURE 8. M-mode echocardiogram and operatively excised mitral valve with morphologic mitral valve prolapse in a 67-year-old man (S80-172) with chronic, severe, isolated pure mitral regurgitation. **Upper,** echocardiogram of mitral valve (MV) with holosystolic prolapse of the posterior leaflet during ventricular systole. VS = ventricular septum. **Lower,** operatively excised valve with an "anular" circumference of 16 cm and a leaflet area of 18 cm².

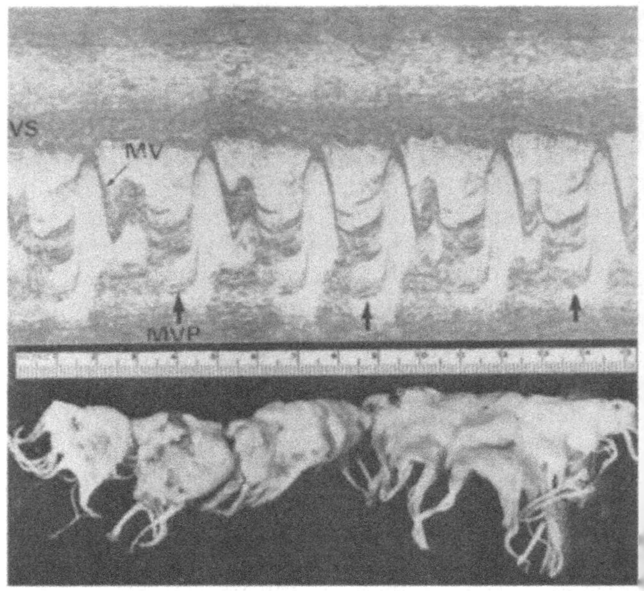

FIGURE 9. M-mode echocardiogram and operatively excised prolapse mitral valve from a 60-year-old man (S79–119) with isolated pure MR **Upper,** echocardiogram of mitral valve (MV) showing holosystolic echocardiographic mitral valve prolapse (MVP) during ventricular systol and thickened leaflets suggesting leaflet vegetation. VS = ventricula septum. **Lower,** operatively excised mitral valve showing an "anular" circumference of 15 cm, leaflet area of 18 cm² and extensive area of leaflet fibrous thickening. No leaflet vegetations or ruptured chorda tendineae were present.

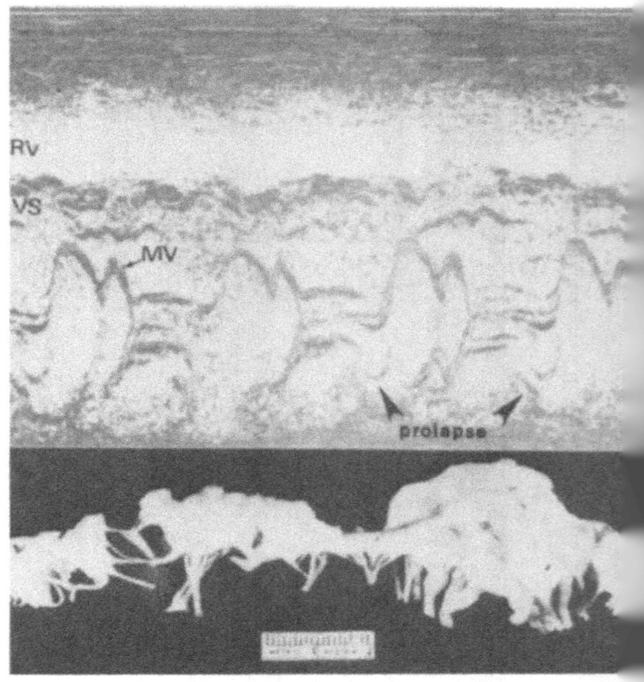

FIGURE 10. M-mode echocardiogram and operatively excised mit valve with morphologic mitral valve prolapse (MVP) from a 45-year- woman (S78–142) with chronic, severe, isolated pure mitral regur tation. **Upper,** echocardiogram of mitral valve (MV) showing late syst MVP of the posterior mitral leaflet during ventricular systole. RV = ri ventricular cavity; VS = ventricular septum. **Lower,** operatively exci valve with an anulus of 14 cm and a leaflet area of 15 cm².

23 cm²) (Fig. 2). Of the 5 false-negative echo patterns, 3 occurred in patients with morphologic MVP and holosystolic echo patterns; the other 2 were in patients without echo or morphologic MVP and without echo patterns of ruptured chordae (Table I).

M-mode echo patterns of leaflet "vegetations" of infective endocarditis were observed in 13 patients (20%) (11 with and 2 without morphologic MVP) (Fig. 9). In none of the 13 were the "vegetations" active. Of the 13 patients, 7 (5 with and 2 without morphologic MVP) had focal areas of leaflet indentation and fibrous thickening at sites of healed ruptured chordae indicative of healed infective endocarditis; the other 6 had mitral valves without morphologic MVP but with intact chordae tendineae, valves similar to the remaining 29 valves with morphologic MVP with intact chordae whose echograms did not have "vegetation" patterns.

Discussion

Considerable variation exists in the sensitivity of echo in detecting morphologic MVP because of the lack of consistent diagnostic criteria of morphologic MVP using auscultatory, angiographic or morphologic standards. Waller et al[5] recently reported a morphologic definition of MVP producing MR severe enough to warrent mitral valve replacement. The definition was based on mitral anular circumference and leaflet area. Operatively excised valves with morphologic MVP had anular circumferences or leaflet areas clearly increased over that of other mitral valve conditions causing severe, pure MR. Except when associated with ruptured chordae tendineae, anular circumferences >11 cm served to separate valves with from those without morphologic MVP. Valves with morphologic MVP and ruptured chordae had mitral circumferences usually increased above normal, but the additional measurement of increased leaflet area was necessary to clearly distinguish the valves with from those without morphologic MVP. With these morphologic criteria established, it became possible to assess the reliability of echo MVP using morphologic standards.

The combined sensitivity of holosystolic (hammocking) and late systolic (buckling) MVP patterns in diagnosing morphologic MVP in the present study was 88%. Of the 48 patients with morphologic MVP, 6 had false-negative M-mode echocardiograms of MVP and

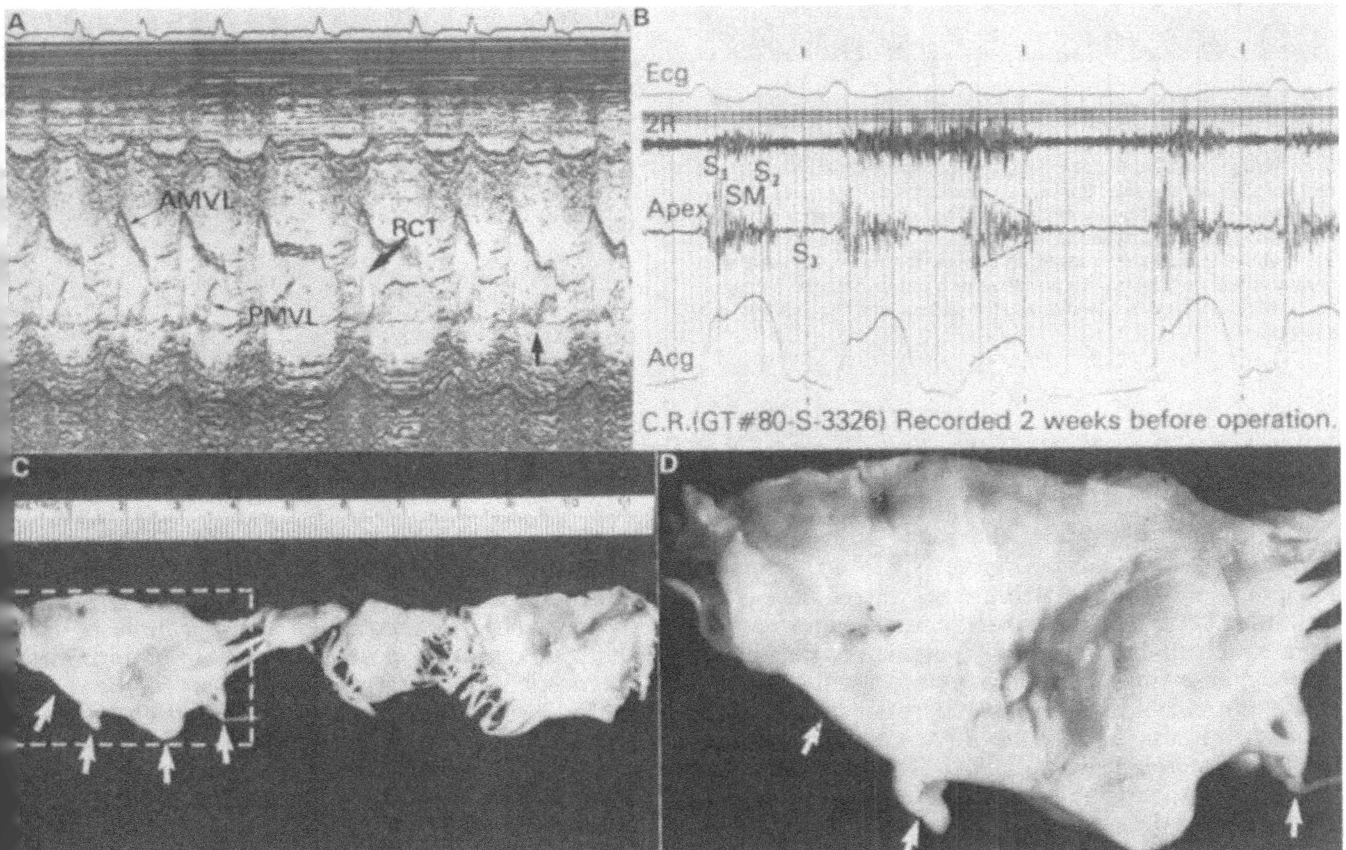

GURE 11. Preoperative noninvasive data and operatively excised prolapsed mitral valve with ruptured chordae tendineae (RCT) from a 63-year-old an with severe, isolated pure mitral regurgitation. **A,** M-mode echocardiogram of anterior (AMVL) and posterior (PMVL) mitral valve leaflet showing ratic and vibratory movements of the PMVL indicating RCT (**arrows**). The echocardiographic pattern of mitral valve prolapse (MVP) is absent. phonocardiogram recorded at the second right sternal border (2R) and apex showing a holosystolic murmur (SM) that decreases in late ventricular stole (**dashed lines**). Acg = apexcardiogram; Ecg = electrocardiogram; S_1, S_2, and S_3 = first, second and third heart sounds. **C,** operatively cised valve with morphologic MVP and an "anular" circumference of 11.5 cm and a leaflet area of 12 cm². Multiple chordae tendineae to an ongated posterior leaflet (**dashed box**) are missing (**arrows**). **D,** blow-up of leaflet in dashed box showing multiple RCT (**arrows**).

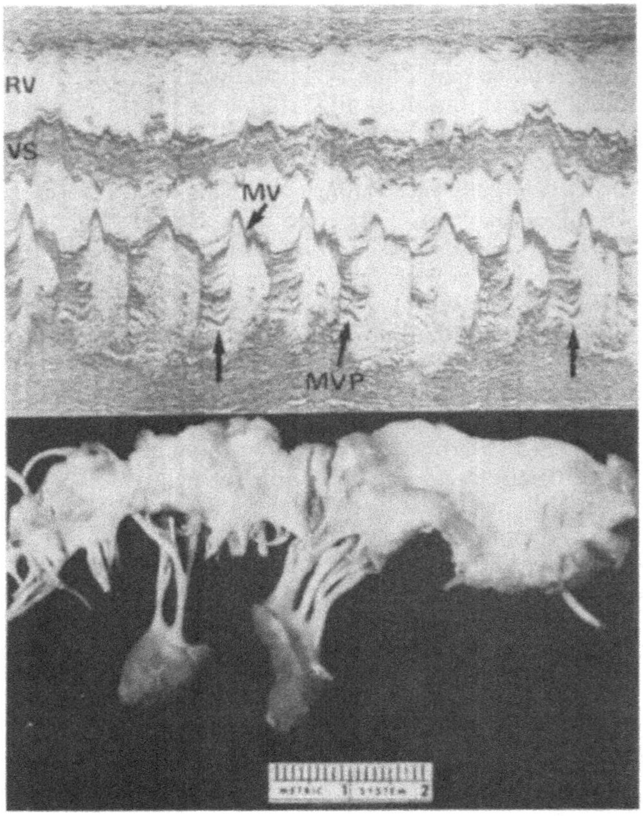

FIGURE 12. M-mode echocardiogram and operatively excised valve without morphologic mitral valve prolapse (MVP) from a 56-year-old man (GT 77S–5736) with chronic, isolated, pure mitral regurgitation from healed infective endocarditis on a previously anatomically and functionally normal valve. **Upper,** echocardiogram of mitral valve (MV) showing MVP and vibratory motion of portions of the posterior leaflet indicating ruptured chordae tendineae. RV = right ventricular cavity; VS = ventricular septum. **Lower,** operatively excised mitral valve with normal mitral "anular" circumference (9.5 cm) and leaflet area (9.8 cm^2). Multiple chordae tendineae are absent and the leaflets are scarred.

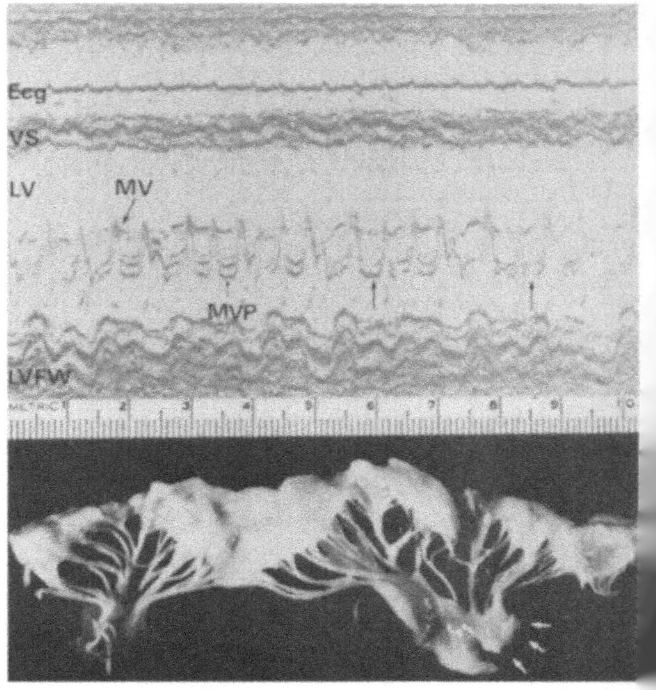

FIGURE 13. M-mode echocardiogram and operatively excised mitra valve without morphologic mitral valve prolapse (MVP) from a 54- year-old man (GT81-S-2186) with severe, chronic, pure mitral regur- gitation from papillary muscle dysfunction secondary to atherosclerotic coronary heart disease. **Upper,** echocardiogram showing a dilated lef ventricular (LV) cavity, increased E-to-septal distance, and holosystolic MVP. Ecg = electrocardiogram; LVFW = left ventricular free wall; MV = mitral valve; VS = ventricular septum. **Lower,** operatively excised valve with normal circumference (10.3 cm) and leaflet area (10.2 cm^2 but scarred and atrophied papillary muscle (**arrows**).

each had ruptured chordae tendineae. In the 42 patients with true-positive echo MVP, the mitral circumference leaflet areas and/or circumference area products were greater than that of the 6 valves with morphologic MVP and false-negative echocardiograms. Previously reported causes of false-negative MVP on M-mode echograms have been attributed to incomplete echo "scanning" of the mitral valve ("single-beam view" of the mitral leaflets), improperly positioned transducer or low-gain settings.[9] The data in the present study indicate that mitral valve anulus and leaflet sizes also are factors in producing false-negative echograms in patients with morphologic MVP. Valves with morphologic MVP but with small anuli and leaflet areas may not produce echo MVP.

The combined diagnostic specificity of the 2 echo MVP patterns in our study was 82%. Two of the 3 false-positive echocardiograms were from patients with ruptured chordae tendineae resulting from infective endocarditis on previously normal valves; each of the 2 valves had normal mitral anuli and leaflet areas. The third patient with false-positive echo MVP had papillary muscle dysfunction from atherosclerotic coronar heart disease and the mitral valve anulus and leafle area also were normal (Fig. 13). Previously reporte causes of false-positive MVP on M-mode echogram have been observed in patients with papillary muscl dysfunction from coronary artery disease,[10] "flail leaf lets" associated with infective endocarditis,[4] mitra anular calcium,[11] inferior transducer angulation[12] an large pericardial effusions.[13] Thus, valves withou morphologic MVP may produce echo MVP that is in distinguishable from that produced by valves wit morphologic MVP.

Previous echo reports[2,17,21] have emphasized th sharp, midsystolic, posterior buckling pattern as th diagnostic cornerstones of morphologic MVP, wherea the holosystolic hammock pattern has been associate with ruptured chordae tendineae ("flail leaflet") an had been less reliable in the diagnosis of morphologi MVP. In the present study, holosystolic MVP was four in 26 (54%) of 48 patients with morphologic MVP: (23%) had ruptured and 20 (77%) had intact chord tendineae. The mitral leaflet area and "anular" ci cumference, however, generally correlated with the echo patterns of morphologic MVP. Valves with mo phologic MVP and very large circumferences (>14.5 cr and leaflet areas (>18 cm^2) had holosystolic echo MV Excluding valves with ruptured chordae, valves wi morphologic MVP and smaller anuli (<12.5 cm) and leaflet areas ($<14.5\ cm^2$) had mid-to-late systolic echo MVP. DeMaria et al[22] also reported holosystolic echo MVP as the most frequent echocardiographic pattern of MVP in 26 patients with angiographic evidence of prolapse, but none of the valves from their patients was studied morphologically.

References

1. **Burgess J, Clark, R, Kamigaki M, Cohn K.** Echocardiographic findings in different types of mitral regurgitation. Circulation 1973;48:97–106.
2. **Popp RL, Brown OR, Silverman JF, Harrison DC.** Echocardiographic abnormalities in the mitral valve prolapse syndrome. Circulation 1974;49:428–433.
3. **Corrigall D, Bolen J, Hancock EW, Popp RL.** Mitral valve prolapse and infective endocarditis. Am J Med 1977;63:215–222.
4. **Child JS, Skorton DJ, Taylor RD, Krivokapich J, Abbasi AS, Wong M, Shah PD.** M-mode and cross-sectional echocardiographic features of flail posterior mitral leaflets. Am J Cardiol 1979;44:1383–1390.
5. **Waller BF, Morrow AG, Maron BJ, Del Negro AA, Ken KM, McGrath FJ, Wallace RB, McIntosh CL, Roberts WC.** Etiology of clinically isolated, severe, chronic, pure mitral regurgitation: analysis of 97 patients over 30 years of age having mitral valve replacement. Am Heart J 1982;104:276–288.
6. **Roberts WC, Virmani R.** Aschoff bodies at necropsy in valvular heart disease. Evidence from analysis of 543 patients over 14 years of age that rheumatic heart disease, at least anatomically, is a disease of the mitral valve. Circulation 1978;57:803–812.
7. **Roberts WC, Buchbinder NA.** Healed left-sided infective endocarditis: a clinicopathologic study of 59 patients. Am J Cardiol 1977;40:876–888.
8. **Haikal M, Alpert MA, Whiting RB, Ahmad M, Kelly D.** Sensitivity and specificity of M-mode echocardiographic signs of mitral valve prolapse. Am J Cardiol 1982;50:185–190
9. **Feigenbaum H.** Echocardiography. 2nd Ed. Philadelphia: Lea & Febiger, 1976:119–130.
10. **Aranda JM, Befeler B, Lazzara R, Embi A, Machado H.** Mitral valve prolapse and coronary artery disease. Circulation 1975;52:245–253.
11. **Dashkoff N, Karacuschansky M, Come PC, Fortuin NJ.** Echocardiographic features of mitral annulus calcification. Am Heart J 1977;94:585–592.
12. **Sahn DJ, Allen HD, Goldberg SJ, Friedman WF.** Echocardiographic spectrum of mitral valve motion in children with and without mitral valve prolapse: the nature of false positive diagnosis. Am J Cardiol 1977;39:422–431.
13. **Levisman JA, Abbasi AS.** Abnormal motion of the mitral valve with pericardial effusion: pseudo-prolapse of the mitral valve. Am Heart J 1976;91:18–20.
14. **Criley JM, Kissel GL.** Prolapse of the mitral valve: the click and late systolic murmur syndrome. In: Goodwin J, Yu PN, eds. Progress in Cardiology. Vol. 4. Philadelphia: Lea & Febiger, 1976:23–26.
15. **Wann LS, Dillon JC, Weyman AE, Feigenbaum H.** Echocardiography in bacterial endocarditis. N Engl J Med 1976;295:135–139.
16. **Chandraratna PAN, Lagevin E.** Limitations of the echogram in diagnosing valvular vegetations in patients with mitral valve prolapse. Circulation 1977;56:436–438.
17. **Dillon JC, Haine CL, Chang S, Feigenbaum H.** Use of echocardiography in patients with prolapsed mitral valve. Circulation 1971;43:503–507.
18. **Kerber RE, Isaeff DM, Hancock EW.** Echocardiographic patterns in patients with the syndrome of systolic click and late systolic murmur. N Engl J Med 1971;284:691–693.
19. **Markiewicz W, Stoner J, London E, Hunt SA, Popp RL.** Mitral valve prolapse in one hundred presumably healthy young females. Circulation 1976;54:464–473.
20. **Higgens CB, Reinke RT, Gosink BB, Leopold GR.** The significance of mitral valve prolapse in middle-aged and elderly men. Am Heart J 1976;91:292–296.
21. **DeMaria AN, Neumann A, Lee G, Mason D.** Echocardiographic identification of the mitral valve prolapse syndrome. Am J Med 1977;62:819–829.
22. **DeMaria AN, King JF, Borgren HJ, Lies JE.** The variable spectrum of echocardiographic manifestations of the mitral valve prolapse syndrome. Circulation 1974;50:33–41.

Aneurysm (Redundancy) of the Atrial Septum (Fossa Ovale Membrane) and Prolapse (Redundancy) of the Mitral Valve

WILLIAM C. ROBERTS, MD

Intracardiac aneurysms involve a cardiac valve or adjacent valvular structure (e.g., sinus of Valsalva aneurysm), ventricular septum or atrial septum. Aneurysm of a valvular leaflet or adjacent valvular structure often is a consequence of infective endocarditis. Prolapse of a tricuspid or mitral valve leaflet is a type of intracardiac aneurysm. A localized protrusion of the ventricular septum usually is either a consequence of myocardial infarction or a result of congenital redundancy of the membranous ventricular septum. Aneurysm of the atrial septum always involves the fossa ovale portion, and may be the consequence of a large pressure difference between the 2 atria (secondary) or it may be unassociated with a significant pressure difference between these 2 chambers (primary). The classic example of secondary protrusion of the fossa ovale membrane toward the left atrium is in association with severe pulmonic valve stenosis with intact ventricular septum.[1] The classic example of secondary protrusion of the fossa ovale membrane toward the right atrium is in association with aortic valve atresia.[2]

Primary aneurysm or redundancy of the fossa ovale membrane was recently recognized by echocardiography.[3–5] The fossa ovale membrane has been shown to move into the right atrium during expiration and into the left atrium during inspiration.[3,4] The cause of primary aneurysmal formation of the fossa ovale membrane is unclear. Its virtual absence during childhood in the absence of major congenital cardiac anomalies—as is the usual circumstance with mitral valve prolapse (MVP)—suggests that a certain amount of time is required for the redundancy of this membrane to become apparent even though the connective tissue of the membrane may be congenitally defective. MVP in most patients probably represents an inherent deficiency of leaflet tissue. Because both fossa ovale membrane and mitral and tricuspid valve leaflet represent

From the Pathology Branch, National Heart, Lung, and Blood Institute, National Institutes of Health, Bethesda, Maryland. Manuscript received and accepted July 23, 1984.

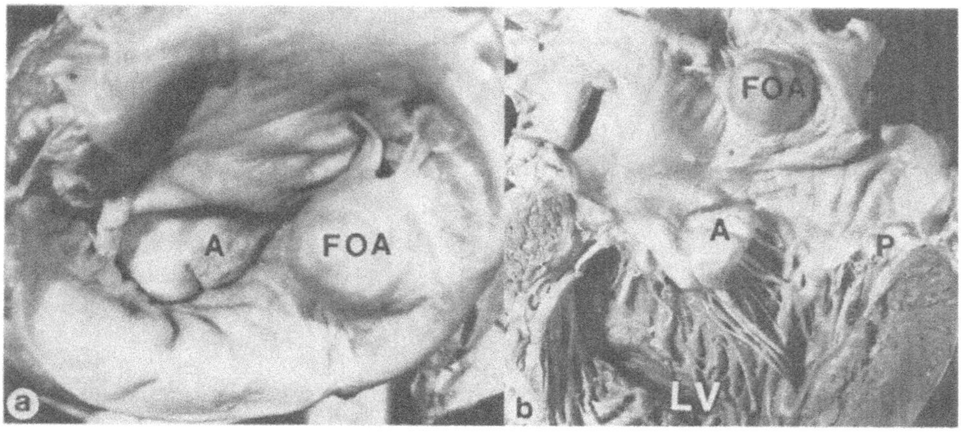

FIGURE 1. Patient 1. Heart. **a,** left atrium from above showing the fossa ovale aneurysm (FOA) and anterior (A) mitral leaflet protruding into the left atrial cavity. **b,** opened left atrium, mitral valve and left ventricle (LV). The posterior half of the anterior (A) mitral leaflet is prolapsed and a small portion of the posterior (P) leaflet is prolapsed.

endocardium, an inherent deficiency in one might be expected to occur frequently in the other. Such was the case in 2 patients described herein.

Patient 1: *A 57-year-old man had been well until age 54 years, when he was found to have islet cell carcinoma. Signs and symptoms attributable to hypoglycemia were his major problem during his last 3 years. Examination 2 months before death disclosed a grade 2/6 precordial systolic blowing murmur, loudest at the apex with radiation into the left axilla. No abnormal cardiac sounds were described. He died from widespread metastatic carcinoma. At necropsy, the posterior half of the anterior mitral leaflet protruded toward the left atrium and the posterior mitral leaflet and some of its chordae tendineae were thickened (Fig. 1). The mural endocardium behind the posterior mitral leaflet was thickened by fibrous tissue. The fossa ovale membrane was aneurysmal and a valvular-competent defect was present in the atrial septum (Fig. 1). The myocardium, semilunar valves and aorta were normal.*

Patient 2: *A 57-year-old woman, who had been told of the presence of a precordial systolic murmur (heard when she was 23 years old), was asymptomatic until 1 week before death, when she had the sudden onset of severe dyspnea. A grade 4/6 systolic murmur (with thrill) was audible, loudest over the left sternal border, and its intensity increased during inspiration. A grade 2/6 diastolic blowing murmur also was audible over, and just to the right and left of, the sternum. Death resulted from rapidly progressing congestive heart failure. At necropsy, the fossa ovale membrane protruded aneurysmally into the left atrial cavity, a large defect (4 cm) was present in the atrial septum (valvular incompetent "patent" foramen ovale), and the posterior mitral leaflet protruded toward the left atrium (Fig. 2). The aortic valve was congenitally bicuspid, the wall of the aorta behind its posterior cusp was aneurysmally dilated, and it had ruptured into the right ventricle. The pulmonic valve was congenitally quadricuspid but functionally normal. Both right atrium and ventricle were considerably dilated and the left-sided chambers were of normal size. Death was clearly the consequence of rupture of the sinus of Valsalva aneurysm into the right side of the heart.*

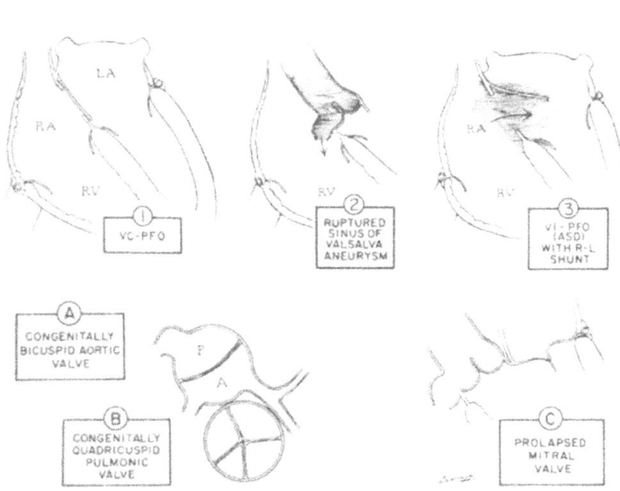

GURE 2. Patient 2. Diagram illustrating the multiple cardiovascular normalities. ASD = atrial septal defect; LA = left atrium; RA = right rium; R-L = right-left; RV = right ventricle; VC/PFO = valvular mpetent patent foramen ovale; VI = valvular incompetent.

The findings in these patients, along with previous echocardiographic evidence,[5] indicate an association between aneurysm of the fossa ovale membrane of the atrial septum and prolapse of the mitral valve. The presence of aneurysm of a sinus of Valsalva and congenital anomalies of both aortic and pulmonic valves in 1 of the 2 patients suggests a developmental association of these additional anomalies with atrial septal aneurysm and MVP.

By auscultation, aneurysm of the fossa ovale membrane may simulate MVP. Alexander et al[3] described a midsystolic click without murmur in a 39-year-old man who had an aneurysm of the fossa ovale membrane and no echocardiographic evidence of MVP. The click, which increased with inspiration and decreased slightly with the Valsalva maneuver, occurred at the point of maximal bulging of the fossa ovale membrane into the right atrium.

References

1. **Roberts WC, Shemin RJ, Kent KM.** Frequency and direction of interatrial shunting in valvular pulmonic stenosis with intact ventricular septum and without left ventricular inflow or outflow obstruction. An analysis of 127 patients treated by valvulotomy. Am Heart J 1980;99:142–148.
2. **Roberts WC, Perry LW, Chandra RS, Myers GE, Shapiro SR, Scott LP.** Aortic valve atresia: a new classification based on necropsy study of 73 cases. Am J Cardiol 1976;37:753–756.
3. **Alexander MD, Bloom KR, Hart P, D'Silva F, Murgo JP.** Atrial septal aneurysm: a cause for midsystolic click. Report of a case and review of the literature. Circulation 1981;63:1186–1188.
4. **Vandenbossche JL, Englert M.** Effects of respiration on an atrial septal aneurysm of the fossa ovale shown by echographic study. Am Heart J 1982;103:922–923.
5. **Iliceto S, Antonelli G, Chiddo A, Rizzon P.** Two-dimensional echocardiographic recognition of an atrial septal aneurysm. Int J Cardiol 1983;2:447–449.

FROM THE EDITOR

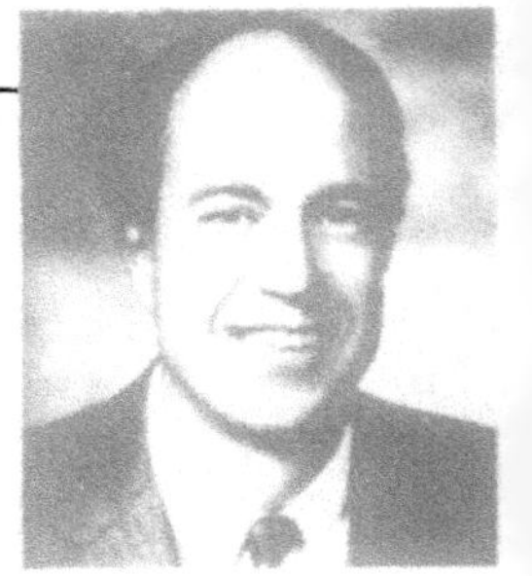

Mitral Valve Prolapse and Systemic Hypertension

In the USA there are approximately 160 million persons over 20 years of age (total population = 238 million). Of the 160 million, an estimated 8 million (5%) have auscultatory evidence of mitral valve prolapse (MVP) and 60 million (37%) have systemic hypertension (SH) (arterial pressure $\geq$140/90 mm Hg). Accordingly, of the 8 million with MVP, nearly 3 million (0.37 $\times$ 8) have SH, and of the 60 million with SH, 3 million (0.05 $\times$ 60) have MVP. The number of persons, therefore, with both MVP and SH in the USA is substantial.

Except in the person with left ventricular outflow obstruction, the systemic peak systolic arterial pressure is identical to the left ventricular peak systolic pressure, which of course is the pressure that closes the mitral valve orifice during ventricular systole. The normal mitral valve withstands elevation of the left ventricular peak systolic pressure without development of mitral regurgitation unless mitral anular calcific deposition is heavy, a process which is more frequent in hypertensive than in normotensive persons.[1] But how well does the defective, i.e., prolapsed or floppy, mitral valve tolerate chronic elevation of the left ventricular peak systolic pressure? My answer is "poorly," and the reason is because the associated SH (specifically, the elevated left ventricular systolic pressure) greatly increases the frequency of spontaneous rupture of mitral chordae tendineae, an occurrence virtually limited to patients with preexisting MVP. Jeresaty and associates[2] found underlying MVP in 23 (92%) of 25 patients with spontaneous rupture of mitral chordae tendineae and Hickey and associates[3] found underlying MVP in 29 (94%) of 31 patients with spontaneous rupture of mitral chordae tendineae. In an earlier study,[4] my colleagues and I examined 60 operatively excised purely regurgitant prolapsed mitral valves: 13 had ruptured chordae tendineae and of these, 11 (85%) had had SH before valve replacement; of the remaining 47 valves, none had ruptured chordae tendineae and only 11 (23%) of them had had SH preoperatively.

The normal mitral leaflets, as with the leaflets of all 4 cardiac valves, consist of 2 components: the fibrosa and the spongiosa. The fibrosa consists of collagen fibrils and the spongiosa, of an acid mucopolysaccharide material. In MVP the collagen fibrils of both the leaflets and chordae tendineae are defective[5] and probably, at least initially, decreased in number, and the spongiosa material, the "weaker" of the 2 components, is present in excessive amounts. It is reasonable to believe that the weaker the mitral leaflet and chordal structures, the greater the effect on them of the left ventricular systolic pressure, and the greater the mitral closing pressure the greater its effect on the defective mitral leaflet and chordal structures.

In summary, the normal mitral valve tolerates elevated left ventricular systolic pressures (mitral closing pressures) well, i.e., without creating mitral regurgitation and without rupturing mitral chordae tendineae. The prolapsed mitral valve, in contrast, contains defective collagen fibrils and excess spongiosa and it appears to withstand elevated left ventricular systolic pressures poorly as manifested by a high frequency of spontaneous rupture of chordae tendineae (and probably also by an increased degree of leaflet prolapse). Thus, proper treatment of SH may prevent or delay the appearance of severe mitral regurgitation that occurs in some patients with MVP.

William C. Roberts

William C. Roberts, MD
Editor in Chief

1. **Roberts WC.** Morphologic features of the normal and abnormal mitral valv Am J Cardiol 1983;51:1005–1028.
2. **Jeresaty RM, Edwards JE, Chawla SK.** Mitral valve prolapse and ruptur chordae tendineae. Am J Cardiol 1985;55:138–142.
3. **Hickey AJ, Wilcken DEL, Wright JS, Warren BA.** Primary (spontaneou chordal rupture: relation to myxomatous valve disease and mitral val prolapse. JACC 1985;5:1341–1346.
4. **Waller BF, Morrow AG, Maron BJ, Del Negro AA, Kent KM, McGrath F Wallace RB, McIntosh CL, Roberts WC.** Etiology of clinically isolated, sever chronic, pure mitral regurgitation: an analysis of 97 patients over 30 yea of age having mitral valve replacement. Am Heart J 1982;104:276–288.
5. **Renteria VG, Ferrans VJ, Jones M, Roberts WC.** Intracellular collagen fibr in prolapsed ("floppy") human atrioventricular valves. Lab Invest 197 35:439–443.

Mechanisms of severe mitral regurgitation in mitral valve prolapse determined from analysis of operatively excised valves

Certain clinical and mitral valvular morphologic findings are described in 83 patients (age 26 to 79 years [mean, 60]; 26 women [31%] and 57 men [69%]) with mitral valve prolapse (MVP) and mitral regurgitation (MR) severe enough to warrant mitral valve replacement. All 83 operatively excised valves were examined by the same person, and all excised valves had been purely regurgitant (no element of stenosis). No patients had hemodynamic evidence of dysfunction of the aortic valve. In each valve a portion of the posterior mitral leaflet was elongated such that the distance from the distal margin to basal attachment of this leaflet was similar to the distance from the distal margin of the anterior leaflet to its basal attachment to the left atrial wall. Two major mechanisms for the severe MR were found: (1) dilatation of the mitral anulus with or without rupture of chordae tendineae and (2) rupture of chordae tendineae with or without dilatation of the mitral anulus. Of the 83 patients, 48 (58%) had both dilated anuli (>11 cm in circumference) and ruptured chordae tendineae; 16 (19%) had dilated anuli without ruptured chordae, and 16 (19%) had ruptured chordae without significant anular dilatation. In three patients the anulus was not dilated, nor were chordae ruptured, and therefore the mechanism of the MR is uncertain. Mitral chordal rupture was nearly as frequent in the 64 patients with clearly dilated anular circumferences as in the 19 patients with normal or insignificantly dilated anular circumferences (≤11 cm). (Am Heart J 1987;113:1316.)

William C. Roberts, M.D., Charles L. McIntosh, M.D., Robert B. Wallace, M.D.,
Bethesda, Md. and Washington, D.C.

Mitral valve prolapse (MVP) is recognized to occur clinically in about 5% of persons over 20 years of age. In the United States, approximately 160 million persons are over 20 years of age, 8 million of whom have MVP. In most persons with clinical evidence of MVP, no symptoms are produced by the prolapsed valve. Although many persons with MVP have auscultatory evidence of minimal or mild mitral regurgitation (MR), the development of severe MR, severe enough to require operative intervention, is uncommon. This article describes certain findings in 83 patients who had MVP and MR severe enough to warrant mitral valve replacement.

PATIENTS STUDIED

The surgical pathology files of the Pathology Branch, National Heart, Lung, and Blood Institute, were searched for persons who had had mitral valve excision for pure MR. All valves had been so classified initially by W.C.R. Nearly 300 cases were so classified. Many cases were eliminated because either the operatively excised valve was no longer available or photographs of the operatively excised valve were unavailable. Some cases were eliminated because it was apparent that the cause of the pure MR was the following: (1) *rheumatic heart disease* (diffuse fibrosis of both mitral leaflets without elongation of the basal to distal margin of the posterior leaflet), (2) *infective endocarditis* involving a previously normal valve or one previously affected by rheumatic heart disease, (3) *papillary muscle dysfunction* from coronary artery disease (necrotic or fibrotic papillary muscle in the absence of either significant mitral anular dilatation or posterior mitral leaflet elongation), (4) *hypertrophic cardiomyopathy* or (5) *systemic lupus erythematosus* or *hypereosinophilic syndrome*. Some cases were eliminated because the aortic valve had also been excised simultaneously or because the aortic valve was found to have functioned abnormally: either stenotic or regurgitant or both. A few cases were eliminated because on review of preoperative hemody-

From the Pathology and Surgery Branches, National Heart, Lung, and Blood Institute, National Institutes of Health, and the Department of Surgery, Georgetown University.

Reprint requests: William C. Roberts, M.D., Pathology Branch, Bldg. 10A, Room 3E-30, National Heart, Lung, and Blood Institute, National Institutes of Health, Bethesda, MD 20892.

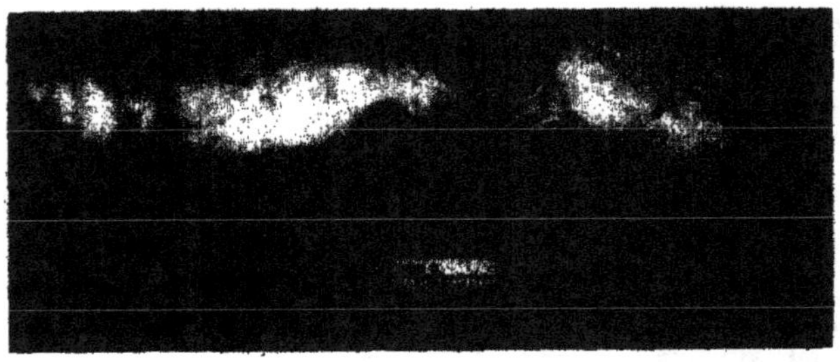

Fig. 1. Operatively excised mitral valve in a 56-year-old man (S68-4175). The anular circumference measures about 11 cm. Some chordae tendineae from the posterior leaflet are missing. The distance from site of attachment (anulus) to distal margin of both posterior and anterior *(A)* leaflets is similar. The atrial surface of the leaflets is shown.

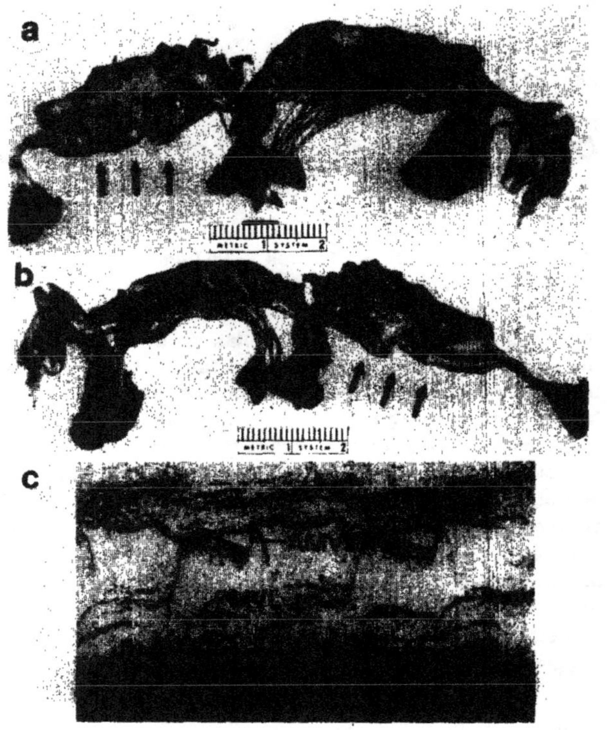

Fig. 2. Operatively excised mitral valve (*a* and *b*) and echocardiogram *(c)* recorded 1 month before valve replacement in a 43-year-old man (S70-3086). *a,* Atrial surface; *b,* Ventricular surface. Chordae are missing from the posterior leaflet *(arrows).* The distance from the site of attachment to distal margin of both anterior *(A)* and posterior leaflets is similar. *c,* The echocardiogram shows prolapse of the posterior leaflet. AMVL = anterior mitral valve leaflet; PMVL = posterior mitral valve leaflet; VS = ventricular septum.

namic data a small mean diastolic gradient had been recorded between the left atrium or pulmonary arterial wedge position and the left ventricle, and therefore the patient did not have "pure" MR.

A total of 83 cases were collected in which preoperative cardiac catheterization had indicated that the hemodynamic lesion involving the mitral valve was *pure* regurgitation, that the aortic valve had functioned normally (no element of either stenosis or regurgitation), and that examination of the operatively excised mitral valve had indicated that it fulfilled the following morphologic definition of MVP: in a portion of the posterior mitral leaflet the distance from its distal margin to its attachment at the mitral anulus was clearly elongated, a finding not observed in patients in whom the MR resulted from other causes, namely, rheumatic, infective endocarditis, coronary artery disease, hypertrophic cardiomyopathy, systemic lupus erythematosus, or hypereosinophilic syndrome. Usually at some point the distance from basal attachment to distal margin of the posterior mitral leaflet was similar to the distance from the distal margin of the anterior mitral leaflet to the point where the left atrial wall contacted it. The elongation of the posterior mitral leaflet caused an increase in the area of this leaflet. Many patients also had dilated mitral anuli, and the chordae in many patients appeared to be longer than usual. This latter finding, however, could not be systematically evaluated because many of the operatively excised mitral valves did not include attached papillary muscles. Photographs of the operatively excised mitral valves were available in 81 (98%) of the 83 patients. Of the 83 cases, 42 (51%) had been included in a previous publication concerning the various causes of pure MR severe enough to warrant mitral valve replacement.[1] Moreover, 25 (30%) of the 83 cases had been included in a previous publication concerning the frequency of calcific deposits in mitral valves excised because of pure MR.[2]

The operation to replace the mitral valve in the 83 patients had been performed at four different medical centers, and the operatively excised valve in each was thereafter submitted to the Pathology Branch of the National Heart, Lung, and Blood Institute for examination. The valve was weighed, its anular circumference was measured, and a determination was made whether chordae tendineae attached to both leaflets were "disrupted" or "missing" or neither. Chordae were considered "disrupted" if detached chordae had rounded or blunted distal ends that were thicker than normal, often thicker than the more proximal portions of the same chordae. Chordae were considered "missing" if none extended caudally beneath the ventricular surfaces of a portion of either or both leaflets. Both "dis-

Fig. 3. Operatively excised mitral valve in a 55-year-old woman (S76-35). The anulus measures about 12 cm in circumference. Most chordae from the posterior leaflet are missing *(arrows)*. *a,* Ventricular aspect of valve. *b,* Ventricular aspect of posterior leaflet. *c,* Atrial aspect of posterior leaflet.

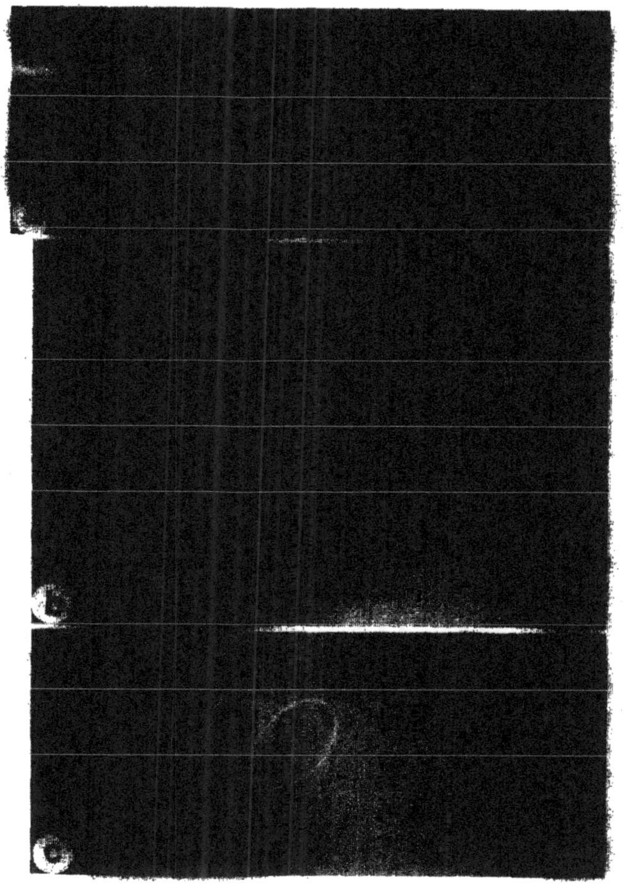

Fig. 4. Operatively excised mitral valve *(a)* showing its atrial aspect and lateral radiographs showing a C-shaped calcific deposit before *(b)* and after *(c)* valve replacement in a 47-year-old woman (S76-156). Some chordae from the posterior leaflet are missing. A = anterior leaflet.

rupted" and "missing" chordae were considered "ruptured" chordae.

RESULTS

The 83 patients included 26 women (31%) and 57 men (69%). The women at the time of mitral valve replacement ranged in age from 42 to 79 years (mean, 61 years) and the men ranged from 26 to 77 years (mean, 59 years). The 26-year-old man had the Marfan syndrome. The next youngest patient was 42 years old. Of the 83 patients, 15 (18%) were younger than 51 years old, and 68 patients (82%) were older than 50 years of age at the time of mitral valve replacement. The excised valves (Figs. 1 to 18) ranged in weight from 4.0 to 14.5 gm (mean, 6.7 gm). The larger weights were in the valves in which one or both papillary muscles had usually been excised. Calcific deposits were present in 28 valves (34%). The calcific deposits involved primarily the mitral anular region in 19 patients (68%), one or both mitral leaflets without anular involvement in three patients (11%), one or more chordae tendineae only in four patients (14%), and papillary muscle only in two patients (7%). The calcific deposits were focal and small in all patients.

The circumference of the mitral anulus in the 26 women ranged from 9 to 15 cm (mean, 12). It was ≤11 cm in 10 patients (38%), and nine (90%) had missing or disrupted chordae tendineae. The circumference was >11 cm in 16 women (62%), and 13 (81%) had missing or disrupted chordae. Of the 26 women, 22 (85%) had ruptured chordae. In the 57 men, the mitral anular circumference ranged from 10 to 18 cm (mean, 14). It was ≤11 cm in nine patients (16%), and seven of the nine had missing or disrupted chordae. It was >11 cm in 48 men (84%), and 35 (73%) had missing or disrupted chordae. Of the 57 men, 42 (74%) had ruptured chordae. Of the entire 83 patients, 64 (77%) had missing or disrupted chordae: in 16 (84%) of the 19 patients in whom the anular circumference was ≤11 cm and in 48 (75%) of the 64 in whom the anular circumference was >11 cm.

Of the 64 (77%) patients with missing or disrupted chordae or both, the missing or disrupted

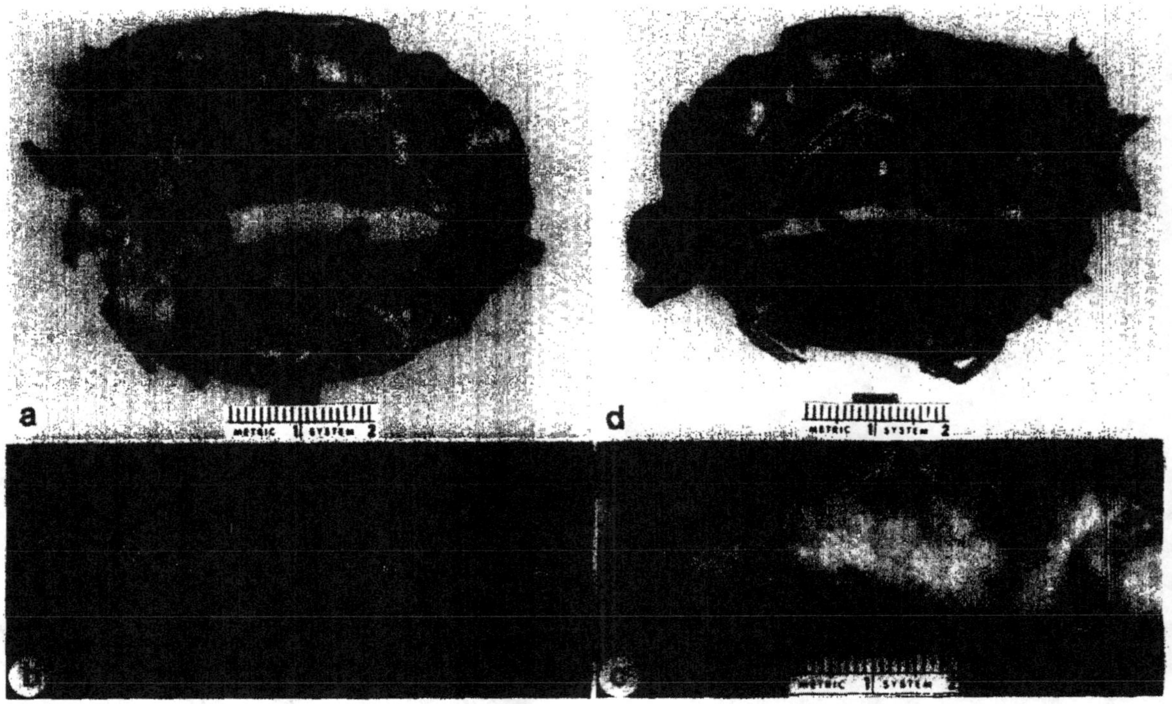

Fig. 5. Operatively excised mitral valve in a 60-year-old man (S77-157). *a-c* Atrial aspect. *d,* Ventricular aspect. Both anterior *(A)* and posterior leaflets are of similar size. Chordae from the posterior leaflet are both missing and disrupted. The disrupted chord is designated by the arrow. *c,* A close-up of the posterior leaflet. (Reproduced with permission from Byram MT and Roberts WC. Frequencies and extent of calcific deposits in purely regurgitant mitral valves: analysis of 108 operatively excised valves. Am J Cardiol 1983;52:1059-61.)

chordae involved the posterior leaflet only in 57 patients (90%), the anterior leaflet only in three patients (5%), and both leaflets in three patients (5%). In all 57 patients in whom only chordae to the posterior leaflet were affected, the chordae were considered missing in each. In the three patients in whom only chordae to the anterior leaflet were affected, the chordae were considered disrupted in one, missing in one, and both disrupted and missing in one. Finally in the three patients in whom chordae from both leaflets were affected, in each some chordae were disrupted and some were missing. No patient with missing chordae had historical evidence of infective endocarditis that had healed, and therefore the chordal rupture in them is considered "spontaneous." Of the eight patients with disrupted chordae with or without missing chordae, five had historical evidence of infective endocarditis that had healed.

DISCUSSION

The above data indicate that there are two major mechanisms for development of severe MR in MVP: (1) dilatation of the mitral anulus with or without rupture of chordae tendineae and (2) rupture of chordae tendineae with or without dilatation of the mitral anulus. Of our 83 patients with MVP, severe MR, and mitral valve replacement, 48 (58%) had both dilated anuli (>11 cm in circumference) and ruptured chordae tendineae; 16 (19%) had dilated anuli without rupture of chordae, and 16 (19%) had ruptured chordae without significant anular dilatation. In three of the 83 patients, the anulus was not dilated, nor were chordae ruptured. Therefore the mechanism of the severe MR in these three patients is unclear. Mitral chordal rupture was nearly as frequent in the 64 patients with clearly dilated mitral anuli (circumference >11 cm) as in the 19 patients with normal or insignificantly dilated anuli (circumference ≤11 cm) (75% [48/64] vs 84% [16/19]).

The reported frequencies of rupture of chordae tendineae in operatively excised prolapsed (floppy) mitral valves have not been as high as in the present study. The explanation almost surely lies in differing definitions of the term "ruptured chordae tendineae." In the present study only nine patients (11%) had easily identifiable, unequivocally disrupted

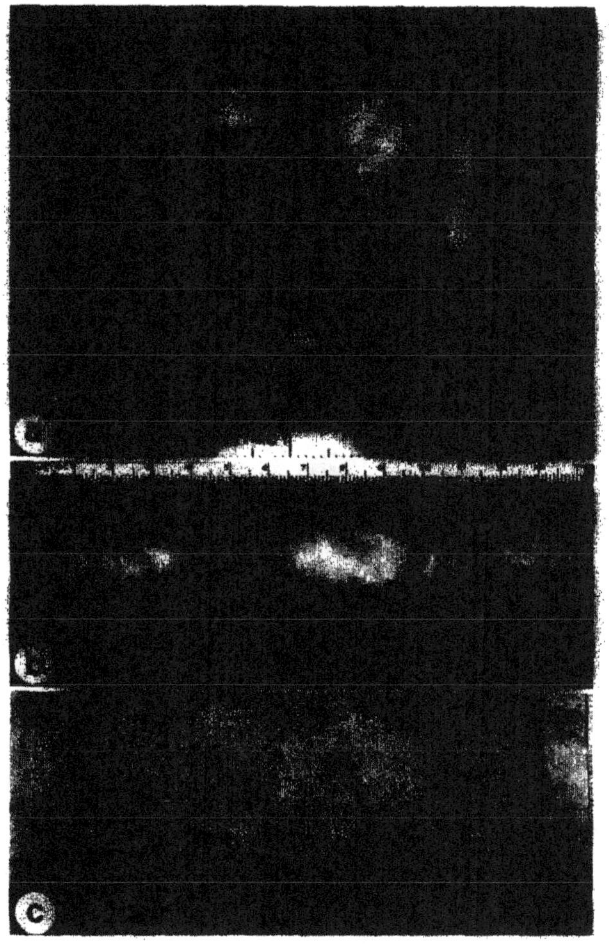

Fig. 6. Operatively excised mitral valve (*a* and *b*) and preoperative echocardiogram *(c)* in a 64-year-old man (S80-64). The anulus is nearly 15 cm in circumference. Chordae from the posterior leaflet are missing *(arrows)*. *c*, Echocardiogram showing prolapse *(arrows)*. A = anterior leaflet; VS = ventricular septum.

Fig. 7. Atrial *(a)* and ventricular *(b)* aspects of the excised mitral valve in a 70-year-old woman (S80-162). The anulus is only about 10 cm in circumference. Many chordae from the posterior leaflet are missing *(arrows)*.

Fig. 8. Intact *(a)* and opened *(b)* operatively excised mitral valve in a 67-year-old man (S80-172). The anulus is enormously dilated (17 cm). Some chordae from the posterior leaflet are missing. A = anterior leaflet.

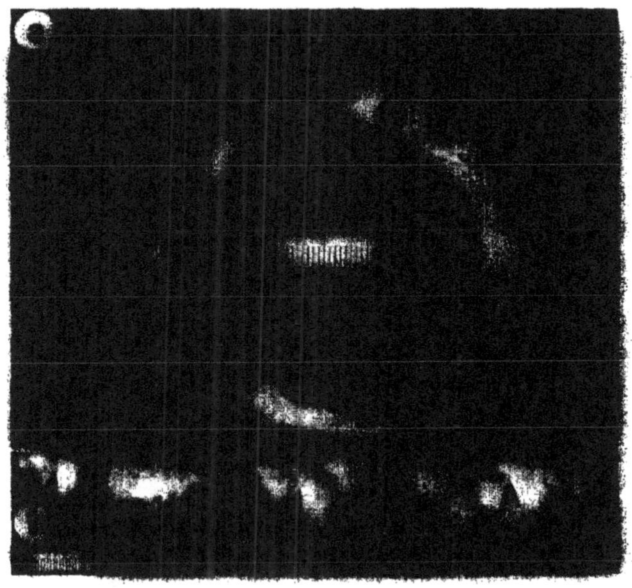

Fig. 9. Intact *(a)* and opened *(b)* operatively excised valve in a 26-year-old man (S82-1) who had the Marfan syndrome. This patient was the youngest in this study. The anulus is enormously dilated (about 18 cm). The chordae appear to be intact. A = anterior leaflet.

chordae. In contrast, 61 (73%) had no identifiable disrupted chordae, but portions of the posterior leaflet were devoid of chordae. These patients were considered to have "missing" chordae, a situation equivalent to disrupted chordae. Of the nine patients with disrupted chordae, seven also had

Fig. 10. Opened mitral valve showing the atrial *(a)* and ventricular *(b)* aspects in a 42-year-old woman (77S-3497). Both anterior *(A)* and posterior leaflets are of similar size. Many chordae from the posterior leaflet are missing. The anulus is about 13 cm in circumference.

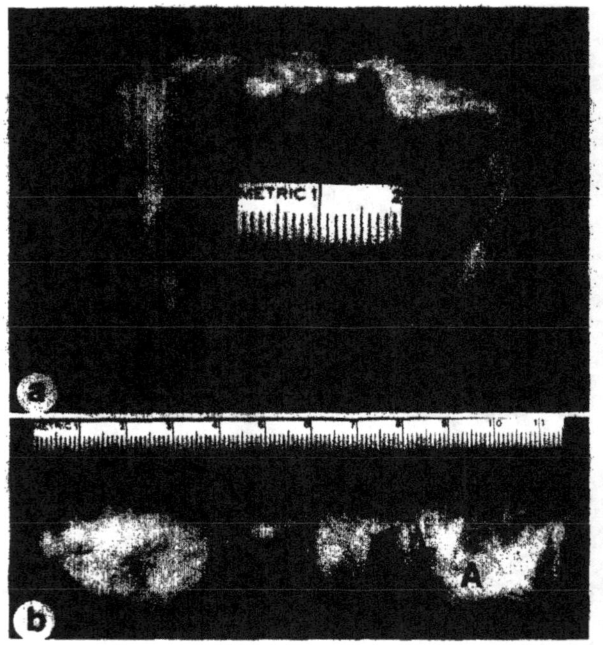

Fig. 11. Intact *(a)* and opened *(b)* mitral valve in a 65-year-old man (80-S-3326). The anulus is about 12 cm in circumference. Most chordae from the posterior leaflet are missing. A = anterior leaflet.

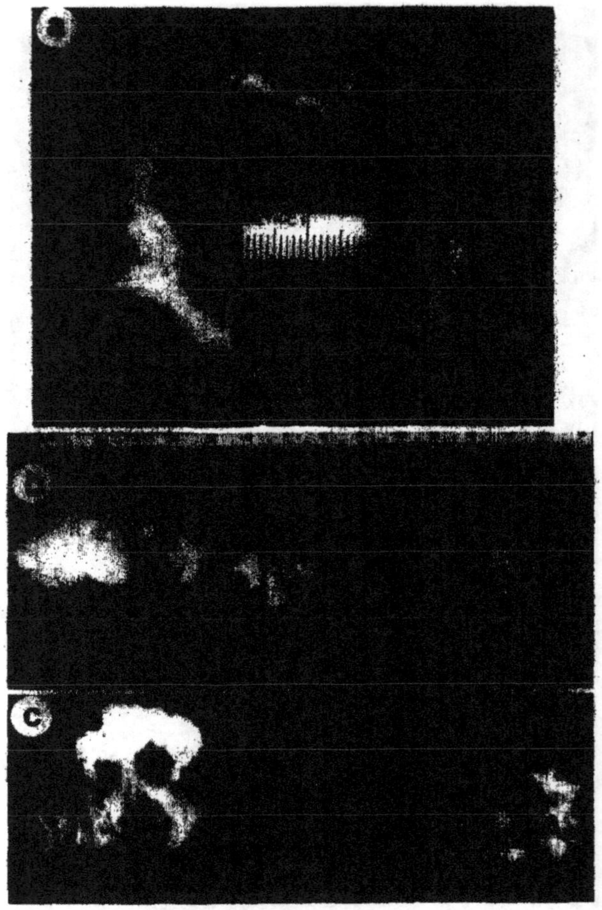

Fig. 12. Intact *(a)* and opened *(b)* mitral valve and a radiograph *(c)* of the valve in a 73-year-old man (81-S-2245). The anulus is about 14 cm in circumference. A large calcific deposit *(arrow)* is located at the anulus (site of attachment) of the largest scallop of the posterior leaflet. Chordae from the posterior leaflet are missing. A = anterior leaflet.

missing chordae. Of the 61 patients with missing chordae, seven also had disrupted chordae. Thus, only two of the 83 patients had disrupted without missing chordae.

The cause of the chordal rupture was not determined in 59 (92%) of the 64 patients, and therefore their chordal rupture is considered "spontaneous." It is now recognized that spontaneous rupture of mitral chordae tendineae is nearly always in the setting of MVP.[3-7] Of the 83 patients studied, at least six had a history of active infective endocarditis that had healed: five had disrupted mitral chordae and one had no disrupted or missing chordae. None of the 54 patients with missing but without disrupted chordae had had a history of active infective endocarditis.

Although MVP appears to be more common in women than in men, severe MR caused by MVP is more common in men. Of our 83 patients with MVR and MR severe enough to warrant mitral replacement, nearly 70% were men. In 23 patients with MVP and MR severe enough to warrant mitral valve replacement and reported by Jeresaty et al.,[3] at least 13 and probably 15 (65%) were men. Of 18 patients

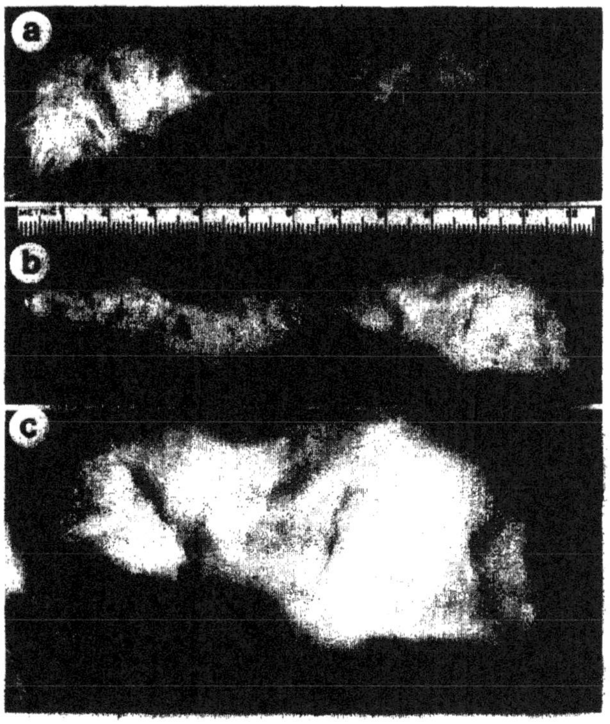

Fig. 13. Opened mitral valve (*a* and *b*) and close-up of portion of posterior leaflet *(c)* in a 58-year-old woman (83-S-3077). *a*, Ventricular aspect. *b*, Atrial aspect. *c*, Atrial aspect. The anulus is about 14 cm in circumference. Many chordae from the posterior leaflet are missing. A = anterior leaflet.

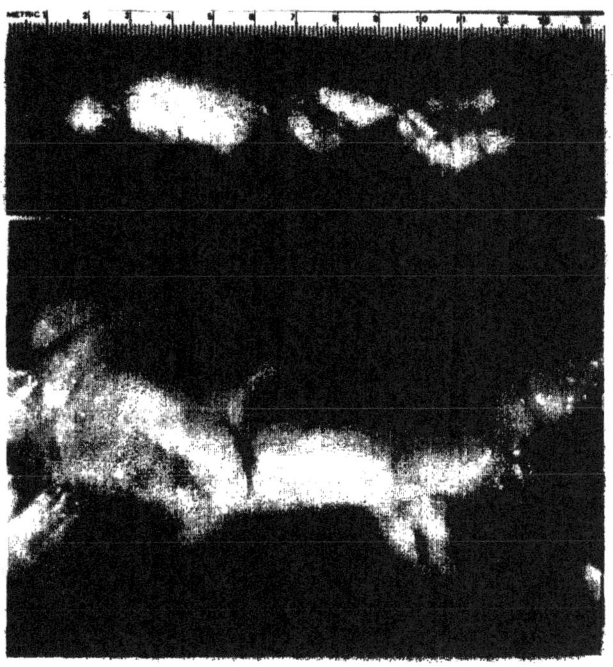

Fig. 14. Opened mitral valve from the atrial aspect in a 64-year-old woman (84-S-325). The anulus is nearly 14 cm in circumference. Many chordae from the posterior leaflet are missing *(arrows)*. A close-up of a portion of posterior leaflet is shown in the lower panel.

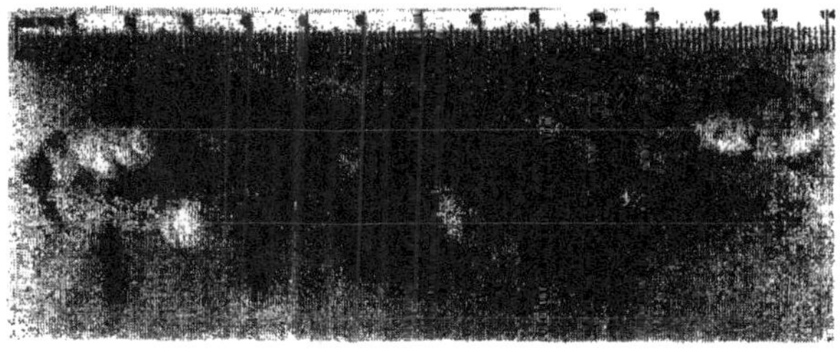

Fig. 15. Opened mitral valve showing its atrial aspects in a 65-year-old woman (84-S-3509). Many chordae from the posterior leaflet are missing *(arrows)*. The anulus is about 14 cm in circumference. A = anterior leaflet.

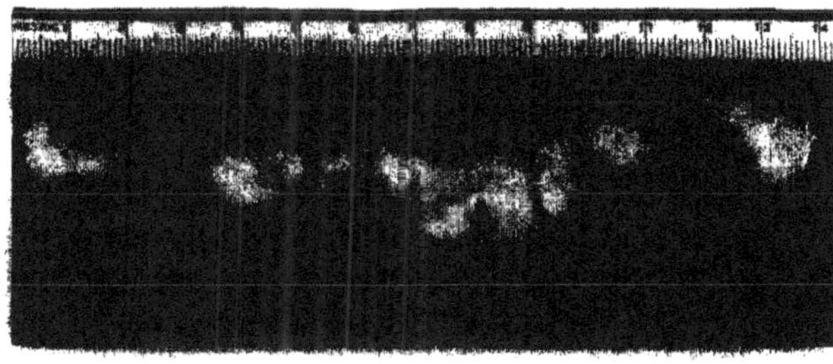

Fig. 16. Opened mitral valve showing its atrial aspect in a 71-year-old woman (84-S-7903). The anulus is about 14 cm in circumference. The chordae appear to be intact. A = anterior leaflet.

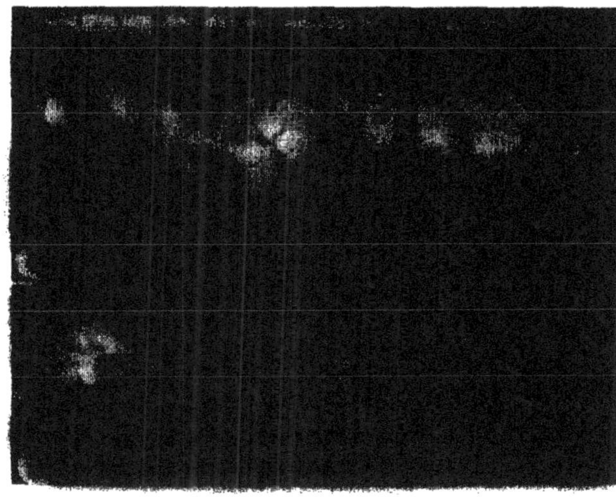

Fig. 17. Opened mitral valve showing its atrial *(a)* and ventricular *(b)* aspects in a 44-year-old man (85-S-971). The anulus is about 15 cm in circumference. Chordae from the posterior leaflet appear to be both missing and others disrupted. A = anterior leaflet.

with MVP and MR severe enough to warrant mitral replacement and reported by Olson et al.,[7] 14 (78%) were men. Of 11 patients ≥60 years of age with MVP and MR severe enough to warrant mitral replacement and reported by Naggar et al.,[8] six (55%) were men.

Finally, opportunities to study systematically

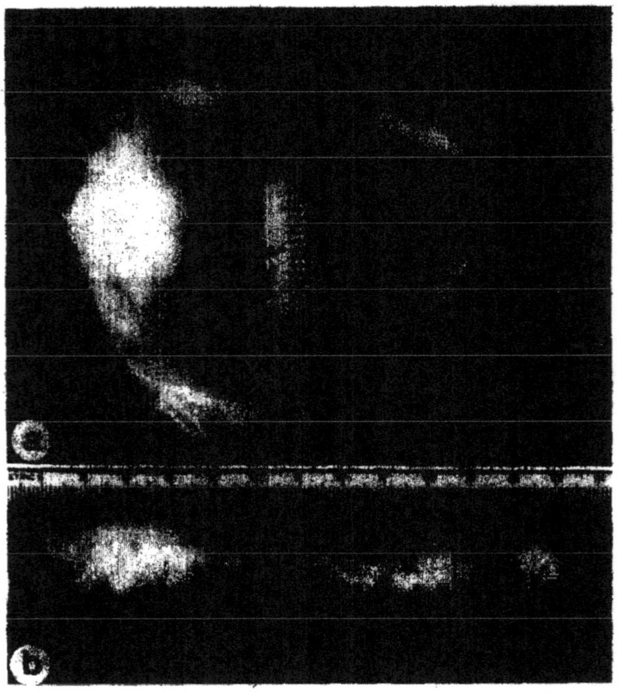

Fig. 18. Unopened *(a)* and opened *(b)* mitral valve in a 66-year-old man (85-S-2575). The anulus is about 14 cm in circumference. Many chordae from the posterior leaflet are missing *(arrows)*. A = anterior leaflet.

operatively excised prolapsed mitral valves in the future will almost surely diminish because of a move away from replacement in favor of repair procedures for patients with severe MR caused by MVP. Thus the data collected in the present study will not likely be collected again in a relatively short period of time.

REFERENCES

1. Waller BF, Morrow AG, Maron BJ, Del Negro AA, Kent KM, McGrath FJ, Wallace RB, McIntosh CL, Roberts WC. Etiology of clinically isolated, severe, chronic, pure mitral regurgitation: Analysis of 97 patients over 30 years of age having mitral valve replacement. AM HEART J 1982;104:276-88.
2. Byram MT, Roberts WC. Frequency and extent of calcific deposits in purely regurgitant mitral valves: analysis of 108 operatively excised valves. Am J Cardiol 1983;52:1059-61.
3. Jeresaty RM, Edwards JE, Chawla SK. Mitral valve prolapse and ruptured chordae tendineae. Am J Cardiol 1985;55:138-42.
4. Hickey AJ, Wicker Del, Wright JS, Warren BA. Primary (spontaneous) chordal rupture: relation to myxomatous valve disease and mitral valve prolapse. J Am Coll Cardiol 1985;5:1341-6.
5. Roberts WC. Mitral valve prolapse and systemic hypertension. Am J Cardiol 1985;56:703.
6. Aronson RJ, Hoffman M, Algueti-Margulis A, Yust I. Spontaneous rupture of mitral chordae tendineae in hypertension. Am J Cardiol (In press, 1987)
7. Olson LJ, Subramanian R, Ackerman DM, Orszulak TA, Edwards WD. Surgical pathology of the mitral valve: a study of 712 cases spanning 21 years. Mayo Clin Proc 1987;62:22-34.
8. Naggar CZ, Pearson WN, Seljan MP. Frequency of complications of mitral valve prolapse in subjects aged 60 years and older. Am J Cardiol 1986;58:1209-12.

Cardiac Valve Replacement for Stenotic Bicuspid Aortic Valve in Husband and for Purely Regurgitant Prolapsed Mitral Valve in Wife

JESSICA M. MANN, MD
CHARLES L. McINTOSH, MD
NEVIN M. KATZ, MD
WILLIAM C. ROBERTS, MD

Congenital heart disease is recognized to occur in families, i.e., in a parent or grandparent and in 1 or more siblings. The occurrence of congenital heart disease in both husband and wife must indeed be rare, and even more so is the occurrence of cardiac valve replacement in both husband and wife. Such was the case, however, in 2 recently studied patients. Each had the most common congenital heart disease that occurs in their sex, namely, mitral valve prolapse in women and bicuspid aortic valve in men.[1]

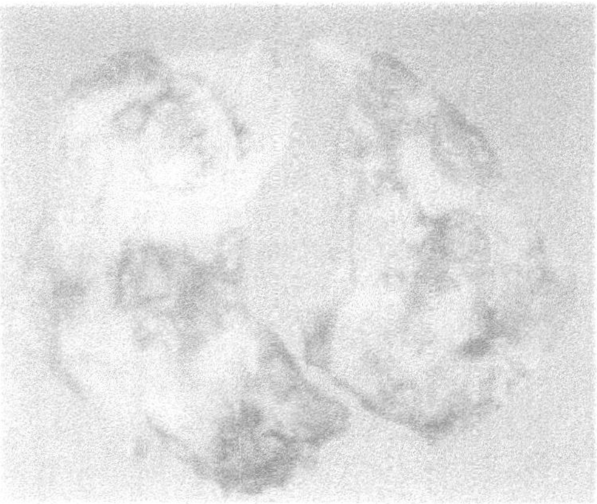

FIGURE 1. View of the operatively excised stenotic bicuspid aortic valve.

From the Pathology and Surgery Branches, National Heart, Lung, Blood Institute, National Institutes of Health, Bethesda, Maryland 20892, and the Department of Surgery, Georgetown University, Washington, D.C. Manuscript received and accepted 18 March 1987.

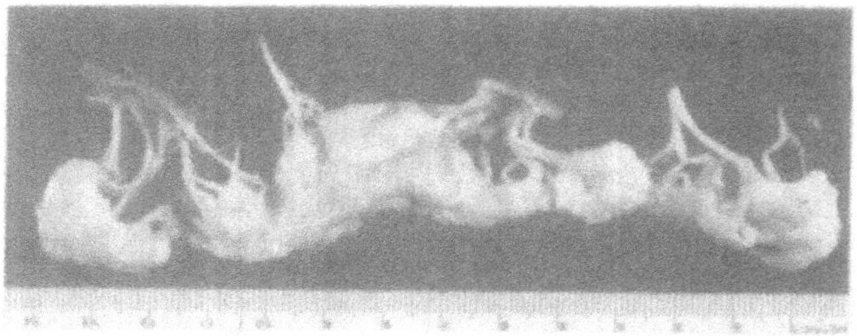

FIGURE 2. View of the operatively excised purely regurgitant and prolapsed mitral valve.

The husband was 63 years old at the time of aortic valve replacement for a congenitally bicuspid stenotic aortic valve (Fig. 1). The wife was 69 years old at the time of mitral valve replacement for mitral regurgitation secondary to a severely prolapsed valve (Fig. 2). The husband's aortic valve was replaced with a Björk-Shiley prosthesis (no. 23). The wife's mitral valve was initially replaced with a porcine aortic valve, which degenerated rapidly because of her oral consumption of calcium supplements.[2] The degenerated porcine bioprosthesis was replaced 18 months after the initial operation by a Medtronic-Hall prosthesis (no. 31). Both husband and wife are on daily warfarin therapy and both are asymptomatic.

The occurrence of cardiac valve replacement in both husband and wife has not been described previously.

1. Roberts WC. *The 2 most common congenital heart diseases. From the editor. Am J Cardiol 1984;53:1198.*
2. Moront M, Katz NM. *Early degeneration of a porcine aortic valve bioprosthesis in the mitral valve position in an elderly woman and its association with long-term calcium carbonate therapy. Am J Cardiol 1987;59:1006–1007.*

Morphologic Comparison of Patients With Mitral Valve Prolapse Who Died Suddenly With Patients Who Died From Severe Valvular Dysfunction or Other Conditions

ALLEN L. DOLLAR, MD,* WILLIAM C. ROBERTS, MD, FACC

Bethesda, Maryland

Clinical and necropsy findings are described in 56 patients with mitral valve prolapse: 15 patients, aged 16 to 69 years (mean 39), died suddenly and mitral valve prolapse was the only cardiac condition found at necropsy (hereafter called isolated mitral valve prolapse); the remaining 41 patients had other conditions that were capable of being fatal. Of the latter 41 patients, 7, aged 17 to 59 years (mean 45), had associated congenital heart disease, and 34 patients, aged 17 to 70 years (mean 52), had no associated congenital cardiac abnormalities.

Compared with the 34 patients without associated congenital heart disease and with nonmitral valve prolapse conditions capable in themselves of being fatal, the 15 patients who died suddenly with isolated mitral valve prolapse were younger (mean age 39 ± 17 versus 52 ± 15 years; p = 0.01), more often women (67% versus 26%; p = 0.008) and had a lower frequency of mitral regurgitation (7% versus 38%; p = 0.02). The 15 patients dying suddenly with isolated mitral valve prolapse also were less likely to have evidence of ruptured chordae tendineae (29% versus 67%; p = 0.04).

The frequency of increased heart weight (67% versus 59%), a dilated mitral valve anulus (80% versus 81%), a dilated tricuspid valve anulus (17% versus 17%), an elongated anterior mitral leaflet (86% versus 54%), an elongated posterior mitral leaflet (79% versus 77%) and fibrous endocardial plaque under the posterior mitral leaflet (73% versus 63%) was similar between the two groups. The severity of the prolapse (mild 20% versus 11%; moderate 27% versus 58%; severe 53% versus 32%) also was similar between the two groups.

Thus, persons with mitral valve prolapse dying suddenly without another recognized condition tend to be relatively young women without mitral regurgitation.

(J Am Coll Cardiol 1991;17:921–31)

Mitral valve prolapse is a common condition affecting an estimated 5% of the U.S. population (1). A rare but much-feared occurrence in persons with mitral valve prolapse is sudden death. Although only a small number of patients with mitral valve prolapse die suddenly (without other potentially fatal conditions), mitral valve prolapse accounts for a substantial proportion of sudden deaths in persons without other clear causes of death. One study (2) of 50 persons, aged 7 to 35 years, dying suddenly and unexpectedly found mitral valve prolapse to be present in 12 (24%). Several necropsy studies (3–23) have reported on individuals or small groups of patients with sudden death associated with mitral valve prolapse.

No study has compared morphologic findings in patients with mitral valve prolapse unassociated with another potentially fatal condition (hereafter called isolated mitral valve prolapse) with those patients with mitral valve prolapse associated with another potentially fatal condition. Such a comparison is the purpose of this study.

From the Pathology Branch, National Heart, Lung, and Blood Institute, National Institutes of Health, Bethesda, Maryland.

*Present address: Division of Cardiology, Department of Medicine, The Washington Hospital Center, Washington, DC.

Manuscript received August 7, 1990; revised manuscript received October , 1990, accepted October 14, 1990.

Address for reprints: William C. Roberts, MD, Pathology Branch, Building 10, Room 2N258, National Institutes of Health, Bethesda, Maryland 0892.

Methods

Inclusion criteria. For a patient to be included in this study, three criteria had to be met: 1) the patient's heart was examined by the Pathology Branch, National Heart, Lung, and Blood Institute, and was classified by us as "mitral valve prolapse"; 2) at death, the patient was 16 to 70 years of age; and 3) the patient's heart (or photographs if the heart was unavailable) possessed morphologic features for the diagnosis of mitral valve prolapse used in this study (to be discussed subsequently). In cases where mitral valve replacement had been performed, the operatively excised mitral valve or photographs of it had to be available to reconfirm the diagnosis of mitral valve prolapse.

Sources of cases. From January 1956 to February 1990, the hearts of 101 patients were classified as "mitral valve prolapse" by the Pathology Branch, National Heart, Lung, and Blood Institute. Of these 101 heart specimens, 81 were available for reexamination by both authors and photographs of the hearts were available in the other 20 cases. Of the 101 cases, review of medical necropsy records disclosed that 21 patients were >70 years of age and that 2 were <16 years of

Table 1. Clinical and Morphologic Features of Mitral Valve Prolapse at Necropsy Unassociated With Other Congenital Cardiovascular Anomalies (49 patients aged 16 to 70 years)

Patient Category	+SCD −MR −CAD	+SCD +MR −CAD	+SCD −MR +CAD	−SCD +MR −CAD	−SCD −MR −CAD	Total (%)
No. of patients	14	3	3	10	19	49
Mean age (yr)	38 ± 17	50 ± 17	65 ± 3	55 ± 13	49 ± 17	48 ± 17
Women/men	10/4	0/3	0/3	3/7	6/13	19/30
Heart weight (g)	379 ± 96	770 ± 105	462 ± 103	577 ± 180	397 ± 131	458 ± 167
MV anulus >10 cm	11/14	1/1	2/3	8/8	6/10	29/36 (81)
TV anulus >14 cm	1/13	1/2	0/3	2/9	1/10	5/37 (14)
AML length >2.0 cm	11/13	1/1	2/3	2/4	3/6	19/27 (70)
PML length >1.5 cm	10/13	1/1	3/3	4/4	3/6	21/27 (78)
Absent chordae	4/12	0/1	2/2	6/8	2/6	14/29 (48)
LV cavity dilated (grade 3/4 or 4/4)	0/14	1/3	0/3	3/9	1/19	5/48 (10)
CA narrowed >75% in CSA	0/14	0/3	3/3	3/9	1/15	7/44 (16)
LV necrosis	0/14	0/3	1/3	0/10	0/18	1/48 (2)
LV fibrosis	0/14	1/3	1/3	2/10	1/18	5/48 (10)
Grade of MVP						
Mild	3/14	0/1	0/3	0/5	2/11	5/34 (15)
Moderate	4/14	0/1	2/3	2/5	7/11	15/34 (44)
Severe	7/14	1/1	1/3	3/5	2/11	14/34 (41)
Endocardial fibrous plaque under PML	10/14	1/1	1/3	6/7	5/9	23/34 (68)
Mitral annular calcium						
Grade 1–2/4	3/14	0/2	1/3	1/7	2/17	7/43 (16)
Grade 3–4/4	1/14	0/2	0/3	2/7	2/17	5/43 (12)
Valvular competent PFO	3/11	1/3	1/3	1/5	1/8	7/31 (23)
Redundant FO membrane	3/11	0/3	1/3	2/5	0/7	6/30 (20)
SCD due to MVP	14/14	1/3	0/3	0/10	0/19	15/49 (31)
The Marfan syndrome	2/14	0/3	0/3	2/10	4/19	8/49 (16)
Mitral valve replacement	0/14	2/3	0/3	1/10	0/19	3/49 (6)

AML = anterior mitral leaflet; CA = coronary artery; CAD = fatal coronary artery disease; CSA = cross-sectional area; FO = fossa ovale; LV = lef ventricular; MR = severe mitral regurgitation; MV = mitral valve; MVP = mitral valve prolapse; PFO = patent foramen ovale; PML = posterior mitral leaflet SCD = sudden cardiac death; TV = tricuspid valve; − = absent; + = present.

age and, therefore, these 23 cases were excluded. The children were excluded because morphologic comparisons with measurements in adults, such as heart weight, leaflet length and anular circumference, would be meaningless. Persons >70 years of age were excluded because some age-related changes in the mitral leaflets of elderly persons are similar to features of mitral valve prolapse, including leaflet thickening, especially in the portions adjacent to the posteromedial commissure, and the thickened portions often protrude toward the left atrium. Although several hearts in the elderly patients clearly had unequivocal features of mitral valve prolapse, many did not. To avoid including patients who did not have mitral valve prolapse, the older patients were excluded.

On reexamination of the remaining 78 patients, 22 were determined not to have morphologic features (to be discussed subsequently) of mitral valve prolapse. After these exclusions, 56 patients, aged 16 to 70 years (mean 48), remained and all had unequivocal morphologic features of mitral valve prolapse.

Definitions. *Sudden cardiac death* was defined as death occurring within 6 h of the onset of symptoms of cardiac dysfunction or myocardial ischemia. *Sudden death* associated with mitral valve prolapse (isolated mitral valve pro lapse) was defined as sudden cardiac death where mitra valve prolapse was present and no other cardiac or noncar diac condition was present at autopsy to explain death Sudden death associated with *coronary artery disease* wa defined as sudden cardiac death with >75% cross-sectiona area luminal narrowing of one or more of the four majo epicardial coronary arteries. If both mitral valve prolaps and significant coronary arterial narrowing was present death was attributed to coronary artery disease.

Significant mitral regurgitation was defined as the pres ence of at least "moderate" or grade 3/4 or 4/4 mitra regurgitation by left ventricular angiography or Dopple echocardiography. If no objective assessment of mitral re gurgitation was made during life, significant mitral regurg tation was presumed to have been present if the left atriu and ventricle were significantly (grade >2/4) dilated in th absence of another cause of chamber enlargement.

Morphologic criteria of mitral valve prolapse. Morpho logic criteria used for the diagnosis of mitral valve prolaps were: 1) elongation of a portion of the posterior mitral leafl such that the distance from distal margin to its attachment

Table 2. Clinical and Morphologic Features in 15 Patients Dying Suddenly Secondary to Mitral Valve Prolapse

Pt No.	Age (yr)	Race	Gender	MVP Diagnosed Clinically	The Marfan Syndrome	Location of Death	Last Activity	Auscultatory Findings SC	Auscultatory Findings SM	SH	CHF	VPCs on ECG	HW (g)	MV Anulus (cm)	TV Anulus (cm)	AML Length (cm)	PML Length (cm)	Chords Missing	Grade of MVP (1–3+)	Plaque Under PML	MAC (0–4+)	VC PFO	Redundant FO Membrane
1	16	W	M	+	+	Basketball court	Sitting after playing	–	+	0	0	+	325	12.5	12	3	2.5	+	2	0	0	–	–
2	18	W	F	+	0	Home	Arguing	–	0	0	0	+*	220	9.6	11.5	2	1.5	0	1	+	0	0	0
3	21	W	F	+	0	Work	Talking on phone	–	–	0	0	–	360	14	—	3	1.5	+	2	0	1	–	–
4	23	W	F	+	0	Work	Drinking water	+	+	0	0	–	280	10	9	2.5	2	0	3	+	0	+	+
5	26	W	F	+	0	Work	Talking	+	+	0	0	0†	265	12	11	3	3	0	3	+	0	+	+
6	30	B	M	0	0	Work	Sitting alone	–	–	–	0	–	570	15.5	13	3	2.5	0	3	+	0	0	0
7	30	W	M	0	0	Golf course	Playing golf	–	–	0	0	–	475	10	11	3	2	0	1	+	0	0	0
8	40	W	F	0	+	Home	Playing with children	–	–	0	0	–	355	13	12	–	–	+	2	0	2	–	+
9	47	W	F	0	0	Home	Gardening	–	–	0	0	+	445	12.5	12.5	2.5	2	0	3	+	0	0	0
10	51	W	M	+	0	Restaurant	Sitting after fast dancing	+	+	0	0	0	500	10.5	12	2	1.5	0	1	0	0	0	0
11	53	W	F	+	0	Church	Sitting	–	–	0	0	+	325	12.6	10.5	2.5	3	0	2	+	3	0	0
12	53	W	F	0	0	Restaurant	Getting up to dance	–	–	–	0	–	390	13.6	11	3.5	3	0	3	+	1	+	+
13	55	W	F	+	0	Home	Standing	+	+	0	0	+	390	13	13	3	2.5	+	3	+	0	0	0
14	55	W	M	+	0	Home	Sleeping	–	+	0	+	+	670	>12	14	3.5	2	0	3	+	0	+	0
15	69	W	F	0	0	Home	—	–	–	–	0	–	400	15.4	14.5	2.5	3	+	3	+	0	0	0

*This patient had survived a cardiac arrest 2 years earlier; †this patient had a history of paroxysmal atrial tachycardia. AML = anterior mitral leaflet; B = black; CHF = congestive heart failure; F = female; FO = fossa ovale; HW = heart weight; M = male; MVP = mitral valve prolapse; MAC = mitral annular calcification; PFO = patent foramen ovale; PML = posterior mitral leaflet; Pt = patient; SC = systolic click; SH = systemic hypertension: SM = systolic murmur; TV = tricuspid valve; VC = valvular competent; VPC = ventricular premature complex; W = white; + = present; 0 = absent; – = no information available.

the mitral anulus was >1.5 cm; or 2) presence of mitral leaflet protrusion toward the left atrium, usually also associated with missing chordae tendineae, and the prolapsed portion of the leaflet involving >50% of the anterior leaflet and >33% of the posterior leaflet. Others (9,23) have referred to this leaflet prolapse as "interchordal hooding."

Morphologic measurements. All morphologic measurements and observations were performed by one or both authors. The length of the mitral leaflets was measured from the line of attachment of the leaflet to its free margin at the longest portion of each leaflet. Chordae tendineae were considered "missing" if none extended caudally from the ventricular surface of a portion of either or both leaflets or if detached chordae that had rounded or blunted distal ends were present. ("Missing" chordae were considered to represent sites of previously ruptured chordae [24]). The severity of mitral valve prolapse was subjectively graded as mild, moderate or severe.

Determination of normal measurement values. Normal values for various morphologic measurements were determined

Figure 1. Patient 1. The heart of a 16 year old boy (Suffolk County Medical Examiner #84-4276, Hauppauge, NY) who had skeletal features of Marfan syndrome (examination of his aorta did not reveal "cystic medial necrosis"). He had a systolic murmur and mitral valve prolapse was diagnosed by echocardiography. His rest electrocardiogram showed occasional uniform premature ventricular complexes that disappeared with exercise. He died suddenly in a locker room after playing basketball. **Top,** View of the opened mitral valve, showing mild changes of mitral valve prolapse in the anterior leaflet (A) and more severe changes in the posterior leaflet. **Bottom,** Close-up view of the posterior leaflet.

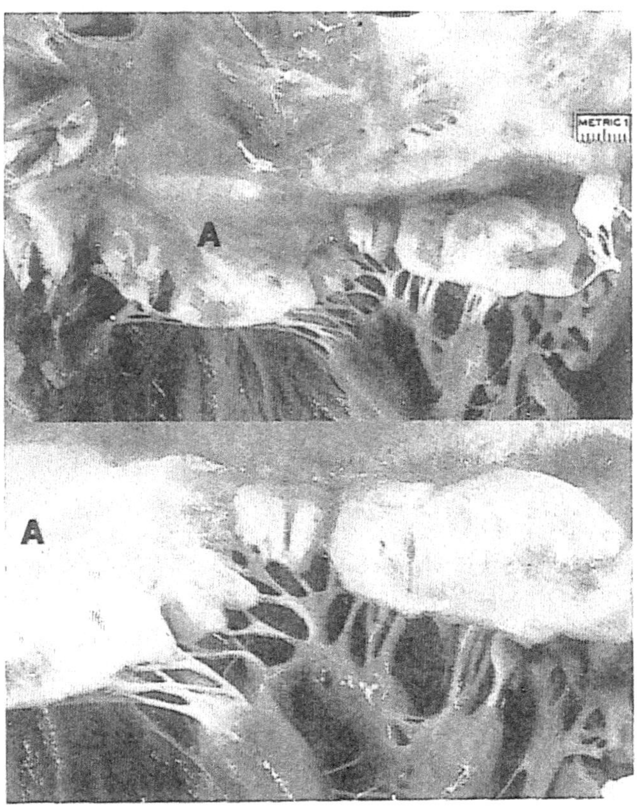

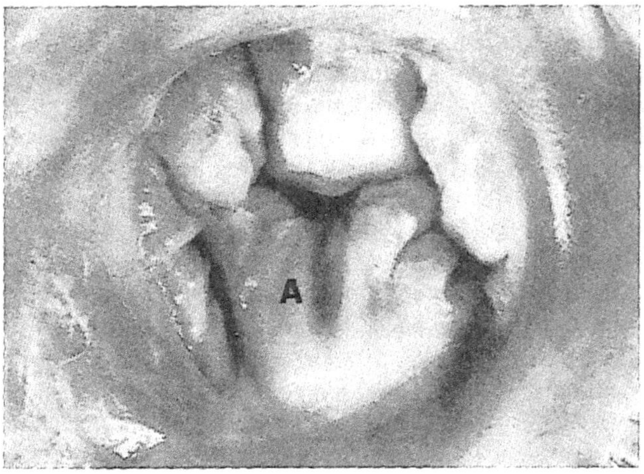

Figure 2. Patient 2. View of the intact mitral valve from the l atrium, showing a normal-appearing anterior leaflet (A) and prolap of the posterior leaflets from the heart of an 18 year old woman (Rockford Memorial Hospital #A85-6, Rockford, IL) who was the daughter of a physician. Twenty-seven months before death, she had a cardiac arrest from which she was resuscitated. Evaluation included electrocardiography, coronary angiography, echocardiography, exercise stress testing, electrophysiologic studies and right ventricular endomyocardial biopsy. These examinations revealed mitral valve prolapse, a slightly prolonged QTc interval (0.46 s) and ventricular premature complexes that became more frequent and complex (couplets and triplets) during the recovery phase after exercise. She did not have mitral regurgitation. She was taking propranolol and mexiletine at the time of death, which occurred during an emotional argument.

by measurements in 20 normal hearts from persons aged 15 to 70 years (mean 47). The 95% confidence intervals derived from these measurements of normal hearts were: mitral anular circumference 7.8 to 8.5 cm, tricuspid valve anulus 8.4 to 11.4 cm, anterior mitral leaflet length 1.5 to 1.8 cm and posterior mitral leaflet length 1.1 to 1.3 cm. The following upper limits therefore were used: mitral anular circumference 10 cm; tricuspid valve anular circumference 14 cm; anterior mitral leaflet length 2 cm and posterior mitral length 1.5 cm.

Histologic studies. One or more of the following histologic sections (stained by hematoxylin and eosin or Movat stain) were prepared from each heart: 1) at least two sections of left ventricular myocardium extending from endocardium to epicardium; and 2) a transverse section of the ascending aorta about 1 cm cephalad to the sinotubular junction.

Results

Subgroupings of the patients with mitral valve prolapse without congenital heart disease. Table 1 summarizes clinical and morphologic findings in the 49 patients without congenital heart disease. The 49 patients were divided into five subgroups on the basis of the presence or absence of sudden cardiac death (SCD) (from any cause), regurgitation (MR) (as determined by objective studies during the patient's life

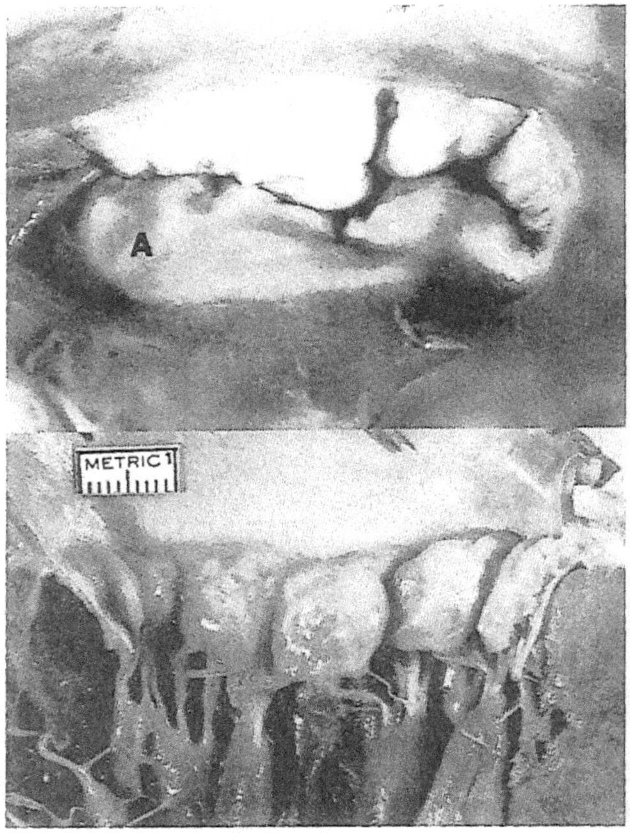

Figure 3. Patient 4. The heart of a 21 year old woman (York Hospital #81AX-132, York, PA) who had the diagnosis of mitral valve prolapse at age 16 years. One year before death, while pregnant, she complained of palpitation and substernal pressure. She died suddenly at a water fountain. **Top,** View of the intact mitra valve from the left atrium, showing prolapse of several scallops o the posterior leaflet, but the valve does not appear regurgitant. **Bottom,** View of the posterior leaflet of the opened mitral valve showing extensive "hooding" and elongation of the leaflet. A = anterior leaflet.

and morphologic evidence of significant mitral regurgitation and fatal coronary artery disease (CAD). Fourteen of the 1 patients who had sudden death associated with mitral valv prolapse (isolated mitral valve prolapse) comprise the cate gory *+SCD, −MR, −CAD,* and the 1 patient with sudde death due to mitral valve prolapse but who had mitr regurgitation is in the category *+SCD, +MR, −CAD.* N patient had a history or morphologic evidence of infectiv endocarditis.

Characteristics of the 15 patients dying suddenly fro mitral valve prolapse. Of the total group of 56 patients, 2 died suddenly from a cardiac cause: 4 had significant coro nary artery disease (>75% cross-sectional area narrowing o at least one major epicardial coronary artery), 2 had ha mitral valve replacement, 1 had cyanotic congenital hea disease and 15 (Table 2) had no explanation for death oth than mitral valve prolapse. The age of the latter 15 patien ranged from 16 to 69 years (mean 39); 10 (67%) were wome

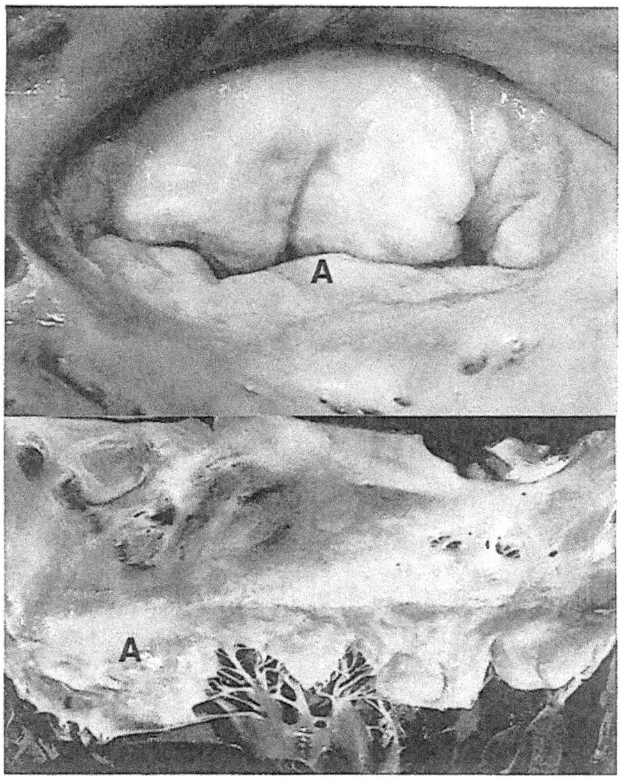

Figure 4. Patient 5. The heart of a 26 year old woman (District of Columbia Medical Examiner's Office #87-07-681) who was a lawyer. She had palpitation associated with paroxysmal atrial tachycardia beginning at age 9 years and had mitral valve prolapse diagnosed by echocardiography at age 15 years. She was started on propranolol therapy at 15 years of age and changed to atenolol 2 years before death. She had an episode of atrial tachycardia about once each 3 months, and it resolved promptly with the Valsalva maneuver. While talking with two colleagues, she collapsed suddenly and died. **Top**, View of the intact mitral valve from the left atrium, showing pronounced prolapse of the posterior leaflet. **Bottom**, View of the opened mitral valve, showing pronounced "hooding" of the posterior leaflet. The anterior leaflet (A) is relatively uninvolved.

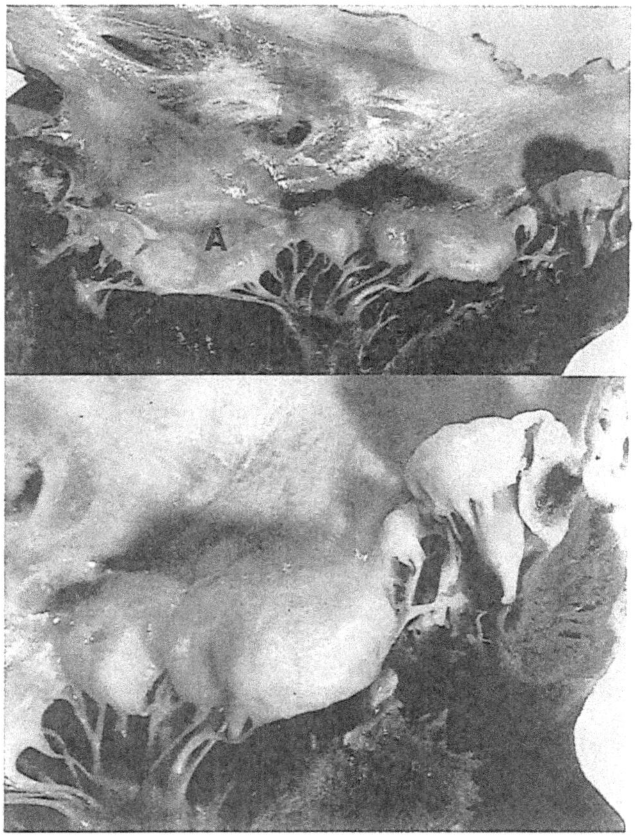

Figure 5. Patient 8. The heart of a 40 year old woman (Suffolk County Medical Examiner #84-4578, Hauppauge, NY) who had Marfan syndrome. She had a history of "valve problems," but no echocardiography was ever done. She was asymptomatic and on no medication. She collapsed suddenly and died while playing with neighborhood children. **Top**, View of the opened mitral valve, showing a mildly abnormal anterior leaflet (A) and a very abnormal posterior leaflet. **Bottom**, Close-up view of a portion of the posterior leaflet, showing a scallop of this leaflet, which is severely prolapsed toward the left atrium. This heart weighed 355 g and no chamber was dilated.

Diagnosis of mitral valve prolapse was made during life in eight (53%); Marfan syndrome was diagnosed in two (13%). Of seven patients whose electrocardiographic (ECG) data were available, six had ventricular premature complexes on their rest ECG, including one patient who had nonfatal cardiac arrest 2 years before death. Four patients were known to be on medication at the time of death: one woman who had nonfatal cardiac arrest was taking propranolol and mexiletine; one woman with paroxysmal atrial tachycardia was taking atenolol; one woman with frequent ventricular premature complexes was taking nadolol and one woman was taking thyroxine. Four patients died suddenly during or shortly after physical exertion and one patient died after an emotional argument.

Certain cardiac morphologic findings in some of the 15 patients who died suddenly from mitral valve prolapse are illustrated in Figures 1 to 7. In the 15 patients, the heart weight ranged from 220 to 670 g (mean 398); in the 5 men, four hearts weighed >400 g; in the 10 women, six hearts weighed >350 g. The mitral valve anulus was dilated (>10 cm in circumference) in 12 of the 15 patients (mean anular circumference 12.4 ± 1.9 cm). The anterior mitral leaflet was elongated (>2 cm from margin of attachment to free margin) in 12 of 14 patients, and the posterior leaflet was elongated (>1.5 cm) in 11 of 14 patients. In none of the 15 hearts was any major epicardial coronary artery narrowed >25% in cross-sectional area and none had gross or microscopic foci of myocardial necrosis or fibrosis. By visual inspection, the cardiac chambers were of normal size in eight patients, only mildly dilated in six and moderately dilated in one. Fibrous thickening of the mural endocardium (endocardial plaque) behind the posterior mitral leaflet was present in 11 of the 15 patients. The presence or absence of mitral

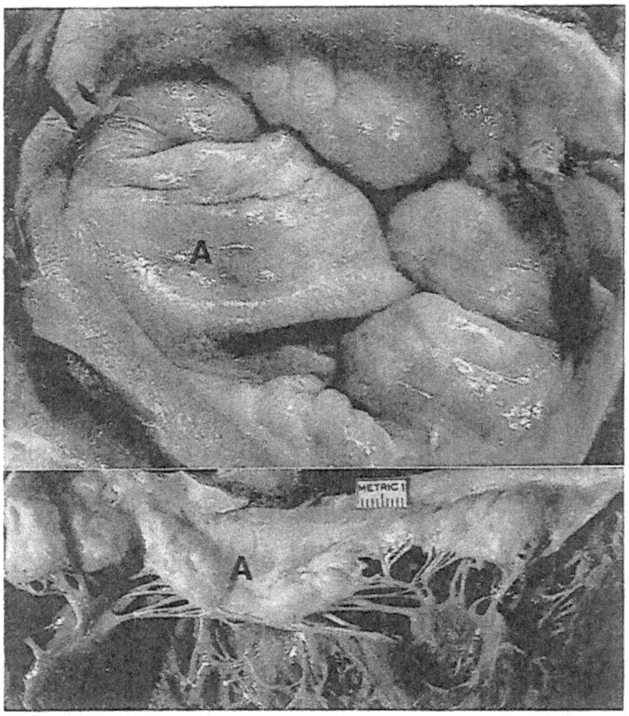

Figure 6. Patient 9. The heart of a 47 year old woman (District of Columbia Medical Examiner's Office #80-06-485) who was a psychiatrist. She had been dieting for 2 weeks before death and was taking thyroid supplements to aid in her weight loss. She was found dead in her yard, dressed in jogging clothes. Her only known cardiac problem was ventricular premature complexes noted by her physician husband. **Top,** View of the intact mitral valve from the left atrium, showing both the anterior (A) and posterior leaflets to be redundant. **Bottom,** The opened mitral valve, showing the posterior leaflet to be elongated.

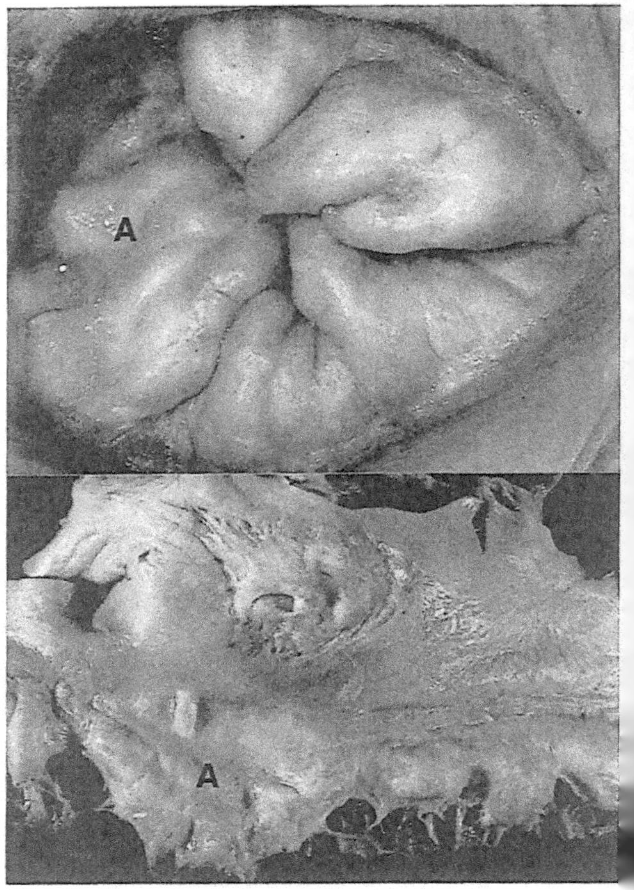

Figure 7. Patient 12. The heart of a 53 year old woman (District of Columbia Medical Examiner's Office #88-09-961) who was the wife of a plastic surgeon. She was out with her husband, got up to dance and suddenly collapsed and died. **Top,** View of the intact mitral valve from the left atrium, showing prolapse of the posterior leaflet above the anterior leaflet (A). **Bottom,** The opened mitral valve, showing a very large anterior leaflet (A) and an elongated redundant posterior leaflet.

regurgitation was documented during life by objective testing in three patients: echocardiography showed trace mitral regurgitation in one patient; left ventricular angiography showed no regurgitation in one patient and moderate regurgitation in another. The latter patient's heart weighed 670 g and all four cardiac chambers were moderately dilated.

Comparison of patients dying suddenly with isolated mitral valve prolapse with other patients with mitral valve prolapse without congenital heart disease. Comparison of the 15 patients in whom sudden death was associated with isolated mitral valve prolapse (14 patients from the group *+SCD, −MR, −CAD* and 1 patient with mitral regurgitation from the group *+SCD, +MR, −CAD*) with the other patients with mitral valve prolapse without associated congenital heart disease (Table 1) disclosed the following differences: 1) a lower mean age at death (39 ± 17 versus 52 ± 15 years; p = 0.01); 2) a preponderance of women (10 [67%] of 15 versus 9 [26%] of 34; p = 0.008); 3) a lower frequency of mitral regurgitation (1 [7%] of 15 versus 13 [38%] of 34; p = 0.02); and 4) a lower frequency of having evidence of ruptured chordae tendineae (4 [29%] of 14 versus 10 [67%] of 15; p = 0.04). No significant differences were noted between the patients dying suddenly with mitral valve prolapse and the other patients with mitral valve prolapse with regard to hear weight, circumference of the mitral or tricuspid anulus length of the anterior or posterior mitral leaflet, presence o missing chordae tendineae, grade of mitral valve prolapse presence of endocardial fibrous plaque under the posterio mitral leaflet or presence of a patent foramen ovale o redundant fossa ovale membrane. Cardiac morphologic findings in two patients from the group *−SCD, +MR, −CAD* ar illustrated in Figures 8 and 9 and two patients from the grou *−SCD, −MR, −CAD* are illustrated in Figures 10 and 11.

Mitral valve prolapse associated with congenital hear disease. Congenital heart disease was present in 7 of the 5 patients (Table 3). These congenital abnormalities include *ostium secundum atrial septal defect* (four patients), *bicus pid aortic valve* (three patients), *coarctation of the aort* (one patient), *Ebstein's anomaly* (one patient), *partial atrio*

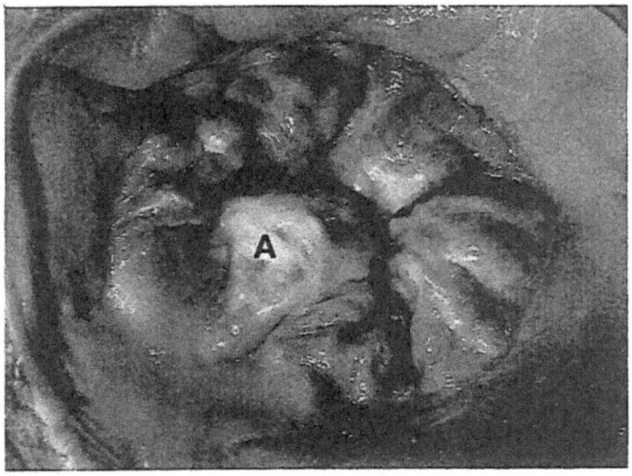

Figure 8. Patient from $-SCD$, $+MR$, $-CAD$ group. The heart of a 65 year old woman (Georgetown University Hospital #81A-122, Washington, DC) who had chronic congestive heart failure and severe mitral regurgitation. She died in cardiogenic shock. View of the intact mitral valve from the left atrium, showing prolapse of both the anterior (A) and posterior mitral leaflets. CAD = fatal coronary artery disease; MR = mitral regurgitation; SCD = sudden cardiac death; – = absent; + = present.

ventricular canal (one patient) and *sinus of Valsalva aneurysm* (one patient). The patient with total anomalous pulmonary venous connection and one patient with a severely stenotic bicuspid aortic valve died suddenly.

Mitral valve prolapse associated with the Marfan syndrome. Eight patients had the Marfan syndrome, two of whom died suddenly without a clear cause. Three had rupture of the ascending aorta, one had congestive heart failure with severe aortic and mitral regurgitation and two died of noncardiac causes. Histologic sections of ascending aorta were available in six of the eight patients: four had

Figure 9. Patient from $-SCD$, $+MR$, $-CAD$ group. The heart of a 54 year old man (District of Columbia Veterans Administration Hospital #83A-84, Washington, DC) with grade 3/4 chronic atrial fibrillation and mitral regurgitation by ventriculography. He died of a cerebral embolic event. **a**, View of the intact mitral valve from the left atrium, showing a patulous mitral valve with a very dilated anulus (15 cm). **b**, Close-up view of the posterior leaflet of the opened mitral valve, showing pronounced hooding of each of the scallops of the leaflet. **c**, The opened mitral valve. **d**, Transverse slices of the ventricles, showing a surprising lack of left ventricular dilation given the degree of mitral regurgitation present. Abbreviations as in Figure 8.

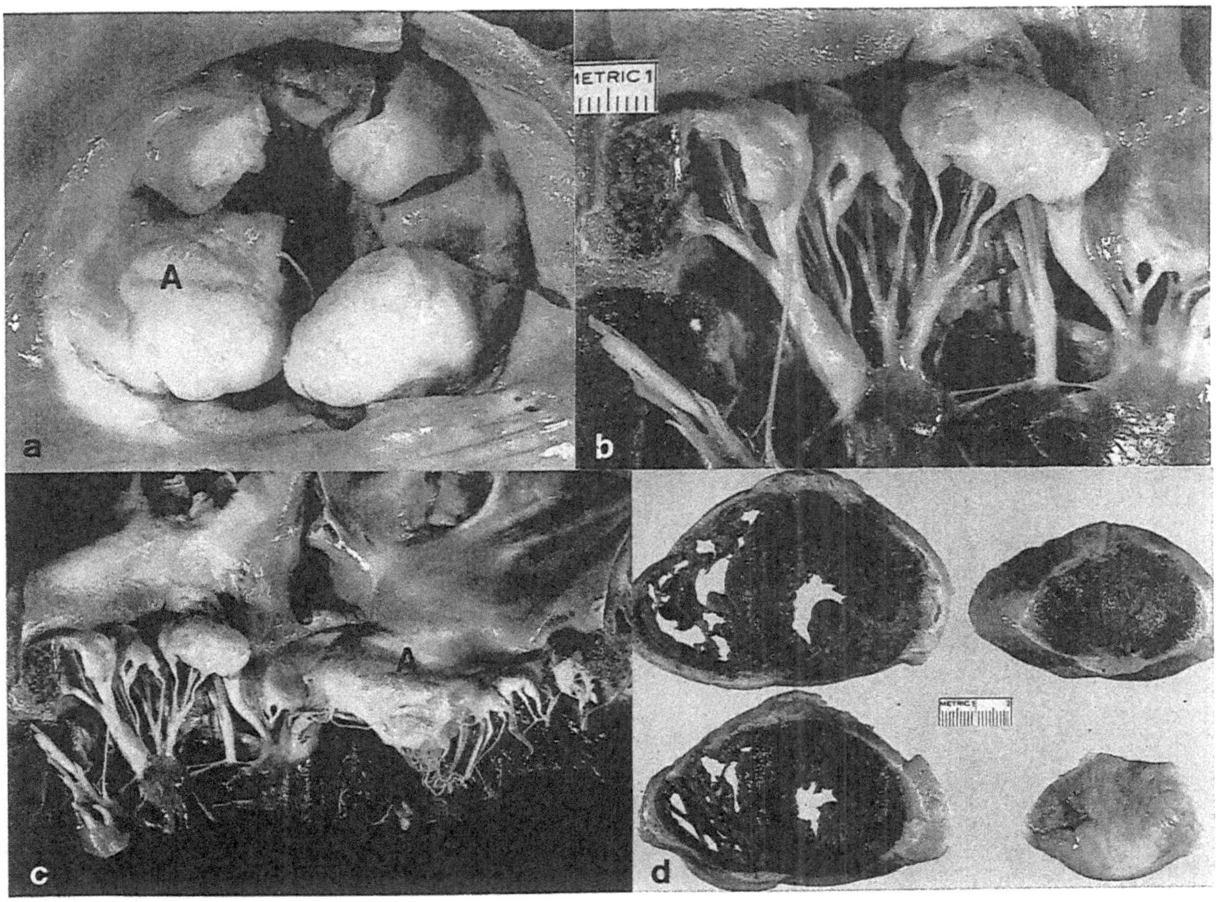

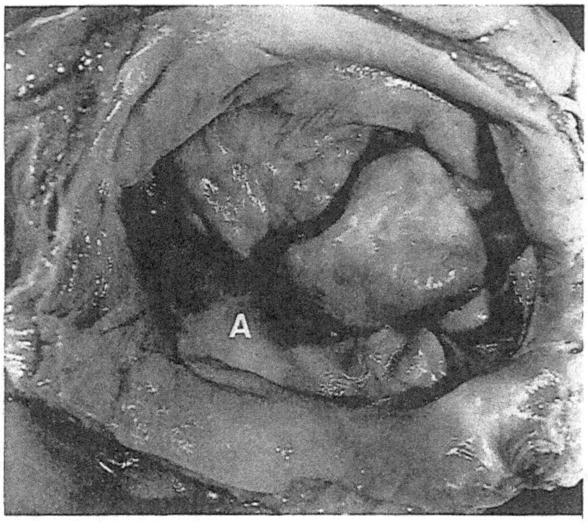

Figure 10. Patient from *−SCD, −MR, −CAD* group. The heart of a 63 year old woman (Georgetown University Hospital #79A-100, Washington, D.C.) who died of cancer. View of the intact mitral valve from the left atrium, showing herniation of the posterior leaflet above the anterior leaflet (A). Abbreviations as in Figure 8.

classic "medial cystic necrosis" with massive degeneration of elastic fibers and two had a normal configuration of elastic fibers in the aortic media. At least one histologic section of ascending aorta stained for elastic fibers was examined in 22 patients with mitral valve prolapse unassociated with the Marfan syndrome, and the aortic media in each appeared normal.

Discussion

Major findings in the present study. Several differences were observed in the 15 patients with sudden death associated with isolated mitral valve prolapse (without the pres-

Figure 11. Patient from *−SCD, −MR, −CAD* group. The heart of a 63 year old man (Georgetown University Hospital #82A-04, Washington, DC) who died of cancer. **a**, View of the heart from above after removal of the atria. **b**, Radiograph of the base of the heart, showing massive calcium deposits in the anulus of the mitral valve, aortic valve and epicardial coronary arteries. **c**, Close-up view of the intact mitral valve as viewed from the left atrium showing pronounced enlargement of the posterior leaflet. **d**, View of the aortic valve from above, showing a stenotic tricuspid valve with calcium deposits and no fusion of the commissures. Abbreviations as in Figure 8.

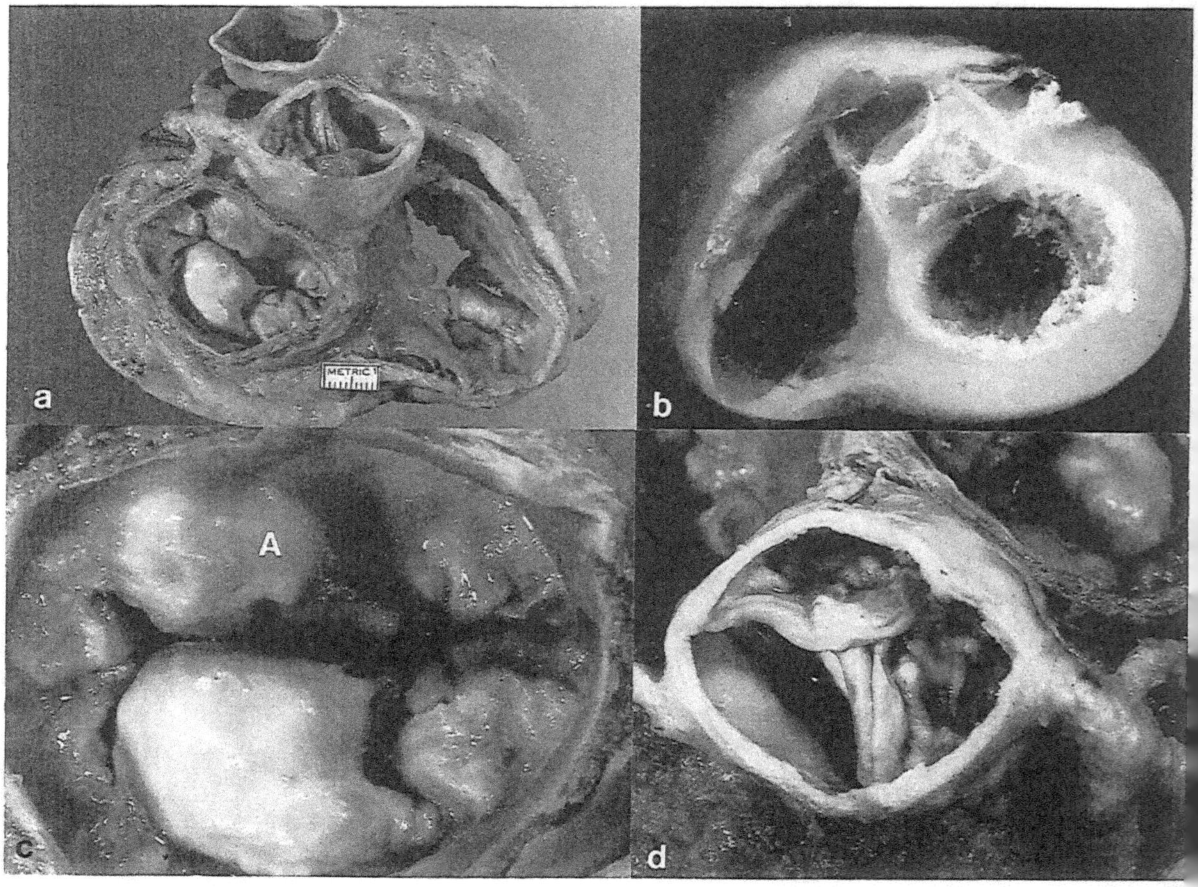

Table 3. Clinical Features of Seven Adult Patients With Congenital Heart Disease With Morphologic Features of Mitral Valve Prolapse Studied at Necropsy

Pt No.	Congenital Abnormality	Age (yr)/ Gender	MVP Diagnosed Clinically	MR	Cardiac Operation	Mode of Death
1	ASD (secundum), Ebstein's anomaly	17/F	0	–	0	Noncardiac (cancer)
2	Aortic coarctation, BAV (AR)	30/M	+	+	Coarctectomy, AVR, MVR	Cardiac operation
3	ASD (secundum), TAPVC	42/M	0	–	0	Sudden (cardiac)
4	Atrioventricular canal (partial)	55/F	+	+	0	Noncardiac (pneumonia)
5	BAV, valvular aortic stenosis	56/M	–	–	Coronary bypass	Sudden (CAD + AS)
6	ASD (secundum), BAV, SV aneurysm	57/F	0	–	0	Rupture of SV aneurysm
7	ASD (secundum)	59/F	+	+	ASD closure, MVR	Cardiac operation

ASD = atrial septal defect; AVR = aortic valve replacement; BAV = bicuspid aortic valve; MVR = mitral valve replacement; SV = sinus of Valsalva; TAPVC = total anomalous pulmonary venous connection; + = present; 0 = absent; – = no information available; other abbreviations as in Tables 1 and 2.

ence of other potentially fatal conditions) compared with the patients with mitral valve prolapse with other potentially fatal causes of death and without other congenital cardiac malformations: the patients who died suddenly with isolated mitral valve prolapse were younger, more likely to be women and less likely to have mitral regurgitation or evidence of ruptured chordae tendineae.

Severe mitral regurgitation was infrequent (1 of 15 patients) in the patients with mitral valve prolapse who died suddenly without associated significant coronary artery disease or other congenital cardiac anomalies. There have been conflicting views regarding the importance of mitral regurgitation as a predisposing factor for sudden death in patients with mitral valve prolapse. Some investigators (25,26) emphasized the importance of mitral regurgitation as a risk factor for sudden death in patients with mitral valve prolapse, going so far as to calculate an estimated annual mortality rate from sudden death due to mitral valve prolapse in patients with and without mitral regurgitation. Their estimates were based primarily on a study by Davies et al. (15), who reported on 13 patients at necropsy who died suddenly and had mitral valve prolapse. At least 4 of their 13 patients, however, had an etiology for the mitral regurgitation and sudden death other than mitral valve prolapse: 2 patients had bacterial endocarditis, 1 had a previous myocardial infarction and 1 patient, a 79 year old man, had chronic lung disease. After reviewing 25 previously reported patients with mitral valve prolapse who died suddenly, Jeresaty (27) concluded that the typical patient with mitral valve prolapse who dies suddenly has only minimal to moderate mitral regurgitation.

Frequency of mural endocardial fibrous plaque in patients dying suddenly with mitral valve prolapse. The presence of mural endocardial fibrous plaque beneath the posterior mitral leaflet has been noted previously in necropsy studies of patients dying suddenly from mitral valve prolapse. Chesler et al. (22) suggested that the friction between chordae tendineae and the underlying left ventricular mural endocardium, presumably the mechanism of formation of this endocardial plaque, may cause ventricular arrhythmias. We found a high frequency of such plaque, both in patients whose death was attributed to isolated mitral valve prolapse (11 of 15) and patients whose death was attributed to other causes (12 of 19).

Abnormalities of the fossa ovale membrane in patients with mitral valve prolapse. Secundum atrial septal defect is associated with mitral valve prolapse (28,29). Four of our seven patients with mitral valve prolapse and congenital heart disease had ostium secundum atrial septal defect. Redundancy (aneurysm) of the fossa ovale membrane also has been noted (30) in association with mitral valve prolapse at necropsy, and a recent report (31) found a higher prevalence of atrial septal aneurysm diagnosed by echocardiography in patients with mitral valve prolapse (9.5%) compared with those without (3.1%). We found a 20% frequency of redundancy of the fossa ovale membrane among the 49 patients with mitral valve prolapse without congenital cardiovascular anomalies. Probe-patent valvular-competent foramen ovale occurred in 7 (23%) of 31 patients among the entire group. This frequency, however, is similar to that of valvular-competent patent foramen ovale in normal adult hearts (30). Neither redundancy of the fossa ovale membrane nor probe-patency of the foramen ovale was more common among the sudden death group compared with the other patients with mitral valve prolapse.

Previously reported studies on patients who died suddenly from mitral valve prolapse. We searched for published reports of patients with mitral valve prolapse who died suddenly and who had no other condition present at autopsy to explain death. A total of 63 patients (3–14,16–23) were found, of whom 39 had individualized clinical data (3–14, 16–22) (Table 4). These previously reported patients were similar in many respects to our group of 15 patients dying suddenly with mitral valve prolapse. The mean age of the previously published patients was 33 ± 14 years; 27 (71%) of 38 were women and the mean heart weight was 306 ± 76 g. Severe mitral regurgitation was uncommon; only one patient had a heart weight above normal (≤350 g for women and ≤400 g for men) and only one other patient (whose heart weighed 340 g) had dilated cardiac chambers. Only six patients had results of cineangiocardiography: mitral regur-

Table 4. Clinical Information in 39 Previously Reported Patients Studied at Necropsy Who Died Suddenly With Mitral Valve Prolapse as the Only Explanation for Death

Reference (first author)	Year	Age (yr)/ Gender	MVP Diagnosed Clinically	P	D	S	CP	Auscultatory Findings: MR	SH	CHF	SC	SM	MR by LV Cine (0–3+)	ECG Findings: Rhythm	QTc (ms)	T Wave Inversion	VPCs	Last Activity	Medication	HW (g)	Abnormal MV Leaflet: AML	PML	Plaque Under PML
Hancock (3)	1966	29/F	+	+	0	0	0	–	0	0	+	+	–	S	45	+(A,I)	+	—	Quinidine	–	–	–	–
Barlow (4)	1968	39/M	+	–	–	–	–		–	–	+	+	–		–	–	+	Mowing lawn	—	–	–	–	–
Trent (5)	1970	63/F	+	+	0	0	+	Y	0	+	0	+	++	S	–	–	0	—	Digoxin	340	+	+	–
Jeresaty (6)	1973	62/F	+	–	–	–	–	–	–	–	0	+	++	AF	N	+(A,I)	+	Sleeping	—	–	–	–	–
Shappell (7)	1973	27/F	+	0	0	+	0	N	0	0	+	+	0	S	45–47	+(I)	0	Arguing	Propranolol	310	+	+	–
Marshall (8)	1974	36/F	+	+	+	0	0	–	0	0	–	–	–	–	–	–	–	Sitting		350	+	+	–
Guthrie* (9)	1976	20/F	+	0	0	0	0		–	0	+	0	–		N	0	+	—	0	–	–	–	–
Guthrie* (9)	1976	25/F	+	+	+	+	+		–	–	+	+	+		–	–	+	—	Quinidine, propranolol	–	–	–	–
Guthrie* (9)	1976	29/M	0	0	0	0	0		–	0	0	+	–		–	–	–	Sitting at desk	—	–	–	–	–
Jeresaty (10)	1976	39/F	+	0	0	0	0	Y	0	0	+	+	+	S	N	+(I)	0	—	Furosemide	–	+	+	–
Kleid (11)	1976	38/F	–	+	0	0	0	N	0	0	0	+	–	S	–	–	+	—	0	–	–	–	–
Koch (12)	1976	9/–	+	–	–	–	–	–	–	–	–	–	–	–	–	–	**	—	—	–	–	–	–
Koch (12)	1976	30/–	+	–	–	–	–	–	–	–	–	–	–	–	–	–	**	—	—	–	–	–	–
Koch (12)	1976	32/–	+	–	–	–	–	–	–	–	–	–	–	–	–	–	**	—	—	–	–	–	–
Koch (12)	1976	50/–	+	–	–	–	–	–	–	–	–	–	–	–	–	–	**	—	—	–	–	–	–
Koch (12)	1976	64/–	+	–	–	–	–	–	–	–	–	–	–	–	–	–	**	—	—	–	–	–	–
Mills (14)	1977	58/M	+	–	+	–	–		–	+	0	+	–		–	+	+	—	Quinidine	–	–	–	–
Mair (16)	1980	25/F	+	+	0	+	0	–	0	0	+	+	–	–	–	–	–	Driving	0	230	+	+	+
Mair (16)	1980	29/F	+	–	–	+	–	–	0	0	+	0	–	–	–	–	–	Lying in bed	0	250	+	+	+
Mair (16)	1980	35/F	–	+	+	0	0	–	0	0	–	–	–	–	–	–	–	Conversing	0	270	+	+	+
Bharati (17)	1981	17/M	0	–	–	–	–	–	–	0	–	–	–	–	–	–	–	Playing football	—	–	–	–	–
Bharati (17)	1981	19/F	0	–	–	–	–	–	–	–	–	–	–	–	–	–	–	—	—	–	–	–	–
Bharati (18)	1981	45/M	+	+	–	–	–	–	–	–	+	+	–	S	N	–	+	—	0	–	–	+	–
Dupasquier (19)	1981	43/M	+	+	–	+	0	Y	0	0	0	+	–	S	N	+(I)	0	Driving	0	550	–	–	–
Salmela (20)	1981	27/M	+	–	+	+	0	–	0	0	+	+	–	S	N	+(I)	+	Watching television	Digoxin	–	–	+	–
Pocock (21)	1984	24/F	+	+	0	0	0	Y	0	0	+	+	+	S	N	+(I)	+	Conversing	Disopromide, acebutolol	–	0	+	+
Chesler (22)	1983	14/F	0	0	0	0	0	0	–	–	–	–	–	–	–	–	–	—	Methyldopa	230	+	+	+
Chesler (22)	1983	19/F	–	–	–	–	–		–	–	–	–	–	–	–	–	–	—	—	230	0	+	+
Chesler (22)	1983	19/M	+	0	0	0	0	0	–	–	+	+	–	–	–	–	–	—	Steroid inhaler	220	+	+	+
Chesler (22)	1983	21/F	+	0	0	0	0	0	–	–	+	0	–	–	–	–	–	—	Primidone	260	0	+	0
Chesler (22)	1983	21/F	+	+	0	0	0	0	–	–	+	+	–	–	–	–	–	—	0	290	+	+	+
Chesler (22)	1983	24/F	–	0	0	0	0	0	–	–	0	+	–	–	–	–	–	—	0	350	+	+	+
Chesler (22)	1983	25/F	+	+	+	0	+		–	–	+	+	–	–	–	–	–	—	Propranolol	220	+	+	+
Chesler (22)	1983	26/F	–	–	–	–	–		–	–	–	–	–	–	–	–	–	—	—	340	+	+	+
Chesler (22)	1983	27/F	–	0	0	0	0	0	–	–	0	+	–	–	–	–	–	—	0	325	+	+	+
Chesler (22)	1983	29/M	–	+	0	0	0	0	–	–	0	+	–	–	–	–	–	—	0	365	+	+	+
Chesler (22)	1983	30/M	+	0	0	0	0	0	–	–	+	0	–	–	–	–	–	—	0	325	+	+	+
Chesler (22)	1983	39/F	0	0	0	0	0	0	–	–	0	0	–	–	–	–	–	—	0	348	+	+	0
Chesler (22)	1983	59/F	0	0	0	0	0	0	–	–	–	–	–	–	–	–	–	—	0	320	0	+	+

*Some of the details of these cases were not in the original report but were provided in Jeresaty (6); †two of these five patients had multiform ventricular premature complexes (VPCs) on their electrocardiogram. A = anterior; AF = atrial fibrillation; CP = chest pain; D = dizziness; I = inferior; LV Cine = left ventricular cineangiogram; N = normal; P = palpitation; QTc = QT interval corrected for rate; S = syncope; Y = yes;

gitation was absent in one, mild in three and moderate in two.

Previously reported patients with mitral valve prolapse who survived potentially lethal ventricular arrhythmias. Several studies (33–35) have detailed the characteristics of patients with mitral valve prolapse who had life-threatening ventricular tachyarrhythmias or who survived cardiac arrest. Winkle et al. (33) reported on seven patients (five women, mean age 49 years) with mitral valve prolapse who had survived one or more episodes of life-threatening ventricular arrhythmias: six patients had a systolic click or systolic murmur, or both. Mitral regurgitation was objectively diagnosed or excluded in only three of the seven patients (by left ventricular angiography): mitral regurgitation was absent in two and moderate in one. Wei et al. (34) reported on 10 patients with mitral valve prolapse (7 women, mean age 47 years) with symptomatic recurrent ventricular tachyarrhythmias refractory to conventional drug therapy. Although left ventricular angiography was performed in all patients, there was no specific mention of mitral regurgitation. Boudoulas et al. (33) reported on nine patients with mitral valve prolapse who had cardiac arrest (seven women, mean age 33 years) of whom seven survived. All seven had cardiac catheterization, but mitral regurgitation was not mentioned.

References

1. Savage DD, Garrison RJ, Devereux RB, et al. Mitral valve prolapse in the general population. I. Epidemiologic features: the Framingham Study. Am Heart J 1983;106:571–6.
2. Topaz O, Edwards JE. Pathologic features of sudden death in children, adolescents, and young adults. Chest 1985;87:476–82.
3. Hancock EW, Cohn K. The syndrome associated with midsystolic click and late systolic murmur. Am J Med 1966;41:183–96.
4. Barlow JB, Bosman CK, Pocock WA, Marchand P. Late systolic murmurs and non-ejection ("mid-late") systolic clicks: an analysis of 90 patients. Br Heart J 1968;30:203–18.
5. Trent JK, Adelman AG, Wigle ED, Silverman MD. Morphology of a prolapsed posterior mitral valve leaflet. Am Heart J 1970;79:539–43.
6. Jeresaty RM. Mitral valve prolapse-click syndrome. Prog Cardiovasc Dis 1973;15:623–52.
7. Shappell SD, Marshall CE, Brown RE, Bruce T. Sudden death and the familial occurrence of mid-systolic click, late systolic murmur syndrome. Circulation 1973;48:1128–34.
8. Marshall CE, Shappell SD. Sudden death and the ballooning posterior leaflet syndrome: detailed anatomic and histochemical investigation. Arch Pathol 1974;98:134–8.
9. Guthrie RB, Edwards JE. Pathology of the myxomatous mitral valve: nature, secondary changes and complications. Minn Med 1976;59:637–47.
10. Jeresaty RM. Sudden death and the mitral valve prolapse-click syndrome. Am J Cardiol 1976;37:317–8.
11. Kleid JJ. Sudden death and the floppy mitral valve syndrome. Angiology 1976;27:734–7.
12. Koch FH, Hancock EW. Ten year follow-up of forty patients with the mid-systolic click/late systolic murmur syndrome (abstr). Am J Cardiol 1976;37:149.
13. Allen H, Harris A, Leatham A. Significance and prognosis of an isolated late systolic murmur: a 9-to-22-year follow-up. Br Heart J 1974;36:525–32.
14. Mills P, Rose J, Hollingsworth J, Amara I, Craige E. Long-term prognosis of mitral-valve prolapse. N Engl J Med 1977;297:13–8.
15. Davies MJ, Moore BP, Braimbridge MV. The floppy mitral valve: study of incidence, pathology, and complications in surgical, necropsy, and forensic material. Br Heart J 1978;40:468–81.
16. Mair WJ. Sudden death in young females with floppy mitral valve syndrome. Aust N Z J Med 1980;10:221–3.
17. Bharati S, Granston AS, Liebson PR, Loeb HS, Rosen KM, Lev M. The conduction system in mitral valve prolapse syndrome with sudden death. Am Heart J 1981;101:667–70.
18. Bharati S, Rosen KM, Miller LB, Strasberg B, Lev M. Sudden death in three teenagers (abstr). Circulation 1981;64(suppl IV):IV-72.
19. Dupasquier E, Berney JL. Le syndrome du prolapsus valvulaire mitral: deux complications rares: la mort subite, l'embolie cerebrale. Schweiz Med Wochenschr 1981;111:73–81.
20. Salmela PI, Ikaheimo M, Juustila H. Fatal ventricular fibrillation after treatment with digoxin in a 27-year-old man with mitral leaflet prolapse syndrome. Br Heart J 1981;46:338–41.
21. Pocock W, Bosman CK, Chesler E, Barlow JB, Edwards JE. Sudden death in primary mitral valve prolapse. Am Heart J 1984;107:378–82.
22. Chesler E, King RA, Edwards JE. The myxomatous mitral valve and sudden death. Circulation 1983;67:632–9.
23. Virmani R, Atkinson JB, Forman MB, Rabinowitz M. Mitral valve prolapse. Hum Pathol 1987;18:596–602.
24. Roberts WC, McIntosh CL, Wallace RB. Mechanisms of severe mitral regurgitation in mitral valve prolapse determined from analysis of operatively excised valves. Am Heart J 1987;113:1316–23.
25. Kligfield P, Levy D, Devereux RB, Savage DD. Arrhythmias and sudden death in mitral valve prolapse. Am Heart J 1987;113:1298–307.
26. Devereux RB, Kramer-Fox R, Kligfield P. Mitral valve prolapse: causes, clinical manifestations, and management. Ann Intern Med 1989;111:305–17.
27. Jeresaty RM. Mitral Valve Prolapse. New York: Raven, 1979:209–21.
28. Betriu A, Wigle ED, Felderhof CH, McLoughlin MJ. Prolapse of the posterior leaflet of the mitral valve associated with secundum atrial septal defect. Am J Cardiol 1975;35:363–9.
29. Leachman RD, Cokkinos DV, Cooley DA. Association of ostium secundum septal defects with mitral valve prolapse. Am J Cardiol 1976;38:167–9.
30. Roberts WC. Aneurysm (redundancy) of the atrial septum (fossa ovale membrane) and prolapse (redundancy) of the mitral valve. Am J Cardiol 1984;54:1153–4.
31. Rahko PS, Xu QB. Increased prevalence of atrial septal aneurysm in mitral valve prolapse (abstr). Circulation 1989;80(suppl II):II-10.
32. Barry A, Patten BM. The structure of the adult heart. In: Gould SE, ed. Pathology of the Heart and Blood Vessels. Springfield, IL: Charles C Thomas, 1968:91–130.
33. Winkle RA, Lopes MG, Popp RL, Hancock EW. Life-threatening arrhythmias in the mitral valve prolapse syndrome. Am J Med 1976;60:961–7.
34. Wei JY, Bulkley BH, Schaeffer AH, Greene HL, Reid PR. Mitral-valve prolapse syndrome and recurrent ventricular tachyarrhythmias. Ann Intern Med 1978;89:6–9.
35. Boudoulas H, Schaal SF, Stang JM, Fontana ME, Kolibash AJ, Wooley CF. Mitral valve prolapse–sudden death with long term survival (abstr). J Am Coll Cardiol 1986;7:29A.

Severe Mitral or Aortic Valve Regurgitation, or Both, Requiring Valve Replacement for Infective Endocarditis Complicating Hypertrophic Cardiomyopathy

WILLIAM C. ROBERTS, MD, FACC, JOAN C. KISHEL, MD, CHARLES L. McINTOSH, MD, FACC, RICHARD O. CANNON III, MD, FACC, BARRY J. MARON, MD

Bethesda, Maryland

Certain clinical and morphologic findings are described in 11 patients with hypertrophic cardiomyopathy complicated by infective endocarditis that produced severe mitral or aortic valve regurgitation, or both, necessitating valve replacement. All 11 patients had changes in the operatively excised valve or valves characteristic of healed infective endocarditis. The infection involved only the mitral valve in seven patients, only the aortic valve in three patients and both valves in one patient.

Study of the operatively excised mitral valves indicated that the healed vegetations were located most commonly on the left ventricular aspects of the anterior mitral leaflet, indicating that vegetation had formed at contact points of this leaflet with mural endocardium of the left ventricular outflow tract. In all 11 patients, the infective endocarditis either worsened preexisting valve regurgitation or initiated valve regurgitation and led to worsened signs and symptoms of cardiac dysfunction, necessitating valve replacement. Functional class improved in the nine patients who survived 7 to 101 months after valve replacement.

Hypertrophic cardiomyopathy appears to be a factor predisposing to infective endocarditis. Patients with hypertrophic cardiomyopathy should receive prophylactic antibiotic therapy during procedures that predispose to infective endocarditis.

(J Am Coll Cardiol 1992;19:365–71)

From 1961 through October 1989, 626 patients with hypertrophic cardiomyopathy underwent a cardiac operation at the Surgery Branch of the National Heart, Lung, and Blood Institute: partial septotomy/septectomy alone in 539 patients (86%); septotomy/septectomy followed later by mitral valve replacement in 19 patients (3%) and mitral valve replacement alone in 68 patients (11%). Of the 87 patients undergoing mitral valve replacement with or without septotomy/septectomy, mitral valve replacement was performed because of severe left ventricular outflow obstruction unassociated with severe thickening of the ventricular septum in 65 patients; damage to either the mitral or aortic valve at the time of earlier septotomy/septectomy in 5 patients; inability to wean the patient from cardiopulmonary bypass after septotomy/septectomy in 3 patients; severe regurgitation of uncertain etiology in 3 patients; and valvular regurgitation caused by or worsened by infective endocarditis in 11 patients. This report describes certain clinical and morphologic cardiac findings in the 11 patients with hypertrophic cardiomyopathy with severe mitral or aortic valvular regurgitation, or both, from infective endocarditis.

From the Pathology, Cardiology and Surgery Branches, National Heart, Lung, and Blood Institute, National Institutes of Health, Bethesda, Maryland.
Manuscript received May 8, 1991; revised manuscript received July 15, 1991, accepted July 29, 1991.
Address for reprints: William C. Roberts, MD, Building 10, Room 2N258, NHLBI-NIH, Bethesda, Maryland 20892.

Methods

Clinical characteristics (Tables 1 to 3). All 11 patients had clear clinical evidence of hypertrophic cardiomyopathy: 1) each had evidence of left ventricular hypertrophy on both the electrocardiogram (ECG) and the M-mode echocardiogram; 2) immediately before cardiac valve replacement, only 1 patient had a dilated left ventricular cavity as determined by left ventricular angiography and the dilation was of mild degree; 3) none had a history of systemic hypertension and, with one exception, all had systemic arterial indirect pressure recordings ≤140 mm Hg systolic and ≤90 mm Hg diastolic (Patient 3 had a systemic arterial direct pressure of 160/90 mm Hg recorded immediately before valve replacement, but other pressures recorded were normal); 4) although cardiac index was normal in only four of nine patients in whom it was recorded, the other five had evidence of severe valvular regurgitation (worsened by infective endocarditis) at the time of the recording; 5) the maximal thickness of the ventricular septum was greater than that of the left ventricular free wall in all patients before either valve replacement or partial ventricular septotomy/septectomy and 6) all patients had hemodynamic documentation of subaortic obstruction at some time.

Characteristics of infective endocarditis. All 11 patients had evidence of active infective endocarditis at some time (Fig. 1 to 7). Ten patients had a typical clinical illness of active infective endocarditis. Of the nine patients with on

Table 1. Clinical and Morphologic Features in 11 Patients Having Valve Replacement for Valvular Regurgitation Due to or Worsened by Infective Endocarditis Complicating Hypertrophic Cardiomyopathy

		Diagnosis of HCM		NYHA Functional Class (I–IV)			Septotomy/Septectomy (7 patients)							Type Valve Prosthesis		Morphology of Operatively Excised Valve				
																MV			AV	
Pt No.	Age (yr) at VR/ Gender	Before IE	After IE	Just Before IE	After IE	Just Before VR	Before IE	After IE	Before VR	With VR	Follow-Up After Valve Replacement (mo)	NYHA Class at Latest Follow-Up	Interval IE to VR (mo)	MV (size)	AV (size)	Calcium	P	RCT	Calcium	P
1	12/M	+	0	II	IV	IV	0	0	0	0	7	I	17	SE	–	+	+	+	–	–
2	25/M	+	0	II	III	III	+	+	0	+	21	I	10	H (27 mm)	–	+	+	+	–	–
3	43/M	+	0	II	III	III	0	0	0	0	10	II	19	H (25 mm)	–	+	+	+	–	–
4	46/M	–	–	–	–	III	0	+	0	+	101	III	–	H (25 mm)	–	0	+	+	–	–
5	63/M	+	0	III	IV	IV	0	0	0	0	90	II	8	H (31 mm)	–	+	+	+	–	–
6	64/M	0	+	II	II	III	0	0	0	0	18	I	156	H (31 mm)	–	+	+	+	–	–
7	71/M	+	0	II	III	IV	0	–	+	0	30 days	Dead	204	H (31 mm)	–	+	+	+	–	–
8	51/M	0	+	I	IV	IV	0	–	0	+	72	I	3	–	SE (9A)	–	–	–	+	+
9	52/F	+	0	II	III	III	0	–	0	+	33	II	7	–	SE (9A)	–	–	–	+	+
10	64/F	0	+	I	III	IV	0	+	0	+	12	I	60	–	H (21 mm)	–	–	–	0	+
11	58/M	+	0	III	IV	IV	0	+	+	0	3 days	Dead	168	H (29 mm)	H (23 mm)	+	+	+	0	+

AV = aortic valve; F = female; H = Hancock; HCM = hypertrophic cardiomyopathy; IE = infective endocarditis; M = male; MV = mitral valve; NYHA = New York Heart Association; P = perforation or indentation (deficiency of leaflet tissue); Pt = patient; RCT = ruptured chordae tendineae; SE = Starr-Edwards; VR = valve replacement; 0 = absent or negative; + = present or positive; – = no information available or not applicable.

clinical episode of active infective endocarditis, the interval between active infective endocarditis and valve replacement ranged from 3 to 204 months (mean 54, median 17). This interval was <1 year in four patients. Patient 11 (Table 1) had two episodes of active infective endocarditis that occurred 168 and 27 months, respectively, before valve replacement (Fig. 7). Only the second episode caused clinical worsening of this patient's cardiac status. Patient 4 apparently never had a clinical illness diagnosed as active infective endocarditis, but examination of the operatively excised mitral valve disclosed a large deficit in the anterior mitral leaflet adjacent to several ruptured chordae tendineae, anatomic findings diagnostic of healed infective endocarditis (1). Of the 11 patients, 9 had active infective endocarditis before they were admitted to the National Institutes of Health; 1 had active infective endocarditis treated at another hospital, but hypertrophic cardiomyopathy had previously been diagnosed at the National Institutes of Health; and 1 patient had active infective endocarditis while hospitalized at the National Institutes of Health. Diagnosis of hypertrophic cardiomyopathy had been established previously in 7 of the 10 patients with a clinical illness diagnosed as active infective endocarditis; it was made in the other 3 patients after active infective endocarditis had healed. In five patients, a factor other than hypertrophic cardiomyopathy predisposing to infective endocarditis was apparent: dental procedures in Patients 4 and 5, cardiac catheterization in Patients 6 and 10 and opiate addiction in Patient 11.

During active infective endocarditis, information regarding the results of blood cultures were known in eight patients: in two, the blood cultures were negative and in six a bacterium was identified (alpha streptococcus in Patients 7, 10 and 11; group D streptococcus in two patients [nonenterococcal in Patient 2 and enterococcus in Patient 6]; and *Cardiobacterium hominis* in Patient 4). All 11 patients, however, had anatomic deficiencies of mitral or aortic valve cusps, and in those with infective endocarditis involving the mitral valve, there were associated ruptured chordae tendineae. The 10 patients with clear clinical evidence of active infective endocarditis received appropriate antibiotic treatment, and by the time of valve replacement, the infection had healed in all 10 patients. The M-mode echocardiogram immediately before valve replacement showed "echo densities" compatible with healed vegetations in four of seven patients in whom healed infective endocarditis involved the mitral valve and two of four in whom it involved the aortic valve.

Valvular regurgitation caused by infective endocarditis. Active infective endocarditis worsened the symptomatic status in nine patients by at least one New York Heart Association functional class. It also increased the intensity of the precordial systolic murmur (mitral regurgitation) in three of three patients in whom this information was known and caused the appearance of a basal diastolic murmur in all four patients with aortic regurgitation. Despite the appearance or worsening of valvular regurgitation, the left ventric-

Table 2. M-Mode Echocardiographic Data Before and After Operation in the 11 Patients With Infective Endocarditis Complicating Hypertrophic Cardiomyopathy and Requiring Valve Replacement

Pt No.	Interval Echo to VR (days)	Wall Thickness (mm)		Cavity (mm)			FS (%)	Echo Density		Flail		SAM
		VSd	LVd	LVd	LVs	LA		MV	AV	MV	AV	
1	9 (MVR)	20	13	41	18	45	56	+	0	+	0	+
	PO	16	10	37	18	35	51	–	0	–	0	–
2												
3	78 (MVR)	17	14	36	16	56	55	0	0	+	0	+
	PO	—	—	—	—	—	—	–	–	–	–	–
4	12 (MVR)	19	15	40	18	40	55	0	0	0	0	–
	PO	15	—*	—*	—*	57	—	–	0	–	0	–
5	65 (MVR)	32	14	46	28	55	39	±	0	0	0	+
	PO	14	—	—	—	57	—	–	0	–	0	–
6	16 (MVR)	26	13	56	38	68	32	+	0	0	0	+
	PO	—	—	—	—	—	—	–	–	–	–	–
7	33 (MVR)	—	—	—	—	72	—	0	0	±	0	–
	PO	—	—	—	—	63	—	–	0	–	0	–
8	8 (AVR)	20	13	40	22	43	45	0	+	0	–	0
	PO	10	10	—*	—*	40	—	0	–	0	–	0
9	37 (AVR)	26	14	44	22	49	50	0	+	0	+	0
	PO†		11	51	29	45	43	0	–	0	–	0
10	41 (AVR)	24	13	53	41	60	23	0	0	0	0	–
	PO	11	11	—*	—*	52	—	0	–	0	–	0
11	10 (MVR, AVR)	—	—	—	—	54	—	0	0	0	0	0
	PO	—	—	—	—	—	—	–	–	–	–	–

*Paradoxical movement; †ventricular septal defect created at operation. AV = aortic valve; AVR = aortic valve replacement; d = end-diastole; Echo = echocardiography; FS = fractional shortening; LA = left atrium; LV = left ventricle; MV = mitral valve; MVR = mitral valve replacement; PO = after operation; s = peak systole; SAM = systolic anterior motion of the anterior mitral leaflet; VS = ventricular septum; – = not applicable; other abbreviations as in Table 1.

Table 3. Hemodynamic and Angiographic Data Immediately Before and ≥6 Months After Valve Replacement in 11 Patients With Infective Endocarditis Complicating Hypertrophic Cardiomyopathy

Pt No.	Time of Cath (mo PO)	PA* (s/d)	RV* (s/d)	RA* (m)	Mean PAW*	LA*		LV* (s/d)	SA* (s/d)	LV-SA psg*	MR by LV Cine (0–4+)	AR by AA Cine (0–4+)	CAD by Cine	CI
						a	v							
1	Pre-VR	66/40	65/16	7	26	36	38	180/25	118/60	62	4+	—	—	3.8
	PO (6)	32/14	32/4	4	9	16	10	130/12	125/65	5	—	—	—	2.1
2	Pre-VR	80/40	80/18	18	45	AF	50	138/24	138/60	0	4+	1+	—	2.1
3	Pre-VR	88/40	88/14	11	32	32	44	140/30	114/65	26	4+	0	0	1.8
	PO (6)	44/20	44/6	4	14	16	12	150/14	158/88	0	0	0	—	3.3
4	Pre-VR	90/40	90/10	8	30	27	40	165/32	120/70	45	3+	—	0	2.0
5	Pre-VR†	50/25	50/10	5	15	—	—	245/40	160/90	85	3+	—	—	3.7
	PO (10)‡	—	120/30	19	35	23	55	130/24	130/65	0	2+	0	—	2.[illegible]
	PO (21)	60/25	60/9	11	24	—	32	—	—	—	—	—	—	2.[illegible]
6	Pre-VR	45/23	45/8	4	20	28	36	110/10	105/70	5	3+	—	—	2.[illegible]
	PO (6)	—	24/5	3	—	—	—	105/6	105/60	0	0	—	—	2.[illegible]
7	Pre-VR	50/25	50/5	6	31	AF	50	120/20	130/75	0	4+	—	§	1.[illegible]
8	Pre-VR	85/35	85/12	—	38	AF	55	120/14	120/60	0	4+	—	—	—
9	Pre-VR	50/25	50/15	6	27	40	45	164/34	86/40	78	1+	3+	0	—
	PO (12)	24/11	24/7	4	6	13	8	115/16	110/65	5	—	—	—	2.[illegible]
10	Pre-VR	60/30	65/15	9	20	10	22	200/28	130/68	70	1+	2+	0	3.[illegible]
	PO (8)	—	—	—	16	20	28	105/20	105/55	0	—	—	—	4.[illegible]
	PO (58)	30/12	30/5	6	12	—	—	—	120/70	—	—	—	—	—
11	Pre-VR	55/30	55/6	5	17	26	20	240/30	100/30	140	3+	3+	0	1.[illegible]
	PO (76)	75/35	75/16	15	31	28	44	150/24	145/85	5	3+	1+	0	2.[illegible]

*Pressures in mm Hg. †Cardiac catheterization (Cath) 36 months before valve replacement; ‡peribasilar bioprosthetic communication found by left ventricul[illegible] cineangiography (Cine) and it was operatively closed after this cardiac catheterization procedure. §This patient was the only one with significant coronar[illegible] narrowing and he had aortocoronary bypass grafting in addition to valve replacement (VR). a = a wave; AA = ascending aorta; AF = atrial fibrillation; AR [illegible] aortic regurgitation; CAD = coronary artery narrowing >50% in diameter of >1 major artery; CI = cardiac index in liters/min per m²; LA = left atrium; LV [illegible] left ventricle; MR = mitral regurgitation; PA = pulmonary artery; PAW = pulmonary artery wedge; PO = after operation (months); Pre = before; psg = pea[illegible] systolic gradient; Pt = patient; RA = right atrium; RV = right ventricle; SA = systemic artery; s/d = peak systole/end-diastole; v = v wave.

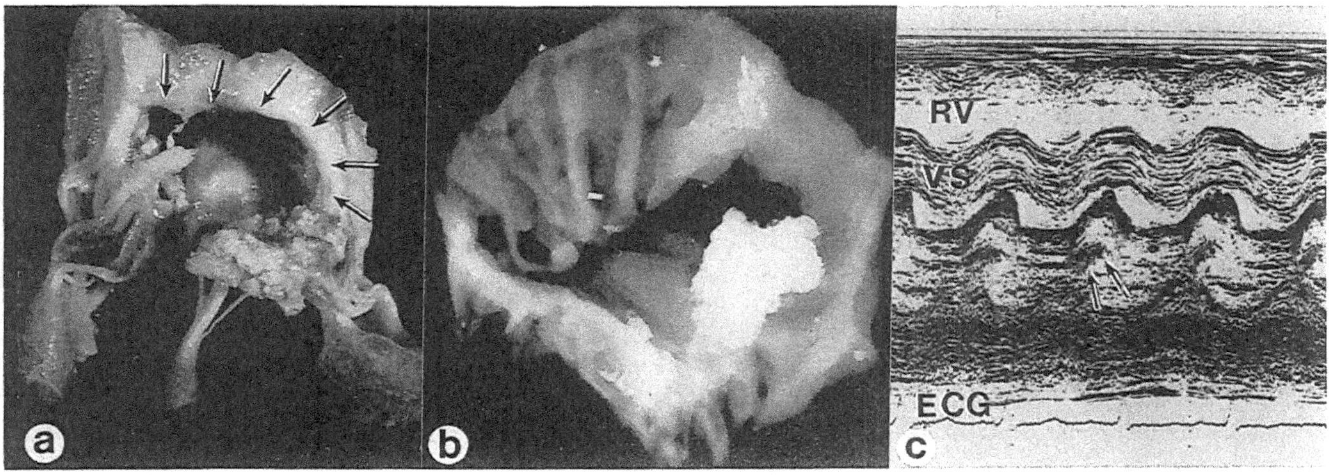

Figure 1 (above). Patient 1. Operatively excised mitral valve. **a,** Leaflets, chordae tendineae and attached papillary muscles showing loss of tissue in the posterior leaflet and absence of chordae tendineae (**arrows**). A large deposit of calcium is present and is better seen in **b**, a radiograph of the excised valve. **c,** M-mode echocardiogram taken shortly before mitral valve replacement, showing thickening and impaired mobility of the anterior mitral leaflet and fluttering (**arrows**) of the posterior leaflet. ECG = electrocardiogram; RV = right ventricular cavity; VS = ventricular septum.

Figure 2 (below). Patient 2. Operatively excised mitral valve (**a, b,** and **c**) and M-mode echocardiogram (**d**). **a,** Radiograph of the opened valve. The **arrows** point to a calcific deposit. **b** and **c,** Close-up views of the atrial aspect of a portion of both leaflets. The anterior leaflet contains two perforations (**solid arrows**) and the posterior leaflet one perforation (**dashed arrow**). **d,** Typical echocardiogram in hypertrophic cardiomyopathy with asymmetric thickening of the anterior ventricular septum (VS). The **arrows** point to dense echoes of the thickened anterior mitral leaflet, which contacts the ventricular septum in diastole. Mild mitral systolic anterior motion is present (*). PW = posterior wall; RV = right ventricular cavity.

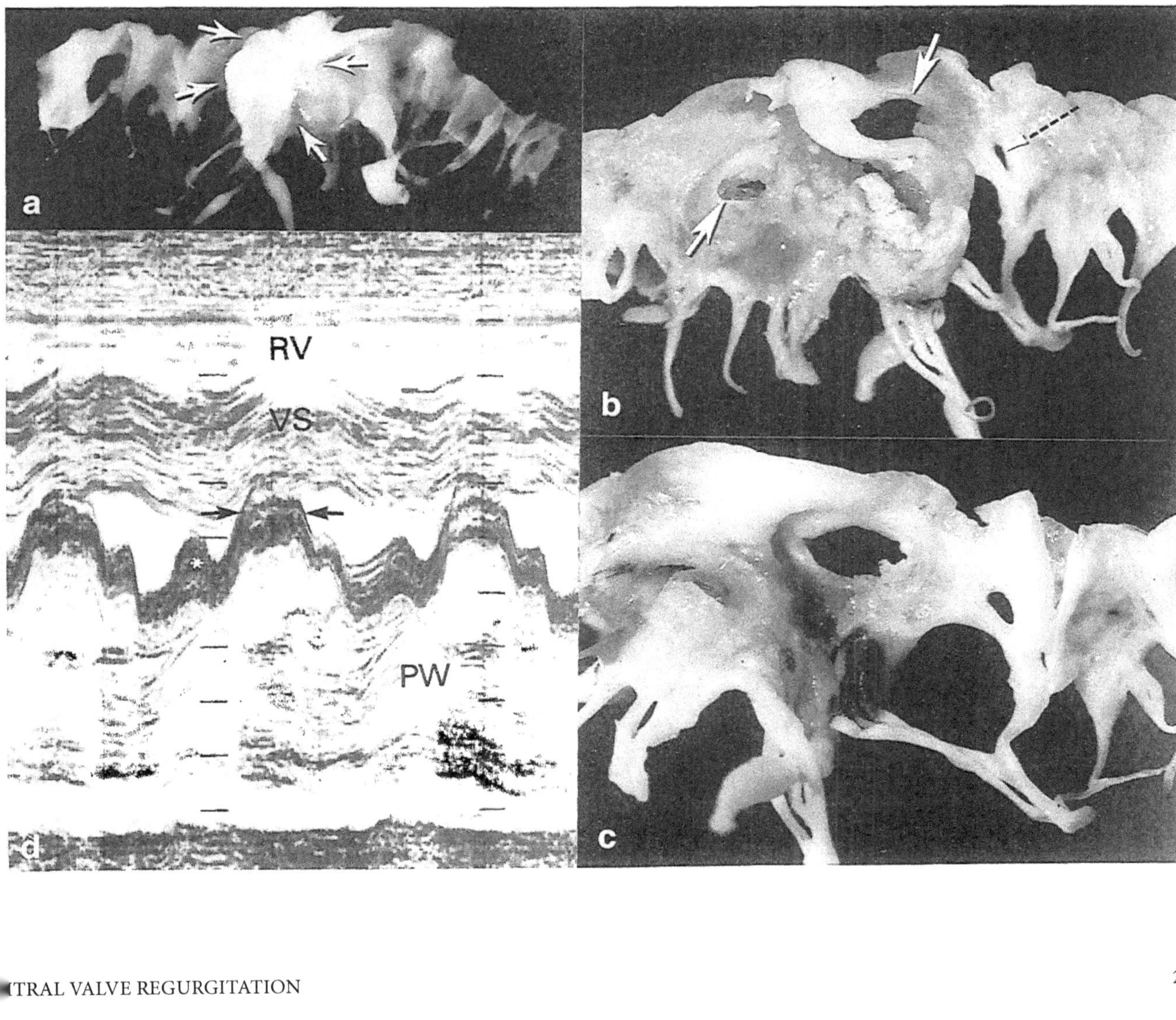

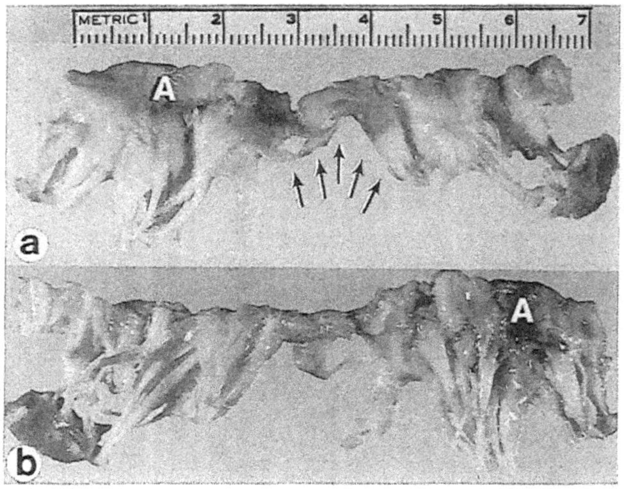

Figure 3. Patient 3. Opened mitral valve. **a**, Atrial surface. **b**, Ventricular surface. The **arrows** designate the area where chordae tendineae are missing (ruptured) and a site where a portion of the leaflet is absent (destroyed by the previous infection). A = anterior mitral leaflet.

ular cavity was of normal size on the echocardiogram immediately before valve replacement in nine of nine patients; left ventricular angiograms in the other two patients disclosed mild left ventricular cavity dilation in one of them. The degree of valvular regurgitation immediately before valve replacement in each of the 11 patients was severe: in the 7 patients with isolated mitral valve replacement, the degree of mitral regurgitation by left ventricular angiography was either 3+/4+ or 4+/4+; in the 3 patients with isolated aortic valve replacement, the degree of aortic regurgitation by aortic root angiography was 3+/4+ in 2 and 2+/4+ in 1; in the single patient with replacement of both left-sided cardiac valves, the degree of mitral regurgitation was 4+/4+ and aortic regurgitation, 1+/4+.

Effect of infective endocarditis on the left ventricular outflow pressure gradient. Active infective endocarditis involving the mitral valve was associated with a decrease in

Figure 4. Patient 5. Opened mitral valve from its atrial aspect, showing a large perforation (**arrow**) in the anterior leaflet (A) with adjacent focal calcific deposits. The perforation represents a site where vegetation had been present.

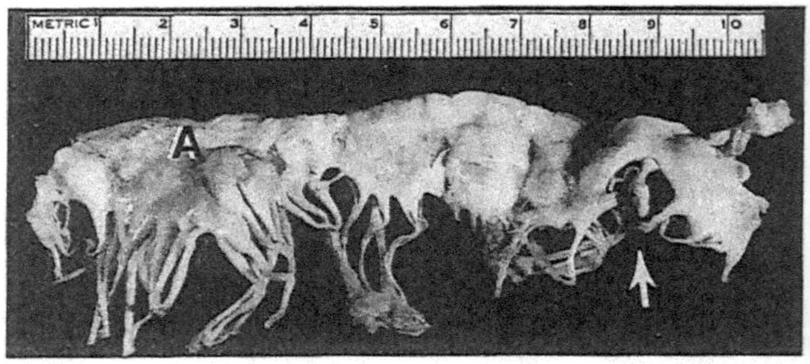

Figure 5. Patient 6. Opened mitral valve from its atrial aspect, showing a large indentation (**arrow**) in the posterior leaflet. Both anterior (A) and posterior leaflets are thickened by fibrous tissue. The indentation represents a site of previous vegetation.

the peak systolic pressure gradient between the left ventricle and a systemic artery. In the three patients who had cardiac catheterization before and after active infective endocarditis, the peak systolic pressure gradient decreased from 90 to 62 mm Hg in Patient 1, from 100 to 5 mm Hg in Patient 4 and from 76 to 55 mm Hg in Patient 6.

Results of cardiac valve replacements. Valve replacement was successful in nine patients. The other two patients (Patients 7 and 11), each of whom died within 30 days of valve replacement, were the only patients who had had partial septectomy and septotomy before cardiac valve replacement. Of the nine hospital survivors after valve replacement (combined with partial septotomy and septectomy in four), eight were in functional class I or II and one was in class III when seen 6 to 21 months after valve replacement, whereas preoperatively three had been in functional class III and five in functional class IV. Cardiac catheterization was performed 6 to 21 months (mean 14 after valve replacement in seven of the nine long-term survivors (Table 3). In three of the seven patients, no lef ventricular outflow tract obstruction was present preopera tively and the postoperative study disclosed no pressure gradient between the left ventricle and a systemic arter during peak systole. In the other four patients, the peak systolic pressure gradient before valve replacement (combined with partial septotomy and septectomy in three patients) decreased from an average of 74 mm Hg (range 62 to 85) preoperatively to ≤5 mm Hg postoperatively.

Discussion

Major findings of present study. Although 30 report describing one or more patients (19 were single case studies with hypertrophic cardiomyopathy and infective endocarditis have appeared (cases tabulated by Alessandri et al. [2]) the presence of infective endocarditis was confirmed anatomically (2–11) only in 15 of the reported 56 cases and i none was the type of valvular damage illustrated. Th present study analyzed 11 patients from the same center wit

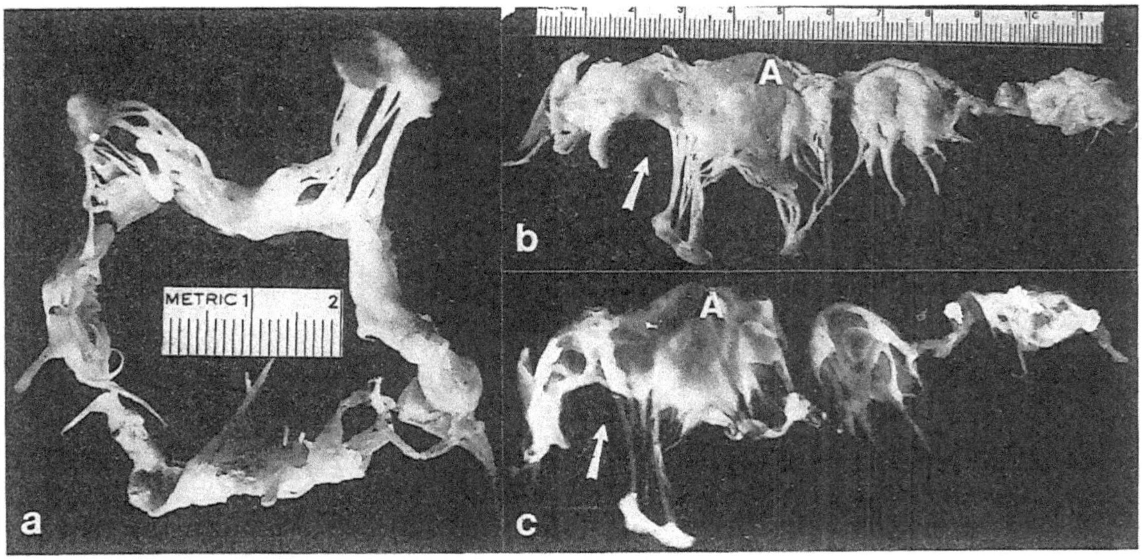

Figure 6. Patient 7. **a,** Unopened mitral valve. **b,** Opened mitral valve showing its atrial aspect. The **arrow** points to an indentation at the junction of the anterior (A) and posterior leaflets. Several chordae tendineae are missing (ruptured) at this site. **c,** Radiograph of the opened mitral valve. Several calcific deposits are present in the annular region of the posterior leaflet.

hypertrophic cardiomyopathy complicated by infective endocarditis necessitating replacement of one or more cardiac valves in each, and in each the operatively excised valve was studied. It is apparent that infective endocarditis should be recognized as a complication of hypertrophic cardiomyopathy and that the latter predisposes to infective endocarditis. The frequency with which the complication occurs is unclear. The present study suggests that among patients with hypertrophic cardiomyopathy with mitral or aortic valve regurgitation, or both, severe enough to warrant valve replacement, infective endocarditis often is responsible for the severe regurgitation. Of the 87 patients with hypertrophic cardiomyopathy who underwent valve replacement at our institution, 11 underwent this procedure because of damage by infective endocarditis. None of the other operatively excised valves had cusp perforations or tears or ruptured chordae tendineae and therefore it is unlikely that any of these other patients had had infective endocarditis at any time.

Location of the vegetations in infective endocarditis complicating hypertrophic cardiomyopathy. The most frequent site of vegetations in patients with hypertrophic cardiomyopathy is the mitral valve and specifically its anterior leaflet. It is this leaflet, of course, which tends to contact the mural endocardium of the ventricular septum during one or both phases of the cardiac cycle and it is likely that vegetations form at these contact sites. Of our 11 patients, 8 had vegetations that left telltale residua of infective endocarditis on the mitral valve (1 also had damage to the aortic valve, but the damage was not diagnostic of healed infective endocarditis [1]) and 3 had both clinical and anatomic evidence of damage to one or more aortic valve cusps by infective endocarditis. The vegetations on the anterior mitral leaflet appear to have been on their ventricular aspects, unlike those in most patients with active infective endocarditis involving the mitral valve. The mechanism of formation of aortic valve vegetations in patients with hypertrophic cardiomyopathy is unclear. In three of our four patients having aortic valve replacement, the left ventricular aortic

Figure 7. Patient 8. Three-cusped aortic valve with severe destruction of one of the three cusps by the infective process.

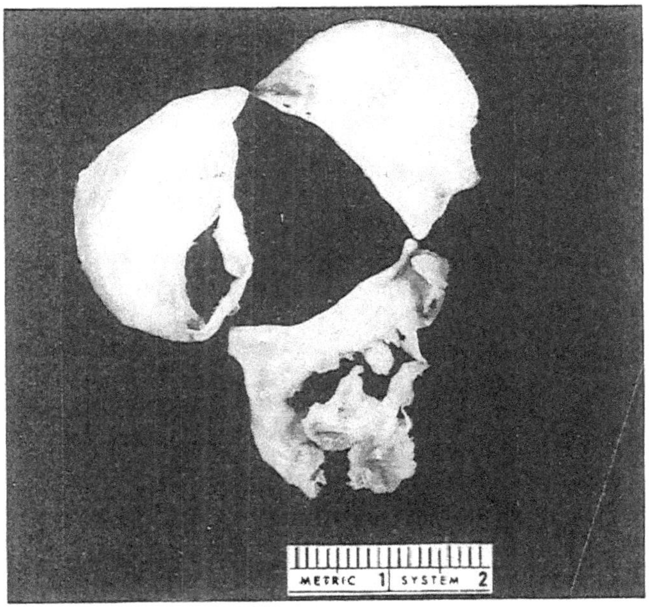

peak systolic pressure gradient was high (70, 78 and 140 mm Hg, respectively), whereas only one of the seven patients with isolated mitral valve replacement had a left ventricular outflow pressure gradient of this magnitude. The vegetations on the aortic valve appear to have been located on the ventricular aspects of these cusps, the usual location of vegetations on this valve.

Valvular regurgitation after infective endocarditis in hypertrophic cardiomyopathy. The present study shows that infective endocarditis complicating hypertrophic cardiomyopathy can result in serious consequences. In all 11 patients, the symptomatic status was unequivocally worsened by active infective endocarditis that healed. Additionally, the intensity of the precordial systolic murmur increased in the patients with infective endocarditis involving the mitral valve, and infective endocarditis involving the aortic valve caused the appearance of a murmur of aortic regurgitation, which was confirmed in each by angiography. The degree of valvular regurgitation was severe in all 11 patients; however, despite the severe degree of regurgitation, the left ventricular cavity immediately before valve replacement was not dilated in any patient on M-mode echocardiography and was only mildly dilated in one of two patients studied by angiography.

Benefit of valve replacement. Despite recognized potential complications of mitral valve replacement in patients with hypertrophic cardiomyopathy (12), the present study indicates that valve replacement for infective endocarditis complicating hypertrophic cardiomyopathy may result in a striking diminution or disappearance of previous symptoms of cardiac dysfunction.

References

1. Roberts WC, Buchbinder NA. Healed left-sided infective endocarditis: a clinicopathologic study of 59 patients. Am J Cardiol 1977;40:876–88.
2. Alessandri N, Pannarale G, del Monte F, Moretti F, Marino B, Reale A. Hypertrophic obstructive cardiomyopathy and infective endocarditis: a report of seven cases and a review of the literature. Eur Heart J 1990;11:1041–8.
3. Nagle JP. Idiopathic hypertrophic subaortic stenosis and bacterial endocarditis. JAMA 1967;200:643–5.
4. Vecht RJ, Oakley CM. Infective endocarditis in three patients with hypertrophic obstructive cardiomyopathy. Br Med J 1968;2:455–9.
5. Caramanian M, Joly F, Fouchard J, Guerinon J. Endocardite infectieuse sur stenose musculaire hypertrophique du ventricule gauche. Arch Mal Coeur 1971;64:1117–31.
6. Chretien EH, Limas C, Garagusi VF. Association of bacterial endocarditis in idiopathic hypertrophic subaortic stenosis. South Med J 1973;66: 269–72.
7. Wang K, Gobel FL, Gleason DF. Bacterial endocarditis in idiopathic hypertrophic subaortic stenosis. Am Heart J 1975;89:359–65.
8. Heret JF, Jandin M, Rigaud M, et al. Endocardite a staphylocoque dore au cours d'une cardiomyopathic obstructive. Arch Mal Coeur 1977;70: 1227–32.
9. Greenland P, Murphy GW. Acute valvular insufficiency complicating hypertrophic obstructive cardiomyopathy. Chest 1979;75:182–3.
10. LeJemtel TH, Factor SM, Koenigsberg M, O'Reilly M, Frater R, Sonnenblick EH. Mural vegetations at the site of endocardial trauma in infective endocarditis complicating idiopathic hypertrophic subaortic stenosis. Am J Cardiol 1979;44:569–74.
11. Pueyo JM, Shahin A, Benazet JM, Camaeno AM, San Miguel JG. Endocarditis infecciosa en estenosis subaortica hipertrofica idiopatica: a proposito de una observacion. Med Clin Barcelona 1981;76:129–31.
12. Roberts WC. Operative treatment of hypertrophic obstructive cardiomyopathy: the case against mitral valve replacement. Am J Cardiol 1973;32: 377–81.

Diversity of Structural Mitral Valve Alterations in Hypertrophic Cardiomyopathy

Heinrich G. Klues, MD; Barry J. Maron, MD;
Allen L. Dollar, MD; and William C. Roberts, MD

Background. **Hypertrophic cardiomyopathy (HCM) is characterized by an asymmetrically hypertrophied left ventricle and is regarded as a disease of cardiac muscle.**

Methods and Results. **To assess the possibility that the mitral valve itself may be involved in the disease process, we studied mitral valves from 94 patients with HCM and 45 normal control subjects. The area of the mitral leaflets was increased in patients with HCM compared with control subjects (12.9±3.7 versus 8.7±2.0 cm²; $p<0.001$). For the overall group of patients, this increase was largely caused by an increase in anterior leaflet length (2.2±0.5 cm for HCM versus 1.8±0.3 cm for control subjects; $p<0.001$), because circumference did not differ between the two groups. Mitral leaflet area was increased (≥12.0 cm²) in 55 (58%) of the 94 valves. In 12 of these 55 valves, both the anterior and posterior leaflets were enlarged; the other 43 valves had asymmetrical or segmental enlargement of either the anterior leaflet (36 patients) or a portion of posterior leaflet (seven patients). In addition, nine patients had a congenital malformation of the mitral apparatus in which one or both papillary muscles inserted directly into anterior mitral leaflet (mitral valve area was normal in seven of the nine).**

Conclusions. **Sixty-two (66%) of 94 mitral valves had a constellation of structural malformations, including increased leaflet area and elongation of the leaflets or anomalous papillary muscle insertion directly into anterior mitral leaflet. These findings expand the morphological definition of HCM by demonstrating that the disease process is not confined to cardiac muscle but rather many patients also have structural abnormalities of the mitral valve that are unlikely to be acquired or secondary to mechanical factors. (*Circulation* 1992;85:1651–1660)**

KEY WORDS • hypertrophy • cardiomyopathies • valves • genetics • left ventricle

Hypertrophic cardiomyopathy (HCM) is considered to be a primary disease of cardiac muscle characterized by a diverse morphological and clinical spectrum.[1–7] It is generally accepted as a basic tenet of HCM that left ventricular hypertrophy represents both the gross anatomic marker and is probably the principal determinant of the clinical and pathophysiological features of the disease.[2–8] Most morphological reports of HCM have described the mitral valve as being intrinsically normal, with only focal secondary thickening of the leaflets and chordae tendineae.[1,2,6,9,10] Anecdotal descriptions, however, have suggested that the mitral valve may be congenitally abnormal in some patients with HCM.[11–16] To resolve this issue, we systematically examined mitral valves in a large number of patients with HCM.

Methods

Selection of Case Material

Patients with HCM. The files of the Pathology Branch from 1982 to 1989 were reviewed. Eighty-two mitral valves previously excised surgically from patients with HCM had been accessioned; 66 had been removed intact and were in suitable condition for study. Of the 66 valves, one had morphological features of mitral prolapse[17–21] and was excluded, reducing the number of operative specimens to 65. These valves had been surgically excised from severely symptomatic patients with HCM undergoing mitral valve replacement to relieve obstruction to left ventricular outflow[15,22–24]; each operation had been performed by the same surgeon (Dr. Charles L. McIntosh). Each mitral valve specimen consisted of both leaflets, the attached chordae tendineae, and in some instances portions of the papillary muscles. To include mitral valves from patients with nonobstructive HCM, as well as patients with obstruction who had not undergone mitral valve replacement, 29 heart specimens with HCM also were selected from the files of the Pathology Branch by virtue of suitable condition for study and a recent complete hemodynamic or echocardiographic evaluation. Of these 29 patients, seven died after ventricular septal myotomy/myectomy (four within 30 days of operation and three later). None of the other 22 had a cardiac operation; 11 died suddenly, seven of progressive congestive heart failure and four of noncardiac causes. Mitral valves were excised from these 29 hearts (as well as 45 controls), with care taken to remove the leaflets from their circumferential attachments along the annular margin, leaving a 2–3-mm border as done by the

From the Pathology and Cardiology Branches, National Heart, Lung, and Blood Institute, National Institutes of Health, Bethesda, Md.

Address for correspondence: Barry J. Maron, MD, Cardiology Branch, National Institutes of Health, Building 10, Room 7B-15, Bethesda, MD 20892.

Received May 13, 1991; revision accepted January 7, 1992.

surgeon in excising the valves at operation. Thus, the 65 mitral valves removed at surgery and the 29 removed after death constitute the overall study group of 94 valves.

In each study patient, diagnosis of HCM was based on the presence of a hypertrophied nondilated left ventricle in the absence of another cardiac or systemic disease capable of producing the magnitude of hypertrophy present in that patient[8]; in addition, each patient had typical necropsy and/or clinical features of HCM.[2–8] The magnitude of the left ventricular outflow gradient was assessed at cardiac catheterization in 89 of 94 patients, including all 65 with mitral valve replacement. In the other five patients, basal left ventricular outflow gradients were estimated by Doppler echocardiography.[25,26] Of these five patients, four had no evidence of basal outflow obstruction; each was also judged to be free of significant provocable obstruction on the basis of the absence of ventricular septal endocardial plaque and the presence of nonthickened mitral leaflets at necropsy.[2,4,6]

Patients were classified as obstructive if the subaortic peak systolic pressure gradient was >30 mm Hg under basal conditions and/or with provocative maneuvers or as nonobstructive if the subaortic gradient was absent under basal conditions and <30 mm Hg with provocation (Table 1).

Control patients. Mitral valves from 45 consecutively studied patients with entirely normal hearts, both functionally and anatomically, were chosen as control subjects (Table 1). All 45 patients died from noncardiac conditions. In each control patient, heart weight was ≤350 g in men and ≤300 g in women. The 45 patients ranged in age from 15 to 74 years (mean, 45); 24 were men, and 21 were women.

Morphometry

Mitral valves were fixed in 10% buffered formalin after their removal at operation. Valves were introduced to the fixative freely without stretching or manipulation. Tissue specimens were placed in an opened position on a cutting board and extended to full length (i.e., circumference) with the atrial aspect exposed. Usually it was necessary to affix the opened valve directly to the board with pins to flatten the specimen.

The following morphological measurements (Figure 1)[27] were made directly from the mitral valve specimen: 1) circumference of the valve annulus measured along its margin of attachment; 2) and 3) maximum lengths of anterior and posterior leaflets (from attachment margin to free edge); 4) thickness of the anterior leaflet; 5) weight of the excised valve; and 6) areas of the leaflets, both together and separately. To assess mitral leaflet area (in square centimeters), borders of the opened valves were traced with a fine-tipped pen on an acetate overlay. The areas of the leaflets were then planimeterized. Maximal thickness of anterior leaflet was measured with an adjustable caliper. Mitral valves were weighed on a scale accurate to 0.1 g.

Reproducibility

Interobserver and intraobserver variability for measurement of mitral leaflet area was tested in a subset of 20 valves (14 with HCM and six normal control subjects). To determine interobserver variability, two observers (H.G.K. and A.L.D.) independently measured the mitral valves. To determine intraobserver variability, one observer (H.G.K.) measured mitral leaflet area on two occasions 4 months apart.

Histology

Twenty-two mitral valves from patients with HCM (10 obstructive and 12 nonobstructive) and 12 from normal control subjects were studied by light microscopy. Longitudinal sections were taken in the midportion of the anterior leaflet as well as in the most elongated portion of the posterior leaflet in 22 valves. Tissue was embedded in paraffin and sectioned at 6 μm. Two histology sections were prepared: one was stained by the Movat method and one with hematoxylin and eosin. The extent of mucopolysaccharide deposition was assessed in qualitative terms from the histological sections.

Statistical Analyses

Data were expressed as mean±SD. Differences in morphological measurements between groups of patients were assessed by unpaired Student's t test. Proportions were compared by the χ^2 test, and other selected comparisons were assessed with one-way ANOVA. Relations between selected parameters or variables were assessed by linear regression analysis. A stepwise regression analysis[28] was used to determine the association between mitral leaflet area and several clinical and morphological variables in patients with HCM and in normal controls (i.e., age, sex, body height and weight, heart weight, previous ventricular septal myotomy/myectomy, left ventricular wall thickness and end-diastolic cavity dimension, magnitude of mitral regurgitation, left ventricular systolic pressure, and outflow gradient).

Results

Group Analysis of Mitral Valve Morphology

Mitral leaflet area. In the 94 patients with HCM, the mitral leaflet area ranged from 6.3 to 23.0 cm^2 (mean, 12.9±3.7 cm^2) and significantly exceeded that of normal control subjects (4.7–13.0 cm^2; mean, 8.7±2.0 cm^2; $p<0.001$) (Figures 2 and 3; Table 1). In 44 (47%) of the 94 valves, total leaflet area exceeded that of the largest control valve. Mitral leaflet area was significantly smaller in valves removed from patients at surgery (12.0±3.5 cm^2) than in those obtained at necropsy (14.6±3.3 cm^2; $p<0.001$) (Tables 2 and 3).

Valve length. In patients with HCM, the lengths of the anterior and posterior leaflets were 1.0–3.4 cm (mean, 2.2±0.5 cm) and 0.7–2.4 cm (mean, 1.4±0.4 cm), respectively, and both significantly exceeded values for normal controls (Figure 4; Table 1).

Valve circumference. Mitral valve circumference was similar in the overall group of 94 patients with HCM (5.5–12.8 cm; mean, 8.5±1.7 cm) and in normal controls (6.4–9.5 cm; mean, 8.2±2.8 cm; $p>0.05$) (Figure 5; Table 1).

Mitral valve weight and thickness. Mitral valves from patients with HCM were thicker and heavier than those from controls (by about 2:1) (Table 1).

Table 1. Clinical, Hemodynamic, and Morphometric Data in Patients With HCM and in Normal Controls

	All HCM patients	Control subjects	p	Obstructive group	Nonobstructive group	p
Patients (n)	94	45	. . .	77 (82%)	17 (18%)	. . .
Surgically excised valves	65	0	. . .	65	0	. . .
Age (mean±SD years) (range)	43±15 (15–77)	45±17 (15–74)	NS	45±15 (15–77)	34±12 (18–54)	NS
Male:female, n (%)	48 (51%): 46 (49%)	24 (53%): 21 (47%)	NS	41 (53%): 36 (47%)	7 (41%): 10 (59%)	NS
Systemic hypertension	6 (6%)	0	NS	5 (6%)	1 (6%)	NS
One or more major coronary arteries narrowed >50% (angiography), n (%)	13 (14%)	0	<0.01	12 (16%)	1 (6%)	<0.01
LV-SA gradient (mm Hg)*						
Basal	52±47	. . .	. . .	69±43	0	<0.001
Provoked	85±55	. . .	. . .	110±36	5±8	<0.001
Operation						
MVR	52 (55%)	0	. . .	52 (68%)	0	. . .
M&M	7 (7%)†	0	. . .	7 (9%)†	0	. . .
M&M plus MVR	13 (10%)†	0	. . .	13 (17%)†	0	. . .
New York Heart Association functional class:						
I	7 (7%)	45	<0.001	1 (1%)	6 (35%)	<0.001
II	8 (9%)	0		6 (8%)	2 (12%)	
III	70 (74%)	0		61 (79%)	9 (53%)	
IV	9 (10%)	0		9 (12%)	0	
Echo measurements (mm)						
Septal thickness	21±6	. . .	. . .	20±5	24±8	<0.05
Free wall thickness	14±4	. . .	. . .	13±4	16±5	<0.05
Mitral valve measurements						
Areas (cm^2)						
Anterior leaflet	5.9±1.7	4.3±1.0	<0.001	5.7±1.7	6.7±1.4	<0.05
Posterior leaflet	2.6±1.1	1.7±0.5	<0.001	2.5±1.1	2.9±1.0	NS
Total leaflet	12.9±3.7	8.7±2.0	<0.001	12.4±3.7	14.4±3.2	<0.05
Circumference (cm)	8.5±1.7	8.2±2.8	NS	8.2±1.6	9.8±1.5	<0.001
Lengths (cm)						
Anterior leaflet	2.2±0.5	1.8±0.3	<0.001	2.1±0.5	2.4±0.3	<0.01
Posterior leaflet	1.4±0.4	1.1±0.2	<0.001	1.4±0.4	1.6±0.4	<0.05
Weight (g)	2.0±0.7	1.0±0.3	<0.001	2.1±0.7	1.3±0.6	<0.001
Thickness, anterior leaflet (mm)	2.1±0.9	1.1±0.4	<0.001	2.4±0.8	1.0±0.4	<0.001
Valves with increased area (>12.0 cm^2), n (%)	55 (59%)	1 (2%)	<0.001	40 (52%)	15 (88%)	<0.01
Valves with papillary muscle insertion, n (%)	9 (10%)	1 (2%)	<0.01	9 (12%)	0	NS
Heart weight (g)‡	597±164	271±45	<0.001	673±127	543±167	<0.05

HCM, hypertrophic cardiomyopathy; LV-SA, left ventricle to systemic artery; MVR, mitral valve replacement; M&M, ventricular septal myotomy/myectomy.

*Determined by cardiac catheterization in 89 patients (95%) and by Doppler echocardiography in five patients (5%).

†Twenty patients with a previous ventricular septal myotomy/myectomy showed no difference in anterior, posterior, and total mitral leaflet area, circumference, lengths of anterior and posterior leaflets, valve weight, and thickness of anterior leaflet compared with the remaining 57 obstructed patients without myotomy/myectomy.

‡Heart weight available only in the 29 necropsy patients.

. . . , Not applicable or complete data not available.

Individual Patient Analysis of Mitral Valve Morphology

Mitral valve size. Mitral leaflet area exceeded the 95th percentile of the normal control valves (≥12.0 cm^2) in 55 (59%) of 94 patients and was <12.0 cm^2 in the other 39 (41%). Consequently, the 55 mitral valves ≥12.0 cm^2 were considered to be increased in size, while the other valves were judged to be of normal size. Also, mitral leaflet area exceeded the greatest value in the control group (i.e., 13.0 cm^2) in 44 (47%) of 94 patients (Figure 3). In 36 of the 55 enlarged valves, only the anterior leaflet was increased in size (area>5.0 cm^2; normal <4.6

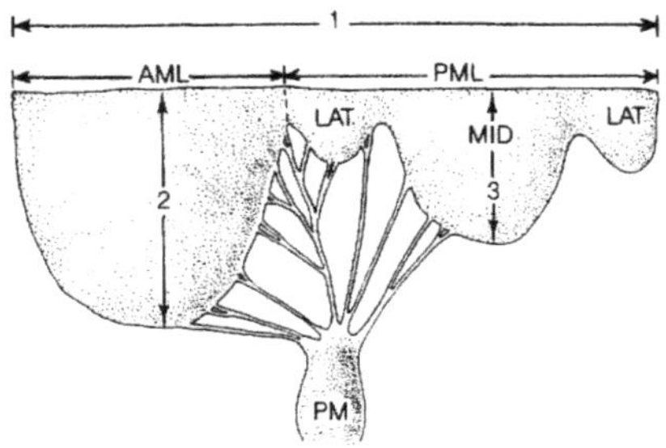

FIGURE 1. *Schematic of an opened normal mitral valve showing anterior (AML) and posterior (PML) mitral valve leaflets. Posterior leaflet is composed of two lateral (LAT) scallops and a middle (MID) scallop. 1, Total circumference of valve along annular margin; 2 and 3, lengths of anterior and posterior leaflets. Anatomic demarcation of anterior mitral leaflet from posterior leaflet was made visually, usually by identification of insertion of a fanlike arrangement of commissural chordae between the two.*[27] *PM, papillary muscle.*

cm²); in seven other valves, only the posterior leaflet was increased in size (area >2.5 cm²; normal <1.9 cm²), often caused by segmental elongation of one scallop of the leaflet (length 85–113% of anterior leaflet length); in the remaining 12 valves both mitral leaflets were enlarged.

Mitral valves were without the morphological features of mitral valve prolapse,[17–21] such as ballooning and redundancy of the leaflets, increased annular circumference, and apparent elongation of the chordae tendineae. Analysis of Movat-stained histological sections showed that none of the patients with HCM studied had increased amounts of mucopolysaccharide compared with normal control subjects.

Anomalous papillary muscle insertion. In nine of the 94 patients with HCM (each with basal outflow obstruction), the head of one or both papillary muscles inserted directly into the ventricular aspect of anterior mitral leaflet, involving the anterolateral or posteromedial commissural region but also extending to adjacent portions of the leaflets (Figure 6).[29] Chordae tendineae were absent in the region of anomalous papillary muscle insertion but appeared normal in other areas. Mitral leaflet size was normal (<12.0 cm²) in seven and mildly increased in two (12.2 and 13.0 cm²).

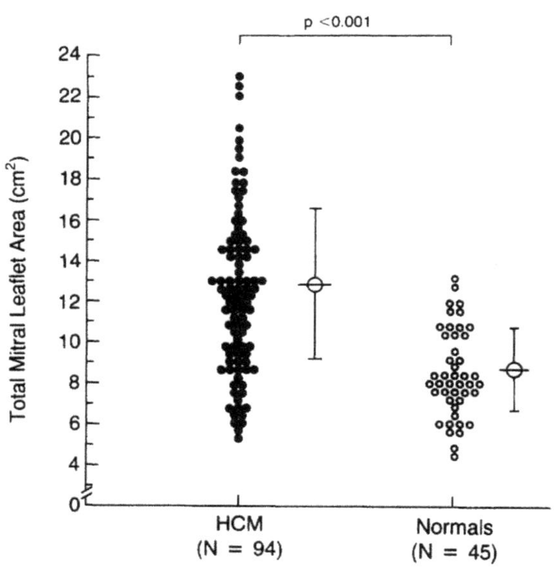

FIGURE 2. *Scatterplot of total area of mitral valve leaflets in patients with hypertrophic cardiomyopathy (HCM) and normal controls.*

Reproducibility

Analysis of interobserver variability showed small differences in mitral leaflet area between the two observers (0.56±1.4 cm²). Linear regression analysis relating the two measurements showed a correlation coefficient of 0.91. Analysis of intraobserver variability also showed small differences in mitral leaflet area between the two observations (0.25±0.9 cm²); linear regression analysis showed a correlation coefficient of 0.97.

Other Valvular Abnormalities

Scallops. Of the 94 mitral valves, 34 (36%) had an increased number of posterior leaflet scallops (either four or five) that were of similar size; the circumference and mitral valve area of these 34 valves (8.9±1.6 cm and 12.9±3.4 cm², respectively) did not differ significantly from those of the other 60 valves (8.4±1.6 cm and 12.3±3.2 cm², respectively). In contrast, only two of the 45 control valves (4%) had more than three posterior leaflet scallops ($p<0.001$).

Fibrous thickening. Of the 94 patients, 38 had no or only focal thickening of the anterior mitral leaflet (usually at the free leaflet edge) that occupied <50% of total leaflet area. In the other 56 valves, the fibrous thickening was more diffuse, often involved most of the leaflet, and was judged to be of secondary origin.[2,6,9]

Markedly different patterns of fibrous thickening were observed in obstructive and nonobstructive patients. The 17 nonobstructive patients had either no or only mild focal thickening; each of the 77 patients with obstruction had mild or diffuse thickening ($p<0.001$). In the subgroup of 38 study patients with no or mild focal anterior leaflet thickening, mitral leaflet area (13.9±3.7 cm²) exceeded that of normal control subjects (8.7±2.0 cm²; $p<0.001$) (Table 4).

Comparison of Obstructive and Nonobstructive Patients

When the 17 patients without outflow obstruction were compared with the combined obstructive group of 77 patients (12 necropsy and 65 surgical), nonobstructive patients proved to have larger leaflet area, circumference, and length (Table 1).

Relation of Mitral Valve Size to Clinical and Morphological Features

The relation of mitral valve area to clinical and pathological variables was analyzed by stepwise regression analysis separately for patients with mitral valve replacement and those studied at necropsy. In patients with mitral valve replacement, leaflet area was inversely related to female sex and directly related to body height ($p=0.041$ and $p=0.014$, respectively; multiple $r^2=0.24$); in necropsy patients, leaflet area was inversely related only to female sex ($p<0.001$). In both analyses, the body

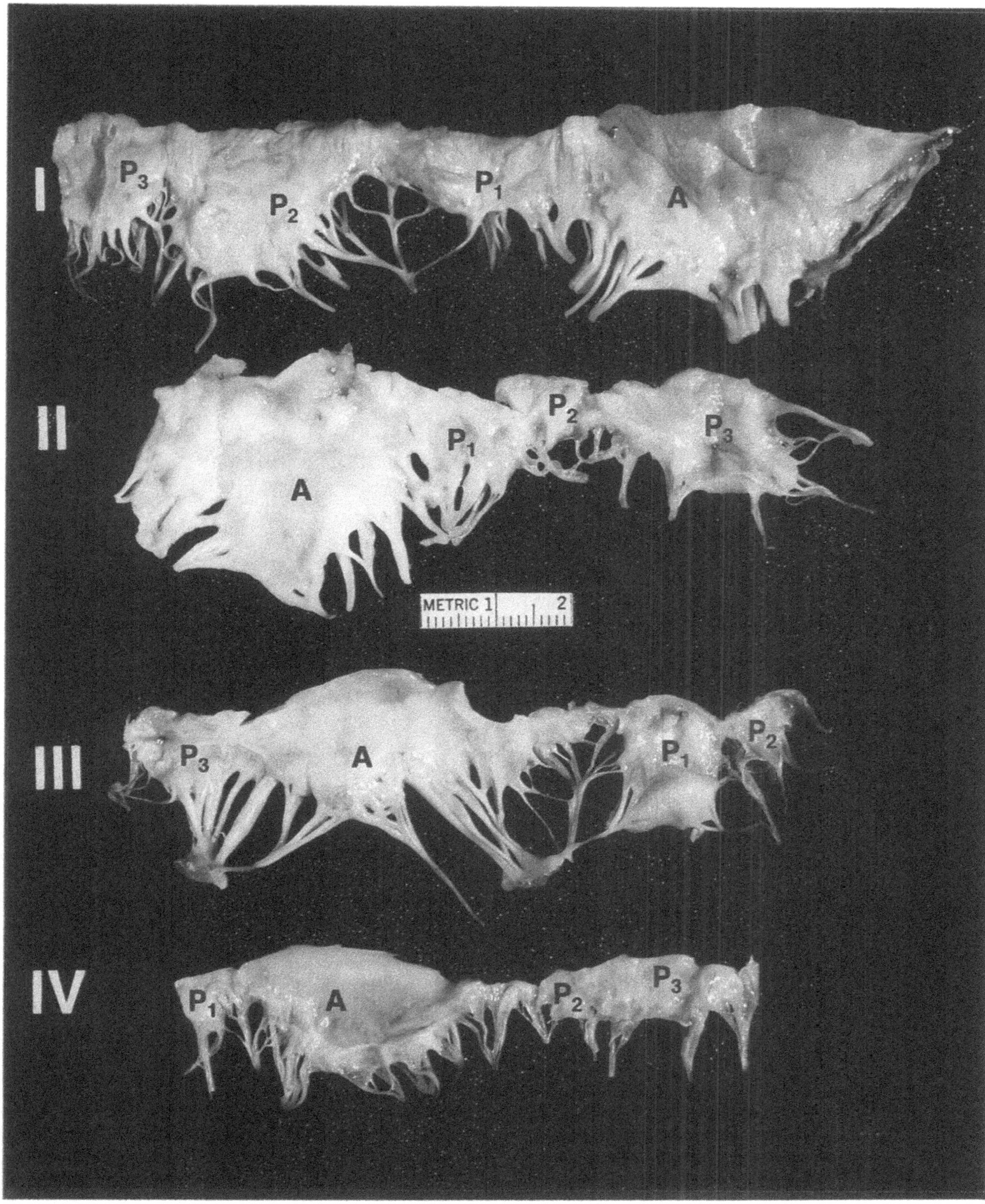

FIGURE 3. *Photographs of mitral valves from three patients with obstructive hypertrophic cardiomyopathy aged 31, 29, and 60 years (I, II, and III) and from a normal control patient without cardiovascular disease (IV) showing variation in valvular size and structure. Valves have been opened with the circumference displayed in a horizontal orientation, exposing the atrial surface. I, Large valve (area, 22 cm²) in which both the anterior (A) and posterior (P) leaflets are greatly elongated and increased in area. II, Large valve in which increased valve size (area, 18 cm²) is caused primarily by elongation and enlargement of the anterior leaflet. III, Segmental elongation and increased area confined to a lateral scallop of posterior mitral leaflet, which has virtually the same length as the normal-size anterior leaflet. IV, Valve is normal in area (i.e., 11 cm²), length, and thickness.*

TABLE 2. Comparison of Patients With HCM Who Had Mitral Valves Removed Surgically With Those With Mitral Valves Removed at Necropsy

	Mitral valves removed surgically	Mitral valves removed at necropsy	p
Patients (n)	65 (69%)	29 (31%)	. . .
Age (mean±SD years)	47±14	36±14	<0.001
Male:female, n (%)	32 (49%):33 (51%)	17 (59%):12 (41%)	NS
LV-SA peak systolic gradient (mm Hg)			
Basal	71±45	24±34	<0.001
Provoked	111±37	33±48	<0.001
New York Heart Association functional class			
I	0	7	<0.001
II	3	5	
III/IV	62	17	
Echo measurements			
Septal thickness (mm)	19±4	25±7	<0.001
Free wall thickness (mm)	13±3	16±5	<0.001
Mitral valve measurements			
Areas (cm^2)			
Anterior mitral leaflet	5.4±1.5	7.0±1.6	<0.001
Posterior mitral leaflet	2.4±1.1	3.0±1.0	<0.02
Total leaflets	12.0±3.5	14.6±3.3	<0.001
Circumference (cm)	8.0±1.5	9.7±1.6	<0.001
Lengths (cm)			
Anterior mitral leaflet	2.0±0.5	2.5±0.3	<0.001
Posterior mitral leaflet	1.3±0.4	1.6±0.4	<0.001
Weight (g)	2.2±0.7	1.6±0.7	<0.001
Thickness (mm) (anterior leaflet)	2.4±0.8	1.4±0.9	<0.001

HCM, hypertrophic cardiomyopathy; LV-SA, left ventricle to systemic artery.
. . . , Not applicable.

height and/or gender accounted for only 24% of the observed variability in mitral valve area.

The relation between mitral leaflet area and heart weight in patients with HCM was not significant; correlation coefficients were 0.36 (p=0.054), although there was a significant correlation between these two parameters in normal controls (correlation coefficient, 0.40; p=0.01). For the overall group, there was no linear relation between mitral leaflet area and either age, magnitude of mitral regurgitation or outflow tract gradient, left ventricular cavity size, or wall thickness. Sixteen female patients >50 years old had the smallest mitral valves, with leaflet areas significantly less than those for the other 78 patients (11.0±2.5 versus 13.2±3.8 cm^2; $p<0.05$).

Histological Findings

Valves from patients with obstructive HCM had histological changes judged to be secondary in origin. Normal leaflet architecture remained largely intact, although the thickness of the fibrosa was markedly increased because of increased amounts of fibrous tissue that appeared in a pattern of parallel layers with varying density. In contrast, the spongiosa layer was decreased in thickness, with reduced amounts of elastic fibers. Patients with nonobstructive HCM had a histological mitral valve structure similar to that of the control subjects.

Discussion

Hypertrophic cardiomyopathy is generally regarded as an inheritable disease of cardiac muscle.[3–5,30] Most pathophysiological consequences of HCM have been ascribed largely to the asymmetrically thickened left ventricular muscle, which is the most characteristic morphological marker of this disease.[1,2,4–6,31–33] For many years, the mitral valve has been known to play an important role in hemodynamic alterations by producing systolic anterior motion, midsystolic contact with the ventricular septum, and consequently dynamic obstruction to left ventricular outflow.[11,16,34–40] The question of whether or not the mitral valve is altered as part of the basic disease process in HCM has never been studied systematically or resolved. Indeed, most previously reported observations made either at necropsy or surgery have described the mitral valve as virtually free of intrinsic disease (although often secondarily thickened).[1,2,6,9,10] Isolated observations in selected patients with HCM, however, have described structural abnormalities of the mitral valve that appear to be congenital and are associated with systolic anterior motion and outflow obstruction.[11–16]

The findings of the present study of almost 100 mitral valves removed at necropsy or at surgery provide substantial evidence for important structural abnormalities of the mitral valve in HCM that do not appear to be of

TABLE 3. Patients With HCM and Obstruction to Left Ventricular Outflow: Comparison of Mitral Valves Removed Surgically With Those Removed at Necropsy

	Mitral valves removed surgically	Mitral valves removed at necropsy	*p*
Patients (*n*)	65	12	. . .
Age (mean±SD years)	47±14	38±16	NS
Male:female, *n* (%)	32 (49%):33 (51%)	9 (75%):3 (25%)	NS
LV-SA peak systolic gradient (mm Hg)			
Basal	71±45	60±26	NS
Provoked	111±37	102±26	NS
New York Heart Association functional class			
I	0	1	<0.01
II	3	3	
III/IV	62	8	
Echo measurements			
Septal thickness (mm)	19±4	27±5	<0.001
Free wall thickness (mm)	13±3	17±5	<0.05
Mitral valve measurements			
Areas (cm^2)			
Anterior mitral leaflet	5.4±1.5	7.4±1.7	<0.001
Posterior mitral leaflet	2.4±1.1	3.1±1.1	NS
Total leaflets	12.0±3.5	14.8±3.7	<0.05
Circumference (cm)	8.0±1.5	9.6±1.8	<0.01
Lengths (cm)			
Anterior mitral leaflet	2.0±0.5	2.6±0.3	<0.001
Posterior mitral leaflet	1.3±0.4	1.6±0.4	<0.05
Weight (g)	2.2±0.7	2.1±0.5	NS
Thickness (mm) (anterior leaflet)	2.4±0.8	2.0±1.0	NS

HCM, hypertrophic cardiomyopathy; LV-SA, left ventricle to systemic artery.
. . . , Not applicable.

acquired origin. Indeed, these observations would appear to expand the basic morphological definition of HCM, and representing an evolution of the precept that this disease is structurally confined to cardiac muscle. Mitral leaflet area was significantly greater in our patients with HCM than in control patients without car-

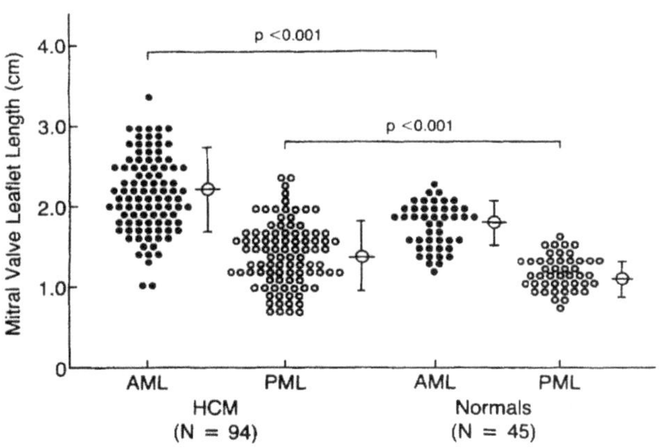

FIGURE 4. *Scatterplot of mitral valve leaflet lengths shown separately for both anterior (AML) and posterior mitral leaflets (PML) in patients with hypertrophic cardiomyopathy (HCM) and normal controls.*

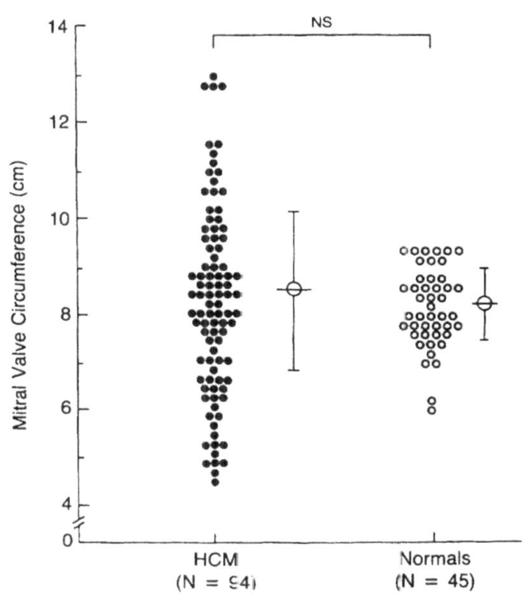

FIGURE 5. *Scatterplot of mitral valve circumference in patients with hypertrophic cardiomyopathy (HCM) and normal controls.*

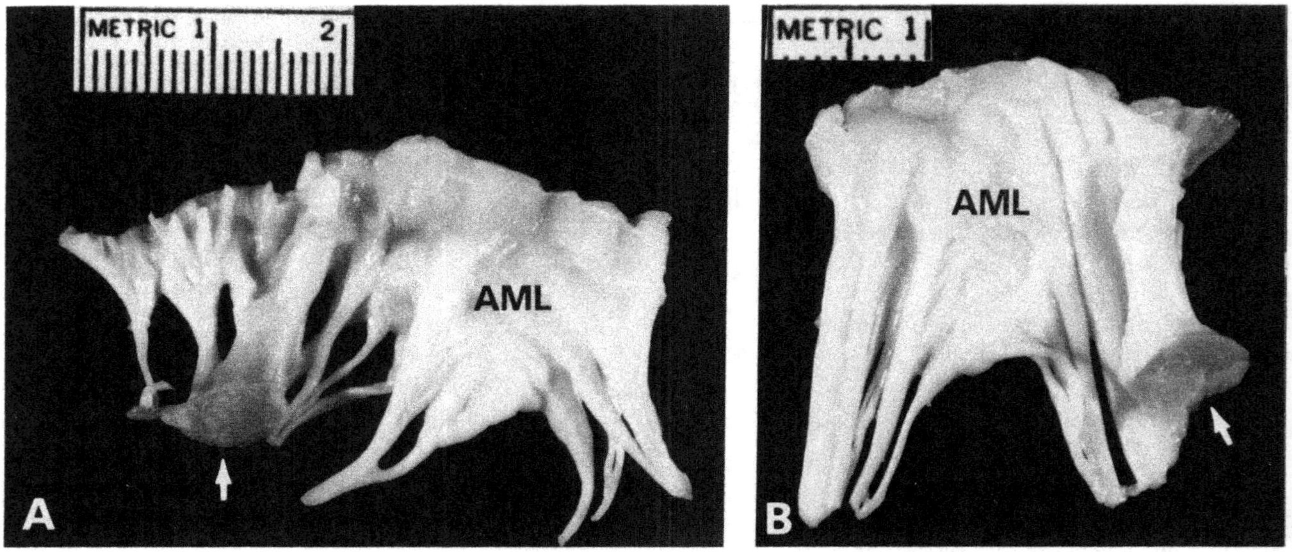

FIGURE 6. *Photographs of mitral valve specimens (with ventricular aspect exposed) excised at operation from a 31-year-old man* (panel A) *and a 62-year-old woman* (panel B), *both with obstructive HCM, showing anomalous papillary muscle insertion directly into anterior mitral leaflet. Panel A: Papillary muscle (arrow) insertion is largely confined to the area of the posteromedial commissure but spares the distal margin of anterior leaflet. Panel B: Papillary muscle (arrow) inserts into the anterolateral commissural region and also occupies substantial portions of the anterior mitral leaflet (AML).*

diovascular disease. The patients with HCM also showed considerable variability with respect to mitral valve structure and size. About 60% of all mitral valves were enlarged (some up to twice the normal leaflet area), and only about 40% were within the 95% confidence limits of the normal control valves (<12.0 cm^2). For the overall group of patients with HCM, the increased mitral leaflet size was largely a result of an increase in leaflet length (from margin of attachment to free margin).

In addition to increased overall mitral valve size, leaflet elongation, and asymmetrical (segmental) enlargement of either the anterior or a portion of the posterior leaflet, other structural malformations of the

TABLE 4. Comparison of Control Subjects and Patients With HCM Having No or Mild Focal Fibrous Mitral Valve Thickening

	Control subjects	HCM with no or mild focal fibrous thickening	*p*
Patients (*n*)	45	38	. . .
Age (mean±SD years)	45±17	38±14	<0.05
Male:female, *n* (%)	24 (53%):21 (47%)	24 (53%):21 (47%)	NS
New York Heart Association functional class			
I	45	6	<0.001
II	0	4	
III/IV	0	28	
Heart weight (g)	271±45	561±161	<0.001
Mitral valve measurements			
Areas (cm^2)			
Anterior mitral leaflet	4.3±1.0	6.5±1.7	<0.001
Posterior mitral leaflet	1.7±0.5	2.8±1.1	<0.001
Total leaflets	8.7±2.0	13.9±3.7	<0.001
Circumference (cm)	8.2±2.8	9.3±1.7	<0.001
Lengths (cm)			
Anterior mitral leaflet	1.8±0.3	2.4±0.5	<0.001
Posterior mitral leaflet	1.1±0.2	1.5±0.4	<0.001
Weight (g)	1.0±0.3	1.6±0.7	<0.001
Thickness (mm) (anterior leaflet)	1.1±0.4	1.3±0.5	NS

HCM, hypertrophic cardiomyopathy; LV-SA, left ventricle to systemic artery.
. . . , Not applicable.

mitral valve were found that are not readily explained as secondary or acquired abnormalities. About 10% of the patients studied had a congenital malformation of the mitral apparatus characterized by direct insertion of one or both papillary muscles into anterior mitral leaflet.[29,41] Thus, two thirds of our study patients had increased mitral leaflet size or a structural valve malformation that is likely to have been present from birth. Furthermore, multiple regression analysis of a variety of clinical, morphological, and hemodynamic parameters that theoretically could have influenced mitral leaflet area and shape showed that the combined impact of all such variables accounted for no more than about 25% of the observed variability in valve size. In addition, mitral leaflet enlargement could not be explained on the basis of fibrous thickening alone (secondary to traumatic septal contact), because our subset of 38 study patients with either no or minimal mitral valve thickening nevertheless had mitral valve areas that were also significantly greater than those of the normal controls.

Although we cannot exclude with absolute certainty the hypothesis that other undefined mechanical factors related to the complex left ventricular geometry in HCM influenced mitral valve structure, it is difficult to conceive of secondary mechanisms by which malformations such as direct anomalous papillary muscle insertion into anterior mitral leaflet or particularly enlarged and elongated mitral leaflets (>13 cm^2 in area) could have been acquired. Even if some of the mitral valve abnormalities described in the present report are not primary, our findings would nevertheless represent a major conceptual departure by expanding the basic morphological definition of HCM beyond the ventricular myocardium to the mitral valve.

The size of the mitral leaflets does not, however, appear to be the sole determinant of outflow obstruction in patients with HCM. Indeed, in those patients without outflow obstruction, mean mitral leaflet area was actually slightly greater than in patients with obstruction; also, more than 70% of the nonobstructive patients had enlarged valves, and there was no identifiable relation between the magnitude of outflow gradient and mitral leaflet area. The explanation for the absence of outflow obstruction in some patients with enlarged valves probably lies with the observation that variables other than mitral leaflet area and length may also be important determinants of obstruction—e.g., increased ejection velocity,[25,26,35] reduced outflow tract area,[39] anterior displacement of mitral valve and papillary muscles within the left ventricular cavity,[40,42–44] and probably also basal ventricular septal thickness.[43] Undoubtedly, mitral valve systolic anterior motion (and outflow obstruction) results from a complex interplay between a number of these variables, in addition to mitral valve size.

In the present study, we have demonstrated considerable variability in mitral valve structure among patients with HCM. However, the mitral valve alterations identified are not unique to this disease. Patients with mitral valve prolapse, for example, also have increased mitral leaflet size.[17–21] Increased leaflet area in "floppy" mitral prolapse valves, however, is associated with distinctive morphological features not present in our HCM valves, such as leaflet ballooning, elongated chordae, and excessive mucopolysaccharide deposition.[17–20] Furthermore, valves producing mitral prolapse also show a marked increase in circumference[21] not characteristic of most mitral valves in HCM. Finally, preoperative echocardiograms recorded in each of our 65 patients with mitral valve replacement did not show evidence of mitral valve prolapse motion pattern. Therefore, there is no convincing evidence that the structurally abnormal mitral valves present in our patients represent examples of the primary floppy mitral valve, itself an uncommon occurrence in patients with HCM.[45]

The findings of the present study also have potentially relevant implications with regard to the pathogenesis of HCM. Recently, mutations in the gene that encodes for the heavy chains of cardiac myosin (localized to chromosome 14) have been identified in members of families with HCM.[46–48] However, to date, not all families with HCM studied appear to show this abnormality,[49] and therefore the broad morphological spectrum and clinical heterogeneity of HCM ultimately may not be explained solely by a myosin defect. Indeed, the findings of the present study that focus on structural valve abnormalities represent an evolution in our understanding of the complex nature of HCM and raise the possibility that the disease process is not limited to myocardium (and a defect in myosin) in all patients.

Acknowledgment

We wish to recognize the expert photographic assistance of Mr. Michael Spencer.

References

1. Teare D: Asymmetrical hypertrophy of the heart in young adults. *Br Heart J* 1958;20:1–8
2. Roberts CS, Roberts WC: Morphologic features, in Zipes DP, Rowlands DJ (eds): *Progress in Cardiology* 2/2. Philadelphia, Pa, Lea & Febiger, 1989, pp 3–32
3. Braunwald E, Lambrew CT, Rockoff SD, Ross J Jr, Morrow AG: Idiopathic hypertrophic subaortic stenosis: I. A description of the disease based upon an analysis of 64 patients. *Circulation* 1964; 30(suppl IV):IV-3–IV-119
4. Wigle ED, Sasson Z, Henderson MA, Rudd TD, Fulop J, Rakowski H, Williams WG: Hypertrophic cardiomyopathy: The importance of the site and the extent of hypertrophy: A review. *Prog Cardiovasc Dis* 1985;28:1–83
5. Maron BJ, Bonow RO, Cannon RO, Leon MB, Epstein SE: Hypertrophic cardiomyopathy: Interrelation of clinical manifestations, pathophysiology, and therapy. *N Engl J Med* 1987;316: 780–789, 844–852
6. Olsen EG: Anatomic and light microscopic characterization of hypertrophic obstructive and nonobstructive cardiomyopathy. *Eur Heart J* 1983;4(suppl F):1–6
7. Maron BJ, Roberts WC: Quantitative analysis of cardiac muscle cell disorganization in the ventricular septum of patients with hypertrophic cardiomyopathy. *Circulation* 1979;59:689–706
8. Maron BJ, Epstein SE: Hypertrophic cardiomyopathy: A discussion of nomenclature. *Am J Cardiol* 1979;43:1242–1244
9. Morrow AG, Roberts WC, Ross J Jr, Fisher RD, Behrendt DM, Mason DT, Braunwald E: Obstruction to left ventricular outflow: Current concepts of management and operative treatment. *Ann Intern Med* 1968;69:1255–1286
10. Roberts WC: Operative treatment of hypertrophic obstructive cardiomyopathy: The case against mitral valve replacement. *Am J Cardiol* 1973;32:377–381
11. Maron BJ, Harding AM, Spirito P, Roberts WC, Waller BF: Systolic anterior motion of the posterior mitral leaflet: A previously unrecognized cause of dynamic subaortic obstruction in patients with hypertrophic cardiomyopathy. *Circulation* 1983;68:282–293
12. Bjork VO, Hutquist G, Lodin H: Subaortic stenosis produced by an abnormally placed anterior mitral leaflet. *J Thorac Cardiovasc Surg* 1969;41:659–669
13. Moro E, ten Cate FJ, Hugenholtz PG, Roelandt J: Genesis of systolic anterior motion of the mitral valve in hypertrophic cardio-

myopathy: An anatomical or dynamic event? *Eur Heart J* 1987;8: 1312–1321
14. Mikami T, Hashimoto M, Kudo T, Sugawara T, Sakamoto S, Yasuda H: Mitral valve and its ring in hypertrophic cardiomyopathy: A mechanism creating surplus mitral leaflet involved in systolic anterior motion. *Jpn Circ J* 1988;52:597–603
15. Ellis JG, Terneny OJ, Winters WL, Leachman RD: The critical role of the mitral valve leaflet in hypertrophic subaortic stenosis and amelioration of the disease by mitral valve replacement. *Chest* 1971;9:378–382
16. Fix P, Moberg A, Soderberg H, Karnell J: Muscular subvalvular aortic stenosis: An abnormal anterior mitral leaflet possibly the primary factor. *Acta Radiol* 1964;2:177–193
17. Angelini A, Becker AE, Anderson RH, Davies MJ: Mitral valve morphology: Normal and mitral valve prolapse, in Boudoulas H, Wooley CF (eds): *Mitral Valve Prolapse and the Mitral Valve Prolapse Syndrome.* New York, Futura Publishing Co, Inc, 1988, pp 13–53
18. Pomerance A: Ballooning deformity (mucoid degenerations) of atrioventricular valves. *Br Heart J* 1969;31:343–351
19. Popp RL, Winkle RA: Mitral valve prolapse syndrome. *JAMA* 1976;236:867–870
20. Davies MJ, Moore BP, Braimbridge MV: The floppy mitral valve: Study of incidence, pathology, and complications in surgical, necropsy, and forensic material. *Br Heart J* 1978;40:468–481
21. Waller BF, Morrow AG, Maron BJ, Del Negro AA, Kent KM, McGrath FJ, Wallace RB, McIntosh CL, Roberts WC: Etiology of clinically isolated, severe, chronic, pure mitral regurgitation: Analysis of 97 patients over 30 years of age having mitral valve replacement. *Am Heart J* 1982;104:276–288
22. McIntosh CL, Greenberg GJ, Maron BJ, Leon MB, Cannon RO III, Clark RE: Clinical and hemodynamic results after mitral valve replacement in patients with obstructive hypertrophic cardiomyopathy. *Ann Thorac Surg* 1989;47:236–244
23. Krajcer Z, Leachman RD, Cooley DA, Ostajic M, Coronado R: Mitral valve replacement and septal myectomy in hypertrophic cardiomyopathy: Ten-year follow-up in 80 patients. *Circulation* 1989;80(suppl I):I-57–I-64
24. Cooley DA, Leachman RD, Wukasch DC: Diffuse muscular subaortic stenosis: Surgical treatment. *Am J Cardiol* 1973;31:1–6
25. Yock PG, Hatle L, Popp RL: Patterns and timing of Doppler-detected intracavitary and aortic flow in hypertrophic cardiomyopathy. *J Am Coll Cardiol* 1986;8:1047–1058
26. Sasson Z, Yock PG, Hatle LK, Aldermann EL, Popp RL: Doppler echocardiographic determination of the pressure gradient in hypertrophic cardiomyopathy. *J Am Coll Cardiol* 1988;11:752–756
27. Ranganathan N, Lam JHC, Wigle ED, Silver MD: Morphology of the human mitral valve: II. The valve leaflets. *Circulation* 1970;41: 459–467
28. Draper N, Smith H: The stepwise regression procedure, in Draper N, Smith H (eds): *Applied Regression Analysis,* ed 3. New York, John Wiley & Sons, Inc, 1981, pp 307–311
29. Klues HG, Roberts WC, Maron BJ: Anomalous insertion of papillary muscle directly into anterior mitral leaflet in hypertrophic cardiomyopathy. *Circulation* 1991;84:1188–1197
30. Maron BJ, Nichols PF III, Pickle LW, Wesley YE, Mulvihill JJ: Patterns of inheritance in hypertrophic cardiomyopathy: Assessment by M-mode and two-dimensional echocardiography. *Am J Cardiol* 1984;53:1087–1094
31. Martin RP, Rakowski H, French J, Popp RL: Idiopathic hypertrophic subaortic stenosis viewed by wide-angle, phased-array echocardiography. *Circulation* 1979;59:1206–1217
32. Shapiro LM, McKenna WJ: Distribution of left ventricular hypertrophy in hypertrophic cardiomyopathy: A two-dimensional echocardiographic study. *J Am Coll Cardiol* 1983;2:437–444
33. Maron BJ, Gottdiener JS, Epstein SE: Patterns and significance of distribution of left ventricular hypertrophy in hypertrophic cardiomyopathy: A wide-angle, two-dimensional echocardiographic study of 125 patients. *Am J Cardiol* 1981;48:418–428
34. Shah PM, Taylor RD, Wong M: Abnormal mitral valve coaptation in hypertrophic obstructive cardiomyopathy: Proposed role in systolic anterior motion of mitral valve. *Am J Cardiol* 1981;48: 258–262
35. Shah PM, Gramiak R, Kramer DH: Ultrasound location of left ventricular outflow obstruction in hypertrophic obstructive cardiomyopathy. *Circulation* 1969;40:3–11
36. Maron BJ, Epstein SE: Clinical significance and therapeutic implications of the left ventricular outflow tract pressure gradient in hypertrophic cardiomyopathy. *Am J Cardiol* 1986;58:1093–1096
37. Spirito P, Maron BJ: Pattern of systolic anterior motion of the mitral valve in hypertrophic cardiomyopathy: Assessment by two-dimensional echocardiography. *Am J Cardiol* 1984;54:1039–1046
38. Rodger JC: Motion of mitral apparatus in hypertrophic cardiomyopathy with obstruction. *Br Heart J* 1976;38:732–737
39. Simon AL, Ross J, Gault JH: Angiographic anatomy of the left ventricle and mitral valve in idiopathic hypertrophic subaortic stenosis. *Circulation* 1967;36:852–867
40. Henry WL, Clark CE, Griffith JM, Epstein SE: Mechanism of left ventricular outflow obstruction in patients with obstructive asymmetric septal hypertrophy (idiopathic hypertrophic subaortic stenosis). *Am J Cardiol* 1975;35:337–345
41. Roberts WC, Cohen LS: Left ventricular papillary muscles: Description of the normal and a survey of conditions causing them to function abnormally. *Circulation* 1972;46:138–154
42. Wigle ED, Adelman AG, Auger P, Marquis Y: Mitral regurgitation in muscular subaortic stenosis. *Am J Cardiol* 1969;24:698–706
43. Spirito P, Maron BJ: Significance of left ventricular outflow tract cross-sectional area in hypertrophic cardiomyopathy: A two-dimensional echocardiographic assessment. *Circulation* 1983;67: 1100–1108
44. Jiang L, Levine RA, King ME, Weyman AE: An integrated mechanism for systolic anterior motion of the mitral valve in hypertrophic cardiomyopathy based on echocardiographic observations. *Am Heart J* 1987;113:633–644
45. Petrone RK, Klues HG, Panza JA, Peterson E, Maron BJ: Coexistence of mitral valve prolapse in a consecutive group of 528 patients with hypertrophic cardiomyopathy assessed by echocardiography. *J Am Coll Cardiol* (in press)
46. Jarcho JA, McKenna WJ, Pare PJA, Solomon SD, Holcombe RF, Dickie S, Levi T, Donis-Keller H, Seidman JG, Seidman CE: Mapping a gene for familial hypertrophic cardiomyopathy to chromosome 14q1. *N Engl J Med* 1989;321:1372–1378
47. Tanigawa G, Jarcho JA, Kass S, Solomon SD, Vosberg HP, Seidman JG, Seidman CE: A molecular basis for familial hypertrophic cardiomyopathy: An α/β cardiac myosin heavy chain hybrid gene. *Cell* 1990;62:991–998
48. Geisterfer-Lowrance AA, Kass S, Tanigawa G, Vosberg HP, McKenna WJ, Seidman CE, Seidman JG: A molecular basis for familial hypertrophic cardiomyopathy: A β cardiac myosin heavy chain gene missense mutation. *Cell* 1990;62:999–1006
49. Solomon SD, Jarcho JA, McKenna WJ, Geisterfer-Lowrance A, Germain R, Salerni R, Seidman JG, Seidman CE: Familial hypertrophic cardiomyopathy is a genetically heterogenous disease. *J Clin Invest* 1990;86:993–999

Morphologic aspects of cardiac valve dysfunction

William C. Roberts, MD. *Bethesda, Md.*

This review focuses on congenital and acquired conditions affecting one or more cardiac valves and causing valvular dysfunction. The focus will be on the mitral and aortic valves.

MITRAL REGURGITATION

Mitral valve prolapse. Although recognized earlier,[1-4] delineation of the click–late systolic murmur syndrome as a consequence of mitral valve prolapse was not appreciated until the 1960s.[5-9] It is now apparent that the click–late systolic murmur is common, probably occurring in 5% or more of persons >15 years of age.[10-12] Although generally not considered as such, the click–systolic murmur syndrome in most persons is probably a form of congenital heart disease and therefore is the most common congenital heart disease.[13] The auscultatory manifestations, however, are usually not evident until adulthood.

The click–murmur syndrome may be viewed from both auscultatory and morphologic standpoints as manifesting three stages: (1) systolic click(s) only, (2) click(s) plus a mid to late systolic murmur, and (3) pansystolic murmur only. Although progression from stage 1 to 3 has been documented in relatively few patients, it appears likely that this is the natural sequence of events in some patients. In others, there may be no progression from stage 1, patients in stage 2 may revert to stage 1, patients in stage 1 may lose their click(s) altogether, and patients appearing in stage 3 (pansystolic murmur) may have had no documentation of stages 1 and 2. With rare exception, stages 1 and 2 are unassociated with symptomatic evidence of cardiac dysfunction. The exception includes patients with arrhythmias or chest pain. Patients in stage 3 have congestive heart failure because of the associated severe mitral regurgitation. The stage 3 floppy mitral valve is the major cause of pure (no element of stenosis) severe, isolated (aortic valve normal anatomically and functionally) mitral regurgitation requiring valve replacement or repair.[14] As a consequence, there is considerable anatomic information available on the floppy mitral valve that produces a pansystolic murmur (stage 3) and causes severe mitral regurgitation.[15] In contrast, there is less anatomic information available in patients with only a systolic click(s) (stage 1) or those with both a click(s) and a late systolic murmur (stage 2).[16]

Several names applied to this syndrome describe to some extent what the valve looks like anatomically, thus the names "prolapsing posterior mitral leaflet," "prolapsing mitral valve," "billowing or ballooning mitral leaflet syndrome," "overshooting or hooded mitral valve," "floppy mitral valve," and "myxomatous or mucinous degeneration of the mitral valve." I prefer the term "mitral valve prolapse."

Defining mitral valve prolapse morphologically has not been easy. Pomerance[17] defined the entity as a ballooning deformity of the mitral leaflets, the affected portions of which were increased in area and protruded into the left atrium in ventricular systole. Waller et al.[14] also utilized either a focal or a diffuse increase in mitral area as a criterion but also required an increased length, either focal or diffuse, from basal attachment of the leaflet to its distal margin. Lucas and Edwards[18] listed the following features for diagnosis: (1) interchordal hooding involving both the rough and the clear zones of the involved leaflet or leaflets, (2) height of the interchordal hooding >4 mm, and (3) interchordal hooding involving >50% of the anterior leaflet or >37% of the posterior leaflet. Dollar and Roberts[16] used two criteria for mitral valve prolapse: (1) elongation of a portion of the posterior mitral leaflet such that the distance from the distal margin to its attachment at the mitral annulus was >1.5 cm or (2) presence of mitral leaflet protrusion toward the left atrium, usually also associated with missing chordae tendineae, and the prolapsed

From the Pathology Branch, National Heart, Lung, and Blood Institute, National Institutes of Health.

Received for publication Oct. 24, 1991; accepted Dec. 10, 1991.

Reprint requests: William C. Roberts, MD, Pathology Branch, NHLBI-NIH, Bldg. 10, Room 2N258, Bethesda, MD 20892.

4/1/36461

portion of the leaflet involving >50% of the anterior leaflet. Others have referred to this leaflet prolapse as "interchordal hooding."

Other useful anatomic findings in identifying mitral valve prolapse including the following:

1. *An increase in the transverse dimension of the leaflets such that the length of the mitral circumference measured on a line corresponding to the distal margin of the posterior leaflet is much larger than the circumference measured at the level of the mitral annulus.* In the normal valve, the two are the same. The result is analogous to an accordion not fully extended, or better, a skirt gathered at the waist. The leaflets of the opened mitral valve are flat or smooth (like the mucosa of the ileum), whereas those of the opened floppy mitral valve are undulating (like those of the duodenum or jejunum)

2. *Excessive thinning and lengthening of chordae tendineae.* Chordal elongation, however, is rare without concomitant leaflet elongation. The chordae also occasionally may be shorter than normal.

3. *Dilatation of the mitral annulus.* This does not occur to any significant degree in the absence of mitral valve prolapse.[19] Annular dilatation is the major cause of the development of severe mitral regurgitation in the presence of mitral valve prolapse (the other is rupture of chordae tendineae).[15] Normally, the mitral annulus in adults averages about 9 cm in circumference. In patients with left ventricular dilatation from any cause with or without mitral regurgitation, the circumference of the mitral annulus usually dilates slightly, usually to about 11 cm or <25% above normal. Among patients with mitral valve prolapse associated with severe mitral regurgitation, the circumference of the mitral annulus generally increases >50% above normal or to circumferences of 14 to 18 cm. When the annulus dilates to this extent, the leaflets may "stretch" or flatten transversely, and this stretching diminishes the amount of scalloping. In addition, the left ventricular dilatation may cause longitudinal stretching of the leaflets. The amount of scalloping in the stage 3 valves therefore appears to be less than that observed in the stage 2 valves. Roberts et al.[15] examined operatively excised mitral valves in 83 patients (aged 26 to 79 years [mean 60]; 26 women [31%] and 57 men [69%]) with mitral valve prolapse and mitral regurgitation severe enough to warrant mitral valve replacement. All 83 operatively excised valves were examined by the same person, and all excised valves had been purely regurgitant (no element of stenosis). No patients had hemodynamic evidence of dysfunction of the aortic valve. In each valve a portion of the posterior mitral leaflet was elongated such that the distance from the distal margin to basal attachment of this leaflet was similar to the distance from the distal margin of the anterior leaflet to its basal attachment to the left atrial wall. Two major mechanisms for the severe mitral regurgitation were found: (1) dilatation of the mitral annulus with or without rupture of chordae tendineae and (2) rupture of chordae tendineae with or without dilatation of the mitral annulus. Of the 83 patients, 48 (58%) had both dilated annuli (>11 cm in circumference) and ruptured chordae tendineae, 16 (19%) had dilated annuli without ruptured chordae, and 16 (19%) had ruptured chordae without significant annular dilatation. In three patients the annulus was not dilated nor were chordae ruptured and therefore the mechanism of the mitral regurgitation is uncertain. Mitral chordal rupture was nearly as frequent in the 64 patients with clearly dilated annular circumferences as in the 19 patients with normal or insignificantly dilated annular circumferences (≤11 cm).

4. *Focal thickening of mural endocardium of left ventricle behind the posterior mitral leaflet and the mitral chordae tendineae.* Salazar and Edwards[20] called these fibrous thickenings "*friction lesions*" to indicate that they are believed to result from friction between the overlying leaflets and chordae and the underlying left ventricular wall. Of the 102 necropsy cases with mitral valve prolapse studied by Lucas and Edwards,[18] 77 (75%) had these friction lesions and in three (3%) the mural endocardial friction lesions had entrapped the overlying chordae. Dollar and Roberts[16] observed these friction lesions in 23 (68%) of 34 patients with mitral valve prolapse in whom each heart was examined specifically for these lesions. The friction lesions therefore are common in patients with mitral valve prolapse and their presence strongly suggests the presence of mitral valve prolapse.

5. *Fibrinous deposits on the atrial surface of the prolapsed portion of mitral leaflet and particularly at the angle formed between the prolapsed leaflet and the left atrial wall* (mitral valve–left atrial angle). These deposits in the angle may be a source of emboli.

Microscopically, the prolapsed mitral leaflet may or may not contain an excessive amount of acid mucopolysaccharide material. Both the normal and the prolapsed mitral leaflets consist of two elements, the fibrosa and the spongiosa. The *fibrosa* consists of fibrous tissue (collagen), and the *spongiosa* consists of mucoid or myxomatous material high in acid mucopolysaccharide material. In most valve diseases, the fibrosal element is increased and it may entirely replace the spongiosal element. In the prolapsed mitral leaflet, the spongiosal element, the more central portion of the leaflet, may increase to a greater extent than the fibrosal element. The resulting increased myxoid or myxomatous stroma, however, does not appear abnormal—i.e., degenerated. Thus the term myxoid or myxomatous "degeneration" for this condition is not appropriate. The amount of fibrous tissue in the mitral leaflets in mitral valve prolapse also is usually increased but perhaps its increase is a secondary phenomenon. The fibrosa element may be subdivided into two components, the *auricularis*, which normally is a thin layer forming the atrial or contact aspect of the leaflet, and the *ventricularis*, which normally is a relatively thick layer that covers the ventricular aspect of the leaflet. The atrial aspect of the prolapsed mitral leaflet often is focally thickened. This change probably is secondary to abnormal friction from contact between the prolapsed segment of the leaflet and its "opposite number," that is, the other leaflet, or between two prolapsed segments of the same leaflet.[21, 22] The changes on the ventricular surface of the leaflet consist of connective tissue "pads" forming primarily in the interchordal segments, and this proliferation of fibrous tissue may extend into adjacent chordae tendineae and onto ventricular endocardium behind the posterior mitral leaflet.[20, 22] The interchordal collections of fibrous tissue are considered responses to the tension and stretching that occur at the undersurface of a prolapsed leaflet or segment of leaflet.[22] This increase in fibrous tissue, particularly on the ventricular surface of the leaflet, has caused, I suspect, the floppy valve in years past to be considered rheumatic in origin. Fibrin deposits also may occur on the atrial aspects of the prolapsed mitral leaflet, and they may not be found on gross examination.[17]

Ultrastructure studies of floppy mitral valves have disclosed alterations of the collagen fibers in the leaflets and in the chordae tendineae.[23] These changes have included fragmentation, splitting, swelling, and coarse granularity of the individual collagen fibers, and in addition, spiraling and twisting of the fibers. Also, some elastic fibers are fragmented and contain cystic spaces. These alterations in the structure of the collagen may be more important than the accumulation of the acid mucopolysaccharide material in that they lead to focal weaknesses in the leaflets. The left ventricular systolic pressure exerted against these weakened areas may lead to prolapse or focal interchordal hooding. Although the actual prolapse of the mitral valve may be acquired and be a consequence of the left ventricular systolic (closing) pressure, the focally weak areas of the leaflets are probably most often congenital in origin, and the later bulging with or without rupture is acquired as a consequence of the high intraarterial pressure. The frequency of mitral valve prolapse also may be higher in persons with elevated left ventricular systolic pressures compared with persons in whom this pressure is at normal levels.[24]

Opportunities for structural study of a mitral valve associated with only a click(s) have been rare. I have studied one such valve. (The child had been examined by John Barlow, MD, of Johannesburg, South Africa.) The child, who had no symptoms of cardiac dysfunction, died of leukemia and at necropsy had a perfectly competent mitral valve but three distinct foci where leaflet overlapped adjacent leaflet. The leaflets otherwise were smooth and specifically were devoid of so-called scallops. There are no reported anatomic descriptions, to my knowledge, of mitral valves producing one or more systolic clicks without an associated precordial systolic murmur. Examination at necropsy of mitral valves of patients who during life had documentation of systolic click(s) plus a mid-late systolic murmur (Barlow syndrome) also are infrequent. Death in stage 2 as in stage 1 is usually from a noncardiac cause. In this stage, the most characteristic feature is leaflet scalloping, which represents excessive leaflet owing to an increase in the transverse or commissure-to-commissure dimension of the leaflet.[16] The mitral annulus, as in stage 1, is not dilated. The chordae tendineae may or may not be elongated.

Just as the frequency of mitral valve prolapse varies clinically depending on the age and sex group being examined and in the clinical criteria employed for diagnosis (ausculatory, echocardiographic, angiographic), its frequency at necropsy is quite variable and the variation is determined by several factors: (1) age and sex group of population being examined; (2) type of institution where necropsy is performed (general hospital, referral hospital for cardiovascular disease, or medical examiner's [coroner's] office); (3) expertise in cardiovascular disease of the physician performing the necropsy or reporting the findings; (4) percent of total deaths having autopsies at the particular hospital; (5) presence or absence of evidence of cardiac disease before death; (6) whether the patient underwent mitral valve replacement or repair; and (7) whether the percentage of patients being examined had a high frequency of the Marfan syndrome, infective endocarditis, atrial septal defect, and so on. No study better shows how bias alters the findings in necropsy studies than the one performed by Lucas and Edwards.[13] These investigators in one portion of their study determined the frequency of and complications of floppy mitral valves observed at necropsy in one community (nonreferral) hospital for adults. Of 1376 autopsies performed, 7.4% or 102 patients at necropsy had morphologically floppy mitral valves. Their mean age at death was 69 ± 12 years; 62 (61%) were men and 40 (39%) were women. Of the 102 patients, mitral valve prolapse was the cause of death in only two. Of the 102 patients, one leaflet had prolapsed in 34 patients, and two leaflets had prolapsed in 68. Only 18 had anatomic evidence of previous mitral regurgitation: seven had infective endocarditis, seven had ruptured chordae tendineae (without infection), one had the Marfan syndrome, and three had secundum atrial septal defect. No patient died suddenly. In contrast, in the other portion of their study, these authors described complications in 69 necropsy patients whose hearts had been sent to Edwards for his opinion and interest. Among these 69 patients, 16 (23%) had died suddenly and unexpectedly; 19 (28%) had ruptured chordae tendineae (without infection), 7 (10%) had infective endocarditis, 20 (29%) had the Marfan syndrome, and nine (13%) had secundum type atrial septal defect. Thus in contrast to their infrequency in their community hospital series, most cases submitted to their cardiovascular registry from other institutions had ruptured chordae, infective endocarditis, sudden unexpected death, or the Marfan syndrome.

Two other necropsy studies can be compared with the community hospital series collected by Lucas and Edwards. Pomerance[17] collected from one general hospital 35 cases at necropsy of "ballooning deformity" of the mitral valve: 23 (66%) were men and 12 (34%) were women; their ages ranged from 51 to 98 years (mean 74). Death was attributed to mitral valve prolapse in only four patients (11%). One leaflet only had prolapsed in 12 patients and two leaflets had prolapsed in 23 (6%). Eight patients had anatomic evidence of mitral regurgitation, only one had atrial septal defect, nine (26%) had anatomic evidence of tricuspid valve prolapse, nine (26%) had mitral annular calcific deposits, and 13 (37%) had hearts of increased weight. Davies et al.[25] gathered 90 necropsy cases of the floppy mitral valve from four general hospitals. This number represented 4.5% of autopsies at the four hospitals during the time. Of the 90 patients, 44 (49%) were men and 46 (51%) were women; they ranged in age from <40 to 100 years. Death in 15 was attributed to mitral valve prolapse (the number dying suddenly was not mentioned). The prolapse involved one leaflet in 69 patients (77%) and both mitral leaflets in 21 (23%); 63 (70%) also had anatomic evidence of tricuspid valve prolapse. Only six (7%) patients had dilated mitral annuli; only three (3%) had mitral annular calcium, and eight had hearts weighing >300 gm.

Dollar and Roberts[16] studied at necropsy 56 patients aged 16 to 70 years (mean 48) with mitral valve prolapse. Fifteen patients, aged 16 to 69 years (mean 39), died suddenly and mitral valve prolapse was the only cardiac condition found at necropsy (hereafter called isolated mitral valve prolapse); the remaining 41 patients had other conditions that were capable of being fatal. On the latter 41 patients, seven, aged 17 to 59 years (mean 45), had associated congenital heart disease and 34 patients, aged 17 to 70 years (mean 52), had no associated congenital cardiac abnormalities. Compared with the 34 patients without associated congenital heart disease and with nonmitral valve prolapse conditions capable in themselves of being fatal, the 15 patients who died suddenly with isolated mitral valve prolapse were younger (mean age 39 ± 17 versus 52 ± 15 years; $p = 0.01$), were more often women (67% versus 26%; $p = 0.008$), and had a lower frequency of mitral regurgitation (7% versus 38%; $p = 0.02$). The 15 patients dying suddenly with isolated mitral valve prolapse also were less likely to have evidence of ruptured chordae tendineae (29% versus 67%; $p = 0.04$). The frequency of increased heart weight (67% versus 59%), a dilated mitral valve annulus (80% versus 81%), a dilated tricuspid valve annulus (17% versus 17%), an elongated anterior mitral leaflet (86% versus 54%), an elongated posterior mitral leaflet (79% versus 77%), and fibrous endocardial plaque under the posterior mitral leaflet (73% versus 63%) was similar between the two groups. The severity of the prolapse (mild 20% versus 11%; moderate 27% versus 58%; severe 53% versus 32%) was also similar between the two groups. Thus persons with mitral valve prolapse dying suddenly without another recognized condition tend to be relatively young women without mitral regurgitation.

The frequency of mitral valve prolapse among patients undergoing mitral valve replacement for *isolated* (aortic valve function normal), pure (no element of stenosis), and *severe* mitral regurgitation is high—indeed, prolapse appears to be the most common etiology of isolated, pure, and severe mitral regurgitation. My associates and I[14] reviewed the records and operatively excised mitral valves of 97 patients (57 men) aged 32 to 78 years (mean 54) who underwent mitral valve replacement because of 3+/4+ or 4+/4+ mitral regurgitation as determined by left ventricular angiography. Of the 97 patients, the cause of the mitral regurgitation was leaflet prolapse in 60 (62%), papillary muscle dysfunction from coronary artery disease in 29 (30%), infective endocarditis involving apparently previously normal mitral valves in five, and rheumatic heart disease in three patients. Of the 60 patients with mitral valve prolapse, 13 had ruptured chordae tendineae, including all four patients with infective endocarditis superimposed on mitral valve prolapse. The circumference of the mitral annulus in patients with mitral valve prolapse without ruptured chordae was significantly larger than that in the patients in other groups and in 18 control subjects, both of which were normal. Likewise, the areas of the excised leaflets in the prolapsed valves were much larger than in the other groups and in the control subjects, both of which were normal. The product of the circumference (in centimeters) multiplied by the area (in square centimeters) calculated for the normal valves ranged from 45 to 140 cm^3 (average 91). The average product was 150 cm^3 in the prolapsed valves with ruptured chordae, and 273 cm^3 in the prolapsed valves with intact chordae. The products were 87, 91, and 106 cm^3, respectively, in the valves regurgitant because of papillary muscle dysfunction, infective endocarditis, or rheumatic disease; these products did not differ from those of the normal valves.

The correct cause of the mitral regurgitation in the 97 patients was usually predictable from the history alone. Of the 29 patients with papillary muscle dysfunction from atherosclerotic coronary artery disease, all had clinical evidence of myocardial ischemia: history of acute myocardial infarction that had healed in 24, left ventricular aneurysm from a silent infarction in one, and angina pectoris in four. Of the five patients with mitral regurgitation secondary to infective endocarditis, four had well-documented episodes of infection that had been cured by antibiotic therapy; none had evidence of valvular dysfunction before the episode of infective endocarditis. Of the three patients with mitral regurgitation secondary to a rheumatic origin, two had a history of acute rheumatic fever, whereas this item was positive in only 5 of the other 94 patients. Clinical diagnosis of mitral valve prolapse was by a process of exclusion. Only 2 (3%) of the 60 patients had historic evidence of previous acute myocardial infarction, five (8%) had a history of acute rheumatic fever, and four (7%) had a history of active infective endocarditis. Compared with the five patients classified as having ruptured chordae tendineae on previously normal values (four of whom had a history of infective endocarditis), the four patients with healed infective endocarditis and mitral valve prolapse were older (mean age 61 years versus 42 years), had previous systolic murmurs of mitral regurgitation before the episode of infective endocarditis (four of four versus none of five), and had a longer mean duration of congestive heart failure (11 versus 4 months). Thus of the 60 patients with mitral valve prolapse, 51 (85%) had no historic evidence of myocardial ischemia, acute rheumatic fever, or infective endocarditis.

The origin of the mitral regurgitation also was suggested preoperatively by more objective means. All 29 patients with mitral regurgitation secondary to coronary artery disease had abnormal Q waves by electrocardiogram, whereas abnormal Q waves were present in only 4 of the 60 patients with mitral valve prolapse and in none of the eight patients with mitral regurgitation from either infective endocarditis or rheumatic disease. Atrial fibrillation was significantly more common in the patients in whom the mitral regurgitation resulted from coronary artery disease: in 7 (24%) of these 29 patients, in only 4 (7%) of the 60 patients with mitral valve prolapse, and in two of the eight patients with either infective endocarditis or a rheumatic origin. Of the 60 patients with mitral valve prolapse, 43 had M-mode echocardiograms, and in 32 (74%) mitral valve prolapse was demonstrated.[26] Of the 29 patients with symptomatic coronary artery disease, M-mode echocardiograms were done in 22; only two (9%) had mitral valve prolapse. Of the eight patients with mitral regurgitation from infective endocarditis or rheumatic etiology, seven had echocardiograms; none had mitral valve prolapse. Left ventriculograms, performed in all 97 patients, indicated mitral valve prolapse in only 16 (27%) of the 60 patients with mitral valve prolapse and in none of the other 37 patients with other causes. Selective coronary angiograms were performed in 53 (55%) of the 97 patients. All 29 with mitral regurgitation secondary to coronary artery disease had significant (>50% diameter reduction) coronary narrowing angiographically in at least two of the three major coronary arteries. Of the 60 patients with mitral valve prolapse, coronary angiograms were performed in 23; only three (13%) had significant coronary arterial narrowing, limited in each to one coronary artery. Auscultation and hemodynamic data at cardiac catheterization were not helpful in delineating the origin of the mitral regurgitation. None of the 97 patients—including the 60 classified as having mitral valve prolapse—had systolic clicks, and the systolic precordial murmurs in all 97 patients were holosystolic. The average pulmonary arterial, left atrial (or pulmonary artery wedge), and left ventricular pressures were similar in the 97 patients irrespective of the origin of the mitral regurgitation. The systolic systemic arterial pressures, however, were significantly higher in the patients with mitral valve prolapse and ruptured chordae tendineae than in those with mitral valve prolapse and intact chordae tendineae.

Mitral valve prolapse appears now to be a more common cause of rupture of mitral chordae tendineae than does infective endocarditis. Among 25 patients having mitral valve replacement for pure mitral regurgitation associated with rupture of chordae tendineae, Jeresaty et al.[27] found mitral valve prolapse (based on "redundancy and marked hooding of the mitral leaflets") to be the cause of the chordal rupture in 23 (92%), only one of whom had had infective endocarditis. Four of the 25 patients had auscultatory and angiographic or echocardiographic evidence of mitral valve prolapse before the chordal rupture. Among patients with ruptured chordae tendineae associated with mitral valve prolapse, it is sometimes actually difficult to identify ruptured chords. The term "rupture," however, is commonly applied to those leaflets where chordal insertions are no longer present but where chordae clearly should be attached.[15]

In addition to mitral regurgitation, rupture of chordae tendineae, and infective endocarditis, other complications of mitral valve prolapse include mitral annular calcium. Pomerance[17] observed mitral annular calcium in 9 (26%) of her 35 necropsy patients with mitral valve prolapse. The cause of the arrhythmias and chest pain is unclear.[28] There is no evidence of a myocardial or coronary arterial factor. Shrivastava et al.[22] have suggested that the friction between mitral chordae tendineae and the underlying left ventricular mural endocardium may be an arrhythmic stimulus. The cause of the acute strokes or transient cerebral ischemic attacks that occur in an occasional patient with mitral valve prolapse also is unclear. It has been suggested that the small fibrin-platelet thrombi occasionally seen at the mitral valve–left atrial angle are sources of emboli for either cerebral or myocardial ischemia.[18]

The cause of mitral valve prolapse, as alluded to earlier, almost certainly in most patients is congenital in origin, or at least the connective tissue of the mitral leaflets, chordae, and annulus appears to be congenitally defective. The finding of classic mitral valve prolapse at birth is evidence for the congenital thesis. The occurrence of mitral valve prolapse in certain clearly hereditary conditions, for example, the Marfan syndrome, is evidence of congenitally defective mitral tissue. Its association with aneurysm of the fossa ovale membrane or atrial septal defect and Ebstein's anomaly of the tricuspid valve also may support this thesis.[29-31]

CLEFT ANTERIOR MITRAL LEAFLET

Partial atrioventricular "defect" includes a spectrum of five anatomic anomalies.[32, 33] Some patients have all five and others have only one or two. The five anomalies are the following: (1) defect in the lower portion of the atrial septum, so-called primum atrial septal defect; (2) defect in, or absence of, the posterobasal portion of ventricular septum; (3) cleft, anterior mitral leaflet; (4) anomalous chordae tendineae from the anterior mitral leaflet to the crest of the ventricular septum; and (5) partial or complete absence of the septal tricuspid valve leaflet. There are at least four potential functional consequences of these five anatomic anomalies: (1) shunt at the atrial level, (2) shunt at the ventricular level, (3) mitral regurgitation, and (4) obstruction to left ventricular outflow. Well over 95% of patients with partial atrioventricular defect have a primum type atrial septal defect, and most of those without a primum defect have a shunt at the ventricular level. The occurrence of mitral regurgitation from a cleft in the anterior mitral leaflet unassociated with a defect in either atrial or ventricular septa is rare, but such has been the finding in several reported patients.[34-36] Indeed, at least 10 patients have been reported at necropsy to have a cleft in the anterior mitral leaflet unassociated with a defect in either the atrial or ventricular septum.[36] Only five were over 10 years of age. Nine of the 10 patients had mitral regurgitation.

LEFT-SIDED ATRIOVENTRICULAR VALVE REGURGITATION ASSOCIATED WITH CORRECTED TRANSPOSITION OF THE GREAT ARTERIES

Corrected transposition is an entity that has produced much confusion.[37] Corrected transposition and complete transposition are quite different; the only thing they have in common is the word "transposition." Complete transposition is essentially one defect: the great arteries are transposed, so that the aorta arises from the right ventricle and the pulmonary trunk arises from the left ventricle. In corrected transposition, the great arteries also are transposed, but in addition, the ventricles, atrioventricular valves, coronary arteries, and conduction system are inverted. Patients with complete transposition die because they have inadequate communications between the two circuits. Patients with corrected transposition theoretically should be able to live a full life span, but usually this is not the case because associated defects—namely, a ventricular septal defect or regurgitation of the left-sided atrioventricular valve, or both—cause the heart to function abnormally. Abnormalities of the left-sided atrioventricular valve, a systemic valve but anatomically a tricuspid valve, are the most common associated anomalies in corrected transposition.[37, 38] Of the anomalies, the most frequent is the Ebstein-type malformation. These valves are intrinsically regurgitant because the chordae are short and the leaflets are closely adherent to the ventricular endocardium.

Most patients with corrected transposition have a defect in the ventricular septum associated with a left-to-right shunt.[37] Thus most patients with corrected transposition present with evidence of excessive pulmonary blood flow. An occasional patient with corrected transposition, however, may have no defects in the cardiac septa and no ductus.[38] These individuals may present with evidence of pure mitral regurgitation and some of them during life have been considered to have rheumatic mitral regurgitation.[38]

MITRAL STENOSIS

The essential hemodynamic fault caused by mitral stenosis is the inability of the left atrium to empty normally. In sinus rhythm, left atrial contraction serves to augment its emptying, but atrial contraction is lost in atrial fibrillation. The obstruction, represented by a pressure gradient across the valve, results in pulmonary venous obstruction that may lead to pulmonary arterial hypertension.

Of the single or combined cardiac valve lesions severe enough to be fatal, mitral stenosis, in my experience, ranks second.[33] Of 1010 patients >14 years of age with functionally severe (class III or IV, New York Heart Association) valvular cardiac disease whom I had studied at necropsy up to 1980, 434 (44%) had mitral stenosis. Only aortic valve stenosis was more common. Mitral stenosis occurred alone in 189 (44%) patients and in combination with other functional valvular lesions in the other 245 (56%) patients. Mitral stenosis was rheumatic in origin in all 434 patients.

Although a functional classification of valvular heart disease is most useful from physiologic and therapeutic standpoints, an anatomic classification is helpful from an etiologic standpoint.[39] Five anatomic categories have proved useful: isolated mitral, isolated aortic, combined mitral and aortic, combined tricuspid and mitral with or without aortic, and both tricuspid and mitral. Anatomically isolated aortic valve disease is never rheumatic in origin. Isolated mitral disease causing mitral stenosis is, with rare exception, rheumatic in origin, but isolated mitral disease causing pure regurgitation is usually nonrheumatic in origin. Anatomic valve disease involving more than one cardiac valve is usually rheumatic in origin. Isolated anatomic disease of the tricuspid or pulmonic valves, or both, is usually congenital or infectious in origin or is associated with the carcinoid syndrome.[40, 41]

A valve may function normally and yet be anatomically abnormal. Only 62% of the 189 patients with isolated mitral stenosis (with or without mitral regurgitation) had anatomic involvement limited to the mitral valve.[33] In contrast, 88% of the 292 patients with clinically isolated aortic valve stenosis (with or without regurgitation) had anatomic disease limited to the aortic valve only.

Rheumatic heart disease may be viewed as a disease of the mitral valve; other valves also may be involved both anatomically and functionally, but anatomically the mitral valve is always involved.[39] To my knowledge, Aschoff bodies have never been found in hearts without anatomic disease of the mitral valve.[42] Of the first 543 patients with severe valvular heart disease whom I studied at necropsy, 11 (2%) had Aschoff bodies, and all had anatomic mitral valve disease.[39] The ages of the 11 patients with Aschoff bodies ranged from 18 to 68 years (mean 38), and nine had a history of acute rheumatic fever earlier in life.[42] Clinical study revealed that 9 of the 11 patients had mitral stenosis with or without dysfunction of one or more other cardiac valves, one had isolated pure aortic regurgitation, and one had both mitral and aortic regurgitation. All 11 patients had diffuse fibrous thickening of the mitral valve leaflets and all but one had diffuse anatomic lesions of at least two other cardiac valves. No patient with anatomic lesions limited to the aortic valve had Aschoff bodies. Thus among patients with chronic valvular heart disease, Aschoff bodies, the only anatomic lesion pathognomonic of rheumatic heart disease, usually indicate diffuse anatomic lesions of the mitral valve with or without involvement of one or more other cardiac valves. The functional mitral lesion is usually stenosis.

Although they are rare at necropsy in patients with fatal chronic valvular heart disease, Aschoff bodies are fairly common in hearts of patients having mitral valve commissurotomy for mitral stenosis.[43] Among 481 patients undergoing various mitral valve operations, Aschoff bodies were found in 40 (21%) of 191 operatively excised left atrial appendages, in 4 (2%) of 273 operatively excised left ventricular papillary muscles (1 per patient), and in 1 (6%) of 17 patients with both the left atrial appendage and papillary muscle operatively excised. Of the 45 patients with Aschoff bodies, 44 had mitral stenosis preoperatively, and only one, a 10-year-old boy, had pure mitral regurgitation. Sinus rhythm was present in 38 (84%), and atrial fibrillation was present in 7 (16%). Perioperatively, only 1 of the 45 patients with Aschoff bodies had clinical or laboratory stigmas compatible with acute rheumatic fever, and 58% had an illness compatible with acute rheumatic fever at any time.

Not only is rheumatic heart disease a disorder of the cardiac valves, it also affects mural endocardium, pericardium, and myocardium. On histologic study, the atrial walls virtually always have increased amounts of fibrous tissue in both myocardial interstitium and in the mural endocardium, atrophy of some and hypertrophy of other myocardial cells, and hypertrophy of smooth muscle cells of the mural endocardium. In all patients with rheumatic mitral stenosis, the leaflets are diffusely thickened, either by fibrous tissue or by calcific deposits or by both; the commissures are usually fused, and the chordae tendineae are shortened and usually fused to some degree. The great obstruction to this funnel-shaped valve occurs at its apex, which is within the left ventricular cavity. The primary orifice, located at the level of the annulus, is far less narrowed. Fusion may involve one or both commissures. When only one is fused or one is fused more than the other, the stenotic orifice is eccentrically located. A centrally located orifice indicates symmetric commissural fusion. In rheumatic mitral stenosis, the chordae tendineae are occasionally so retracted that the leaflets appear to insert directly into the papillary muscles. When this occurs, the mitral stenosis is always severe because the interchordal spaces are almost entirely obliterated. Sometimes chordae inserting into one papillary muscle are well preserved, whereas those inserting into the other papillary muscle are partially or completely fused. Mitral commissurotomy on a valve in which the leaflets insert almost directly into the papillary muscle(s) usually must include a splitting of the papillary muscle(s) as well as the commissure(s). If there are normally about 120 third-order chordae and about 24 first-order chordae, in mitral stenosis these numbers are usually halved and, on occasion, even reduced to just one chordae.[33]

The amount of calcium in the leaflets of stenotic mitral valves varies considerably.[44] Generally, calcium is more frequent and is larger in quantity in men than in women, in older than in younger patients, and in patients with higher compared with those with lower pressure gradients between the left atrium and the left ventricle.[44] The rapidity with which calcium develops also varies considerably; it is present at a younger age in men than in women. Lachman and I[44] determined the presence or absence and the extent of calcific deposits in operatively excised stenotic mitral valves by radiography of the excised valve in 164 patients aged 26 to 72 years. The extent of the mitral calcific deposits was determined by the percentage of the valvular circumference containing the deposits: grade 0 (14 patients); grade I = 1% to 25% (43 patients); grade II = 26% to 50% (34 patients); grade III = 51% to 75% (39 patients); and grade IV = 76% to 100% (34 patients). The amount of calcific deposits in the stenotic mitral valves correlated with sex and with the mean diastolic pressure gradient across the mitral valve but it did not correlate with the patient's age (after age 25 years), cardiac rhythm, pulmonary arterial or pulmonary arterial wedge pressure, previous mitral commissurotomy, presence of thrombus in the body of the left atrium, or the presence of disease of one or more other cardiac valves.

Among the 164 patients with mitral stenosis having mitral valve replacement and roentgenography of the excised mitral valve, 14 had no mitral calcium and 43 had only trace or minimal mitral calcific deposits.[45] Thus we wondered why these 57 patients had mitral replacement rather than mitral commissurotomy. Of the 57 patients, 37 had moderate to severe mitral regurgitation and therefore they clearly deserved mitral valve replacement. The remaining 20 had absent or minimal calcific deposits but nevertheless they too had mitral replacement. Although in the prevalve replacement era all 20 patients almost surely would have been considered good or ideal candidates for mitral commissurotomy, other factors swung the surgeon to valve replacement rather than to commissurotomy. These factors included the need to replace one or more other cardiac valves (13 patients), the utilization of cardiopulmonary bypass allowing visual inspection rather than simple palpation of the diseased mitral valve (all 20 patients), relatively little experience with mitral commissurotomy in four of the five surgeons (17 patients), displeasure with attempted commissurotomy (three patients), previous mitral commissurotomy (11 patients), and incorrect identification of mitral calcific deposits (two patients). Even though mitral commissurotomy has been in use for 30 years, the mere alternative of valve replacement may have altered the definition of the stenotic mitral valve previously considered ideal for mitral commissurotomy.

A major complication of mitral stenosis is thrombus formation in the left atrial cavity. The thrombus may be limited to the atrial appendage (most common) or be located in both left atrial appendage and body. The latter group hereafter will be referred to as "left atrial body thrombus." Left atrial body thrombus was observed in 5% of 1010 personally studied necropsy patients with fatal valvular heart disease; all had severe mitral stenosis.[33] Left atrial body thrombus was not observed in any of the 165 patients with pure mitral regurgitation with or without aortic valve dysfunction. All patients with left atrial body thrombi had atrial fibrillation. Comparison of these necropsy patients with 46 patients with mitral stenosis operated upon at the National Heart, Lung, and Blood Institute and in whom thrombus was found at operation in the left atrial body disclosed that 42 (91%) patients had atrial fibrillation. In contrast, of 40 living patients undergoing mitral valve replacement for pure mitral regurgitation and operated upon at the National Heart, Lung, and Blood Institute, none had thrombus in the body of the left atrium, although 75% had atrial fibrillation. Thrombus appears to occur in the body of the left atrium only in patients with mitral stenosis, and atrial fibrillation without mitral stenosis is incapable of forming a thrombus in the left atrial body.

Calcific deposits on the mural endocardium of the left atrium are indicative of previous organization with calcification of left atrial thrombi.[46,47] Histologically, the "calcific thrombi" also contain cholesterol clefts and are identical to atherosclerotic plaques. The observation that left atrial thrombi can organize into lesions identical to atherosclerotic plaques supports the view that atherosclerotic plaques may be the result of organization of thrombi. If calcific deposits form on left atrial body endocardium before the left atrial cavity has had time to dilate, this cavity may thereafter be prevented from dilating.[48] The elevated left atrial pressure may lead more rapidly to pulmonary venous, pulmonary arterial, and right ventricular dilatation with subsequent tricuspid regurgitation and development of huge right atrial dilatation.

Nonrheumatic causes of mitral stenosis include congenital anomalies; neoplasms (particularly myxoma) protruding through the mitral orifice from the left atrium (but malignant neoplasms primary or secondary in the lung may grow in the mitral orifice by way of the pulmonary veins[49]); large vegetations from active infective endocarditis[50]; and massive mitral annular calcific deposits,[51] particularly when associated with small-sized left ventricular cavities and left ventricular outflow tract obstruction. A relatively new, acquired cause of mitral stenosis is a mechanical prosthetic or bioprosthetic cardiac valve.[52-54] Since the native mitral valve is within the left ventricle, a prosthetic mitral valve also is located within this cavity. The prosthesis must be small enough for the contracting left ventricular wall not to interfere with movement of the prosthetic poppet or disc. When the prosthesis is too large for the cavity into which it was inserted, the poppet may be prevented from moving adequately and may therefore obstruct left atrial emptying. The latter state is far more common than obstruction to left ventricular emptying by the prosthesis. Thrombus formation on a mitral prosthesis also may obstruct left atrial emptying.

AORTIC VALVE STENOSIS

If papillary muscle dysfunction is excluded, valvular aortic stenosis is the most common fatal cardiac valve lesion, making up 49% of 1010 personally studied necropsy patients >15 years of age with valvular heart disease.[33] Of the 495 necropsy patients with aortic stenosis (with or without aortic regurgitation), the lesion was isolated in 59%, and in the other 41% the mitral valve was stenotic or regurgitant or both. The evidence is substantial that the cause of aortic stenosis, when associated with mitral valve disease, is rheumatic.[39] In contrast, the evidence is substantial that isolated (mitral valve anatomically normal) aortic stenosis (with or without associated aortic regurgitation) is nonrheumatic in origin.[39] This section focuses on patients with isolated aortic stenosis.

In contrast to what was generally believed 30 or so years ago,[55] at least three factors indicate that anatomically isolated aortic valve disease (actually either stenosis or pure regurgitation) is nonrheumatic in origin[39]: (1) the low frequency (about 10%) of a positive history of acute rheumatic fever; (2) the absence of Aschoff bodies; and, most important, (3) the frequency of an underlying congenital malformation of the aortic valve.

The structure of the aortic valve in aortic stenosis can be correlated to some extent with the age of the patient.[56] In patients <15 years old, the aortic valve most commonly (60%) is congenitally unicuspid and unicommissural[57,58]; in patients 16 to 65 years of age, the valve is most commonly (60%) congenitally bicuspid; and in patients age >65 years, the valve is most commonly (90%) tricuspid.[39] The stenosis is either caused by or superimposed on the congenitally malformed aortic valve in virtually all patients <15 years of age, and in about 70% of patients aged 16 to 65 years. A congenitally malformed—in this case congenitally bicuspid—valve appears to be the underlying condition in about 10% of patients >65 years old with aortic stenosis.

The unicommissural valve, the only type of unicuspid valve observed in the aortic valve position, was described initially by Edwards[59] in 1958. Although this valve, like all other congenitally malformed aortic valves, tends to get progressively more stenotic with time, the unicuspid aortic valve is almost certainly stenotic from the time of birth, whereas this usually is not the case with the congenitally bicuspid valve. Actually, the fewer the number of aortic valve cusps and commissures, the greater the likelihood that the valve is stenotic from birth.

Next to the floppy mitral valve, the congenitally biscuspid aortic valve is the most frequent major congenital malformation of the heart or great vessels.[60-62] Although its exact frequency is uncertain, this malformation appears to occur in about 1% of human births. Osler[63] found 10 apparently normally functioning congenitally bicuspid aortic valves in 800 autopsies (750 of which were performed by him), a frequency of 1%. Eight additional patients had infective endocarditis involving congenitally bicuspid aortic valves. Thus 18 (2%) of 800 had either normally functioning or infected congenitally bicuspid aortic valves. Grant et al.[64] found apparently normally functioning congenitally bicuspid aortic valves in 12 (1%) of 1350 necropsy patients. Osler,[63] Lewis and Grant,[65] and Grant et al.[64] do not appear to have appreciated that the bicuspid condition of this valve may underlie severe stenosis at this site. Thus if congenitally bicuspid aortic valves that develop complications (stenosis or regurgitation with or without infection) are added to those that function normally during the entire lifetime, the frequency of congenitally bicuspid aortic valves may exceed 1% in the entire population.

Among the complications of the bicuspid condition of the aortic valve, stenosis is by far the most frequent[60, 62]; pure regurgitation is next,[61] and the latter lesion is most frequently the result of its being the site of infective endocarditis.[66] Among 200 patients (75% male) with congenitally bicuspid aortic valves studied personally at necropsy, 157 (79%) had aortic stenosis, 22 (11%) had pure aortic regurgitation (in 19 from infective endocarditis), and 21 (10%) had normally functioning bicuspid valves.[62] The latter 21 patients died of noncardiac causes, and the presence of the congenitally bicuspid aortic valve was a surprise finding at necropsy. Of the 157 patients with aortic stenosis, calcific deposits were present on both aortic valve cusps in 155 (99%); the two patients without calcific deposits were <30 years of age. Calcific deposits, in contrast, were rare in the patients with pure aortic regurgitation. Infective endocarditis occurred in 14 (9%) of the 157 patients with aortic stenosis and in 19 (86%) of the 22 with pure aortic regurgitation, and the infection was the prime cause of the regurgitation in all 19 patients. Infective endocarditis usually affects the normally functioning or only mildly dysfunctioning bicuspid aortic valve.[66] It infrequently affects a significantly stenotic aortic valve. The infection usually causes considerable destruction of one or both aortic valve cusps, leading to severe aortic regurgitation. Rarely, perforation of a cusp may occur without superimposed infective endocarditis.[67] The presence of a bicuspid aortic valve in an intravenous drug user is particularly devastating.[68]

Congenitally bicuspid aortic valves also are commonly observed in patients having aortic valve replacement for isolated (mitral valve function normal) aortic stenosis with or without associated aortic regurgitation.[61] Among 393 patients aged 17 to 74 years with aortic stenosis with or without aortic regurgitation having aortic valve replacement at the National Heart, Lung, and Blood Institute from 1962 to 1982, 28 (7%) had unicommissural, unicuspid aortic valves; 203 (52%) had congenitally bicuspid aortic valves; 101 (26%) had tricuspid aortic valves; and in 61 (15%) the number of cusps could not be determined by examination of the operatively excised valve. Subramanian et al.[69] determined the number of aortic valve cusps present in 338 patients (most aged 50 to 70 years) undergoing aortic valve replacement for isolated (I excluded their 36 patients with associated mitral stenosis or regurgitation) "pure" aortic stenosis during 4 different years (1965, 1970, 1975, and 1980). Of the 338 patients, 21 (6%) had unicommissural, unicuspid valves; 171 (51%) had congenitally bicuspid valves; 94 (28%) had tricuspid aortic valves; and in 14 patients (4%) the number of cusps present was not discernible.

Congenitally bicuspid aortic valves also are found commonly among patients undergoing aortic valve replacement for isolated (normal mitral valve function), pure (no element of stenosis) aortic regurgitation. Of 190 patients having aortic valve replacement for pure, chronic aortic regurgitation (mitral valve normal) at the National Heart, Lung, and Blood Institute, 21 (11%) had congenitally bicuspid aortic valves.[62] Of the 21 patients, 14 (67%) never had infective endocarditis, and therefore the regurgitation was on the basis of the congenital malformation only; the other seven (33%) had infective endocarditis superimposed on the bicuspid condition, and severe aortic regurgitation in each resulted primarily from the infection, which in each was healed by antibiotics. Olson et al.[70] also determined the frequency of bicuspid aortic valves in 145 patients having isolated aortic valve replacement for pure aortic regurgitation or severe regurgitation associated with only mild aortic stenosis. (The basis of the presence or absence of associated aortic stenosis was by "clinical" means, which apparently did not mean hemodynamic studies.) Of the 145 patients, 49 (34%) had congenitally bicuspid aortic valves. Of these 49 patients, 41

(84%) apparently never had infective endocarditis, and the regurgitation primarily was on the basis of the bicuspid state of the valve; the other eight (16%) had had infective endocarditis, which was the major cause of the regurgitation. Of the remaining 96 patients (66%), 94 (65% of the total) had tricuspid aortic valves, and two (1% of the total) had quadricuspid valves. Of the 94 patients with tricuspid aortic valves, the cause of the aortic regurgitation in 34 (36%) was "postinflammatory" (presumably rheumatic in at least 31—each of the aortic valve cusps in these patients was diffusely fibrotic with or without cuspal retraction or commissural fusion); was associated with aortic root dilatation in 44 (47%) (idiopathic in 43 [98%] and syphilitic in one [2%]); was associated with infective endocarditis in 12 (13%); and was associated with ventricular septal defect in four (4%).

The reason one congenitally bicuspid aortic valve becomes stenotic, another becomes purely regurgitant, and another becomes the site of infective endocarditis is unknown. It is clear, however, that stenosis, regurgitation, and infection are complications of the bicuspid condition of the aortic valve, and none of these conditions are present at birth. It appears likely that a congenitally bicuspid aortic valve becomes stenotic only as its cusps become fibrotic and calcified; neither cusp of a congenitally bicuspid aortic valve is severely thickened by fibrous tissue or by calcific deposits at the time of birth.

The frequency of the development of stenosis or pure regurgitation at the site of a congenitally bicuspid aortic valve also is unknown. Lewis and Grant[65] concluded that vegetations develop at these sites in about 23% of adults (16 of 69) with congenitally bicuspid valves. Of 31 patients with "subacute infective endocarditis" studied at necropsy by Lewis and Grant,[65] eight (26%) had congenitally bicuspid aortic valves. Two (9%) of 22 patients studied at necropsy by Fulton and Levine[71] had congenitally bicuspid aortic valves. None of these investigators apparently was aware that congenitally bicuspid aortic valves could also become stenotic.

The mechanism by which a congenitally bicuspid aortic valve becomes stenotic or purely regurgitant is uncertain. There is no evidence that the valve is stenotic or regurgitant at birth. Likewise, there is no evidence that superimposed rheumatic fever or rheumatic heart disease is the cause of the stenosis or pure regurgitation. The explanation advanced by Edwards[72] is attractive. He proposed that it is not mechanically possible for a congenitally bicuspid aortic valve to open and close properly. The distances between the lateral attachments of normal aortic valvular cusps along their free margins are curved lines. The extra length allows the cusps to move freely during opening and closing of the orifice. In contrast, the distances between the lateral attachments of congenitally bicuspid aortic valves along their free margins approach straight lines. If these distances were exactly straight lines, the valve could not open during ventricular systole. Consequently, at least one cusp is larger than the other. But the excessive length of one or both cusps of a congenitally bicuspid aortic valve produces abnormal contact between the cusps. This abnormal contact in turn causes focal fibrous thickening that with time becomes diffuse, and dystrophic calcification thereafter occurs. Thus stenosis of a congenitally bicuspid aortic valve may be the result of trauma to these cusps produced by their abnormal contact with each other. Although this explanation is appealing, it does not explain why one congenitally bicuspid aortic valve becomes stenotic, another becomes entirely regurgitant with or without infection, and another remains free of complications.

It is well recognized that patients with aortic isthmic coarctation often have congenitally bicuspid aortic valves. Of 200 patients with aortic ischemic coarctation studied at necropsy by Abbott,[73] 27% had congenitally bicuspid aortic valves. Of 104 patients with aortic isthmic coarctation studied at necropsy by Reifenstein et al.,[74] 62% had congenitally bicuspid aortic valves. These authors also pointed out that ascending aortic tears with or without dissection also were common (about 20%) in patients with aortic isthmic coarctation, but similar aortic lesions have an increased frequency among patients with congenitally bicuspid aortic valves unassociated with aortic isthmic coarctation. It is less well appreciated that an occasional patient may present with clinical features of aortic stenosis but by aortogram be found to have aortic isthmic coarctation. Among 157 personally studied necropsy patients with stenotic congenitally bicuspid aortic valves, seven (4%) had aortic isthmic coarctation.[62]

Patients with bicuspid aortic valves have an increased frequency of aortic dissection compared with persons with a tricuspid aortic valve. A bicuspid aortic valve was found in 11 (13%) of 85 patients with aortic dissection reported by Gore and Seiwert,[75] in 11 (9%) of 119 cases reported by Edwards et al.,[76] and in 14 (7.5%) of 186 necropsy patients with aortic dissection reported by Roberts and Roberts.[77] Aortic dissection was found in 8 (5%) of 152 necropsy patients ≥20 years of age with a bicuspid aortic valve by Fenoglio et al.[78] Larson and Edwards[79] observed aortic dissection in 18 (6%) of 293 necropsy patients with a bicuspid aortic valve and in 141 (0.67%) of 21,105 persons with a tricuspid aortic valve, a ninefold difference. Roberts and Roberts[77] found aortic dissection in 14 (4%) of 328 patients studied at necropsy with a congenitally bicuspid aortic valve. Of the 16 patients with congenitally malformed aortic valves (14 bicuspid and 2 unicuspid) studied by Roberts and Roberts,[77] the entrance tear was in the ascending aorta in all 16. The aortic valve was stenotic in six and two had associated aortic isthmic coarctation. Histologic sections of aorta disclosed severe degeneration of the elastic fibers of aortic media in 90% of the patients studied. Thus a congenitally malformed aortic valve appears to be present at least five times more frequently in adults with than in those without aortic dissection.

The use of echocardiography and magnetic resonance imaging allows detection of the presence of a bicuspid aortic valve before symptoms or signs of cardiac dysfunction appear.[80, 81] In a person found to have a bicuspid aortic valve, the following advice may be useful in preventing the development of complications[82]:

(1) *Avoid infection.* Prophylactic antibiotics obviously are required during dental and other operative procedures. Sir William Osler[83] was the one who pointed out in 1885 the extreme propensity of the bicuspid aortic valve to be the site of infective endocarditis. Certainly, one with a bicuspid aortic valve should not use illicit drugs intravenously.[84]

(2) *Maintain a normal systemic blood pressure.* Although the bicuspid aortic valve probably is not affected adversely by the left ventricular systolic pressure irrespective of its level, the level of the valve's closing pressure—i.e., the aortic diastolic pressure—probably plays a prominent role in determining whether the bicuspid valve becomes stenotic or purely regurgitant (without superimposed infective endocarditis) or functions normally throughout life.

(3) *Keep the heart rate relatively slow.* It is reasonable to believe that if the aortic valve closes only 55 times a minute rather than 75 times a minute (a 27% heart rate reduction), the wear and tear received by the aortic valve from the aorta's closing pressure would be reduced. The best way to produce a relatively slow heart rate is by various aerobic exercises. Although the heart rate increases during exercise, the total 24-hour heart beats probably would be reduced substantially. β-Blocker therapy could be useful to achieve this objective.

(4) *Keep the total serum cholesterol level relatively low.* The major reason a bicuspid aortic valve becomes stenotic is because large calcific deposits develop on the aortic aspects of the cusps and the large deposits impart an immobility to the cusps that prevents their opening adequately during ventricular systole. Thus prevention of calcific deposits is essential for prevention of stenosis. In older persons in the Western world it is common to develop calcific deposits on the aortic aspects of the aortic valve cusps, on the ventricular aspects of the posterior mitral leaflet (mitral "annular" calcium), and in atherosclerotic plaques in the coronary arteries (as well as in plaques in other arteries). The development of calcific deposits on the aortic valve, mitral annulus, and coronary arteries with age occurs only in those populations with total serum cholesterol levels >150 mg/dl, and usually in those persons with levels >200 mg/dl. Thus maintaining a low total serum cholesterol level prevents calcific deposits on a normally formed aortic valve, and therefore it is reasonable to believe that maintaining a low level would have a similar effect on a bicuspid aortic valve. Calcific deposits are never present on the aortic valve at birth; they are always acquired. Calcific deposits are less common on stenotic mitral valves (rheumatic origin) in persons residing in the undeveloped nations of the world (where the total serum cholesterol levels often are <150 mg/dl) than in persons in the Western world where these levels are usually >150 mg/dl. Thus maintaining a relatively low total serum cholesterol level might deter calcific deposition on a bicuspid aortic valve and, if no calcium, usually no stenosis. Preventing calcific deposits, however, would not prevent the development of pure aortic regurgitation or infective endocarditis.

(5) *Try to forget that the aortic valve is bicuspid.* As long as the bicuspid valve functions normally there is nothing to worry about, and no one can predict which bicuspid aortic valve will function normally for a full lifetime and which one will become stenotic, purely regurgitant (without superimposed infective endocarditis), or infected. In other words, the natural history of a congenitally bicuspid aortic valve is unknown. It appears that about 1% of live births have a congenitally bicuspid valve. If that be the case, about 50 million (of 5 billion) persons on planet earth have a congenitally bicuspid aortic valve, and about 2.5 million persons in the USA have a bicuspid aortic valve. What percentage of them in a lifetime will develop stenosis, pure regurgitation, infection, or no complications is unknown. Thus life must continue and the focus must be on things other than the bicuspid aortic valve. Even with the worst scenario, aortic valve replacement is usually highly successful.

In contrast to the congenitally bicuspid aortic valve, the congenitally unicuspid aortic valve is far less common (about 15 times less common). At least two varieties of the unicuspid aortic valve exist. In one, the orifice is located in the center of the cusp and there are no attachments or only rudimentary attachments to the wall of the aorta. Edwards[59] referred to this valve as the simple-dome type. Another name might be *acommissural valve*. This type of valve is commonly found in patients with congenital pulmonic stenosis—indeed, it is the most frequent type of valve seen in that setting but it is exceedingly uncommon in the aortic valve position. A second type of unicuspid valve is the *unicommissural valve*. This valve, described by Edwards[59] in 1958, is characterized by an eccentrically located orifice and only one lateral attachment to the aortic wall and that at the level of the orifice. From above, this valve has the appearance of an exclamation mark. In contrast to the bicuspid aortic valve, the unicuspid valve is nearly always stenotic from the time of birth.

Tricuspid aortic valves rarely appear to be stenotic at birth. If stenosis is present at birth and the aortic valve has three cusps, the stenosis is usually the result of a very small aortic "annulus" rather than the result of fusion of the cusps. Acquired stenosis of a tricuspid aortic valve, in contrast, is common. Of necropsy patients aged 16 to 65 years studied personally with clinically isolated aortic stenosis (with or without regurgitation), 25% had tricuspid valves, and among those aged >65 years of age, 90% had tricuspid valves.[56] In the age group 16 to 65 years, about 50% of these patients with clinically isolated aortic stenosis and tricuspid aortic valves also had diffuse fibrous thickening of the mitral leaflets. The associated diffuse mitral leaflet thickening is strong evidence that the etiology of the aortic stenosis in this group is rheumatic.[39] Also, nearly 75% of this group had positive histories of acute rheumatic fever, whereas 10% of the other group, that is, those with anatomically normal mitral valves with aortic stenosis, had positive histories.[39] The etiology of the aortic stenosis in patients ≤65 years with tricuspid aortic valves and anatomically normal mitral valves is unsolved. Possibly, minor abnormalities in the sizes of the aortic valve cusps from birth set the stage for abnormal contact of the cusps with one another, with resultant fibrosis and finally stenosis.[85]

Stenosis of the aortic valve in patients over age 65 is usually characteristic.[86-88] The valves are tricuspid, calcific deposits are rather uniformly distributed on the aortic aspects of the cusps, and the commissures are not fused. Obstruction is entirely the result of the presence of large calcific deposits that prevent the cusps from retracting adequately during ventricular systole. Because the commissures are usually not fused, associated aortic regurgitation is infrequent.

Clinically, aortic stenosis in the elderly is characterized by several features that are either absent or more prominent than in a younger subject with this valvular lesion[86]: (1) the systemic arterial pulse pressure may be increased because of a systolic hypertension; (2) a harsh right basasl systolic murmur may be relatively inconspicuous while a pure musical systolic murmur may be prominent at the apex; (3) a coexisting apical systolic murmur of mitral regurgitation may be related to mitral annular calcium and not to left ventricular failure; and (4) systemic systolic hypertension can result in a comparatively small pressure gradient despite severe left ventricular outflow obstruction.

Auscultatory signs that accompany aortic stenosis in the elderly may differ from those in younger subjects. Ejection sounds are characteristically absent since the cusps are rigid and ejection sounds depend upon abrupt movement of mobile valves. Atrial sounds (fourth heart sounds) are useful signs for judging the severity of aortic stenosis in the younger adult but are of little help in the elderly patient, since they may occur normally in the older age group. Ordinarily, the systolic murmur of valvular aortic stenosis is harsh, rough, grunting, and is loudest at the right base with radiation upward and to the right. In elderly patients with aortic stenosis, the harsh murmur at the right base may persist but may be of less intensity, and auscultation may be dominated instead by a loud, pure-frequency, musical systolic murmur maximal at or near the cardiac apex. At least three reasons account for these patterns. First, older persons tend to have increased upper thoracic chest dimensions that soften the basal murmurs. Second is the effect of the morphology of the stenotic aortic valve. A rigid, calcified valve with commissural fusion provides a suitable mechanism for a high velocity jet into the ascending aorta; the noisy murmur at the right base appears to originate within the ascending aorta because of turbulence caused by the high velocity jet. A calcified, stenotic, trileaflet aortic valve without commissural fusion, the most common type in the elderly, behaves differently. Ejection into the ascending aorta may take the form of a "spray" instead of a jet, so that the harsh murmur at the right base may be comparatively inconspicuous. Since the cusps are not fused, they may vibrate during ventricular ejection and this may account for the pure-frequency, musical "cooing" murmur recordable within the left ventricle. Third, calcium in the mitral annulus, itself a producer of precordial murmurs, in elderly patients frequently accompanies calcium of the aortic valve. Mitral regurgitation can result from inability of the calcified annulus to decrease its circumference during ventricular contraction. Accordingly, the holosystolic murmur of mitral regurgitation may be present at the apex and may be difficult to distinguish from the coexisting pure-frequency aortic stenotic apical murmur. Although mitral annular calcium tends to complicate the auscultatory diagnosis of aortic stenosis, the radiologic identification of these calcific deposits implies that coexisting aortic stenosis is likely to be caused by calcific deposits on a trileaflet valve without commissural fusion.

The degree of left ventricular systolic hypertension in elderly patients may be considerably higher than that occurring in younger subjects with similar degrees of aortic stenosis, since the peripheral systolic systemic pressure ususally rises with age. The degree of systolic hypertension that the elderly left ventricle is capable of achieving can be astonishingly high, particularly since this chamber seldom maintains a systolic pressure in excess of 250 mm Hg even in younger subjects. Systemic hypertension may reduce the aortic gradient, and the degree of obstruction may be underestimated in the elderly patients if the peak systolic pressure difference is taken as the only index of severity. As the gradient diminishes in the presence of systemic systolic hypertension, the murmur at the right base may soften and shorten. Even if this auscultatory change does not occur with systemic hypertension, the modification of the systemic arterial pulse may be misleading, since the rate of rise can be relatively normal and the pulse pressure may be increased despite severe obstruction to the left ventricular outflow.

The frequency of atrial fibrillation is higher in older compared with younger patients with aortic stenosis. This arrhythmia, however, is common in elderly persons without valvular cardiac disease. The left atrial cavities are dilated in patients with aortic stenosis, but left atrial dilatation commonly accompanies old age in the absence of functionally significant valvular lesions. The left ventricular wall becomes less compliant with age, and the superimposed left ventricular hypertrophy (without left ventricular dilatation) of aortic stenosis may further impede left atrial emptying. The only common anatomic feature in elderly patients with atrial fibrillation is left atrial dilatation. The combination of atrial fibrillation, a long apical systolic murmur, and left atrial dilatation can obscure the diagnosis of aortic stenosis and lead to a mistaken diagnosis of isolated mitral regurgitation. Atrial fibrillation is especially undesirable in aortic stenosis, since the left ventricle requires the help of augmented left atrial contraction that increases end-diastolic fiber length and permits the left ventricle to contract with greater force.

The cause of the aortic stenosis in elderly patients has been considered the "wear-and-tear" of aging. My own view is that the calcific deposits are a form of atherosclerosis because they occur only in societies where the total serum cholesterol level is >150 mg/dl.[89] Most patients >65 years of age with aortic stenosis also have calcific deposits in the mitral annular region and virtually 100% have calcific deposits in the coronary arteries (within plaques). The latter lesions are of course the result of atherosclerosis, a fact that suggests that calcific deposits in both aortic valve cusps and the mitral annular region are atherosclerotic in nature.

Although relatively few patients with valvular aortic stenosis have positive histories of acute rheumatic fever, the occurrence of a positive history in a patient presenting clinically with apparently pure aortic stenosis (with or without regurgitation) should caution the examining physician to the possibility of accompanying mitral valvular disease. Usually in this situation the mitral leaflets are diffusely, although mildly, thickened but mitral valvular function is normal. On rare occasions, however, mitral stenosis may be an accompanying lesion and of such severity that it is clinically silent. Mitral stenosis should be ruled out, however, before operative therapy is undertaken in any patient presenting with apparently isolated valvular aortic stenosis (with or without regurgitation) and a positive history of acute rheumatic fever.

AORTIC REGURGITATION

In contrast to valvular aortic stenosis, which basically has only three etiologies (congenital, atherosclerotic, and rheumatic), there are numerous causes of pure aortic regurgitation.[88] The causes may be subdivided into those resulting from conditions affecting primarily the valvular cusps, and into those affecting primarily the aorta. This discussion will include only the major causes of fatal aortic regurgitation. Those affecting primarily the cusps include rheumatic disease, infective endocarditis, and congenital malformations. Those causing aortic regurgitation primarily by affecting the aorta include syphilis, the Marfan syndrome and its forme fruste varieties, and ankylosing spondylitis.

Rheumatic heart disease. Rheumatic heart disease is primarily a disease of the mitral valve.[33] Other valves may be affected, but the mitral valve is always involved anatomically, although it may function normally. Rheumatic heart disease never affects only the aortic valve, and if this valve is the only one involved anatomically, the cause is a condition other than rheumatic. The aortic valve, however, may be made seriously incompetent (or stenotic) by rheumatic involvement and yet the mitral valve may show only mild fibrous scarring but no dysfunction. Most patients with serious rheumatic aortic valve disease have some aortic stenosis as well as incompetency. Less frequently encountered is the aortic valve made purely incompetent by rheumatic involvement unless the mitral valve also is made to function improperly by this condition.

Among the causes of pure aortic regurgitation, rheumatic disease is still an important one. Clinically, the clue to a rheumatic etiology is a positive history of acute rheumatic fever, which was present in 8 of the 10 necropsy patients studied personally. The purely incompetent rheumatic aortic valve is diffusely thickened by fibrous tissue and one or more of the three cusps is severely retracted. A cusp may be so contracted by the rheumatic process that only a small residue of the original cusp is identifiable. The commissures are only mildly fused if at all. Most valves associated with significant commissural fusion have elements of stenosis and therefore are not purely regurgitant. Calcific deposits are either absent or present in small amounts. The major feature of the rheumatic process therefore is diffuse fibrous thickening of the three cusps with retraction of one or more of them. The ascending aorta may be dilated, but it is of normal thickness and the intima is not affected. The mitral valve cusps are diffusely thickened by fibrous tissue.

INFECTIVE ENDOCARDITIS

Infective endocarditis is the most common cause of fatal isolated pure aortic regurgitation, and the aortic valve is the valve most commonly affected by fatal infective endocarditis.[66] Not all patients with active infective endocarditis involving the aortic valve, however, develop aortic regurgitation. The aortic regurgitation results from perforations or tears of one or more of the cusps. Usually vegetations are present on each aortic valve cusp when the valve is regurgitant. Although it is well appreciated that the congenitally bicuspid aortic valve has a particular propensity to become the site of vegetations, the aortic valve in most patients with infective endocarditis consists of three cusps.

Fatal infective endocarditis is more often observed when the infection involves a previously normal rather than a previously abnormal aortic valve.[66] Because infection of previously anatomically normal valves is nearly always by virulent organisms, and because the infective process can more easily destroy a thin, delicate (normal) valve as opposed to a thick, tough (abnormal) valve, the frequency of involvement by infective endocarditis of previously anatomically normal valves in a necropsy study might be abnormally high. The frequency of infective endocarditis is clearly higher in persons with underlying cardiac disease than in persons with previously normal hearts. Among cases of infective endocarditis, however, there is more involvement of previously normal than previously abnormal valves. This fact may be explained simply by the larger number of normal than abnormal valves.

An unfortunate consequence of infective endocarditis affecting the aortic valve is the frequency with which ring abscesses develop. Ring abscesses of the mitral valve, in contrast, occur infrequently. Ring abscesses are the result of the spreading of the infective process from the valve cusps into the adjacent tissue. Although the material within the abscess can be made sterile by antibiotics, the presence of a ring abscess can prevent successful valve replacement were this procedure necessary during the period of activity.

Considerable destruction to an aortic valve by active infective endocarditis does not prevent healing of the infective process. Relatively little information, however, is available on the morphologic aspects of healed infective endocarditis. The only anatomic abnormality definitely indicative of healed infective endocarditis of the aortic valve is the presence of cuspal perforations.[90]

CONGENITAL MALFORMATIONS

Aortic regurgitation commonly occurs in patients with congenitally malformed aortic valves, particularly those that are bicuspid. The aortic regurgitation may be severe and unassociated with any element of stenosis or any signs of previous infective endocarditis.[61]

SYPHILIS

Syphilis remains an important cause of severe aortic regurgitation.[87, 88] The luetic process causes the aortic wall to be as much as four times thicker than normal. The thickening is the result of both intimal and adventitial scarring. The aortic media, in contrast, is not thickened, and many of its elastic fibers are replaced by scar tissue. The walls of the vasa vasora are thickened and their lumens are narrowed. Collections of lymphocytes and plasma cells surround many vasa vasora. Arteriosclerotic plaques are superimposed on the diseased aorta in all patients. No spirochetes are found on special stains of aorta. The aortic "annuli" are dilated and this root dilatation may prevent coaptation of the aortic valve cusps. The distal margins of the aortic cusps are thickened but the cusps are freely mobile and otherwise grossly and histologically normal. The commissures are usually not "widened."

Aortic regurgitation occurs in about 30% of patients with cardiovascular syphilis. The aortic regurgitation results primarily from aortic root dilatation, the consequence of the destructive aortitis. Stretched by the dilated aortic root, the cusps are unable to meet in ventricular diastole and a central regurgitant stream results. The fibrosis of the rolled free margins of the aortic valve cusps appears to be a consequence of the aortic regurgitation and not the result of valvulitis per se. Syphilitic aortitis may involve the entire ascending aorta, or some portions may be spared. The site of disease in the aorta is the major determinant of valvular dysfunction. Extensive destruction of the ascending aorta, even with aneurysm, may occur in the absence of aortic regurgitation if the aortic wall immediately behind the sinuses is spared. Thus the aortic root is the important determinant of aortic valve function, and involvement of it by the leutic process usually prevents valve closure during ventricular diastole.

Ankylosing spondylitis. Bulkley and Roberts[91] studied at necropsy eight patients with ankylosing spondylitis and aortic regurgitation. All were men aged 34 to 55 years. All had severe congestive cardiac failure and signs and symptoms of joint involvement consistent with akylosing spondylitis. In all eight patients, the joint symptoms antedated those of congestive cardiac failure, in seven of them by 10 to 20 years. In five of the eight patients, however, precordial murmurs of aortic regurgitation were noted at the same time or within 1 year of the onset of joint symptoms. Serologic tests (Venereal Disease Research Laboratories [VDRL]) for syphilis were negative in all patients. Conduction disturbances were present in six patients. At catheterization, the left ventricular and systemic arterial diastolic pressures were equal in five of seven patients studied. Aortic valve replacement was carried out in five patients. Death in seven patients was directly related to the aortic valvular disease and occurred at an average of 6 years from the onset of congestive cardiac failure.

At necropsy, the hearts weighed 520 to 1100 gm (average 756). The aortic valve cusps were shortened and always thickened at their basal attachments and distal margins, and frequently in between. Focal calcific deposits were present along the bases of the cusps in four patients, and in one they extended to the anterior mitral leaflet and membranous septum. The ascending aorta was diffusely dilated in all eight patients. The thickening was limited to the most caudal 3 cm of the ascending aorta, and the wall behind the sinuses of Valsalva was always involved. The thickening resulted from dense connective tissue in the adventitia of the aorta. The adventitial scarring was continuous with similar scarring in the groove between the anterior mitral leaflet and the aortic valve cusps, producing a fibrous ridge between the base of the aortic valve cusps and the anterior mitral leaflet. In four patients the fibrous tissue also infiltrated the membranous ventricular septum. A few mononuclear cells were present in the adventitia of the aorta, and the lumens of the vasa vasora were narrowed by extensive intimal fibrous proliferation and medial hypertrophy (just as in syphilis). The media of the aorta behind the sinuses showed evidence of severe degeneration, and the overlying intima was thickened by proliferated fibrous tissue.

Although aortic regurgitation had been described previously in ankylosing spondylitis, the distinctive morphologic features of the cardiovascular lesion were described by Bulkley and Roberts.[91] The aortic valve cusps, particularly their basal attachments and margins, are thickened by fibrous tissue. The extension of the dense adventitial fibrosis below the attachments of the aortic valve cusps to the anterior mitral leaflet and the membranous ventricular septum distinguished these patients morphologically from those with aortic regurgitation of other etiologies. The extension of the scarring process below the aortic valve also explains the frequency of conduction disturbances in ankylosing spondylitis and their infrequency in patients with syphilis.

Although the aortic valve cusps are abnormal in as high as 20% of patients, aortic regurgitation is said to occur clinically in only about 3% of patients with ankylosing spondylitis. Symptoms of arthritis usually antedate the cardiac disease by 10 to 20 years. In five of the eight patients studied by Bulkley and Roberts[91] and in patients described by others, precordial murmurs were noted within 2 years of the onset of joint symptoms. Symptoms of cardiac dysfunction, however, developed much later. This observation suggests that the joints and the aortic root area may be attacked at the same time, but that it takes many years for the sclerosing process to produce aortic regurgitation.

Ankylosing spondylitis has been described as a benign disease. Seven of the eight patients studied by Bulkley and Roberts, however, died of consequences of aortic regurgitation at a mean age of 46 years, with death occurring within 6 years of the first symptoms of cardiac disease. The age at death in the 16 patients with ankylosing spondylitis and aortic regurgitation reported by Clark et al.[92] was 45 years, and the interval from the onset of symptomatic heart disease to death was also 6 years. In contrast, the overall mortality of patients with ankylosing spondylitis has been reported to be similar to that of the general population. Thus the presence of aortic regurgitation appears to be a prime determinant of whether or not ankylosing spondylitis shortens life.

THE MARFAN SYNDROME

The Marfan syndrome generally involves the bones, joints, eyes, heart, and blood vessels. The extremities are long and thin (dolichostenomelia), the ligaments and joint capsules are redundant, the lenses are dislocated (ectopia lentis), the ascending aorta often is dilated, and one or both left-sided cardiac valves frequently are regurgitant. Cardiovascular disease is by far the most common cause of death in patients with the Marfan syndrome. Of 18 personally studied necropsy patients fulfilling McKusick's criteria for this syndrome, all died from cardiovascular disease and death in each was premature (mean age = 34 years [range 15 to 52]).[93] Of 56 deceased patients with this syndrome studied during life by Murdoch et al.,[94] cardiovascular disease was the cause of death in 52 (93%), and the mean age at death was 32 years. Of the 151 previously reported necropsy patients with the Marfan syndrome, the mean age at death was 23 years and ranged from stillbirth to 65 years. (The 91 articles in which these 151 patients were described are listed in the article by Roberts and Honig.[93])

A variety of cardiovascular lesions has been observed in the great arteries and hearts of patients with the Marfan syndrome. My personally studied 18 necropsy patients with this syndrome readily separated into three groups on the basis of their cardiovascular lesions. Group I included 13 patients with fusiform aneurysms of the ascending aorta. All 13 patients had aortic regurgitation, and six also had associated mitral regurgitation. In each, the aneurysm involved the sinus and the proximal tubular portions of the ascending aorta; two also had fusiform aneurysms in the descending thoracic aorta. Histologic study of the wall of the ascending aorta disclosed the typical lesion of this syndrome, that is, massive loss of elastic fibers and increased amounts of mucoid material in the media. Group II included three patients with dissection of the entire aorta. Before dissection, the aorta in each was of normal size, and histologically the wall of the aorta was normal. None of these three patients had either aortic or mitral regurgitation before the aortic dissection. Two, however, had had systemic hypertension. Group III included two patients with isolated mitral regurgitation with floppy mitral leaflets and markedly dilated mitral annuli. In each, the aortic lumen was of normal size and its wall was normal histologically.

In contrast to the predominant occurrence of fusiform ascending aortic aneurysm in my personally studied patients (13 of 18) and the relatively infrequent occurrence of aortic dissection (3 of 18), aortic dissection was the most frequent gross cardiovascular abnormality observed in the previously reported necropsy patients with the Marfan syndrome (57 [38%] of 151 patients), followed by aortic root aneurysm without dissection (53 patients [38%]), then mitral regurgitation without aortic root aneurysm or dissection (33 patients [22%]); and finally, eight patients (5%) did not have aortic dissection or root aneurysm or mitral regurgitation and were placed in a miscellaneous group. Analysis of the previously reported necropsy patients disclosed that those with either fusiform ascending aortic aneurysm or aortic dissection had similar mean ages (28 and 27 years), males were slightly more frequent in both groups (3:2), and only 10% of the 110 patients were aged $\leq$15 years. Sisk et al.[95] observed similar findings in 15 patients with the Marfan syndrome diagnosed at <15 years of age.

As in all our 13 patients with fusiform ascending aortic aneurysms (or "annuloaortic ectasia"), evidence of aortic regurgitation was present in almost all (95%) of the previously reported necropsy patients with fusiform ascending aortic aneurysm. As an indication of the severity of the aortic regurgitation in the reported patients with fusiform ascending aortic aneurysm, the average indirect peak systolic systemic arterial pressure in the 29 (of the 53) patients in whom this information was available was 146 mm Hg (range 100 to 195), and the average end-diastolic systemic arterial pressure was 43 mm Hg (range 0 to 90), yielding an average pulse pressure of just over 100 mm Hg (range 40 to 170). Of the 29 patients with fusiform root aneurysm and reported blood pressure measurements, 18 (62%) had systemic arterial systolic pressures <140 mm Hg, 26 (90%) had systemic diastolic pressures <60 mm Hg, and 23 (79%) had pulse pressures >60 mm Hg.

In contrast to their frequent recording in the reported necropsy patients with fusiform ascending aortic aneurysms, blood pressure values before the dissection occurred were virtually undisclosed in the 57 previously reported necropsy patients with aortic dissection (see Roberts and Honig[93]). Nevertheless, evidence of the presence of aortic regurgitation before the aortic dissection was rare. The reason that aortic regurgitation before dissection is rare in the patients with aortic dissection is because dissection in infrequent in the patients with fusiform ascending aortic aneurysm, and it is the latter which primarily is responsible for the severe aortic regurgitation (in the absence of healed dissection). With few exceptions, aortic dissection in patients with the Marfan syndrome tends to affect the previously normal-sized aorta or the aorta only slightly dilated. None of 13 personally studied necropsy patients with fusiform ascending aortic aneurysm had aortic dissection, and none of three personally studied patients with dissection of the entire aorta had evidence of fusiform ascending aortic aneurysm or aortic regurgitation before the dissection. Of the reported patients with aortic dissection, those with dilated ascending aortas over a long period of time usually had healed dissections, and the dilatation in them appeared to be the result of aneurysm of the false channel. In at least 14 of the 57 previously reported patients with aortic dissection, the dissection had healed (see Roberts and Honig[93]).

The reason that fusiform ascending aortic aneurysm occurs in some patients with the Marfan syndrome and aortic dissection occurs in others appears to lie in the status of the aortic media. In each of the 13 personally studied necropsy patients with fusiform aneurysm of the ascending aorta, histologic study of the wall of the aorta disclosed severe degrees of "cystic medial necrosis." In contrast, none of three patients with dissection involving the entire aorta had cystic medial necrosis by histologic examination. Furthermore, in 44 of the 53 previously reported necropsy patients with fusiform ascending aortic aneurysm cystic medial necrosis was described, and in the other nine patients its presence or absence was simply not mentioned. It was not mentioned as being absent in any patient, and in those in whom photomicrographs were illustrated, the degree of cystic medial necrosis was nearly always severe. Among the 57 previously reported necropsy patients with aortic dissection, cystic medial necrosis was described as being present in 35 and as being absent in seven. In the patients, however, in whom photomicrographs of the aorta were illustrated, the degree of cystic medial necrosis was usually minimal or mild, and rarely was the degree of cystic medial necrosis as severe as that observed routinely in the patients with fusiform ascending aortic aneurysm.

Thus the aortic media appears to be quite different in the patient with fusiform ascending aortic aneurysm and in those with aortic dissection, particularly when the latter involves the entire aorta. In the patients with fusiform ascending aortic aneurysm, there is usually "massive" degeneration or loss of the elastic fibers of the media and increased quantities of collagen and mucoid material. The increased quantities of collagen would appear to prevent longitudinal aortic dissection. The aortic media in the patients with aortic dissection, in contrast, tends to be normal or to have only a mild degree of cystic medial necrosis, just as in patients with aortic dissection and systemic hypertension who do not have the Marfan syndrome.[96] Two of the three patients with aortic dissection studied by me had evidence of diastolic systemic hypertension, whereas none of the other 16 patients had diastolic hypertension.

In none of the previous reports describing necropsy patients with the Marfan syndrome was the degree of cystic medial necrosis graded. In 1970, however, Carlson et al.[96] graded the severity of cystic medial necrosis from 1 to 4 among patients with systemic hypertension and among others with normotension. They found that the frequency of cystic medial necrosis increased progressively from 10% in the first two decades of life to 60% and 64% in the seventh and eighth decades, respectively. The frequency and extent of cystic medial necrosis were higher in the hypertensive than in the normotensive patients of similar age. Schlatmann and Becker[97] confirmed the observation that certain degrees of cystic medial necrosis are observed in the normal aorta and that the degrees of cystic medial necrosis increase with age. Schlatmann and Becker[98] also compared the ascending aortic media in patients with dilated aortas with those in patients with complete or incomplete dissection and found only quantitative differences between the normal aging aorta and the overtly abnormal aorta. Thus these newer observations regarding the frequency, extent, and significance of cystic medial necrosis must be taken into account when one is evaluating its presence in patients with the Marfan syndrome. Probably many of the Marfan patients with aortic dissection have no more cystic medial necrosis than might be expected for their age or level of systemic arterial pressure.

The term "cystic medial necrosis," incidentally, has certain defects because "cysts" are relatively infrequent and "necrosis" is difficult to identify. Furthermore, the striking histologic aortic lesion, when full blown, is massive degeneration of elastic fibers, and this feature is ignored by the term "cystic medial necrosis." When Gsell[99] in 1928 first used the term "medionecrosis" and a year later Erdheim[100, 101] used the term "cystic medial necrosis," stains for elastic fibers were apparently infrequently employed and loss or degeneration of elastic fibers may be difficult to appreciate on hematoxylin-eosin-stained sections.

When elastic fibers disappear from the aortic wall in this condition, the space previously occupied by them appears to be replaced by collagen fibrils and mucoid material. Although the increased acid mucopolysaccharide material has been considered an inherent defect in this condition, it is just as reasonable to believe that this material serves simply as "a filler" for the lost elastic fibers. Normally, the media of aorta in the ascending portion contains approximately 58 elastic lamellae.[102] It is not clear whether the numbers of the elastic lamellae are normal or decreased at the time of birth in patients with the Marfan syndrome. Whether normal or decreased, however, fusiform ascending aortic aneurysm, with or without tears, has not been described in newborns with this syndrome. Thus it appears that although the composition of the aortic media may be defective at birth, the aneurysms form later, presumably the consequence of the intraaortic pressure's effect on an inherently weak wall.

Although most fusiform aneurysms in the Marfan syndrome involve the ascending aorta (both sinus and tubular portions), aneurysm also may involve the descending thoracic aorta (as it did in two personally studied patients) and, as reported by others, the abdominal aorta. Because the numbers of elastic fibers in the abdominal aorta are only about one half of those present in the ascending aorta with intermediate numbers in between,[102] and because the major histologic finding in the medial portion of the aneurysmal wall is massive loss of elastic fibers, it is logical of course that the ascending aorta is the most common location of fusiform aneurysm in the Marfan syndrome. The ascending portion also moves ("stretches") the most with each heart beat ("hypermobile aorta"), and this factor also may play a role in this preferential location of aneurysms in this syndrome.[103]

Although the major consequence of fusiform ascending aortic aneurysm in the Marfan syndrome is aortic regurgitation (100% of 13 personally studied patients and 95% of 42 previously reported patients where this information was recorded), rupture of the aneurysm is of course also a danger. This event occurred in 2 of 13 personally studied patients and in at least 14 (25%) of the 57 previously reported necropsy patients with aortic dissection. Thus treatment of Marfan patients with fusiform ascending aortic aneurysms must be directed at elimination or prevention of aortic regurgitation and at prevention of aneurysmal rupture, not at prevention of dissection, because the latter is an infrequent complication in such patients.

Mitral regurgitation also is frequent in patients with the Marfan syndrome. At least six factors may be important in causing the mitral regurgitation: (1) dilatation of mitral annuli; (2) floppiness or prolapse of mitral leaflets or elongation of chordae tendineae; (3) calcification of mitral annuli; (4) rupture of mitral chordae tendineae; (5) infective endocarditis; and (6) papillary muscle dysfunction. Of these six factors, numbers 1,2,3, and 5 appear most important in causing severe degrees of mitral regurgitation. Of my 18 personally studied necropsy patients, nine had mitral regurgitation, isolated in two and combined with aortic regurgitation in seven. Of these nine patients, four had floppy mitral valves, whereas none of the nine patients without mitral regurgitation had floppy valves. The "floppiness" involved the posterior mitral leaflet in all four patients. Of the nine patients with mitral regurgitation, the circumference of the mitral annulus ranged from 10 to 17 cm (mean = 15; normal = 9), and of the nine patients without mitral regurgitation, the circumference ranged from 9 to 13 cm (mean 11). Thus the mean circumference of the mitral annulus in the nine patients with mitral regurgitation was dilated 67% over normal (15 compared with 9), and that in the nine patients without mitral regurgitation was dilated only 22% over normal (12 compared with 9). Thus both mitral leaflet prolapse and annular dilatation play significant roles in causing mitral regurgitation in these patients.

Calcification of the mitral annulus is known to cause or at least to be associated with mitral regurgitation. The degree of regurgitation produced by this mechanism alone, however, is nearly always mild or minimal, and in addition, the mitral annuli in patients not having the Marfan syndrome with mitral annular calcium are nearly always of normal or near-normal circumference. Of the 18 personally studied necropsy patients, five had mitral annular calcific deposits; all five had associated mitral regurgitation, but in addition, four had prolapsing mitral leaflets and in four the circumference of the mitral annulus was quite dilated (range 13 to 17 cm [mean = 15]). Evidence for rupture of mitral chordae tendineae was found in five of nine personally studied patients with, and in none of the nine patients without, mitral regurgitation. Two of these five patients had histories of infective endocarditis that had healed. All five patients with evidence of mitral chordal rupture had prolapsing mitral leaflets, and four had dilated mitral annuli (range 15 to 17 cm [mean = 16]).

The role played by "papillary muscle dysfunction" in causing mitral regurgitation in these patients is less clear. Among the 18 personally studied patients, the left ventricle was dilated in each and the left ventricular mass was increased in each. The hearts of the 18 patients ranged in weight from 375 to 850 gm (mean = 654). In 13 of the 18 patients, the mitral leaflets were increased in length from their basal attachments to their distal margins. This "stretching" was probably in part the result of the elongation (apex to base) of the left ventricular cavities, resulting primarily from the associated aortic regurgitation. The resulting left ventricular dilatation may have altered the normal angulation between the papillary muscles and the mitral leaflets. Whether or not mitral regurgitation was increased in any patient by this mechanism, however, is uncertain.

In contrast to fusiform ascending aortic aneurysm

and dissection, which generally become manifest after childhood, mitral valve abnormalities in the Marfan syndrome may be present at birth. I have studied at necropsy the heart of a 2-day-old child who at birth was found to have a loud murmur typical of mitral regurgitation and, at necropsy was found to have floppy mitral and tricuspid valve leaflets. Although this child had the typical musculoskeletal features of the Marfan syndrome, the eyes were not examined and there was no family history of the Marfan syndrome in other family members; therefore, this child was not included among the 18 personally studied necropsy patients because the definition of the syndrome was not fulfilled. Nevertheless, it is likely that the child did have the Marfan syndrome. Others also have described abnormalities of the mitral or tricuspid valves in patients <1 year of age with the Marfan syndrome.

Although most reports describing necropsy observations in patients with the Marfan syndrome have not mentioned the status of the mitral or tricuspid valves, it must be recalled that the floppy or prolapsing mitral valve was not recognized clinically until 1963,[5] and at necropsy was not recognized until a year or so later. Thus morphologic descriptions of floppy or prolapsing mitral or tricuspid valves would not be expected in the Marfan patients until about 1965, and most of the detailed reported necropsy descriptions were before that date. Nevertheless, it is now clear that prolapse of one or both mitral leaflets is common at necropsy in the Marfan syndrome and that clicks, late systolic murmurs, and echocardiographic evidence of prolapse are common in these patients. Spangler et al.[104] found mitral valvular abnormalities by echocardiogram in 16 (62%) of 26 patients with the Marfan syndrome, and late or pansystolic apical murmurs or clicks or both in 16 (62%). Of 50 consecutive patients with the Marfan syndrome examined and reported by Pyeritz and McKusick,[105] 24 (48%) had midsystolic clicks with or without late systolic murmurs, and 29 (58%) had echocardiographic evidence of mitral valve prolapse. Although necropsy studies demonstrate abnormalities of the aorta with or without aortic regurgitation to be the most frequent cardiovascular abnormality in the Marfan syndrome, recent clinical and echocardiographic studies show that mitral valve dysfunction is even more common. Even among the previously reported necropsy patients aged ≤ 15 years, however, mitral regurgitation was the most frequent type of cardiovascular dysfunction.

Relatively little information on the circumference of the mitral and tricuspid valve annuli has been provided in the previously reported necropsy patients with the Marfan syndrome with or without mitral regurgitation. Of the reported patients with mitral regurgitation, the mitral or tricuspid annular circumference was described as "increased" in several patients. In the 21-year-old man with severe mitral regurgitation reported by Van Buchem,[106] the mitral annulus was reported to be 18 cm and the tricuspid annulus was 23 cm in circumference. These are the largest annular circumferences encountered.

Marfan patients with fusiform ascending aortic aneurysms also may have mitral valvular abnormalities with or without mitral regurgitation. Seven of 13 personally studied patients with fusiform ascending aortic aneurysms had mitral regurgitation, but none of the three patients with aortic dissection had mitral regurgitation. Of the 53 previously reported necropsy patients with fusiform ascending aortic root aneurysms, at least nine (17%) had anatomic mitral valve abnormalities, but only one definitely had evidence of mitral regurgitation and that patient was only 7 months old, by far the youngest of any of the reported patients with aortic root aneurysm and the Marfan syndrome (see reference 79). Of the 57 reported necropsy patients with aortic dissection, nine (16%) had anatomic abnormalities of the mitral valve, with mitral regurgitation in at least three.

The Marfan syndrome may be associated with mitral annular calcium at a young age. Mitral annular calcific deposits were described in 5 of the 151 previously reported necropsy patients with the Marfan syndrome, and their ages ranged from 15 to 35 years (mean 27)[102]; three were female and two were male. Only two definitely had evidence of mitral regurgitation.

Infective endocarditis involving the mitral valve was described in 6 and possibly in 7 of the 151 previously reported necropsy patients with the Marfan syndrome. Five of the six definite cases were among the 33 patients in the mitral regurgitation group. In all seven patients, the infection involved the mitral valve, and in one it also involved the aortic valve. Thus the mitral valve is the usual site of vegetations when infective endocarditis occurs in patients with the Marfan syndrome. The floppy or prolapsing valve is the one most likely to be the site of infection. Because rupture of the chordae tendineae is a frequent complication of infection involving the mitral valve, the degree of mitral regurgitation resulting from the infection can be severe.[107]

Although the heretofore discussion concerned only patients with typical features of the Marfan syndrome, the cardiovascular features described in them also occur in patients without skeletal or ocular features of this syndrome or in those without histories of this syndrome in other family members.[108] In addition, the characteristic histologic features in the wall of the ascending aorta also have been observed in the aorta of patients with congenitally malformed aortic valves, particularly the bicuspid condition, and in patients with aortic stenosis superimposed on a congenitally malformed valve.[109, 110]

REFERENCES

1. Griffith JP. Mid-systolic and late systolic mitral murmurs. Am J Med Sci 1892;104:285-94.
2. Levine SA, Thompson WP. Systolic gallop rhythm. A clinical study. N Engl J Med 1935;213:1021-5.
3. Brigden W, Leatham A. Mitral incompetence. Br Heart J 1953;15:55-73.
4. Reid JVO. Mid-systolic clicks. S Afr Med J 1961;35:353-5.
5. Barlow JB, Pocock WA, Marchand P, Denny M. The significance of late systolic murmurs. AM HEART J 1963;66:443-52.
6. Segal BL, Likoff W. Late systolic murmur of mitral regurgitation. AM HEART J 1964;67:757-63.
7. Barlow JB, Bosman CK. Aneurysmal protrusion of the posterior leaflet of the mitral valve. An auscultatory-electrocardiographic syndrome. AM HEART J 1965;71:166-78.
8. Criley JM, Lewis KB, Humphries JO, Ross RS. Prolapse of the mitral valve: clinical and cine-angiocardiographic findings. Br Heart J 1966;28:488-96.
9. Barlow JB, Bosman CK, Pocock WA, Marchand P. Late systolic murmurs and non-ejection ("mid-late") systolic clicks. An analysis of 90 patients. Br Heart J 1968;30:203-18.
10. Markiewicz W, Stoner J, London E, Hunt SA, Popp RL. Mitral valve prolapse in one hundred presumably healthy young females. Circulation 1976;53:464-73.
11. Procacci PM, Savran SV, Schreiter SL, Bryson AL. Prevalence of clinical mitral-valve prolapse in 1169 young women. N Engl J Med 1976;294;1086-8.
12. Savage DD, Garrison RJ, Devereux RB, Castelli WP, Anderson SJ, Levy D, McNamara PM, Stokes J III, Kannel WB, Feinleib M. Mitral valve prolapse in the general population. I. Epidemiologic features. The Framingham study. AM HEART J 1983;106:571-6.
13. Roberts WC. The 2 most common congenital heart diseases. Am J Cardiol 1984;53:1198.
14. Waller BF, Morrow AG, Maron BJ, Del Negro AA, Kent KM, McGrath FJ, Wallace RB, McIntosh CL, Roberts WC. Etiology of clinically isolated severe, chronic, pure mitral regurgitation: analysis of 97 patients over 30 years of age having mitral valve replacement. AM HEART J 1982;104:276-88.
15. Roberts WC, McIntosh CL, Wallace RB. Mechanisms of severe mitral regurgitation in mitral valve prolapse determined from analysis of operatively excised valves. AM HEART J 1987;113:1316-23.
16. Dollar AL, Roberts WC. Morphologic comparison of patients with mitral valve prolapse who died suddenly with patients who died from severe valvular dysfunction or other conditions. J Am Coll Cardiol 1991;17:921-31.
17. Pomerance A. Ballooning deformity (mucoid degeneration) of atrioventricular valves. Br Heart J 1969;31:343-51.
18. Lucas RV Jr, Edwards JE. The floppy mitral valve. Curr Probl Cardiol 1982;7:1-48.
19. Bulkley BH, Roberts WC. Dilatation of the mitral annulus. A rare cause of mitral regurgitation. Am J Med 1975;59:457-63.
20. Salazar AE, Edwards JE. Friction lesions of ventricular endocardium. Relation to chordae tendineae of mitral valve. Arch Pathol 1970;90:364-76.
21. Guthrie RB, Edwards JE. Pathology of the myxomatous mitral valve: nature, secondary changes and complications. Minn Med 1976;59:637-47.
22. Shrivastava S, Guthrie RB, Edwards JE. Prolapse of the mitral valve. Mod Concepts Cardiovasc Dis 1977;46:57-61.
23. Renteria VG, Ferrans VJ, Jones M, Roberts WC. Intracellular collagen fibrils in prolapsed ("floppy") human atrioventricular valves. Lab Invest 1976;35:439-43.
24. Roberts WC. Mitral valve prolapse and systemic hypertension. Am J Cardiol 1985;56:703.
25. Davies MJ, Moore BP, Bainbridge MV. The floppy mitral valve. Study of incidence, pathology, and complications in surgical, necropsy, and forensic material. Br Heart J 1978; 40:468-81.
26. Waller BF, Maron BJ, Del Negro AA, Gottdiener JS, Roberts WC. Frequency and significance of M-mode echocardiographic evidence of mitral valve prolapse in clinically isolated pure mitral regurgitation. Analysis of 65 patients having mitral valve replacement. Am J Cardiol 1984;53:139-47.
27. Jeresaty RM, Edwards JE, Chawla SK. Mitral valve prolapse and ruptured chordae tendineae. Am J Cardiol 1985;55:138-42.
28. Savage DD, Levy D, Garrison RJ, Castelli WP, Kligfield P, Devereux RB, Anderson SJ, Kannel WB, Feinleib M. Mitral valve prolapse in the general population. 3. Dysrhythmias: the Framingham Study. AM HEART J 1983;106:582-6.
29. Roberts WC, Glancy DL, Seningen RP, Maron BJ, Epstein SE. Prolapse of the mitral valve (floppy valve) associated with Ebstein's anomaly of the tricuspid valve. Am J Cardiol 1976;38:377-82.
30. Cabin HS, Roberts WC. Ebstein's anomaly of the tricuspid valve and prolapse of the mitral valve. AM HEART J 1981; 101:177-80.
31. Roberts WC. Aneurysm (redundancy) of the atrial septum (fossa ovale membrane) and prolapse (redundancy) of the mitral valve. Am J Cardiol 1984;54:1153-4.
32. Roberts WC, Perloff JK. Mitral valvular disease. A clinicopathologic survey of the conditions causing the mitral valve to function abnormally. Ann Intern Med 1972;77:939-75.
33. Roberts WC. Morphologic features of the normal and abnormal mitral valve. Am J Cardiol 1983;51:1005-28.
34. Braunwald E, Ross RS, Morrow AG, Roberts WC. Differential diagnosis of mitral regurgitation in childhood: Ann Intern Med 1961;54:1223-42.
35. Brockenbrough EC, Braunwald E, Roberts WC, Morrow AG. Partial persistent atrioventricular canal simulating pure mitral regurgitation. AM HEART J 1962;63:9-17.
36. Barth CW III, Dibdin JD, Roberts WC. Mitral valve cleft without cardiac septal defect causing severe mitral regurgitation but allowing long survival. Am J Cardiol 1985;55:1229-31.
37. Berry WB, Roberts WC, Morrow AG, Braunwald E. Corrected transposition of the aorta and pulmonary trunk. Clinical, hemodynamic and pathologic findings. Am J Med 1964; 36:35-53.
38. Roberts WC, Ross RS, Davis FW Jr. Congenital corrected transposition of the great vessels in adulthood simulating rheumatic valvular disease. Bull Johns Hopkins Hosp 1964; 114:157-72.
39. Roberts WC. Anatomically isolated aortic valvular disease. The case against its being of rheumatic etiology. Am J Med 1970;49:151-9.
40. Roberts WC, Sjoerdsma A. The cardiac disease associated with the carcinoid syndrome (carcinoid heart disease). Am J Med 1964;36:5-34.
41. Ross EM, Roberts WC. The carcinoid syndrome: comparison of 21 necropsy subjects with carcinoid heart disease to 15 necropsy subjects without carcinoid heart disease. Am J Med 1985;79:339-54.
42. Roberts WC, Virmani R. Aschoff bodies *at necropsy* in valvular heart disease. Evidence from an analysis of 543 patients over 14 years of age that rheumatic heart disease, at least anatomically, is a disease of the mitral valve. Circulation 1978;57:803-7.
43. Virmani R, Roberts WC. Aschoff bodies in operatively excised atrial appendages and in papillary muscles. Frequency and clinical significance. Circulation 1977;55:559-63.

44. Lachman AS, Roberts WC. Calcific deposits in stenotic mitral valves. Extent and relation to age, sex, degree of stenosis, cardiac rhythm, previous commissurotomy and left atrial body thrombus from study of 164 operatively-excised valves. Circulation 1978;57:808-15.
45. Roberts WC, Lachman AS. Mitral valve commissurotomy versus replacement. Considerations based on examination of operatively excised stenotic mitral valves. AM HEART J 1979;98:56-62.
46. Roberts WC. Does thrombosis play a major role in the development of symptom-producing atherosclerotic plaques? Circulation 1973;48:1161-6.
47. Roberts WC. Coronary thrombosis and fatal myocardial ischemia. Circulation 1974;49:1-3.
48. Roberts WC, Humphries JO, Morrow AG. Giant right atrium in rheumatic mitral stenosis. Atrial enlargement restricted by mural calcification. AM HEART J 1970;79:28-35.
49. MacLowry JD, Roberts WC. Metastatic choriocarcinoma of the lung. Invasion of pulmonary veins with extension into the left atrium and mitral orifice. Am J Cardiol 1966;18:938-41.
50. Roberts WC, Ewy GA, Glancy DL, Marcus FI. Valvular stenosis produced by active infective endocarditis. Circulation 1967;36:449-51.
51. Hammer WJ, Roberts WC, deLeon AC Jr. "Mitral stenosis" secondary to combined "massive" mitral anular calcific deposits and small, hypertrophied left ventricles. Am J Med 1978;64:371-6.
52. Shepard RL, Glancy DL, Stinson EB, Roberts WC. Hemodynamic confirmation of obstruction to left ventricular inflow by a caged-ball prosthetic mitral valve. Case report. J Thorac Cardiovasc Surg 1973;65:252-4.
53. Jones AA, Otis JB, Fletcher GF, Roberts WC. A hitherto undescribed cause of prosthetic mitral valve obstruction. J Thorac Cardiovasc Surg 1977;74:116-7.
54. Roberts WC. Complications of cardiac valve replacement: characteristic abnormalities of prostheses pertaining to any or specific site. AM HEART J 1982;103:113-22.
55. Karsner HT, Koletsky S. Calcific disease of the aortic valve. Philadelphia: JB Lippincott, 1947:111.
56. Roberts WC. The structure of the aortic valve in clinically-isolated aortic stenosis. An autopsy study of 162 patients over 15 years of age. Circulation 1970;42:91-7.
57. Roberts WC, Morrow AG. Congenital aortic stenosis produced by a unicommissural valve. Br Heart J 1965;27:505-10.
58. Falcone MW, Roberts WC, Morrow AG, Perloff JK. Congenital aortic stenosis resulting from unicommissural valve. Clinical and anatomic features in twenty-one adult patients. Circulation 1971;44:272-80.
59. Edwards JE. Pathologic aspects of cardiac valvular insufficiencies. Arch Surg 1958;77:634-49.
60. Roberts WC. The congenitally bicuspid aortic valve. A study of 85 autopsy cases. Am J Cardiol 1970;26:72-83.
61. Roberts WC, Morrow AG, McIntosh CL, Jones M, Epstein SE. Congenitally bicuspid aortic valve causing severe, pure aortic regurgitation without superimposed infective endocarditis. Analysis of 13 patients requiring aortic valve replacement. Am J Cardiol 1981;47:206-9.
62. Roberts WC. Congenital cardiovascular abnormalities usually silent until adulthood. Adult congenital heart disease. Philadelphia: FA Davis Company, 1987:631-91.
63. Osler W. The bicuspid condition of the aortic valves. Trans Assoc Am Physicians 1886;2:185-92.
64. Grant RT, Wood JE, Jones TD. Heart valve irregularities in relation to subacute bacterial endocarditis. Heart 1928; 14:247-61.
65. Lewis T, Grant RT. Observations relating to subacute infective endocarditis. Part 1. Notes on the normal structure of the aortic valve. Part 2. Bicuspid aortic valves of congenital origin. Part 3. Bicuspid aortic valves in subacute infective endocarditis. Heart 1923;10:21-99.
66. Arnett EN, Roberts WC. Active infective endocarditis: a clinicopathologic analysis of 137 patients. Curr Probl Cardiol 1976;1:1-76.
67. Roberts WC, McIntosh CL, Wallace RB. Aortic valve perforation with calcific aortic valve stenosis and without infective endocarditis or significant regurgitation. Am J Cardiol 1987;59:476-8.
68. Dressler FA, Roberts WC. Infective endocarditis in opiate addicts: analysis of 80 cases studied at necropsy. Am J Cardiol 1989;63:1240-57.
69. Subramanian R, Olson LJ, Edwards WD. Surgical pathology of pure aortic stenosis: a study of 374 cases. Mayo Clin Proc 1984;59:683-90.
70. Olson LJ, Subramanian R, Edwards WD. Surgical pathology of pure aortic insufficiency: a study of 225 cases. Mayo Clin Proc 1984;59:835-41.
71. Fulton MN, Levine SA. Subacute bacterial endocarditis, with special reference to the valvular lesions and previous history. Am J Med Sci 1932;183:60-77.
72. Edwards JE. The congenital bicuspid aortic valve. Circulation 1961;23:485-8.
73. Hamilton WF, Abbott ME. Coarctation of the aorta of the adult type. II. A statistical study and historical retrospect of 200 recorded cases, with autopsy, of stenosis or obliteration of the descending arch in subjects above the age of two years. AM HEART J 1928;3:392-421, 574-618.
74. Reifenstein GH, Levine SA, Gross RE. Coarctation of the aorta. A review of 104 autopsied cases of the "adult type," 2 years of age or older. AM HEART J 1947;33:146-68.
75. Gore I, Seiwert VJ. Dissecting aneurysm of the aorta: pathologic aspects. An analysis of eighty-five fatal cases. Arch Pathol 1952;53:121-41.
76. Edwards WD, Leaf DS, Edwards JE. Dissecting aortic aneurysm associated with congenital bicuspid aortic valve. Circulation 1978;57:1022-5.
77. Roberts CS, Roberts WC. Dissection of the aorta associated with congenital malformation of the aortic valve. J Am Coll Cardiol 1991;17:712-6.
78. Fenoglio JJ Jr, McAllister HA Jr, DeCastro CM, Davia JE, Cheitlin MD. Congenital bicuspid aortic valve after age 20. Am J Cardiol 1977;39:164-9.
79. Larson EW, Edwards WD. Risk factors for aortic dissection: a necropsy study of 161 cases. Am J Cardiol 1984;53: 849-55.
80. Brandenburg RO Jr, Tajik AJ, Edwards WD, Reeder GS, Shub C, Seward JB. Accuracy of 2-dimensional echocardiographic diagnosis of congenitally bicuspid aortic valve. Echocardiographic-anatomic correlation in 115 patients. Am J Cardiol 1983;51:1469-73.
81. Stewart WJ, King ME, Gillam LD, Guyer DE, Weyman AE. Prevalence of aortic valve prolapse with bicuspid aortic valve and its relation to aortic regurgitation: a cross-sectional echocardiographic study. Am J Cardiol 1984;54:1277-82.
82. Roberts WC. Living with a congenitally bicuspid aortic valve. Am J Cardiol 1989;64:1408-9.
83. Osler W. Maligant endocarditis. Lancet 1885;1:445,459,505.
84. Dressler FA, Roberts WC. Modes of death and types of cardiac diseases in opiate addicts: analysis of 168 necropsy cases. Am J Cardiol 1989;64;909-20.
85. Silver MA, Roberts WC. Detailed anatomy of the normally functioning aortic valve in hearts of normal and increased weights. Am J Cardiol 1985;55:454-61.
86. Roberts WC, Perloff JK, Costantino T. Severe valvular aortic stenosis in patients over 65 years of age. A clinicopathologic study. Am J Cardiol 1971;27:497-506.
87. Roberts WC, Dangel JC, Bulkley BH. Non-rheumatic valvular cardiac disease. A clinicopathologic survey of 27 different conditions causing valvular dysfunction. Cardiovasc Clin 1973;5:333-446.
88. Roberts WC. Left ventricular outflow tract obstruction and aortic regurgitation. In: Edwards JE, Lev M, Abell MR, eds. The heart. Baltimore: The Williams & Wilkins Co, 1974: 110-75.

89. Roberts WC. The senile cardiac calcification syndrome. Am J Cardiol 1986;58:572-4.
90. Roberts WC, Buchbinger NA. Healed left-sided infective endocarditis: a clinico-pathologic study of 59 patients. Am J Cardiol 1977;40:876-88.
91. Bulkley BH, Roberts WC. Ankylosing spondylitis and aortic regurgitation. Description of the characteristic cardiovascular lesion from study of eight necropsy patients. Circulation 1973;48:1014-27.
92. Clark WS, Kulka P, Bauer W. Rheumatoid aortitis with aortic regurgitation. An unusual manifestation of rheumatoid arthritis (including spondylitis). Am J Med 1957;22:580-90.
93. Roberts WC, Honig MS. The spectrum of cardiovascular disease in the Marfan syndrome: a clinico-morphologic study of 18 necropsy patients and comparison to 151 previously reported necropsy patients. AM HEART J 1982;104:115-35.
94. Murdoch JL, Walker BA, Halpern BL, Kuzma JW, McKusick VA. Life expectancy and causes of death in the Marfan syndrome. N Engl J Med 1972;286:804-8.
95. Sisk ME, Zahka KG, Pyeritz RE, with the technical assistance of Cathy Hensley. The Marfan syndrome in early childhood: analysis of 15 patients diagnosed at less than 4 years of age. Am J Cardiol 1983;52:353-8.
96. Carlson RG, Lillehei CW, Edwards JE. Cystic medial necrosis of the ascending aorta in relation to age and hypertension. Am J Cardiol 1970;25:411-5.
97. Schlatmann TJM, Becker AE. Histologic changes in the normal aging aorta: implications for dissecting aortic aneurysm. Am J Cardiol 1977;39:13-20.
98. Schlatmann TJM, Becker AE. Pathogenesis of dissection aneurysm of aorta. Comparative histopathologic study of significance of medial changes. Am J Cardiol 1977;39:21-6.
99. Gsell O. Wandnekrosen der aorta als selbst ändige Erkrankung und ihre Beziehung zur spontanruptur. Virchows Arch Pathol Anat Physiol 1928;270:1-36.
100. Erdheim J. Medionecrosis aortae idiopathica. Virchows Arch Pathol Anat Physiol 1929;273:454-79.
101. Erdheim J. Medionecrosis aortae idiopathica cystica. Virchows Arch Pathol Anat Physiol 1930;276:187-229.
102. Wolinsky H, Glagov S. A lamellar unit of aortic medial structure and function in mammals. Circ Res 1967;20:99-111.
103. Benchimol A, Dresser KB, Neese TC. Hypermobility of the aorta in Marfan's syndrome. Angiology 1972;23:103-4.
104. Spangler RD, Nora JJ, Lorfscher RH, Wolfe RR, Okin JT. Echocardiography in Marfan's syndrome. Chest 1976;69: 72-8.
105. Pyeritz RE, McKusick VA. The Marfan syndrome: diagnosis and management. N Engl J Med 1979;300:772-7.
106. VanBuchem FSP. Cardiovascular disease in arachnodactyly. Acta Med Scand 1958;161:197-205.
107. Roberts WC, Braunwald E, Morrow AG. Acute severe mitral regurgitation secondary to ruptured chordae tendineae. Clinical, hemodynamic, and pathologic considerations. Circulation 1966;33:58-70.
108. Waller BF, Reis RL, McIntosh CL, Epstein SE, Roberts WC. Marfan cardiovascular disease without the Marfan syndrome. Fusiform ascending aortic aneurysm with aortic and mitral valve regurgitation. Chest 1980;77:533-40.
109. Fukuda T, Tadavarthy SM, Edwards JE. Dissecting aneurysm of aorta complicating aortic valvular stenosis. Circulation 1976;53:169-75.
110. Roberts CS, Roberts WC. Dissection of the aorta associated with congenital malformation of the aortic valve. J Am Coll Cardiol 1991;17:712-6.

Usefulness of Total 12-Lead QRS Voltage in Diagnosing Left Ventricular Hypertrophy in Clinically Isolated, Pure, Chronic, Severe Mitral Regurgitation

Brian N. Glick, MD,* and William C. Roberts, MD

Electrocardiographic criteria for diagnosing left ventricular (LV) hypertrophy are known to be relatively nonspecific and insensitive. Several studies from this laboratory[1–7] and elsewhere[8–10] have described total 12-lead QRS voltage in various cardiac diseases, and most have found this criterion to be more sensitive than previously described criteria. We examined total 12-lead QRS voltage in 24 necropsied patients with chronic, pure, isolated mitral regurgitation, and compared its sensitivity to the Sokolow-Lyon and Romhilt-Estes criteria for diagnosis of LV hypertrophy.

From the Pathology Branch, National Heart, Lung, and Blood Institute, National Institutes of Health, Bethesda, Maryland 20892. Manuscript received April 24, 1992; revised manuscript received and accepted May 28, 1992.

*Cardiology Fellow, Georgetown University Medical Center, Washington, D.C.

The 24 patients ranged in age from 21 to 84 years (mean 42); 13 (54%) were women and 11 (46%) were men (Table I). All 24 patients had clinical evidence of mitral regurgitation for >5 months. None had clinical or hemodynamic evidence of associated mitral stenosis, and none had evidence of aortic valve dysfunction. Additionally, all 24 patients had New York Heart Association functional class III or IV congestive heart failure, and 9 (38%) had mitral valve replacement or repair from 1 to 120 days (mean 25) before death. Cardiac catheterization was performed in 19 (79%) of the 24 patients and the recorded pressures are listed in Table I. To be included in this study, 1 or more 12-lead electrocardiograms recorded within 400 days of death (always before a mitral valve operation) had to be available for examination. The amplitude of the QRS was measured from the peak of the R wave to the nadir of either the Q wave or

TABLE I Clinical and Hemodynamic Data in the 24 Patients with Clinically Isolated, Pure, Chronic Mitral Regurgitation

Case No.	Necropsy No.	Age (yr)	Gender	Valvular Etiology	Duration of Cardiac Symptoms (yrs)	MVR	Interval MVR to Death (days)	Pressures (mm Hg) LA m	LA v	LV (s/d)	SA (s/d)	RV (s/d)
1	A63–234	21	F	Rheumatic	11	+	2	15	30*	—	120/70	40/3
2	A56–200	23	F	Rheumatic	12	0	—	31	55*	—	125/75	60/7
3	A60–208	23	F	Rheumatic	8	0	—	30	45*	—	125/75	48/12
4	A70–221	24	M	Rheumatic	5	+	17	16	28*	90/8	100/60	30/6
5	A69–240	30	F	Rheumatic	6	+	2	30	65*	102/14	110/78	58/12
6	A60–131	30	M	Rheumatic	5	+	1	30	48	115/20	135/80	—
7	A57–150	31	F	Rheumatic	7	0	—	23	44*	—	118/74	—
8	A58–213	33	F	Rheumatic	3/4	0	—	—	—	—	115/80	—
9	A60–270	38	F	Rheumatic	9	0	—	32	60	115/15	120/70	—
10	A62–232	38	M	Rheumatic	2	+	7	20	39	108/16	120/84	48/8
11	A59–39	39	F	Rheumatic	6	0	—	30	55	125/20	150/65	35/4
12	A64–98	41	F	Rheumatic	6	+	1	—	—	106/15	106/60	34/10
13	A67–178	43	M	Rheumatic	3	0	—	16	28	148/13	150/84	43/4
14	A54–21	49	M	Rheumatic	3	0	—	26	60*	—	170/100	64/0
15	A63–24	28	M	MVP-RCT	1	0	—	—	—	—	130/80	23/5
16	312579	60	F	MVP-RCT	6	0	—	—	—	—	120/70	—
17	A69–62	65	M	MVP-RCT	3/4	+	120	—	—	—	—	—
18	226434	84	M	MVP-RCT	20	0	—	—	—	—	135/80	—
19	A56–59	41	M	MVP+RCT	2	0	—	32	39*	—	150/70	110/21
20	A70–244	56	M	MVP+RCT	7	+	28	25	40	100/12	110/65	42/6
21	A70–280	60	M	MVP+RCT	4	+	50	17	20*	118/17	120/80	110/21
22	A62–19	24	F	IE+RCT	3/4	0	—	27	66	108/11	108/85	—
23	A75–63	54	F	IE+RCT	2	0	—	—	—	110/15	120/70	50/10
24	A72–8	64	F	IE+RCT	12	0	—	38	50*	120/20	120/70	85/18
	Mean	42	—	—	6	—	25	23	43	113/14	125/75	55/9

*Pulmonary arterial wedge rather than left atrial pressures.

ECG = electrocardiogram; IE = infective endocarditis; LA = left atrium; LV = left ventricle; m = mean; MVP = mitral valve prolapse; MVR = mitral valve replacement; RCT = ruptured chordae tendineae; RV = right ventricle; SA = systemic artery; s/d = peak systole/end-diastole; v = v wave.

the S wave, whichever was deeper, according to the method of Siegel and Roberts[1] (Figure 1). The electrocardiographic criteria used to diagnose LV hypertrophy included the Sokolow and Lyon Index[11] (sum of SV_1 plus the larger of RV_5 or RV_6 >35), the Romhilt-Estes point score[12] (a system using ST-T-segment changes, QRS axis, left atrial abnormality, QRS duration and duration of the intrinsicoid deflection in addition to electrographic voltage criteria), and a method using a sum of the amplitudes of the QRS complexes of all 12 leads. Amplitudes were standardized to 10 mm equaling 1 mV.

The hearts at necropsy were examined by WCR and the etiologic classification was made by him.[13] In no patient was the mitral regurgitation the result of myocardial ischemia. Although 3 patients (nos. 13, 17 and 21, Table I) had narrowing (in each case by atherosclerotic plaque) of a single (left anterior descending in each) major epicardial coronary artery, none had LV fibrosis or necrosis as a result. Only 1 (no. 20) of the 24 patients at necropsy had a grossly visible myocardial lesion, namely necrosis; the lesion was secondary to a coronary embolus in the early postmitral valve replacement period, and the electrocardiogram analyzed was that recorded just before the mitral valve operation. Therefore, none of the 24 patients had grossly visible LV lesions when the electrocardiograms used in this study

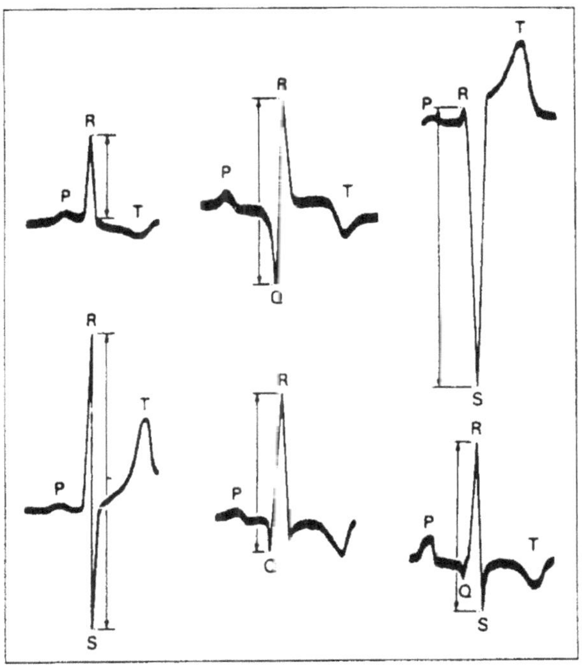

FIGURE 1. Various electrocardiographic QRS complexes showing how the voltage (in mm) was measured. (Reproduced with permission from *Am Heart J.*[1])

TABLE II Electrocardiographic Findings in the 24 Patients with Clinically Isolated, Pure, Chronic Mitral Regurgitation

Case No.	Days ECG Recorded Before Death	Chronic AF	VR (beats/min)	QRS Axis	Leads I	II	III	AVR	AVL	AVF	V_1	V_2	V_3	V_4	V_5	V_6	Total QRS	R-E Score	S-L Index	S Wave V_1	R Wave V_5 or V_6	HW (g)
1	5	+	85	30	10	12	16	6	15	13	8	27	28	24	37	23	219	4	38	8	30	400
2	14	+	85	120	14	16	10	16	11	13	13	40	42	40	38	37	290	4	30	4	26	600
3	15	+	60	60	5	17	18	8	7	17	7	15	33	32	33	36	228	4	39	6	33	400
4	68	+	75	75	5	25	27	15	13	26	12	38	39	30	44	42	316	4	44	10	34	520
5	3	+	140	45	7	9	10	7	8	10	10	15	26	25	23	13	163	1	33	10	23	480
6	13	+	70	30	5	15	11	8	4	11	20	40	50	18	54	58	294	5	78	20	58	600
7	50	+	85	90	4	10	9	5	6	10	8	14	33	34	35	19	187	4	33	7	26	675
8	9	0	90	60	7	18	13	14	8	18	30	40	30	26	36	30	270	5	55	22	33	490
9	213	+	80	60	5	12	17	5	7	15	9	15	32	18	38	32	205	4	44	6	38	450
10	43	+	80	30	5	17	15	10	5	15	24	50	62	40	80	41	364	5	87	7	80	675
11	39	+	60	90	4	15	15	7	7	16	15	30	24	20	30	18	201	4	40	14	26	450
12	2	+	70	60	4	14	17	6	7	15	8	23	31	33	25	13	196	1	25	3	22	470
13	154	+	65	80	2	5	7	5	4	6	5	21	40	22	18	14	149	1	25	7	18	550
14	16	+	65	0	5	15	10	8	5	12	10	17	38	35	45	30	230	4	48	10	38	700
15	11	0	120	120	10	17	26	4	17	21	5	26	43	52	44	24	289	4	15	5	10	600
16	330	+	70	60	4	8	6	5	4	7	5	12	15	35	28	25	154	4	36	6	25	440
17	400	0	110	−45	10	8	8	7	8	9	28	38	26	23	46	48	259	9	70	22	48	640
18	50	+	75	60	5	13	8	8	4	9	12	9	11	18	18	17	111	1	29	12	17	400
19	5	+	140	110	14	25	18	16	12	20	22	20	40	50	40	33	310	3	26	4	22	775
20	30	+	90	−45	6	6	8	4	7	8	14	19	19	10	14	14	129	4	28	14	14	750
21	57	0	65	120	10	10	12	6	9	10	8	44	40	34	36	21	240	4	25	5	20	710
22	9	0	120	90	3	7	8	5	7	8	6	17	23	10	9	11	114	1	14	4	10	350
23	260	+	70	45	6	8	5	7	5	7	9	10	22	27	28	15	149	1	29	9	20	500
24	8	+	100	120	4	12	14	6	7	11	10	26	44	40	24	10	208	4	18	10	8	430
Mean	75		86		6.4	13.1	12.8	7.8	7.8	12.8	12.4	25.3	33.0	29.0	34.3	26.0	220	3.5	38	9	28	544

AF = atrial fibrillation; ECG = electrocardiogram; HW = heart weight; R–E = Romhilt-Estes; S-L = Sokolow-Lyon; VR = ventricular rate.

were recorded. The hearts of the 11 men ranged in weight from 400 to 750 g (mean 629) (normal ≤400), and those of the 13 women, 350 to 675 g (mean 472) (normal ≤350).

The electrocardiographic findings are summarized in Table II. Nineteen patients (79%) had chronic atrial fibrillation. Left atrial abnormality was present in 1 of the 5 patients in sinus rhythm. The QRS complex width was ≥0.12 second in 1 patient (no. 19, Table II), and he had a right bundle branch pattern. All 24 patients were being treated with digoxin at the time of the study electrocardiogram. The total 12-lead QRS amplitude in the 24 patients ranged from 111 to 364 mm (mean 220). (The upper limit of normal for total QRS amplitude of 175 mm was first suggested by Roberts and Day[3] and validated by Odom et al[5] who found that the upper limit yielded a specificity of 100% in subjects whose hearts weighed <400 g.) Of the criteria examined, the total 12-lead QRS amplitude had the highest sensitivity (71%) (Table III). Although the 12-lead QRS amplitude was more sensitive than the other 2 criteria examined, heart weight did not correlate with the total 12-lead QRS amplitude (Figure 2).

TABLE III Sensitivity of Electrocardiographic Criteria for Diagnosing Left Ventricular Hypertrophy in 24 Necropsy Patients with Clinically Isolated, Pure, Chronic, Severe, Mitral Regurgitation

Electrocardiographic Criteria	No. (%) of Patients Above Normal Limit
Total 12-lead QRS amplitude <175 mm	17 (71%)
Sokolow-Lyon index (SV_1 + RV_5 or RV_6 (larger) >35mm)	11 (46%)
Romhilt-Estes point score ≥5	4 (17%)

This study examined total 12-lead QRS voltage and other more standard electrocardiographic criteria for diagnosing LV hypertrophy in patients with clinically isolated, pure, chronic, severe mitral regurgitation. The highest sensitivity among the criteria for LV hypertrophy in our study group was the total 12-lead QRS voltage (71%). In these patients, the criteria of Romhilt and Estes and Sokolow-Lyon index were relatively insensitive (17 and 46%, respectively).

This study is the first to examine total 12-lead QRS voltage in patients with mitral regurgitation. Several

TABLE IV Comparison of the Sensitivity of Total QRS Voltage in Identifying Left Ventricular Hypertrophy of Various Etiologies

	Normal (n = 17)*	Aortic Stenosis (n = 50)	Aortic Regurgitation (n = 30)	Hypertrophic Cardiomyopathy (n = 57)	Idiopathic Dilated Cardiomyopathy (n = 49)	Amyloid (n = 30)	Mitral Regurgitation (n = 24)
Age (years) (mean)	41–74 (54)	16–65 (48)	19–65 (45)	14–87 (49)	19–75 (48)	21–93 (58)	21–84 (42)
Heart weight (g) (range)	288–392	380–880	375–1110	290–1230	400–940	370–900	350–900
Mean	351	606	696	593	614	532	550
Total QRS voltage (mm) (range)	84–159	144–417	109–428	66–339	74–281	58–199	111–364
Mean	124	257	270	197	153	104	220
Patients with 12-lead QRS voltage >175 mm	0 (0%)	47 (94%)	27 (90%)	30 (53%)	20 (41%)	2 (7%)	17 (71%)

*Patients with heart weights <400 g.

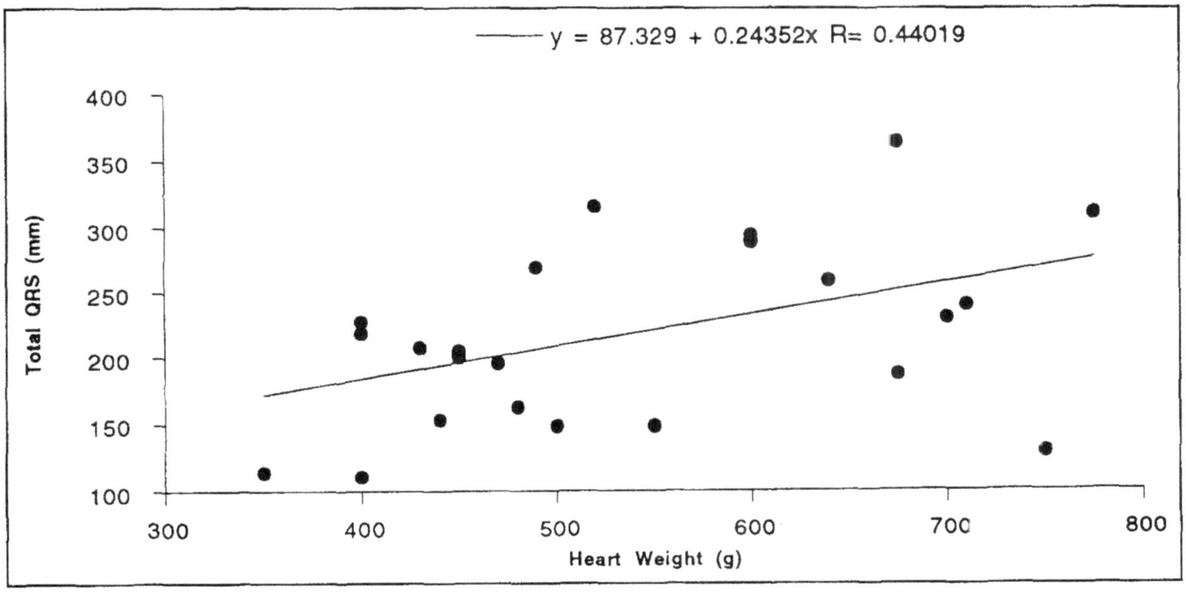

FIGURE 2. Relation between total QRS amplitude and heart weight at necropsy in 24 patients with isolated pure, chronic, severe mitral regurgitation.

studies, however, have evaluated the relation between the total 12-lead QRS voltage and heart weight at necropsy in other cardiac diseases (Table IV).[1-3,5-7]

1. Siegel RJ, Roberts WC. Electrocardiographic observations in severe aortic valve stenosis: correlative necropsy study to clinical, hemodynamic, and ECG variables demonstrating relation of 12-lead QRS amplitude to peak transaortic pressure gradient. *Am Heart J* 1982;103:210–221.

2. Roberts WC, Waller BF. Cardiac amyloidosis causing cardiac dysfunction: analysis of 54 necropsy patients. *Am J Cardiol* 1983;52:137–146.

3. Roberts WC, Day PJ. Electrocardiographic observations in clinically isolated, pure, chronic, severe aortic regurgitation: analysis of 30 necropsy patients aged 19 to 65 years. *Am J Cardiol* 1985;55:432–438.

4. Ross E, Roberts WC. The carcinoid syndrome: comparison of 21 necropsy subjects with carcinoid heart disease to 15 necropsy subjects without carcinoid heart disease. *Am J Med* 1985;79:339–354.

5. Odom H II, Davis JL, Dinh H, Baker BJ, Roberts WC, Murphy ML. QRS voltage measurements in autopsied men free of cardiopulmonary disease: a basis for evaluating total QRS voltage as an index of left ventricular hypertrophy. *Am J Cardiol* 1986;58:801–804.

6. Roberts WC, Siegel RJ, McManus BM. Idiopathic dilated cardiomyopathy: Analysis of 152 necropsy patients. *Am J Cardiol* 1987;60:1340–1355.

7. Dollar A, Roberts WC. Usefulness of total 12-lead QRS voltage compared with other criteria for determining left ventricular hypertrophy in hypertrophic cardiomyopathy: analysis of 57 patients studied at necropsy. *Am J Med* 1989;87: 377–381.

8. Lanti M, Puddu PE, Menotti A. Voltage criteria of left ventricular hypertrophy in sudden and nonsudden coronary artery disease mortality: the Italian section of the Seven Countries Study. *Am J Cardiol* 1990;66:1181–1185.

9. Pelliccia F, Critelli G, Cianfrocca C, Nigri A, Reale A. Electrocardiographic correlates with left ventricular morphology in idiopathic dilated cardiomyopathy. *Am J Cardiol* 1991;68:642–647.

10. Rodriguez P. Usefulness of total 12-lead QRS voltage for determining the presence of left ventricular hypertrophy in systemic hypertension. *Am J Cardiol* 1991;68:261–262.

11. Romhilt DW, Estes EH Jr. A point score system for the ECG diagnosis of left ventricular hypertrophy. *Am Heart J* 1968;75:1752–1758.

12. Sokolow M, Lyon TP. The ventricular complex in left ventricular hypertrophy as obtained by unipolar precordial and limb leads. *Am Heart J* 1949;37:161–186.

13. Roberts WC. Morphologic aspects of cardiac valve dysfunction. *Am Heart J* 1992;123:1610–1632.

Clinicopathologic Features of Active Infective Endocarditis Isolated to the Native Mitral Valve

Daniel J. Fernicola, MD, and William C. Roberts, MD*

Although a number of clinicopathologic studies in patients with active infective endocarditis (IE) have been reported, none have focused on patients studied at necropsy with active IE isolated to the mitral valve. We studied at necropsy 63 patients (aged 12 to 88 years [mean 50], 44 males [70%]) with active IE limited to the native mitral valve: 21 (33%) had preexisting mitral valve disease (rheumatic in 8, prolapse in 3, hypertrophic cardiomyopathy in 1, and mitral annular calcium in 9), and the other 42 patients (67%) had previously normal mitral valves. Of the latter 42 patients, 22 (52%) had recognized predisposing factors to IE: opiate addiction in 14, habitual alcoholism in 6 and/or chronic hemodialysis in 4. *Staphylococcus aureus* or *epidermidis* was the responsible organism in 32 patients (51%), and the active IE was associated with an infection elsewhere in the body in 31 patients (50%). The active IE caused rupture of mitral chordae tendineae in 11 patients (18%), perforation of the anterior mitral leaflet in 7 patients (11%), and mitral ring abscess in 10 patients (16%). Grossly visible systemic emboli were found in 44 patients (70%) and 33 (52%) had infarcts in 1 or more body organs.

Thus, active IE isolated to the mitral valve in necropsied patients appears to be more common in males than females (2 to 1); the infection more commonly than not involves a preexisting anatomically normal valve rather than a preexisting abnormal one (2 to 1); the vegetations often do not cause or worsen valvular dysfunction; a predisposing factor is commonly present (2 of 3 patients), and the IE commonly is part of a generalized or systemic infection (1 of 2 patients).

(Am J Cardiol 1993;71:1186–1197)

From the Pathology Branch, National Heart, Lung, and Blood Institute, National Institutes of Health, Bethesda, Maryland. Manuscript received November 10, 1992; revised manuscript received and accepted December 4, 1992.

*Present address: Baylor Cardiovascular Institute, Baylor University Medical Center, 3701 Junius Street, P.O. Box E010, Dallas, Texas 75246.

Address for reprints: Pathology Branch, National Heart, Lung, and Blood Institute, National Institute of Health, Building 10, Room 2N258, Bethesda, Maryland 20892.

Although numerous reports from this laboratory and elsewhere have described clinical and morphologic features of active infective endocarditis (IE) involving native left-sided cardiac valves,[1–12] surprisingly, few have focused on patients with active IE limited to the mitral valve, and none have described both clinical and morphologic features in patients with active IE limited to the mitral valve. Such is the purpose of the present report.

METHODS

Patients studied: The files of patients in the Pathology Branch, National Heart, Lung, and Blood Institute, were searched for cases coded as active IE on 1 or more native cardiac valves (active infection involving patients with prostheses or bioprostheses and those in patients with congenital cardiovascular shunts were excluded). A total of 217 cases were retrieved. Of this number, 74 (34%) had vegetations limited to the aortic valve,[12] 27 (12.5%) had vegetations on both aortic and mitral valves,[12] 67 (30.5%) had vegetations limited to the mitral valve, and 49 (23%) had vegetations on 1 or both right-sided cardiac valves with or without involvement of 1 or both left-sided cardiac valves. This report is limited to the patients with vegetations limited to the mitral valve. Of the 67 patients, 3 were eliminated from this study because 2 with mitral stenosis had had mitral commissurotomy, and 1 patient, who had hypertrophic cardiomyopathy, had had ventricular septal myotomy and myectomy.

Inclusion criteria: To be included in this study the following criteria were met: (1) age at death >10 years; (2) 1 or more vegetations on the mitral valve at necropsy and no vegetations on any of the other 3 cardiac valves; and (3) never a cardiac operation. Of the 63 patients, 52 (82%) had received 1 or more antibiotics shortly before death, and 11 (17%) had not received antibiotics during the last month of life.

Sources of cases: The 63 patients had necropsies performed at 16 different medical institutions and the hearts were subsequently submitted to the Pathology Branch, National Heart, Lung, and Blood Institute, for examination. The medical records from the submitting medical center subsequently were examined. Of the 63 cases, 12 had the necropsy performed at the Clinical Center of the National Institutes of Health; 9 at Georgetown University Medical Center; 8 at the District of Columbia Medical Examiners' Office; 7 at the District of Columbia General Hospital; 5 at the District of Columbia Veterans' Administration Hospital; 5 at Howard University Hospital; 5 at the Washington Hospital Center; 3 at George Washington University Hospital; 2 at Suburban Hospital (Bethesda, Maryland), and 1 each from 7 different medical centers. The hearts in all 63 patients were

TABLE I Clinical and Morphologic Features of 21 Patients with Anatomically Abnormal Mitral Valves Prior to Infective Endocarditis

Case	Age (years)	Race	Sex	RHD	HC	MVP	MAC	Predisposing Factors					Infecting Organism	Mode of Death			HW (g)	LV		Ring Abscess	RCT	PAML	SE	Gross Organ Infarcts				
								O	HA	H	P	Mn		Sepsis	Embolus	CHF		Fi	N					Brain	Spleen	Kidney	Heart	Other
1	21	B	F	+	0	0	0	0	0	0	0	0	Beta streptococcus	0	+	0	400	0	0	0	+	0	+	+	+	+	0	0
2	37	B	M	+[1]	0	0	0	+	0	0	+	+	—	+	0	0	350	0	0	0	0	0	+	+	+	+	0	+
3	49	W	M	+[1]	0	0	0	0	+	0	0	0	Alpha streptococcus	0	0	0[2]	530	+	0	0	+	0	+	—	—	—	0	—
4	58	W	M	+	0	0	0	0	0	0	0	0	*Staphylococcus aureus*	+	0	0	450	0	0	0	0	0	+	+	+	+	0	+
5	59	W	M	+[1]	0	0	0	0	0	0	0	0	*Pseudomonas aeruginosa*	0	+	0	350	0	0	0	0	0	+	—	—	—	0	—
6	62	W	M	+	0	0	0	0	—	0	—	—	Beta streptococcus	0	+	0	—	+	0	0	0	0	+	—	—	—	0	—
7	66	W	F	+[1]	0	0	0	0	0	0	0	0	Group D streptococcus	0	0	+	600	0	0	0	0	0	+	0	+	0	0	+
8	72	W	F	+[1]	0	0	0	0	0	0	0	0	*Staphylococcus aureus*	+	0	0	480	0	0	+	0	0	—	—	—	—	0	—
9	49	W	M	0	+	0	0	0	0	0	0	0	*Staphylococcus aureus*	0	0	+	650	0	+	0	0	0	+	0	0	+	+	0
10	52	W	M	0	0	+	0	0	0	0	0	0	*Staphylococcus aureus*	0	+	0	—	0	0	0	0	0	+	+	+	+	0	+
11	54	W	M	0	0	+	0	0	0	0	+	+	*Staphylococcus aureus*	0	+	0	500	0	0	0	0	0	+	+	+	+	0	0
12	64	W	F	0	0	+	0	0	0	0	0	0	Alpha streptococcus	0	+	0	275	0	0	0	0	0	+	+	0	0	0	0
13	45	B	F	0	0	0	+	0	0	+	0	0	*Staphylococcus aureus*	—	—	—	—	0	0	0	0	0	—	—	—	0	0	—
14	50	B	M	0	0	0	+	0	0	+	0	0	*Staphylococcus aureus*	0	0	0[3]	520	0	0	0	0	0	0	0	0	0	0	0
15	55	B	F	0	0	0	+	0	0	+	0	0	*Staphylococcus aureus*	+	0	0	360	0	0	+	0	0	+	0	0	+[4]	0	+
16	58	W	F	0	0	0	+	0	0	+	0	0	*Staphylococcus aureus*	—	—	—	—	0	+[5]	0	0	0	—	—	—	—	0	—
17	63	W	M	0	0	0	+	0	0	+	0	0	*Staphylococcus aureus*	0	+	0	530	0	+[5]	0	0	0	+	0	0	0	0	0
18	79	W	M	0	0	0	+	0	0	0	0	0	*Staphylococcus aureus*	—	—	—	530	+	+	0	0	0	—	—	—	—	+	—
19	83	W	M	0	0	0	+	0	0	0	0	0	Beta streptococcus	0	—	0	535	0	0	0	0	0	—	—	—	0	—	—
20	84	W	M	0	0	0	+	0	0	0	+	0	*Staphylococcus aureus*	0	0	0	505	+	0	0	0	0	0	0	0	0	0	0
21	85	W	M	0	0	0	+	0	0	0	+	0	Beta streptococcus	+	0	0	540	0	+	+	0	0	+	0	+	+	+	+
Total or mean	59			8	1	3	9	1	1	5	4	2		5	7	2	479	4	5	3	2	0	14	6	7	8	3	6

[1]Mitral stenosis present; [2]sudden cardiac death without coronary artery embolus but atherosclerotic coronary artery disease; [3]died from hyperkalemia; [4]abscesses of transplanted kidney; [5]myocardial abscess.
B = black; CHF = congestive heart failure; CT = chordae tendineae; F = female; Fi = fibrosis; H = hemodialysis; HA = habitual alcoholism; HC = hypertrophic cardiomyopathy; HW = heart weight; LV = left ventricular; M = male; MAC = mitral annular calcium; Mn = meningitis; MVP = mitral valve prolapse; N = necrosis; O = opiate addict; P = pneumonia; PAML = perforated anterior mitral leaflet; RCT = ruptured chordae tendineae; RHD = rheumatic heart disease; SE = systemic emboli; W = white.

examined initially by WCR, and in 27 patients the hearts were reexamined by DJF. Photographs of the heart were available in 43 cases (68%).

Year of necropsy: Of the 63 cases, 2 (3%) died in the decade 1951–1960; 8 (13%), from 1961–1970; 22 (35%) from 1971–1980; and 31 (49%) from 1981–1990.

Methods of examining the hearts: After "cleaning" each heart of extraneous tissue, the heart was weighed. All portions of the heart including epicardial coronary arteries, valves, and myocardium were carefully examined for lesions (abnormalities) and those observed were recorded. Histologic sections were prepared of myocardium and valvular vegetations and often of epicardial coronary arteries.

Statistical analysis: Data were analyzed using StatView 512+ statistical software package. Categorical comparisons were made with 2-tailed chi-squared analysis. Numerical comparisons were made using a 2-tailed, unpaired *t* test. Statistical significance was defined as $p < 0.05$.

RESULTS

CLINICAL FINDINGS

Age, sex, race: The 63 patients ranged in age from 12 to 88 years (mean 50); 31 were white, 28 were black, and 1 was Hispanic; 19 (30%) were female and 44 (70%) were male. Two patients (3%) were in their teens and 7 patients (11%) were over 70 years of age.

Underlying heart disease: Of the 63 patients, 21 (33%) had underlying cardiac valve disease before active IE: rheumatic heart disease in 8 patients (13%) (mitral stenosis in 5)[13]; mitral valve prolapse in 3 patients (5%)[14]; hypertrophic cardiomyopathy in 1 (2%)[15]; and mitral annular calcium in 9 patients (15%).[16] Certain clinical and necropsy findings in each of the 21 patients with underlying heart disease are tabulated in Table I and illustrated in Figures 1 to 7, and the findings in each of the 42 patients without underlying structural heart disease are listed in Table II and illustrated in Figures 8 to 16.

Other risk factors to infective endocarditis: In addition to underlying structural heart disease (21 patients), other predisposing factors to IE were present in 29 patients (46%), 7 of whom also had underlying structural valvular heart disease: opiate addiction in 15 patients (24%)[11]; habitual alcoholism in 7 patients (11%),[5] and chronic hemodialysis in 9 patients (14%).[16] Four patients (cases 29, 31, 34 and 33, Table I) had ≥2 episodes of active IE. The initial episode appeared to predispose to a subsequent one. The data recorded in the table concerns only the last episode of active IE. One patient (no.

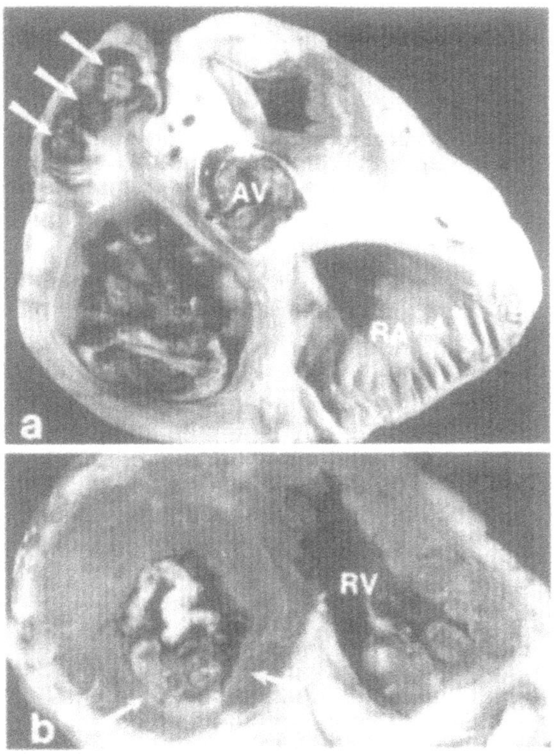

FIGURE 1. (Case 5, Table I.) Views of the base of the heart in a 66-year-old woman with mitral stenosis (NIH# A76-175) who developed infective endocarditis due to group D enterococcus 3 months before death. *a*, the opened left atrial cavity discloses vegetation attached to the atrial aspect of the mitral leaflet and also thrombi *(arrows)* in the left atrial appendage. *b*, vegetation *(arrows)* on the ventricular aspect of the mitral leaflets. The mitral orifice is diminished by the vegetative material and the mitral leaflets are considerably thickened. AV = aortic valve; RA = right atrium; RV = right ventricle.

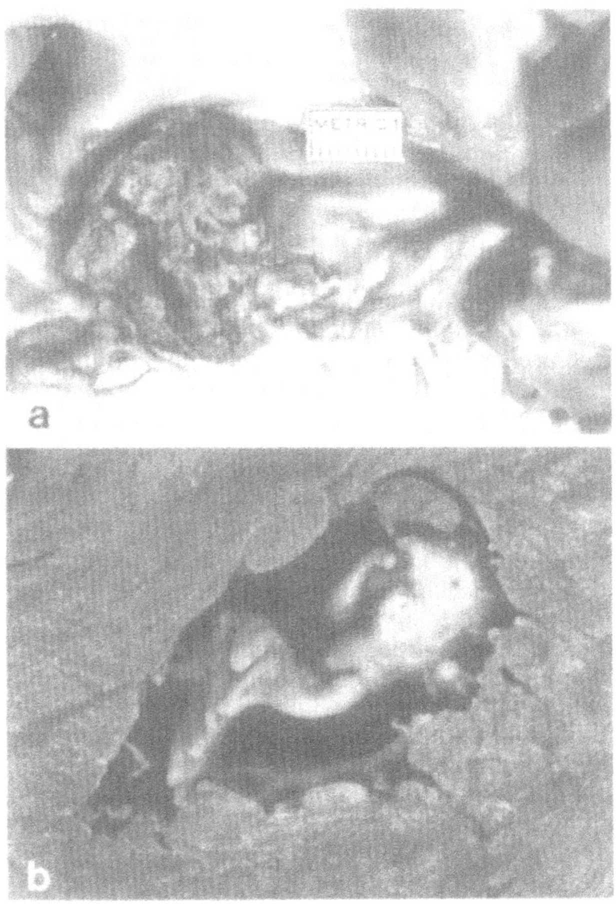

FIGURE 2. (Case 7, Table I.) Mitral valve with superimposed vegetation in a 59-year-old man (NIH# A84-134) with mitral stenosis. *a*, view of vegetation on the opened mitral valve. *b*, stenotic valve from the left ventricular aspect.

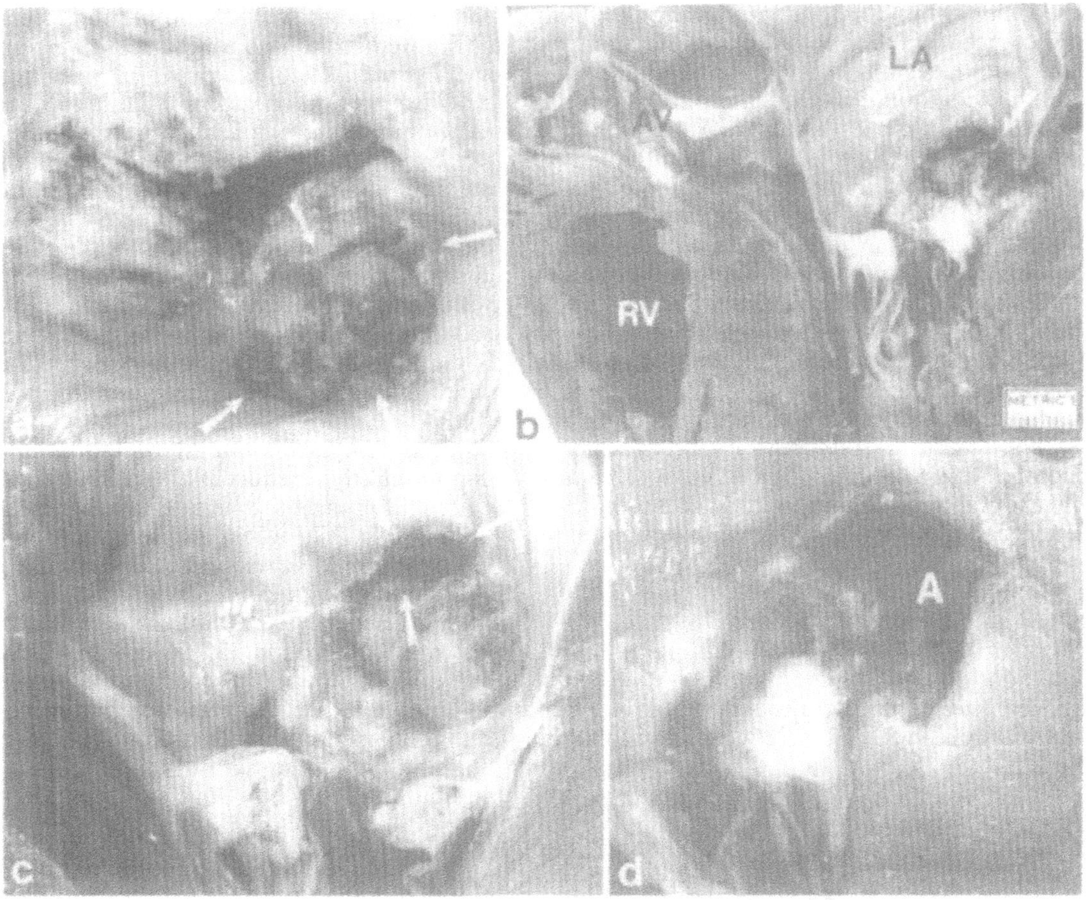

FIGURE 3. (Case 9, Table I.) Mitral valve in a 72-year-old woman with severe mitral stenosis. *a*, view from left atrium showing a vegetation *(arrows)* and the stenotic orifice. *b*, view of valve after longitudinal cut showing the thickened mitral leaflets and the vegetation *(arrow)*. *c*, close-up view of entrance *(arrows)* into a ring abscess. *d*, view of the ring abscess (A). AV = aortic valve; LA = left atrium; RV = right ventricle.

18, Table II), who had structurally normal cardiac valves, had idiopathic dilated cardiomyopathy.[17]

Organisms causing the infective endocarditis: The microorganisms responsible for the active IE are listed in Tables I and II. *Staphylococcus aureus* or *epidermidis* was responsible in 32 patients (51%); streptococcus species in 11 patients (17%); a gram-negative organism in 6 patients (10%); fungal species in 3 patients[1] (5%); and *Streptococcus pneumoniae* in 2 patients (3%). In 7 patients (11%), no information was available regarding the results of blood cultures. In 2 patients (3%) repeated blood cultures were negative but antibiotics were being administered at the time.

Infection in noncardiac organs and tissues: Infection involving organs other than the heart occurred in at least 31 (49%) of the 63 patients. Of the 31 patients, 25 had associated acute pneumonia or meningitis or both, 3 had huge renal abscesses, and 3 had systemic fungal infections involving 1 or more noncardiac organs.[1]

NECROPSY FINDINGS

Heart weight: At necropsy, the hearts in the 63 patients ranged in weight from 195 to 715 g (mean 432). Those in the 19 women ranged from 195 to 600 g (mean 333), and those in the 44 men from 270 to 715 g (mean 471) ($p < 0.05$). The heart weights in the 42 patients without preexisting heart disease ranged from 195 to 715 g (mean 410) (women = 289 g, men = 459 g), and in the 21 with preexisting heart disease from 275 to 650 g (mean 479) (women = 423 g, men = 499 g).

Mitral valve consequences: The active IE caused rupture of mitral chordae tendineae in 11 patients (18%), perforation of the anterior mitral leaflet in 7 patients (11%), and mitral ring abscess in 10 patients (16%).

Systemic emboli and infarcts: Grossly visible systemic emboli were found in 44 patients (70%) and 33

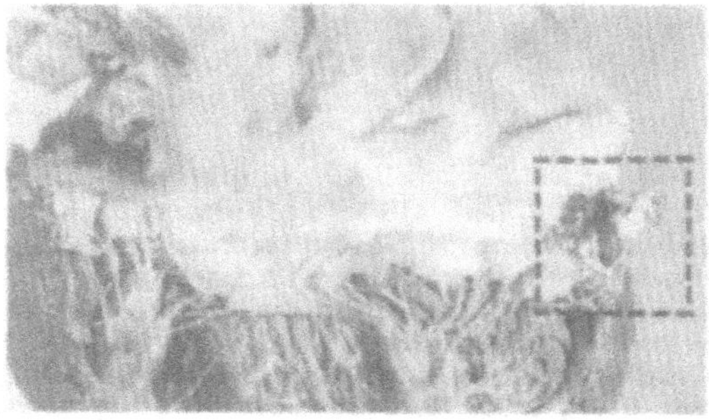

FIGURE 4. (Case 11, Table I.) Opened mitral valve showing a vegetation *(box)* on the posterior leaflet in a 54-year-old man (NIH# A60-27) with preexisting mitral regurgitation from prolapse.

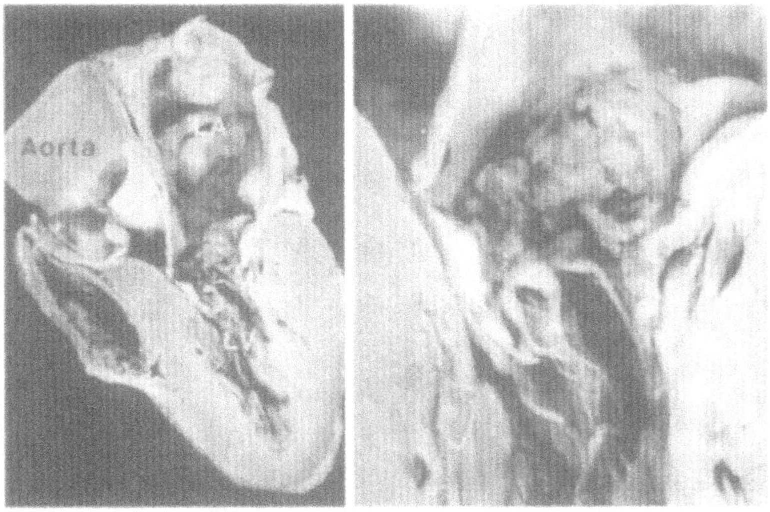

FIGURE 5. (Case 12, Table I.) Mitral valve in a 64-year-old woman (GT# 83A-173) whose first symptom of infective endocarditis was a cerebrovascular accident. *a*, longitudinal view showing a huge vegetation on a "floppy" mitral valve. *b*, close-up view. LA = left atrium; LV = left ventricle.

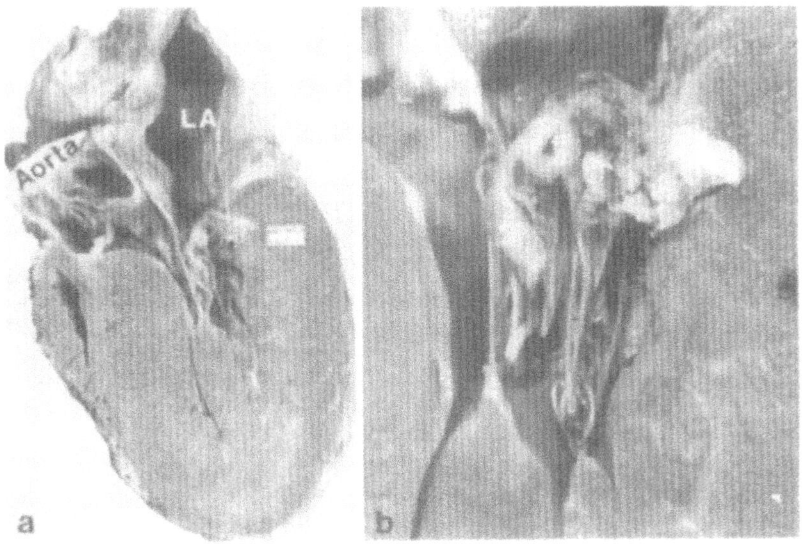

FIGURE 6. (Case 19, Table I.) Infective endocarditis involving a calcified mitral valve annulus in an 83-year-old man (GT# 85A-11) with bullous pemphigoid. *a*, longitudinal cut showing the vegetation on the mitral valve and mitral annular calcium extending into left ventricular myocardium. *b*, close-up view of the mitral valve showing vegetative material and "annular" calcium. At no time before or during the episode of active infective endocarditis were signs or symptoms of heart disease present. The diagnosis of infective endocarditis was not made until autopsy. LA = left atrium.

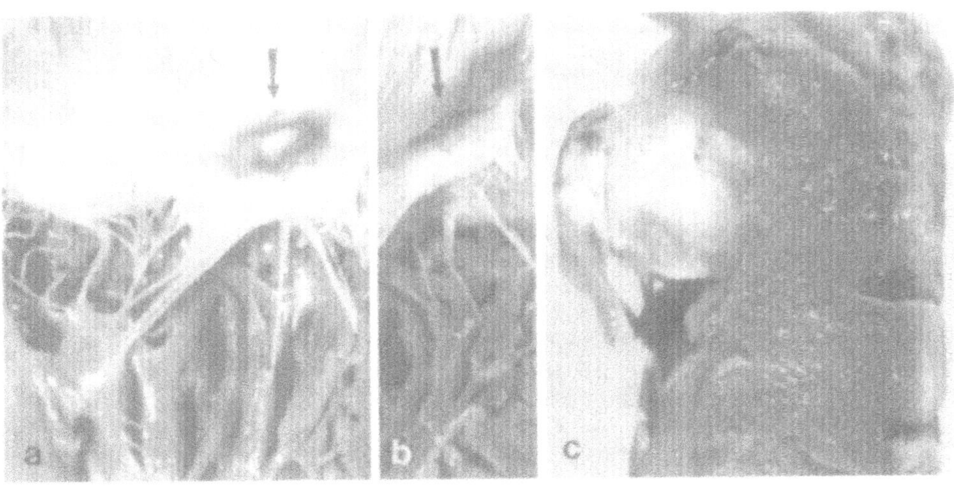

FIGURE 7. (Case 20, Table I.) Mitral valve with infective endocarditis superimposed on mitral annular calcium in an 84-year-old man (DCGH# 82A-34) who presented with pneumonia and was found to have *Staphylococcus aureus* in blood cultures. *a*, view of opened valve showing infection on the atrial aspect of the posterior leaflet. *b*, similar view but underlying annular calcium is now visible. *c*, longitudinal view of calcified mitral "annulus" with superimposed infection.

TABLE II Clinical and Morphologic Features of 42 Patients with Previously Normal Mitral Valves Prior to Active Infective Endocarditis

Case	Age (years)	Race	Sex	Predisposing Factors: O	HA	H	P	Mn	Infecting Organism	MR	Mode of Death: Sepsis	Embolus	CHF	HW (g)	LV: Fi	N	Ring Abscess	RCT	PAML	SE	Gross Organ Infarcts: Brain	Spleen	Kidney	Heart	Other
1	12	W	F	0	0	0	0	0	*Staphylococcus aureus*	0	0	+	0	205	0	+[1]	+	0	0	+	+	—	0	0	—
2	20	B	F	+	0	0	0	+	*Staphylococcus aureus*	0	+	0	+	210	0	0	0	0	0	+	—	—	+	0	—
3	28	W	F	0	0	0	0	+	*Staphylococcus aureus*	0	+	0	0	280	0	0	0	0	0	+	+	+	+	0	+
4	28	B	F	+	0	+	+	0	*Staphylococcus aureus*	0	+	0	0	390	0	+[1]	0	0	0	+	—	+	—	+	+
5	32	B	M	+	0	0	0	0	—	0	0	—	—	335	0	0	0	+	0	0	0	0	0	0	0
6	36	B	M	+	0	+	+	0	Alpha streptococcus	0	+	0	0	715	0	0	0	0	0	0	0	0	0	0	0
7	43	B	M	0	+	0	+	+	*Streptococcus pneumoniae*	0	0	0	0[3]	440	0	+	0	0	+	+	—	—	—	+	—
8	43	His	M	+	0	0	0	0	—	0	0	+	0	535	0	+	0	0	0	+	—	—	—	+	—
9	46	B	M	0	0	0	0	0	*Escherichia coli*[4]	0	0	0	0[5]	620	0	0	+	0	0	+	+	0	0	0	0
10	49	W	M	0	0	0	0	0	*Staphylococcus aureus*[4]	0	0	0	0[3]	280	0	0	0	0	0	0	0	0	0	0	0
11	52	B	M	0	0	+	0	0	*Aspergillus fumigatus*	0	+	0	0	—	0	0	0	0	0	+	+	+	+	0	0
12	54	W	F	0	0	0	+	0	*Pseudomonas aeruginosa*	0	0	+	0	195	0	0	+	0	0	+	0	+	+	0	0
13	54	B	M	0	0	0	0	0	—	0	0	+	0	520	0	0	0	0	0	+	+	—	—	0	—
14	55	—	M	0	0	0	0	0	—	0	—	—	—	—	0	0	0	0	0	+	—	+	+	0	—
15	58	W	M	0	+	0	+	0	*Staphylococcus aureus*	0	+	0	0	420	0	+[1]	0	0	0	+	0	0	+	0	—
16	58	W	M	0	0	0	0	0	*Mucormycosis*	0	0	+	0	340	0	+[1]	0	0	0	+	+	+	+	0	0
17	58	W	M	0	0	0	+	0	*Staphylococcus epidermis*	0	0	+[6]	0	370	0	0	0	0	+	+[2]	0	0	0	0	0
18	60	B	M	0	+	0	0	0	*Staphylococcus aureus*	0	+	0	0	600	0	0	0	0	0	—	—	—	—	0	—
19	62	W	F	0	0	0	0	+	*Staphylococcus aureus*	0	0	—	—	—	0	0	0	0	0	—	—	—	—	0	—
20	63	W	F	0	0	0	0	0	*Escherichia coli*	0	0	0	0[3]	380	0	0	0	0	0	0	—	0	0	0	0
21	64	B	M	0	+	0	+	+	*Streptococcus pneumoniae*	0	+	0	0	—	0	0	0	0	0	—	—	—	—	0	—
22	74	W	M	0	0	0	+	0	*Staphylococcus aureus*	0	+	0	0	390	0	0	0	0	0	+	+	0	0	0	0
23	88	—	F	0	0	0	+	0	Klebsiella species	0	+	0	0	—	0	0	0	0	0	—	—	—	—	0	—
24	15	W	F	0	0	0	+	+	*Staphylococcus aureus*	+	+	0	0	200	0	+[1]	0	0	0	+	—	+	+	0	0
25	15	W	M	0	0	0	0	+	*Staphylococcus aureus*	+	0	+	0	440	0	+[1]	+	0	0	+	+	+	+	0	+
26	22	B	M	+	0	0	0	0	*Staphylococcus aureus*	+	+	0	0	540	0	0	0	0	0	+	+	+	+	0	0
27	27	B	M	+	0	0	0	0	—[7]	+	0	+	0	345	0	+	0	+	0	+	+	+	+	+	0
28	27	B	F	0	0	0	0	0	Negative[8]	+	+	0	0	360	0	+	0	+	0	—	—	—	—	+	—
29	28	B	M	+	0	0	+	0	Alpha streptococcus	+	0	+	0	380	0	0	+	0	0	+[2]	0	0	0	0	+
30	29	B	F	+	0	0	0	0	*Staphylococcus aureus*	+	0	+	0	320	0	+[1]	0	0	0	+	+	+	+	0	—
31	29	B	M	0	0	0	0	0	*Staphylococcus aureus*	+	+	0	0	270	0	0	+	0	0	—	—	—	—	0	—
32	34	B	M	+	0	0	0	0	*Staphylococcus aureus*	+	0	+	0	485	0	0	0	+	0	+	+	+	+	0	0
33	36	B	M	+	0	0	0	0	Group D streptococcus	+	0	0	+	500	0	+	0	+	+	+	0	+	+	0	0
34	39	B	M	+	0	0	—	—	*Staphylococcus aureus*	+	0	+	0	485	0	+[1]	0	0	+	+	+	+	+	+	—
35	41	B	F	+	0	0	+	0	*Staphylococcus aureus*	+	+	0	0	350	0	0	0	+	0	0	0	0	0	0	0
36	42	B	M	—	—	0	0	0	Negative[8]	+	0	0	+	620	+	0	0	+	+	+	+	—	—	+	—
37	43	B	M	+	0	0	0	0	—	+	0	+	0	—	+	0	0	+	0	+[2]	+	0	+	0	+
38	54	W	M	0	+	0	0	0	Group D streptococcus	+	0	0	+	510	0	+[9]	0	0	0	—	—	—	—	0	—
39	59	B	M	0	+	0	0	0	*Serratia marcescens*[4]	+	+	0	0	360	0	0	0	0	+	+	—	+	0	0	0
40	58	—	M	0	0	+	0	0	*Staphylococcus aureus*	+	0	+	0	670	0	+	0	+	+	+	+	0	0	+	0
41	66	W	M	0	0	0	0	0	*Staphylococcus aureus*	+	0	+	0	300	0	0	+	0	0	+	+	0	0	0	0
42	68	W	M	0	0	0	0	0	*Candida parapsilosis*	+	+	0	0	480	+	0	0	0	0	+	0	+	0	0	0
Total or mean	44			14	6	4	12	7		19	17	15	4	412	3	15	7	9	7	30	17	16	16	8	5

[1]Myocardial abscess; [2]pulmonary emboli also; [3]death due to cancer; [4]endocarditis not diagnosed (postmortem blood cultures positive); [5]death due to chronic renal failure 2° to systemic hypertension; [6]pulmonary embolus 2° hypercoagulable state; [7]sudden death before cultures obtained; [8]cultured while on antibiotics; [9]necrosis limited to papillary muscle.

A = alcoholism; B = black; CHF = congestive heart failure; F = female; Fi = fibrosis; H = hemodialysis; His = Hispanic; HW = heart weight; LV = left ventricle; M = male; Mn = meningitis; MR = mitral regurgitation; N = necrosis; O = opiate addict; P = pneumonia; PAML = perforated anterior mitral leaflet; RCT = ruptured chordae tendineae; SE = systemic emboli; + = present; 0 = absent; — = no information available.

(52%) had infarcts in 1 or more body organs (Tables I and II).

Comparison of cases without to those with mitral valve structural abnormalities before the active infective endocarditis: The 42 patients with normal mitral valves before the active IE compared to those with previously structurally abnormal valves were significantly (p <0.05) younger (mean age 44 vs 59 years); were more likely to be opiate addicts (33% vs 5%); were less likely to have beta streptococcus as the infecting organism

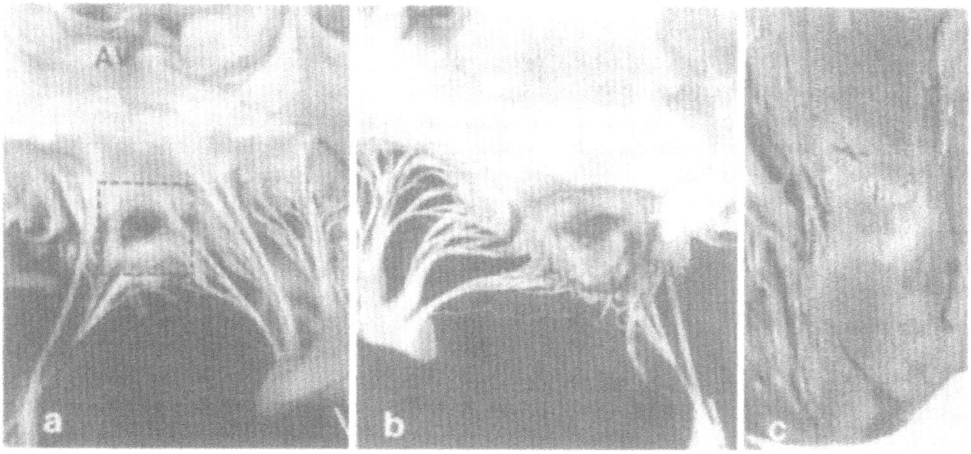

FIGURE 8. (Case 8, Table II.) Active infective endocarditis involving a previously normal valve in 43-year-old man (DCGH# 71A-70). *a*, view of ventricular side of the anterior mitral leaflet showing a perforation *(dashed box)* filled with vegetative material. *b*, view of atrial side of anterior mitral leaflet. The vegetation covers the perforation. *c*, close-up view of left ventricular free wall showing an area of necrosis, the result of a coronary artery embolus. (Reproduced with permission from *The American Journal of Medicine* 1972;53:20–35.[4])

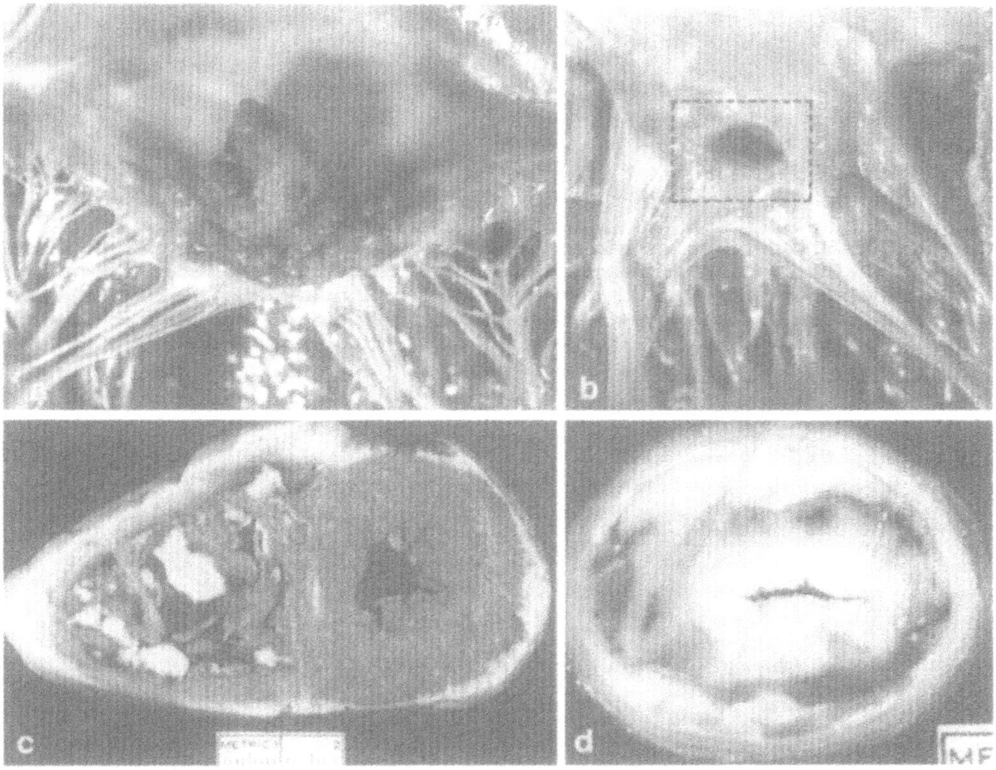

FIGURE 9. (Case 19, Table II.) Active infective endocarditis involving a previously normal valve in a 58-year-old man (NIH# A85-34) who had metastatic colonic carcinoma. *a*, opened mitral valve with a vegetation on the atrial aspect of the anterior mitral leaflet. *b*, view of the ventricular side of the anterior mitral leaflet showing a perforation *(dashed box)* that is filled with vegetative material. *c*, transverse section of the cardiac ventricles showing multiple thrombi in the right ventricular cavity. The patient was in a hypercoagulable state. He died from a pulmonary embolus. *d*, thromboembolic material filling the lumen of a portion of descending thoracic aorta. Apparently no clinical consequences resulted from the near total occlusion of a portion of aorta. The material filling the aorta is different from that of the vegetation on the mitral valve.

(0 of 35 vs 4 of 20 patients), and were more likely to have a perforation of the anterior mitral leaflet (7 of 41 [17%] vs 0 of 21). No significant differences in the 2 groups were observed in sex; the type of infecting organism other than beta streptococcus; or the frequency of habitual alcoholism, hemodialysis, systemic emboli, ring abscess, or ruptured chordae tendineae.

Comparison of patients with and without ruptured chordae tendineae: The 11 patients with compared to the 52 patients without ruptured chordae tendineae were significantly younger ($p < 0.05$) (mean age 37 vs 52 years), and had a higher frequency of opiate addiction (60% vs 15%).

Comparison of patients with and without perforation of the anterior mitral leaflet: The 7 patients with compared to the 56 patients without a perforation in the anterior mitral leaflet had a significantly higher frequency of previously normal mitral leaflets (100% vs 63%), a history of habitual alcoholism (33% vs 9%), and of ruptured chordae tendineae (50% vs 14%).

Comparison of patients with and without ring abscess: Comparison of the 10 patients with to the 53 patients without mitral valve ring abscess disclosed no significant differences in the variables listed in Tables I and II. Complete heart block, however, was present in 3 of the 10 patients with ring abscess and in 1 of the 53 patients without ring abscess. One other patient with ring abscess had right bundle branch block, but the latter patient had clear evidence of digitalis toxicity.

Comparison of patients with to those without mitral annular calcium: The 9 patients with mitral annular calcium compared to the 54 without were significantly (p

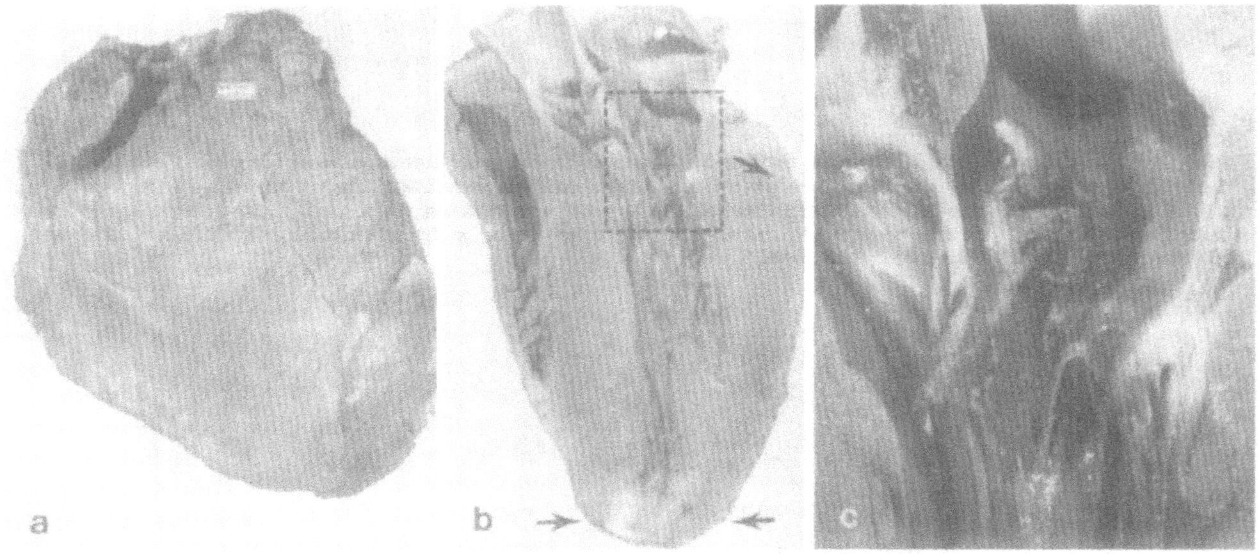

FIGURE 10. (Case 25, Table II.) Active infective endocarditis involving a previously normal valve in a 15-year-old boy (GT# 81A-186). *a*, exterior of the heart showing a diffuse purulent pericarditis but without colonies of microorganisms on histologic study. *b*, longitudinal view showing a partially destroyed mitral valve by the infection. An abscess *(arrows)* is present in the ventricular wall at the apex. *c*, close-up of mitral valve. This boy had been well until he cut his finger while repairing his bicycle 3 weeks before death. The infecting organism was *Staphylococcus aureus*.

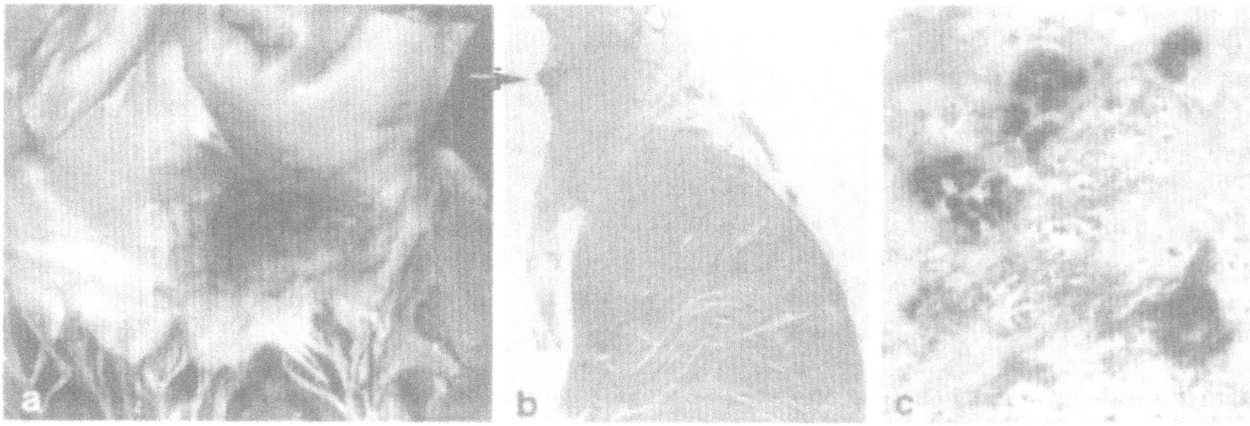

FIGURE 11. (Case 27, Table II.) Active infective endocarditis involving a previously normal valve in a 22-year-old opiate addict (DCGH# 75A-65). *a*, opened mitral valve showing vegetative material on both the posterior leaflet and left atrial endocardium. *b*, histologic section after longitudinal cut through posterior mitral leaflet. The infection also involves mural endocardium of left atrium *(arrow)*. *c*, close-up of colonies of organisms in the vegetation. This man died of a ruptured mycotic aneurysm in the brain. (Hematoxylin-eosin stains × 4 *(b)*, and × 530 *(c)*; reduced by 25%.)

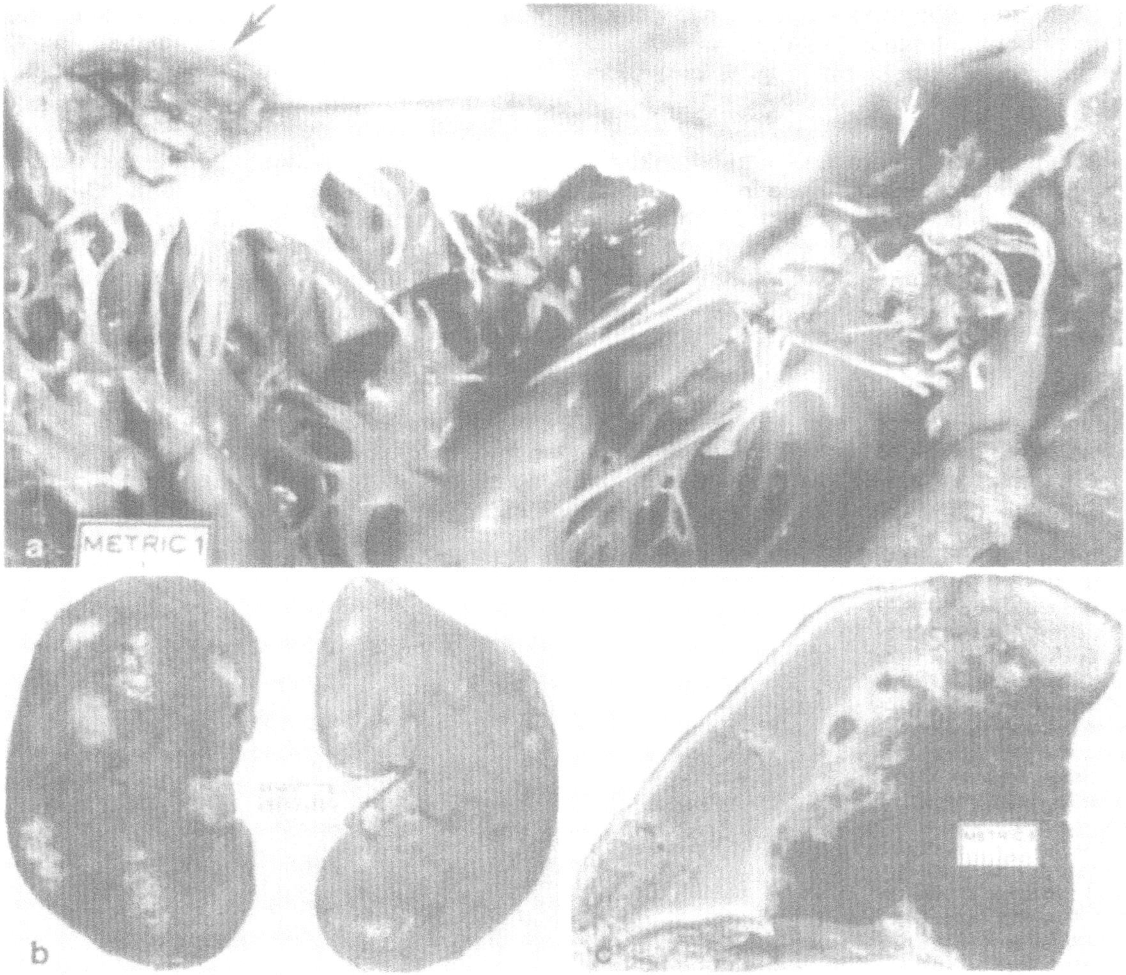

FIGURE 12. (Case 28, Table II.) Opened mitral valve with superimposed vegetations *(arrows) (a)*, exterior of kidneys showing multiple infarcts *(b)*, and cut surface of spleen showing a huge infarct *(c)* in a 27-year-old opiate addict (DCMEO# 83-08-574) who developed signs and symptoms consistent with active infective endocarditis 26 days before death. Despite antibiotic therapy he developed evidence of mitral regurgitation but died from consequences of multiple systemic emboli. The mitral valve was normal before the infection.

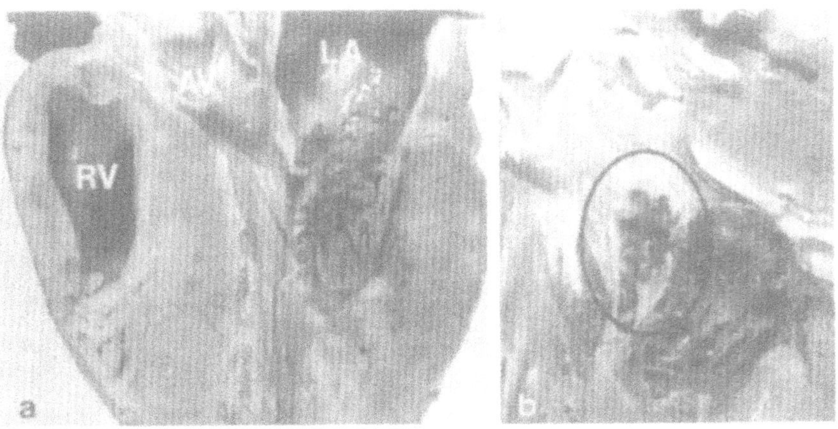

FIGURE 13. (Case 33, Table II.) Infective endocarditis involving a previously normal valve in a 36-year-old opiate addict (DCGH# 75A-159) who died 34 days after onset of congestive heart failure. The infection virtually destroyed the mitral valve which was severely incompetent. *a*, view after a longitudinal cut of the heart. Large vegetations are visible. Multiple abscesses without colonies of organisms were present in the left ventricular wall and the lumens of several intramural coronary arteries contained embolic material. *b*, close-up view showing a perforation in the anterior mitral leaflet *(circle)*.
AV = aortic valve; LA = left atrium; RV = right ventricle.

<0.05) older (mean age 66 vs 46 years); had a higher frequency of chronic hemodialysis (56% vs 18%); and a lower frequency of systemic emboli (60% vs 88%) and cerebral infarcts (0 of 9 vs 21 of 54 [61%]).

Comparison of patients with and without systemic emboli: No significant differences were observed in mean age, sex, infecting organism, and frequency of perforated anterior mitral leaflet, ruptured chordae tendineae, ring abscess, grossly visible organ infarcts, and presence of or type of underlying heart disease in the 44 patients with morphologic evidence of systemic emboli compared to the 7 patients without such evidence.

DISCUSSION

The heretofore described findings in necropsied patients with active IE limited to the mitral valve without operative intervention showed that more patients were males than females (2 to 1); that the infection more commonly involved a previously anatomically normal than a previously anatomically abnormal mitral valve (2 to 1); that vegetations on previously normal mitral valves often did not cause severe valvular dysfunction and that vegetations on previously abnormal valves did not cause or worsen valvular dysfunction; that a predisposing factor to IE (previously abnormal mitral valve, opiate addiction, habitual alcoholism and/or chronic hemodialysis) was common (2 of 3 patients); and that the IE often was simply part of a generalized or systemic infection (1 of 2 patients).

One of the more difficult evaluations in the present study was the determination of the presence or absence of mitral regurgitation as a consequence of vegetations on the mitral valve. When the vegetations are small (≤5 mm in maximal diameter), it is unlikely that mitral regurgitation would result unless chordae tendineae are ruptured and the latter event is infrequent when vegeta-

FIGURE 14. (Case 34, Table II.) Active infective endocarditis involving a mitral valve in a 39-year-old opiate addict (DCMEO# 88-08-887). This man had clinical evidence of active infective endocarditis involving the tricuspid valve 9 months before death. Another episode of infective endocarditis probably occurred 4 months before death when he had a stroke during a febrile period. He again had evidence of cerebral problems including seizures 7 days before death and blood cultures were positive for *Staphylococcus aureus*. At necropsy, a vegetation was present on the mitral valve bordering a leaflet perforation. The perforation probably was produced during an earlier episode of active infective endocarditis.

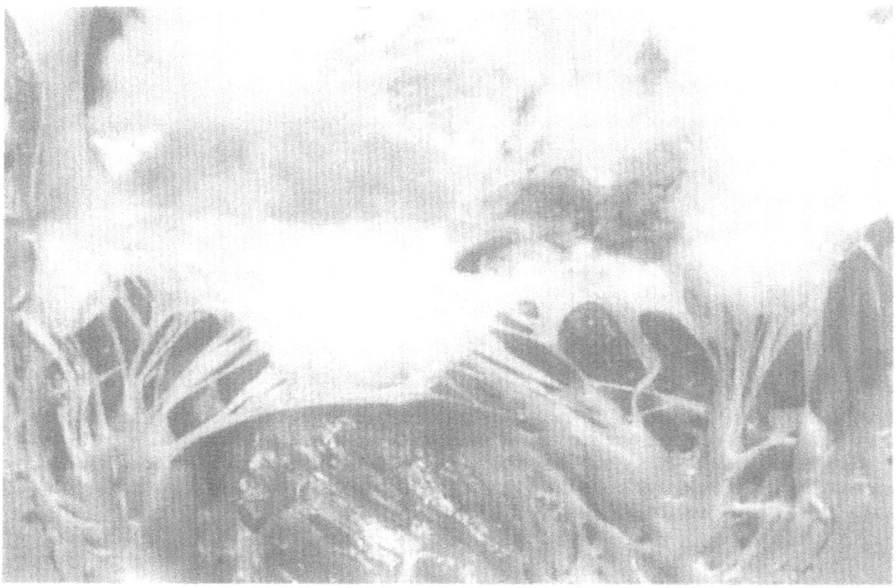

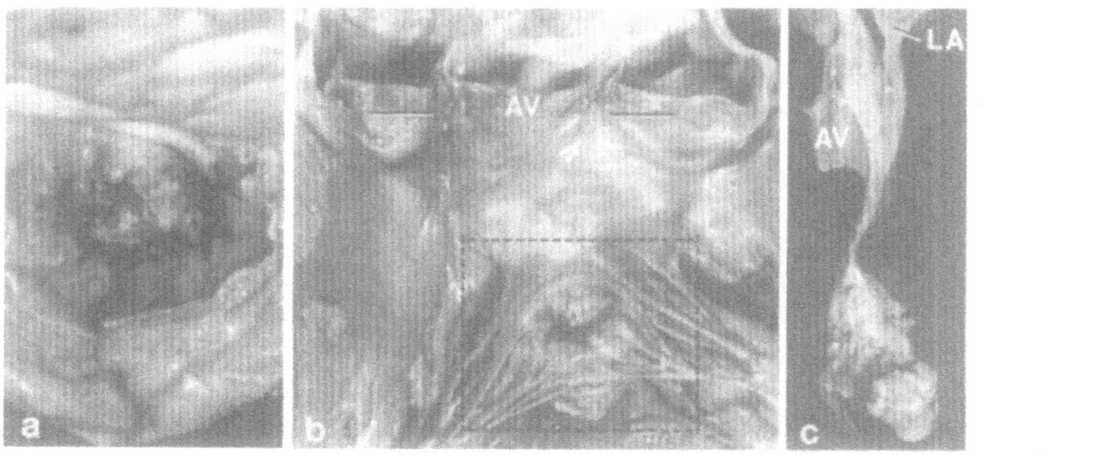

FIGURE 15. (Case 39, Table II.) Active infective endocarditis involving a previously normal valve in a 59-year-old man (DCGH# 75A-123). *a*, left atrium showing a large vegetation on the mitral valve. *b*, opened aortic valve (AV) and ventricular aspect of anterior mitral leaflet showing a perforation *(dashed box)*. *c*, longitudinal section of anterior mitral leaflet, aortic valve and left atrial (LA) wall showing the vegetation in the caudal two thirds of the anterior leaflet. The diagnosis of active infective endocarditis was not suspected in life. The patient presented with pneumonia.

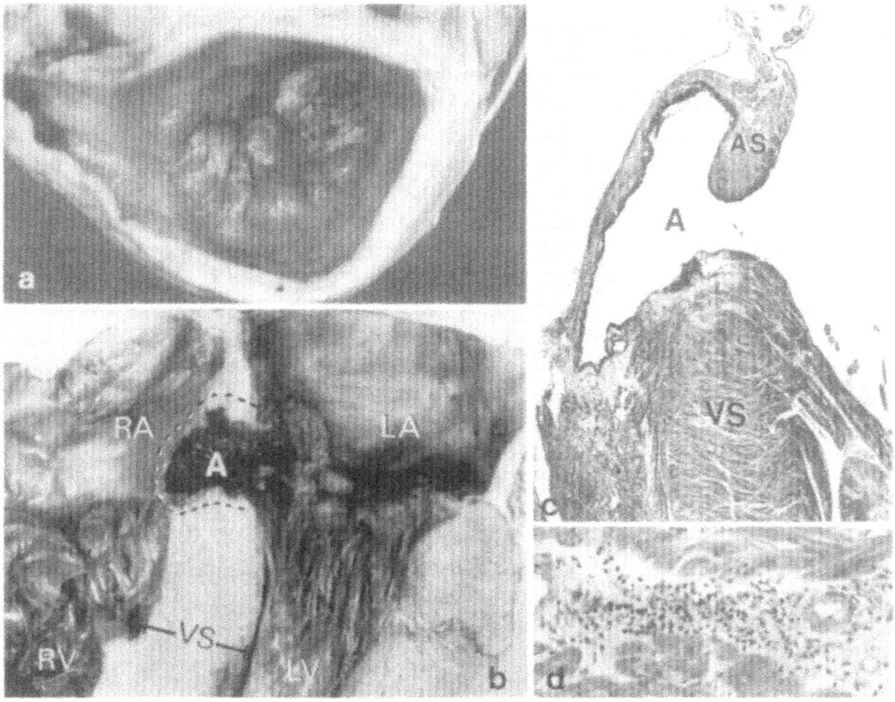

FIGURE 16. (Case 41, Table II.) Active infective endocarditis involving a previously normal mitral valve in a 66-year-old man (MHCMH# A4826) who developed symptoms of active infective endocarditis 20 days before death and complete heart block 14 days before death. *a*, view of left atrium (LA) showing a vegetation at the posteromedial commissure. *b*, 4-chamber view showing a huge ring abscess *(dashed area)* in the caudal half of the atrial septum (AS). *c*, photomicrograph through the area of the ring abscess (A) (Movat stain × 3; reduced by 30%). *d*, foci of acute inflammation were present in the ventricular walls (hematoxylineosin stain × 220; reduced by 30%). LV = left ventricle; RA = right atrium; RV = right ventricle; VS = ventricular septum. (*a* and *b* are reproduced with permission from *Circulation* 1976;54:140–145.[6])

tions are small. Large vegetations, however, even in the absence of ruptured chordae tendineae or perforation of a valvular leaflet probably often cause mitral regurgitation because of their interfering with leaflet coaptation during ventricular systole.

One anatomic finding that usually indicates mitral regurgitation is rupture of chordae tendineae.[2] In the present study 11 patients (18%) had ruptured chordae: 9 (22% of 41 patients) had active IE complicating previously anatomically normal mitral valves and 8 of them had clinical and morphologic evidence of mitral regurgitation; 2 patients (10% of 21 patients) had active IE complicating previously anatomically abnormal valves: 1 of them had preexisting mitral stenosis and no evidence of mitral regurgitation; the other patient had convincing evidence of regurgitation.

The other anatomic finding suggesting the presence of mitral regurgitation (at some time) is the presence of a perforation in a valve leaflet or actual tears or major indentations of a leaflet. In the present study 7 patients had a perforation in the anterior mitral leaflet and all of them had infection on a previously anatomically normal valve. At necropsy in 2 of the 7 patients the perforation was filled with vegetative material so that no regurgitation was occurring through the cuspal "perforation" shortly before death. At least 5 of these 7 patients, however, had clinical evidence of mitral regurgitation.

It is less difficult to determine if a mitral valve, which had previously been anatomically normal, was made incompetent by vegetations than when vegetations are superimposed on mitral leaflets that had previously been abnormal. In the present study 21 patients (34%) had previously abnormal mitral valves: rheumatic in 8, prolapse in 3, hypertrophic cardiomyopathy in 1, and mitral annular calcium in 9. Of the 8 rheumatic patients, 5 had preexisting mitral stenosis and the vegetations in them did not appear to cause mitral regurgitation, but they may have worsened the mitral stenosis because of the orifice space occupied by the vegetation.[3] Although 3 other patients had rheumatic heart disease as evidenced by diffuse fibrosis of the valve leaflets, none of them had clinical evidence of valvular dysfunction before the active IE. Of the 3 patients with prolapse, 2 were believed to have had some mitral regurgitation before the onset of active IE which did not appear to worsen the regurgitation. In the 1 patient with hypertrophic cardiomyopathy, it was not possible to determine if the preexisting mitral regurgitation was worsened by the mitral vegetations. And finally, active IE complicating mitral annular calcium did not cause chordal rupture or leaflet perforation in any patient, and none of these 9 patients were considered to have significant mitral regurgitation either before or after the active IE.

Acknowledgment: We wish to thank Vivian Norman and Rodger Marks for manuscript preparation, Michael Spencer for photography, and Leslie Berry for artwork preparation.

1. Andriole VT, Kravetz HM, Roberts WC, Utz JP. Candida endocarditis: clinical and pathologic studies. *Am J Med* 1962;32:251–285.
2. Roberts WC, Braunwald E, Morrow AG. Acute severe mitral regurgitation secondary to ruptured chordae tendineae: clinical, hemodynamic and pathologic considerations. *Circulation* 1966;33:58–70.
3. Roberts WC, Ewy GA, Glancy DL, Marcus FI. Valvular stenosis produced by active infective endocarditis. *Circulation* 1967;36:449–451.
4. Roberts WC, Buchbinder NA. Left-sided valvular active infective endocarditis: a study of forty-five necropsy patients. *Am J Med* 1972;53:20–35.
5. Buchbinder NA, Roberts WC. Alcoholism: an important but unemphasized factor predisposing to infective endocarditis. *Arch Intern Med* 1973;132:689–692.
6. Arnett EN, Roberts WC. Valve ring abscess in active infective endocarditis: frequency, location, and clues to clinical diagnosis from the study of 95 necropsy

cases. *Circulation* 1976;54:140–145.
7. Arnett EN, Roberts WC. Active infective endocarditis: a clinicopathologic analysis of 137 necropsy patients. *Curr Probl Cardiol* 1976;1:1–76.
8. Andy JJ, Sheikh MU, Ali N, Barnes BO, Fox LM, Curry CL, Roberts WC. Echocardiographic observations in opiate addicts with active infective endocarditis: frequency of involvement of the various valves and comparison of echocardiographic features of right- and left-sided cardiac valve endocarditis. *Am J Cardiol* 1977;40:17–23.
9. Roberts WC. Characteristics and consequences of infective endocarditis (active or healed or both) learned from morphologic studies. In: Rahimtoola SH, ed. Infective Endocarditis. New York: Grune & Stratton, 1978:55–123.
10. Sheikh MU, Covarrubias EA, Ali N, Lee WR, Sheikh NM, Roberts WC. M-mode echocardiographic observations during and after healing of active bacterial endocarditis limited to the mitral valve. *Am Heart J* 1981;101:37–45.
11. Dressler FA, Roberts WC. Infective endocarditis in opiate addicts: analysis of 80 cases studied at necropsy. *Am J Cardiol* 1989;63:1240–1257.
12. Roberts WC, Oluwole BO, Fernicola DJ. Comparison of active infective endocarditis involving a previously stenotic versus a previously nonstenotic aortic valve. *Am J Cardiol* 1993;71:1082–1088.
13. Roberts WC. Morphologic aspects of cardiac valve dysfunction. *Am Heart J* 1992;123:1610–1632.
14. Dollar AL, Roberts WC. Morphologic comparison of patients with mitral valve prolapse who died suddenly with patients who died from severe valvular dysfunction or other conditions. *J Am Coll Cardiol* 1991;17:921–931.
15. Roberts CS, Roberts WC. Morphologic features. In: Zipes DP, Rowlands DJ eds. Progress in Cardiology (2/2), Philadelphia: Lea & Febiger 1989:3–32.
16. Roberts WC, Waller BF. Effect of chronic hypercalcemia on the heart. An analysis of 18 necropsy patients. *Am J Med* 1981;71:371–384.
17. Silver MA, Roberts WC. Active infective endocarditis complicating idiopathic dilated cardiomyopathy. *Am J Cardiol* 1983;52:651–652.

Clinical and Morphologic Features of Mitral Valve Prolapse in Octogenarians

Jamshid Shirani, MD,* and William C. Roberts, MD†

The frequency of mitral valve prolapse (MVP) in women decreases progressively from the third to the ninth decade of life; in men, in contrast, its frequency remains the same from the third to the ninth decade.[1] Of 264 patients with MVP detected by M-mode echocardiography and reported by Savage and associates,[1] only 4 (1.5%) were aged 80 years or over. A previous clinicopathologic study from this laboratory by Dollar and Roberts[2] included 56 patients aged 16 to 70 years. The present study examines clinical and morphologic findings in 12 octogenarians with MVP at necropsy. Al-

From the Pathology Branch, National Heart, Lung, and Blood Institutes, National Institutes of Health, Bethesda, Maryland 20892. Manuscript received February 16, 1993; revised manuscript received and accepted May 20, 1993.

*Present address: Medical College of Virginia, Department of Medicine, Division of Cardiology, Box 128, MCV Station, Richmond, Virginia 23298-0128.

†Present address: Baylor Cardiovascular Institute, Baylor University Medical Center, 3500 Gaston Avenue, Dallas, Texas 75246.

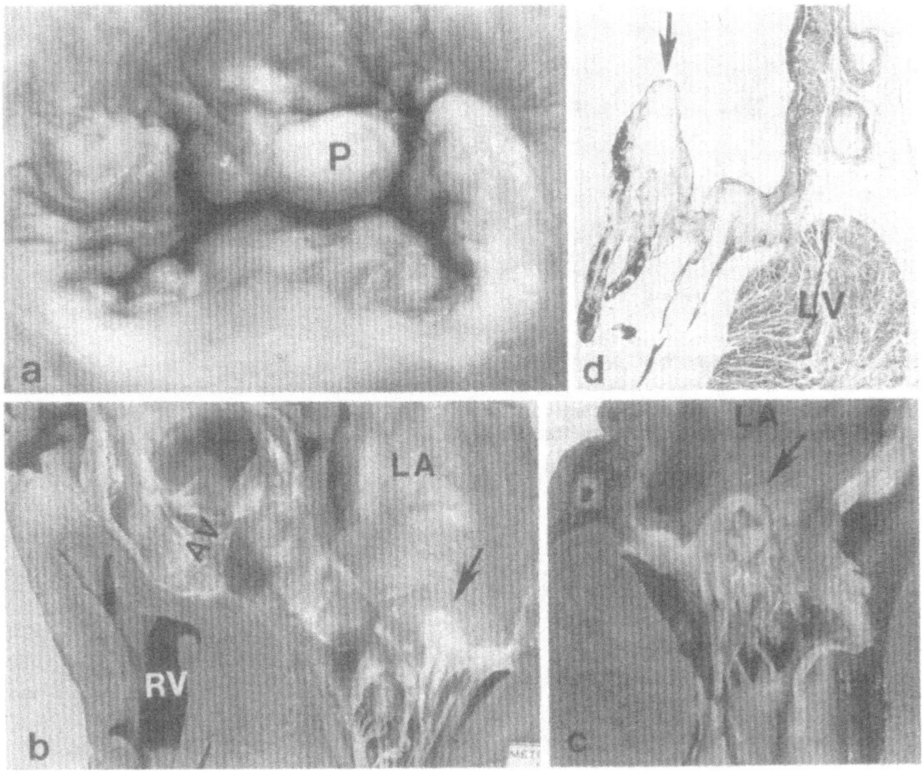

FIGURE 1. The heart of an 80-year-old man (patient 2, GT# 80A-86) who died of gastric lymphoma. On his last hospital admission, a grade 5/6 holosystolic murmur was audible and mitral valve prolapse was diagnosed by echocardiogram. *a*, view of the intact mitral valve from the left atrium (LA) showing prolapsed posterior (P) leaflet. *b*, longitudinal cut showing the posterior one half of the left ventricular outflow tract. The prolapsed portion of posterior mitral leaflet is indicated by the *arrow*. *c*, longitudinal cut showing the anterior one half of the mitral valve. The arrow again designates the prolapsed portion of the posterior leaflet. *d*, photomicrograph of a histologic section through the prolapsed portion *(arrow)* of the posterior mitral leaflet. The distal two thirds of the leaflet is prolapsed. (Movat stain, original magnification × 2, reduced 35%.) AV = aortic valve; LV = left ventricular wall; RV = right ventricular cavity; VS = ventricular septum.

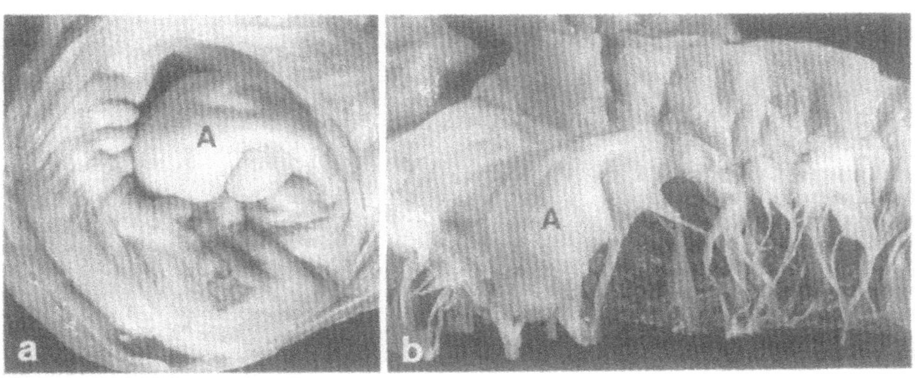

FIGURE 2. The heart of an 81-year-old woman (patient 3, SH #ME-03-1990) who died of pancreatic carcinoma. She never had any signs or symptoms of cardiac dysfunction. On her last admission, a 3/6 holosystolic murmur was heard. *a*, intact mitral valve viewed from the left atrium showing prolapse of the anterior (A) leaflet. *b*, the opened mitral valve showing prominent hooding of the posterior one half of the anterior leaflet.

though patients aged 80 to 89 years have been included in previous necropsy studies of MVP,[3,4] a study focusing exclusively on this age group has not been reported previously.

The necropsy files of the Pathology Branch, National Heart, Lung, and Blood Institute, National Institutes of Health, from January 1956 to February 1993 contain 125 patients coded as having "mitral valve prolapse" or "floppy mitral valve." Twelve of them were 80 to 89 years old at the time of death and are the sub-

TABLE I Certain Clinicopathologic Findings in 12 Octogenarians with Mitral Valve Prolapse

Patient	Age (yr) & Sex	AP	AMI	CHF	SD	SH	MVP Diagnosed Clinically	MR	MVR	Cause of Death	HW (g)	LV Fibrosis	Dilated RV	Dilated LV	CAD	Chords Missing	Grade of MVP (1-3+)	Plaque Under PML	MVAC (cm)	MAC (0-4+)	VC-PFO	Redundant FO Membrane
1	80M	0	0	0	+	0	0	0	0	Sudden death	420	0	0	0	0	0	+++	+	–	0	0	0
2	80M	0	0	+	0	0	+*	+	0	Cancer	415	0	+	0	0	+	+++	0	9.5	0	0	0
3	81F	0	0	0	0	0	0	+	0	Cancer	240	0	0	0	0	+	+++	0	10.5	0	+	0
4	82F	0	0	+	0	+	+†	+	+	Operation‡	360	0	0	0	0	+	+++	0	–	0	0	0
5	82F	0	0	+	0	0	+*	+	0	CHF	390	0	0	+	0	+	+++	0	–	+	0	0
6	82M	+	+	0	0	+	0	0	0	AAA	410	+	0	0	+	0	+	0	9.7	0	0	0
7	82M	0	0	0	0	0	0	0	0	Cancer	460	0	0	0	0	0	++	0	–	0	0	0
8	83M	0	0	+	0	+	0	+	0	Cancer	690	0	0	0	0	0	+	0	12.0	0	0	0
9	84M	+	+	+	0	0	0	+	0	HC§	515	+	0	0	+	+	+++	0	–	+	0	0
10	85F	0	0	+	0	+	0	0	0	Pneumonia	370	0	0	0	0	+	+	+	11.5	++	+	+
11	85F	0	0	+	0	+	0	+	0	IE	330	0	0	0	0	0	++	0	–	0	ASD	0
12	88F	0	0	0	+	0	0	0	0	Car accident	–	0	0	0	0	0	+++	0	–	0	0	0
Totals or (mean)	(83)	2	2	7	2	5	3	7	1		(420)	2	1	1	2	6		2	(10.6)	3	2	1

*Diagnosed by echocardiogram on last hospital admission. †Diagnosed at operation 1 day before death for acute severe mitral regurgitation. ‡Died 1 day after mitral valve replacement. §Not diagnosed during life.

AAA = abdominal aortic aneurysm; AMI = acute myocardial infarction; AP = angina pectoris; ASD = atrial septal defect; CAD = ≥ 1 major epicardial coronary arteries > 75% ↓ in cross-sectional area by plaque; CHF = congestive heart failure; F = female; FO = fossa ovalis; HC = hypertrophic cardiomyopathy; HW = heart weight; IE = infective endocarditis; LV = left ventricle; M = male; MAC = mitral annular calcium; MR = mitral regurgitation; MVAC = mitral valve annular circumference; MVP = mitral valve prolapse; MVR = mitral valve replacement; PML = posterior mitral leaflet; RV = right ventricle; SD = sudden death; SH = systemic hypertension; VC-PFO = valvular-competent patent foramen ovale.

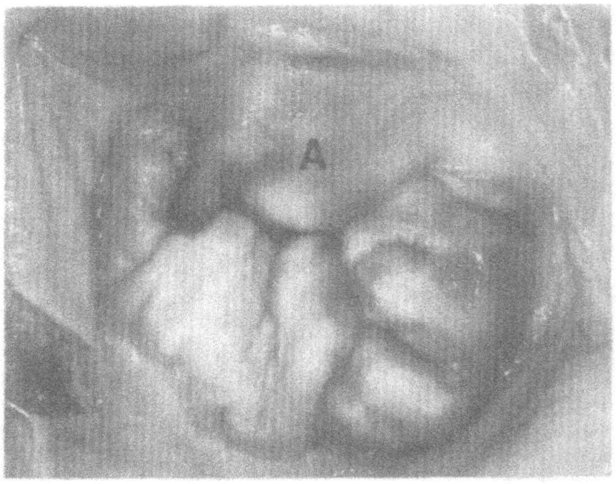

FIGURE 3. View of the intact mitral valve from the left atrium in an 82-year-old man (patient 7, NNMC #A85-127) who died of metastatic adenocarcinoma of the prostate gland. He never had signs or symptoms of cardiac dysfunction. The prolapse involves the posterior leaflet. A = anterior leaflet.

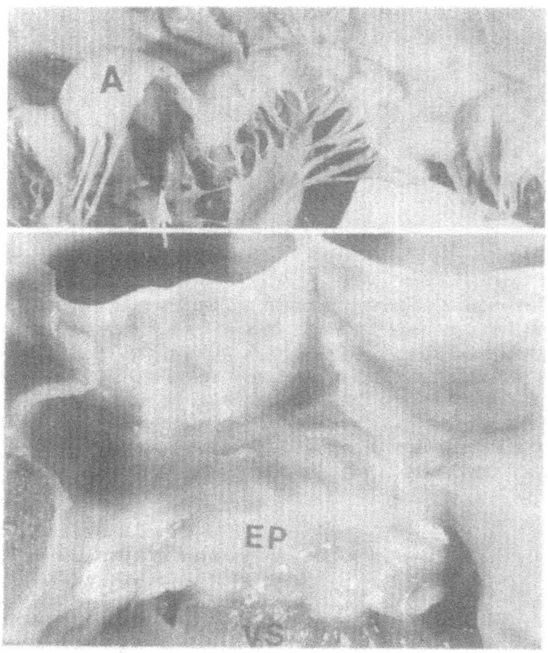

FIGURE 4. The heart of an 84-year-old man (patient 9, WHC #A86-17) with hypertrophic cardiomyopathy. He died during an operation for presumed constrictive pericarditis. *Top,* opened mitral valve showing thickened leaflets with marked hooding of the anterior (A) leaflet and missing chordae tendineae *(arrow)*. *Bottom,* portion of the opened aortic valve and left ventricular outflow tract showing fibrous thickening of the mural endocardium (endocardial plaque). EP = endocardial plaque; VS = ventricular septum.

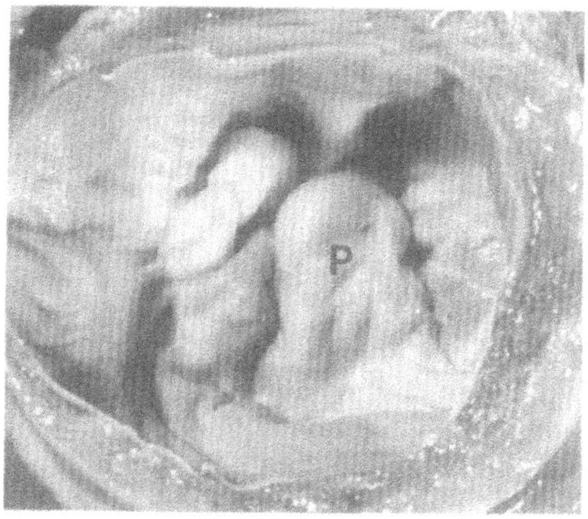

FIGURE 5. Intact mitral valve from left atrium of an 85-year-old woman (patient 10, SH #A87-18) who died of pneumonitis while taking tocainide for symptomatic ventricular tachycardia. Portions of the posterior (P) leaflet are prolapsed. A precordial murmur consistent with mitral regurgitation was audible. Echocardiogram on her last hospital admission did not show mitral prolapse but it did show mitral regurgitation.

jects of this study. They are among 384 patients aged 80 to 89 years at death studied at necropsy in this laboratory.

The following criteria were used to diagnose MVP: (1) the distance from the margin of attachment to distal margin of a portion of posterior mitral leaflet >1.5 cm; and (2) a portion of mitral leaflet protruding into left atrium, i.e., cephalad to the level of the mitral valve annulus.

Certain clinical and morphologic findings in the 12 patients are summarized in Table I and illustrated in Figures 1 to 6. The patients ranged in age from 80 to 88 years (mean 83); 6 were men and 6 were women. Signs and symptoms of congestive heart failure were present in 7 patients, and in 6 of the 7, MVP was the only reasonable cause of the failure. Although a murmur consistent with mitral regurgitation had been heard during life in 7 patients, MVP was diagnosed clinically in only 3 patients (2 by echocardiography during their last hospital admission and 1 at operation for acute severe mitral regurgitation). Death appeared to be related to the MVP in 4 patients (numbers 1, 4, 5 and 11, Table I). At necropsy, the left and right ventricular cavities were of normal size by gross inspection in 11 patients. The mural endocardium behind the posterior mitral leaflet was thickened by fibrous tissue in 2 patients. Calcium was present in the mitral annulus in 3 patients, but its quantity was only mild in each (1–2+/4+). Two patients had a probe-patent valvular-competent foramen ovale which in 1 was associated with redundancy of the fossa ovalis membrane, and 1 patient (number 11) had a secundum atrial septal defect.

Although 7 of the 12 patients in our study had mitral regurgitation by auscultation, and 7 were treated for congestive heart failure, MVP was diagnosed in life in only 3 patients. In all 3, the diagnosis was made during their last hospital admission. Death appeared to be related to the MVP in 4 of the 12 patients. Death was sudden and at home in 1 patient who never had any symptoms or signs of cardiac dysfunction during life, and in whom, except for MVP, no anatomic abnormalities were found at necropsy. Two patients died of congestive heart failure (patients 4 and 5), and a cause other than MVP was not apparent. Death in 1 patient resulted from complications of alpha Streptococcus endocarditis involving the prolapsed mitral valve. In addition to these 4 fatal cases, 2 other patients had congestive heart failure associated with mitral regurgitation. In the remaining 6 patients, MVP caused no cardiac dysfunction and was an incidental finding at necropsy.

This study indicates that MVP may be present in persons aged 80 to 89 years at death, and that the MVP in them may be asymptomatic or cause fatal or nonfatal symptoms of cardiac dysfunction.

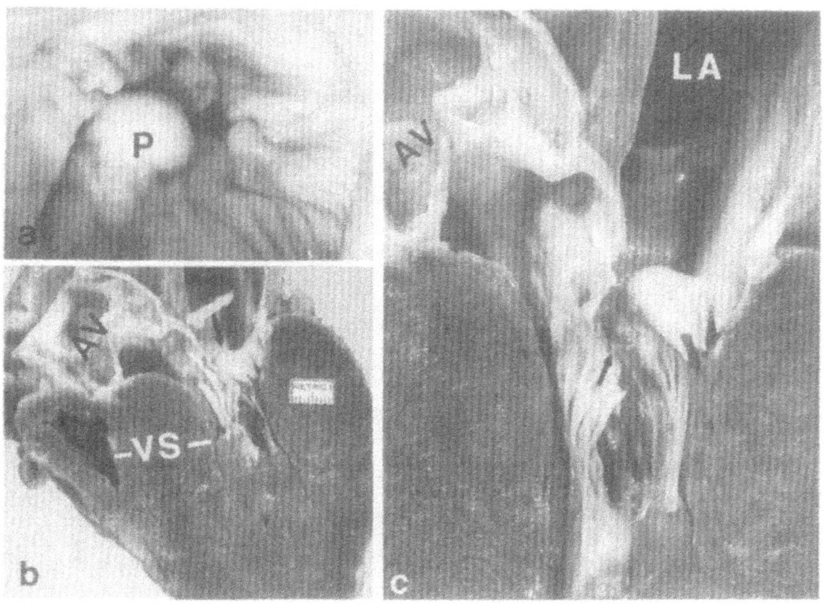

FIGURE 6. Heart of an 85-year-old woman (SH #A84-16) who died of complication of alpha Streptococcus endocarditis involving the prolapsed mitral valve. Mitral valve prolapse was not diagnosed during life. *a*, view of the intact mitral valve from the left atrium (LA) showing prolapse mainly of the posterior (P) leaflet. *b*, longitudinal section of the heart showing prolapsed *(arrow)* posterior mitral leaflet. The left ventricular cavity is small. *c*, close-up view of the mitral valve showing vegetation *(arrow)* on the posterior mitral leaflet. AV = aortic valve; VS = ventricular septum.

1. Savage DD, Garrison RJ, Devereux RB, Castelli WP, Anderson SJ, Levy D, McNamara PM, Stokes J, Kannel WB, Feinleib M. Mitral valve prolapse in the general population. I. Epidemiologic features: the Framingham study. *Am Heart J* 1983;106:571–576.

2. Dollar AL, Roberts WC. Morphologic comparison of patients with mitral valve prolapse who died suddenly with patients who died from severe valvular dysfunction or other conditions. *J Am Coll Cardiol* 1991;17:921–931.

3. Pomerance A. Balooning deformity (mucoid degeneration) of atrioventricular valves. *Br Heart J* 1969;31:343–351.

4. Davies MJ, Moore BP, Braimbridge MV. The floppy mitral valve. Study of incidence, pathology, and complications in surgical, necropsy, and forensic material. *Br Heart J* 1978;40:468–481.

Pure Mitral Regurgitation Associated with a Malfunctioning Congenitally Bicuspid Aortic Valve Necessitating Combined Mitral and Aortic Valve Replacement

Daniel J. Fernicola, MD,* and William C. Roberts, MD†

Some patients with clinically significant aortic valve dysfunction have associated pure mitral regurgitation (no element of mitral stenosis), but usually the mitral regurgitation is of minimal or mild degree. On occasion, however, the degree of pure mitral regurgitation associated with clinically significant aortic valve dysfunction is considerable (i.e., severe enough to result in associated mitral valve repair or replacement at the time of aortic valve replacement). In the present study, we sought to determine the etiology of pure mitral regurgitation in a group of patients who had aortic valve replacement because of a dysfunctioning congenitally bicuspid aortic valve and simultaneous mitral valve replacement because of associated mitral regurgitation.

From the Pathology Branch, National Heart, Lung, and Blood Institute, National Institutes of Health, Bethesda, Maryland. Manuscript received January 4, 1994; revised manuscript received and accepted March 21, 1994.

*Division of Cardiology, Department of Medicine, Georgetown University, Washington, D.C. 20058.
†Baylor Cardiovascular Institute, Baylor University Medical Center, 3500 Gaston Avenue, Dallas, Texas 75246.

The surgical files of the Pathology Branch, National Heart, Lung, and Blood Institute, were reviewed to identify patients who had simultaneous replacement of both native mitral and aortic valves. A total of 115 cases were identified. Of them, 103 patients (90%) had 3-cuspid aortic valves, and 12 (10%) had congenitally bicuspid aortic valves. Of the latter 12 patients, 1 had associated congenital mitral stenosis and was therefore excluded from this study.[1] The other 11 patients with congenitally bicuspid aortic valves had associated pure mitral regurgitation. The 11 operatively excised congenitally bicuspid aortic valves and the simultaneously excised mitral valves were retrieved and reexamined. Certain clinical and cardiac morphologic features in each of the 11 patients are tabulated in Table I and illustrated in Figures 1 to 8.

All 11 patients were men, aged 25 to 77 years (mean 56). Four (cases 1 to 4, Table I) had pure aortic regurgitation and their mean age was younger than that of the 7 patients (cases 5 to 11, Table I) with some degree of aortic valve stenosis (with or without associated aortic regurgitation) (45 vs 63 years). Of the 7 patients with aortic stenosis, 6 had cardiac catheterization, and their

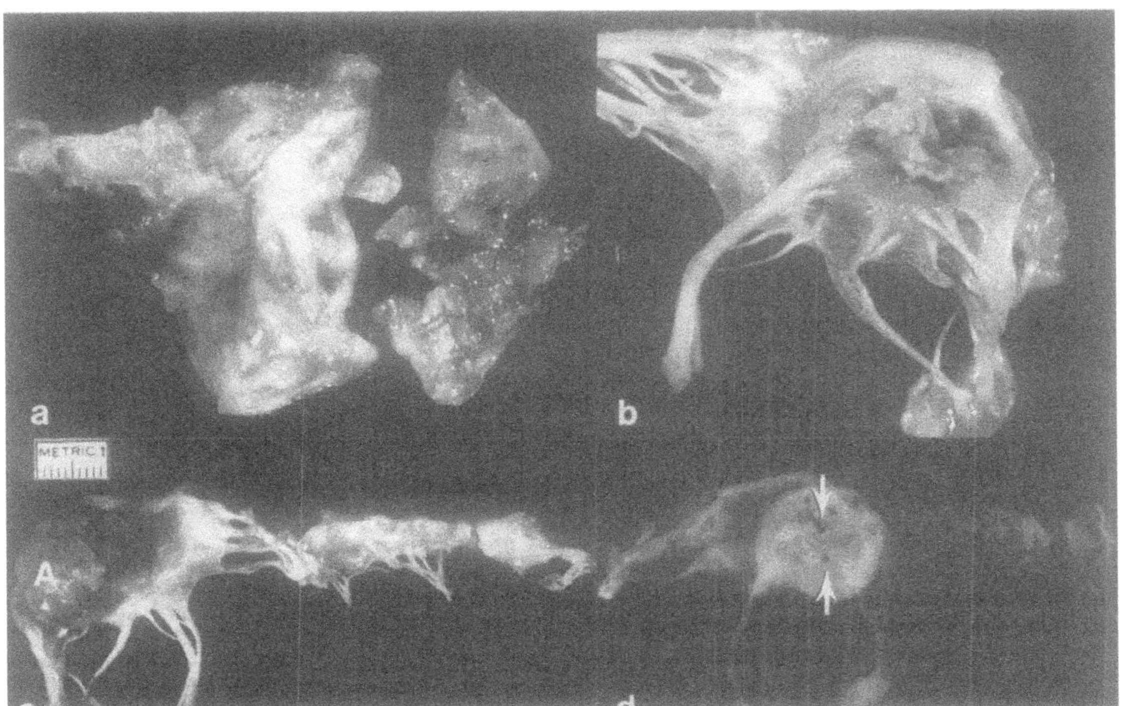

FIGURE 1. Patient 1. G. H. (GT #83-S-1910), a 25-year-old man, developed signs and symptoms of *Streptococcus bovis* endocarditis 4 months before valve replacement. Later he developed acute pulmonary edema due to severe aortic and mitral regurgitation. Both native left-sided cardiac valves were replaced with Carpentier-Edwards bioprostheses. *a*, excised aortic valve. Infective material is located on both cusps. *b*, ventricular aspect of anterior mitral leaflet. Infective material fills an aneurysm of the leaflet. *c*, opened mitral valve showing both leaflets. The large aneurysm (A) bulges toward the left atrium. *d*, radiograph of the mitral valve showing 2 perforations *(arrows)* in the aneurysm.

peak systolic pressure gradient ranged from 10 to 130 mm Hg (average 60). All 11 patients had pulmonary hypertension, with peak systolic pressures ranging from 37 to 90 mm Hg (average 64). Ten of the 11 patients had elevated mean pulmonary artery wedge pressures ranging from 24 to 35 mm Hg (average 29). The pulmonary artery V wave was >35 mm Hg in 7 of the 8 patients in whom this datum was available. The left ventricular angiogram in 8 patients indicated that the mitral regurgitation was 4+/4+ in 3, 3+/4+ in 3, and 2+/4+ in 2. In 4 patients with pure aortic regurgitation, aortic root angiogram indicated the regurgitation to be either 3+/4+ or 4+/4+. The left ventricular cavity was dilated, either by echocardiogram or left ventriculogram, in 9 of the 10 patients in whom either of these procedures

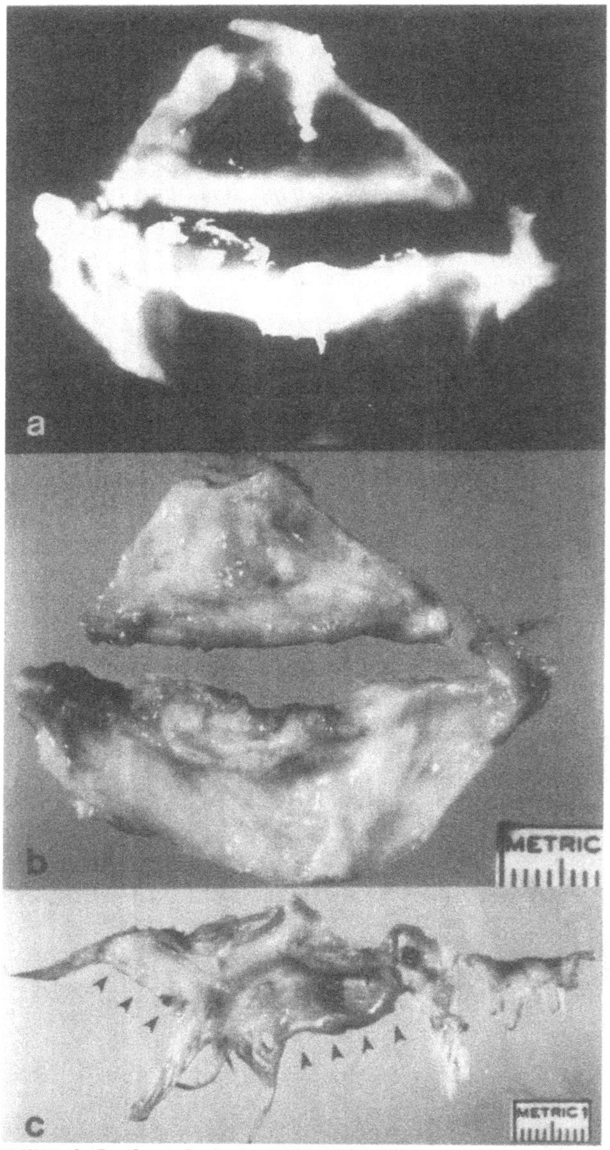

FIGURE 2. Patient 2. A. L. (NIH #S84-105), a 48-year-old man, had aortic regurgitation noted at age 38 years. He developed active infective endocarditis at age 44. A second episode of active infective endocarditis occurred 4 months before valve replacement. Within 3 months, the patient went from New York Heart Association functional class II to functional class IV. *a*, radiograph of the excised aortic valve showing small calcific deposits. *b*, excised aortic valve. The 2 cusps are of unequal size. *c*, excised mitral valve. Most chordae tendineae to the anterior mitral leaflet are ruptured (missing) *(arrowheads)*.

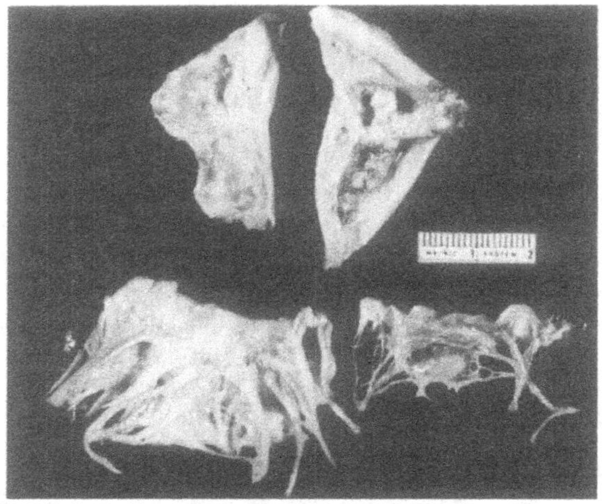

FIGURE 3. Patient 3. D. U. (NIH #S72-4111), a 51-year-old man, was first noted to have a precordial murmur at age 23 years. Symptoms began at age 50 years, approximately 1 year before valve replacement. The excised aortic valve *(top)* is diffusely thickened with a focal calcific deposit limited to the raphe. The excised mitral valve leaflets *(bottom)* are essentially normal.

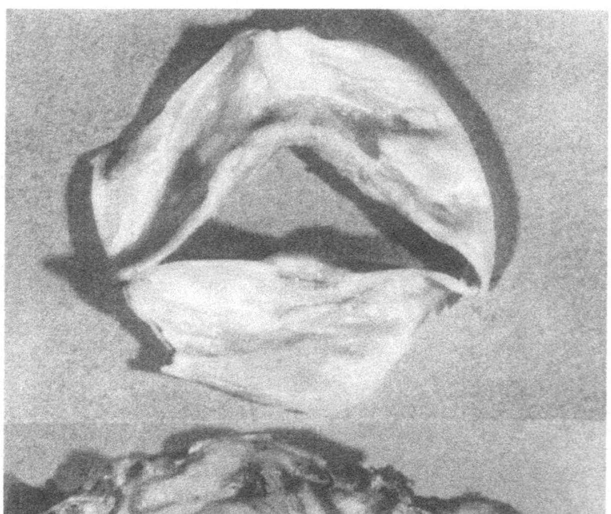

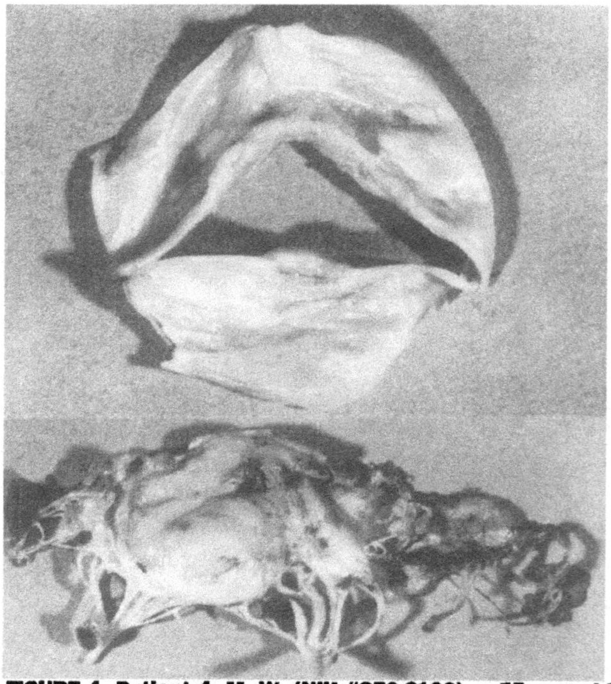

FIGURE 4. Patient 4. M. W. (NIH #S70-3100), a 55-year-old man, was noted to have a murmur of aortic regurgitation at the age of 47. The patient remained asymptomatic until 6 weeks before surgery when he developed acute pulmonary edema. The excised aortic valve *(top)* is mildly and diffusely fibrotic and purely regurgitant. The anterior leaflet of the mitral valve *(bottom)* is greatly thickened by fibrous tissue. The chordae tendineae to the anterior mitral leaflet are thickened by fibrous tissue and are very short. The commissure between the anterior and posterior leaflets is abnormal but not fused.

TABLE I Clinical and Morphologic Features of 11 Men with a Malfunctioning Bicuspid Aortic Valve and Associated Pure Mitral Regurgitation and Operative Excision of Both Valves

Case No.	Age at operation (years)	Interval (days) CC to VR	Pressures (mm Hg) RV (s/d)	PA (s/d)	PAW Mean	PAW V Wave	LV (s/d)	SA (s/d)	LV-SA psg	Angiogram MR (1+–4+)	Angiogram AR (1+–4+)	No. CA >50%
1	25	1	—	50/20	25	—	120/30	120/60	0	2+	4+	—
2	48	30	50/12	45/24	29	41	100/35	110/45	0	3+	4+	0
3	51	4	80/10	80/35	30	65	125/22	125/55	0	3+	3+	—
4	55	21	65/10	65/25	25	65	120/24	120/55	0	4+	4+	—
5	52	30	56/10	55/30	30	36	120/25	110/65	10	2+**	2+	0
6	54	5	70/11	70/30	30	—	220/30	110/60	100	—	—	—
7	56	—	38/11	37/15	24	—	145/10	95/65	50	4+	0	0
8	58	4	—	70/25	35	45	—	118/50	—	—	—	1
9	71	14	90/4	90/40	35	38	210/20	90/60	130	—	—	0
10	71	—	80/15	80/25	10	16	140/16	100/70	40	4+	0	0
11	77	18	44/12	44/19	25	41	126/12	99/57	27	3+	—	3§§

Case No.	Cavity Size (mm) by Echocardiogram LV_s	LV_d	LA	Year of VR	Prosthesis in AV Position Type	Size	Prosthesis in MV Position Type	Size	Calcium (0–4+) AV	MV	BA-DM Length (cm) AML	PML	Etiology of MR IE	MVP	Ruptured MV CT
1	—		—	1983	CE	25	CE	29	0	0	1.4	0.7	+ (A)	0	0
2	51	75	45	1984	SE	24A*	SE	30M†	1+	0	2	—	+ (H)	0	+
3	—‡		—	1972	SE	27A§	SE	32M‖	1+	0	2	1.5	0	0	0
4	—‡		—	1970	SE	26A¶	SE	30M†	0	1+	2.5	1.0	+ (H)	0	0
5	60	65	53	1986	SE	24A*	SE	30M†	3+	1+	1.4	—	0††	0††	0††
6	—		33	1979	Ha	21	Ha	31	4+	0	2.2	1.7	0	0	0††
7	42	61	63	1989	SJM	21	SJM	29	2+	1+	1.8	—	+ (H)††	0††	0
8	62	69	56	1980	SE	24A*	SE	32M‖	3+	0	2.0	1.0	0	0	0
9	60	70	56	1983	Ha	21	Ha	29	4+	0	2.2	1.0	+ (H)	0	+
10	34	52	58	1991	MH	25	MH	31	3+	1+	2	2	0	+	+
11	—	58	40	1992	CE	23	CE	31	2+	1+	2	—	0	0	0

*Old terminology is 10A.
†Old terminology is 3M.
‡Left ventricle very large by left ventricular angiogram.
§Old terminology is 12A.
‖Old terminology is 4M.
¶Old terminology is 11A.
**No mitral regurgitation, however, by Doppler echocardiogram.
††Only the anterior mitral leaflet excised at operation.
§§Coronary artery bypass surgery performed at time of valve replacement.
A = active; AML = anterior mitral leaflet; AR = aortic regurgitation (by aortic root cineangiogram); AV = aortic valve; BA = basal attachment; CA = coronary artery; CC = cardiac catheterization; CE = Carpentier-Edwards bioprosthesis; CT = chordae tendineae; DM = distal margin; H = healed; Ha = Hancock bioprosthesis; IE = infective endocarditis; LA = left atrium; LV = left ventricle; LV_s = left ventricular (cavity size in systole); LV_d = left ventricular (cavity size in diastole); MH = Medtronic-Hall mechanical prosthesis; MR = mitral regurgitation (by left ventriculogram); MV = mitral valve; MVP = mitral valve prolapse; PA = pulmonary artery; PAW = pulmonary artery wedge; PML = posterior mitral leaflet; psg = peak systolic gradient; RV = right ventricle; SA = systemic artery; SE = Starr-Edwards mechanical prosthesis; s/d = peak systole/end-diastole; SJM = Saint Jude mechanical prosthesis; VR = valve replacement.

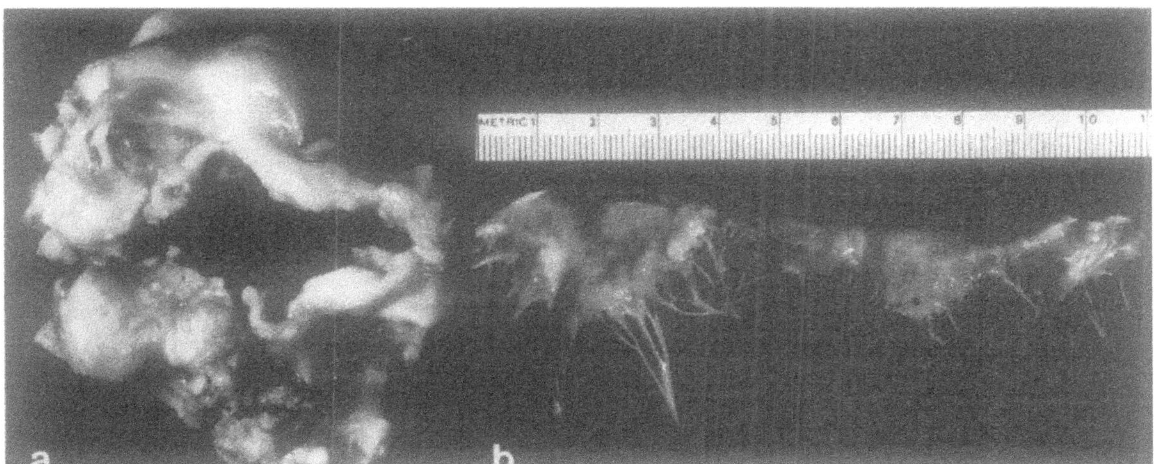

FIGURE 5. Patient 6. B. O. (NIH #S79-142) was a 54-year-old man in whom a precordial murmur was noted at age 43 years. At age 51, the peak systolic pressure gradient between left ventricle and aorta was 65 mm Hg. Over the next 2 years, congestive heart failure progressed. At the time of valve replacement, the peak systolic gradient across the aortic valve was 100 mm Hg. The patient died 12 days after operation from sepsis. *a*, excised heavily calcified aortic valve. *b*, opened mitral valve. Some segments of the posterior mitral leaflet are elongated.

was performed; the 1 patient (case 1, Table I) without cavity dilation had aortic regurgitation secondary to active infective endocarditis of short duration. The 1 patient who did not have either an echocardiogram or a left ventriculogram had an ejection fraction of 20%, and chest radiogram showed a large cardiac silhouette.

Infective endocarditis, either active (case 1) or healed (cases 2, 4, 7, and 9), was the etiology of the mitral regurgitation in 5 patients (45%). In 2 of the 4 patients with healed infective endocarditis, several chordae tendineae in each had ruptured (Figures 2 and 7). In the other 2 patients the diagnosis of infective endocarditis was made by a history of positive blood cultures. In 1 patient (case 4) the excised anterior mitral leaflet was diffusely thickened by fibrous tissue without calcific deposits, the attached chordae tendineae were thickened and short, and the posterior mitral leaflet was smaller than expected. The etiology of this distorted anatomy is uncertain, but infective endocarditis that healed and was not diagnosed clinically may have caused the local fibrous thickening. In 1 patient mitral valve prolapse was present and some chordae tendineae from the posterior mitral leaflet had ruptured. In 4 patients the excised mitral leaflets and chordae tendineae were anatomically normal, but the left ventricular cavities were very dilated.

In the 4 patients with purely regurgitant aortic valves, calcific deposits, determined by x-ray of the excised valves, were either absent or minute. In each of the 7 stenotic aortic valves, large calcific deposits were present. Of the 11 excised mitral valves, 5 had minute calcific deposits, confined to the annular region in 4.

Although most persons with a congenitally bicuspid aortic valve have a normally functioning mitral valve, the present study indicates that associated mitral regurgitation not only may occur, but also may be severe enough to warrant mitral valve replacement at the time of aortic valve replacement. It is well appreciated that the congenitally bicuspid aortic valve has a high propensity to be the site of infective endocarditis.[1–12] Furthermore, when active endocarditis of the aortic valve leads to aortic regurgitation, vegetations on the aortic valve may be dislodged retrogradely by the regurgitant jet and the vegetations may adhere to mitral chordae tendineae causing their rupture, or to the anterior mitral leaflet causing it to perforate or to become aneurysmal. The latter scenario appears to have been responsible for the mitral regurgitation in 5, and possibly 6, of the 11 patients in the present study.

Mitral valve prolapse without superimposed infective endocarditis was responsible for the mitral regurgitation

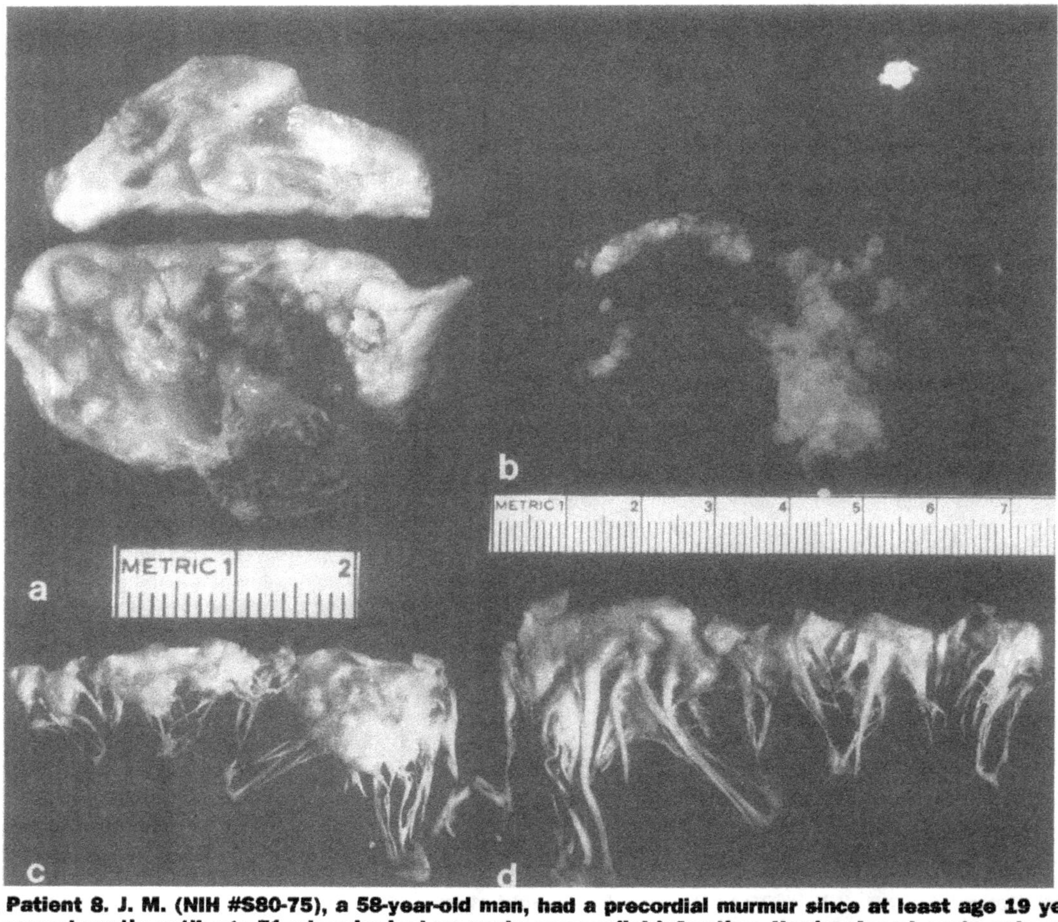

FIGURE 6. Patient 8. J. M. (NIH #S80-75), a 58-year-old man, had a precordial murmur since at least age 19 years. He remained asymptomatic until age 51 when he had an acute myocardial infarction. He developed acute pulmonary edema 2 weeks before valve replacement. *a,* excised aortic valve. *b,* radiograph of the aortic valve. The cusps are of different sizes and calcium is virtually limited to the largest cusp. *c and d,* excised mitral valve. Atrial *(c)* and ventricular *(d)* views of the excised mitral leaflets. Both leaflets are moderately thickened. Portions of the posterior leaflet are elongated.

in only 1 patient.[13–16] It is surprising that mitral valve prolapse (unassociated with infective endocarditis) is not seen more often in patients with congenitally bicuspid aortic valves, because mitral valve prolapse may occur in as many as 5% of the adult population, and the bicuspid aortic valve in as many as 1% of the population.[17] In 4 patients, the mitral leaflets and chordae tendineae were normal but the mitral annulae were quite dilated. Today, these latter 4 patients would probably have had mitral annuloplasty rather than replacement.

Although all 11 patients had pure mitral regurgitation, the type of aortic valve dysfunction was variable. Four patients had pure aortic regurgitation, in 3 due to superimposed infective endocarditis or at least worsened by the endocarditis, and in 1 patient due entirely to the bicuspid condition of the valve. Seven patients had stenotic aortic valves. Of the 4 purely regurgitant aortic valves, 3 had superimposed infective endocarditis; of the 7 stenotic aortic valves, 2 had superimposed infective endocarditis.

In summary, some patients with severely dysfunctioning congenitally bicuspid aortic valves develop pure mitral regurgitation severe enough to warrant mitral valve replacement or repair. The most common cause of the associated mitral regurgitation is leaflet and chordal damage from infective endocarditis.

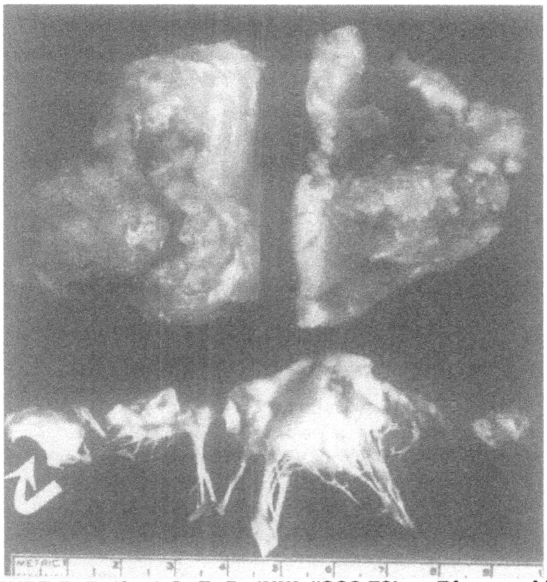

FIGURE 7. Patient 9. E. P. (NIH #S83-56), a 71-year-old man who developed congestive heart failure 9 months before valve replacement. Four months before valve replacement, he was treated with ampicillin for bronchitis. *Top,* excised aortic valve showing heavy calcific deposits. *Bottom,* excised mitral valve. A portion of posterior leaflet is indented *(arrow)* with missing chordae tendineae at this site. These latter findings are consistent with healed infective endocarditis.

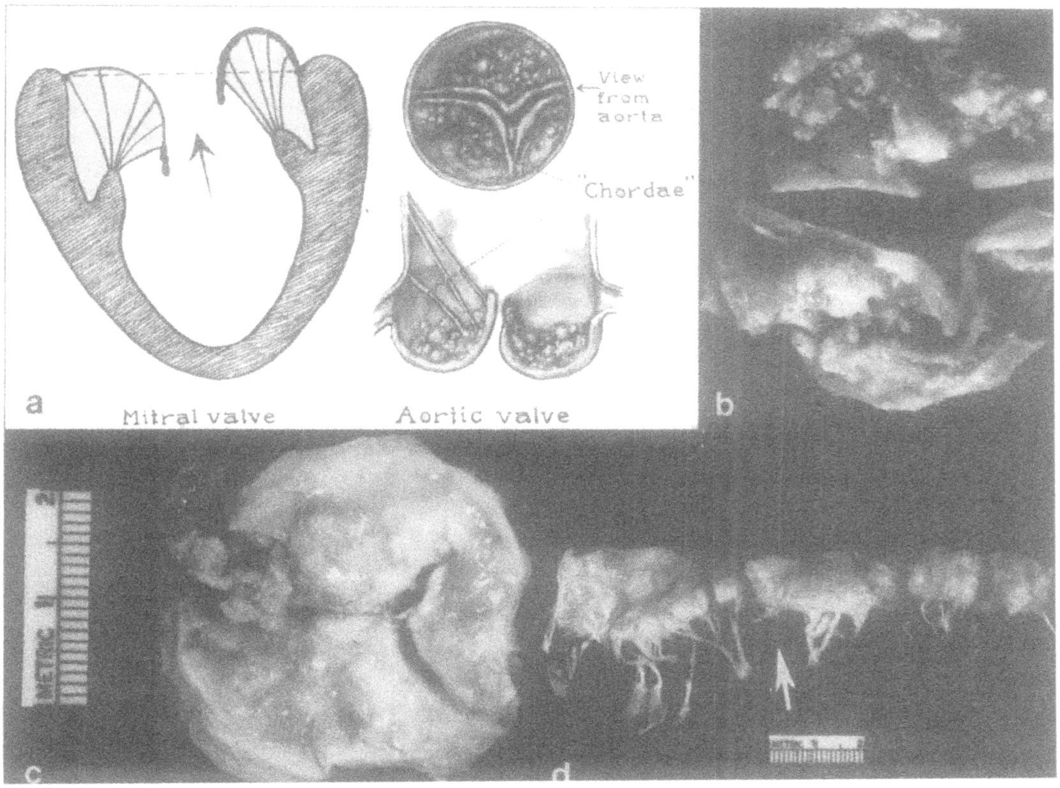

FIGURE 8. Patient 10. A. S. (GT #91S-6903), a 71-year-old man, developed acute pulmonary edema and severe mitral regurgitation 2 weeks before valve replacement. The patient had been in New York Heart Association functional class II before the development of severe mitral regurgitation. *a,* illustration of the mitral and aortic valves as they probably appeared in life. "Chordae" were present from the raphe of the aortic valve cusps to the wall of the aorta. *b,* excised aortic valve from the aortic aspect. *c,* aortic valve from the ventricular side. *d,* excised mitral valve showing "missing" chordae tendineae *(arrows).* An adjacent portion of posterior leaflet is hooded.

1. Roberts WC. The congenitally bicuspid aortic valve. A study of 85 autopsy cases. *Am J Cardiol* 1970;26:72–83.
2. Arnett EN, Roberts WC. Valve ring abscess in active infective endocarditis. Frequency, location, and clues to clinical diagnosis from the study of 95 necropsy patients. *Circulation* 1976;54:140–145.
3. Arnett EN, Roberts WC. Prosthetic valve endocarditis. Clinicopathologic analysis of 22 necropsy patients with comparison of observations in 74 necropsy patients with active infective endocarditis involving natural left-sided cardiac valves. *Am J Cardiol* 1976;38:281–292.
4. Arnett EN, Roberts WC. Active infective endocarditis: a clinicopathology analysis of 137 necropsy patients. *Curr Probl Cardiol* 1976;1:1–76.
5. Roberts WC, Buchbinger NA. Healed left-sided infective endocarditis: a clinicopathologic study of 59 patients. *Am J Cardiol* 1977:72:757–761.
6. Roberts WC, Morrow AG, McIntosh CL, Jones M, Epstein SE. Congenitally bicuspid aortic valve causing severe, pure aortic regurgitation without superimposed infective endocarditis. Analysis of 13 patients requiring aortic valve replacement. *Am J Cardiol* 1981;47:206–209.
7. Roberts WC, McIntosh CL, Wallace RB. Aortic valve perforation with calcific aortic valve stenosis and without infective endocarditis or significant aortic regurgitation. *Am J Cardiol* 1987;59:476–478.
8. Dressler FA, Roberts WC. Infective endocarditis in opiate addicts: analysis of 80 cases studied at necropsy. *Am J Cardiol* 1989;63:1240–1257.
9. Roberts WC. Living with a congenitally bicuspid aortic valve. *Am J Cardiol* 1989;64:1408–1409.
10. Brown PS Jr, Roberts CS, McIntosh CL, Roberts WC, Clark RE. Combined obstructive hypertrophic cardiomyopathy and stenotic congenitally bicuspid aortic valve. *Am J Cardiol* 1990;66:1273–1275.
11. Roberts WC. Morphologic aspects of cardiac valve dysfunction. *Am Heart J* 1992:123:1610–1632.
12. Roberts WC, Oluwole BO, Fernicola DJ. Comparison of active infective endocarditis involving a previously stenotic versus a previously nonstenotic aortic valve. *Am J Cardiol* 1993;71:1082–1088.
13. Rippe JM, Slors LJ, Angoff G, Alpert JS. Mitral valve prolapse in adults with congenital heart disease. *Am Heart J* 1979;97:561–573.
14. Chisholm JC. Mitral valve prolapse syndrome associated with congenital bicuspid aortic valve. *JAMA* 1981;73:921–923.
15. Roberts WC, McIntosh CL, Wallace RB. Mechanisms of severe mitral regurgitation in mitral valve prolapse determined from analysis of operatively excised valves. *Am Heart J* 1987;113:1316–1323.
16. Dollar AL, Roberts WC. Morphologic comparison of patients with mitral valve prolapse who died suddenly with patients who died from severe valvular dysfunction or other conditions. *J Am Coll Cardiol* 1991;17:921–931.
17. Roberts WC. The 2 most common congenital heart diseases. *Am J Cardiol* 1984;53:1198.

Late (≥6 Years) Results of Combined Coronary Artery Bypass Grafting and Mitral Valve Replacement for Severe Mitral Regurgitation Secondary to Acute Myocardial Infarction

Kevin Paul Theleman, MD, Phillip James Stephan, MD, Michael G. Isaacs, MD, Robert F. Hebeler, Jr., MD, A. Carl Henry III, MD, and William Clifford Roberts, MD

Analysis of outcomes in 31 patients who had combined mitral valve replacement (MVR) and coronary artery bypass grafting (CABG) for ischemic mitral regurgitation (MR) disclosed that 12 patients had MR because of papillary muscle rupture and that 19 patients had MR because of papillary muscle necrosis or fibrosis without rupture. Of the 12 patients with rupture, 6 died within 2 months of operation and the other 6 lived ≥6 years postoperatively; of the 19 patients without rupture, none died within 2 months of operation and 11 (58%) lived at least 6 years.

(Am J Cardiol 2003;92:1086–1090)

From the Departments of Internal Medicine (Cardiology), Cardiothoracic Surgery, and Pathology, and the Baylor Heart and Vascular Institute, Baylor University Medical Center; and Department of Surgery, Parkland Hospital, Southwestern Medical School, Dallas, Texas. Dr. Roberts' address is: Baylor Heart & Vascular Institute, Baylor University Medical Center, 3500 Gaston Avenue, Dallas, Texas 75246. E-mail: wc.roberts@baylorhealth.edu. Manuscript received June 11, 2003; revised manuscript received and accepted July 29, 2003.

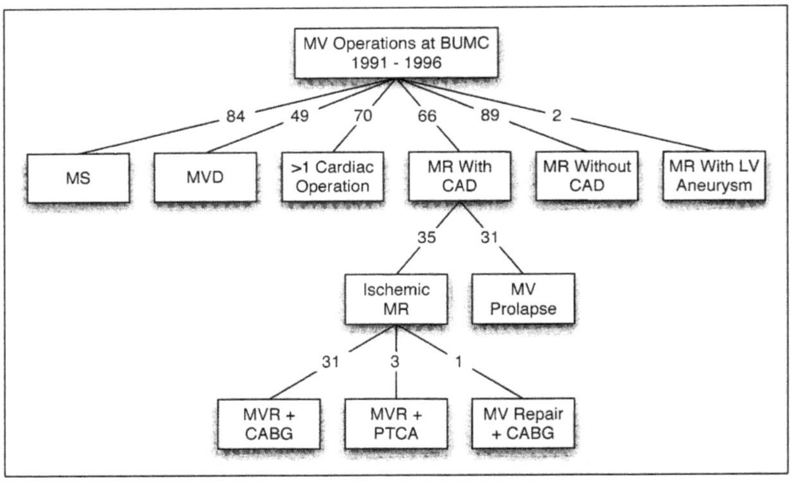

FIGURE 1. Diagram showing origin of the 31 patients with ischemic MR and combined MVR and CABG. BUMC = Baylor University Medical Center; CAD = coronary artery disease; LV = left ventricular; MS = mitral stenosis; MV = mitral valve; MVD = multivalvular disease; PTCA = percutaneous coronary angioplasty.

Mitral regurgitation (MR) is a major complication of acute myocardial infarction (AMI). When MR is severe, mitral valve replacement (MVR) or repair has proved beneficial, whether or not the mitral valve operation was performed during the period of AMI or after healing of the AMI. This report analyzes findings in 31 patients with MVR for severe MR that occurred during or after AMI with simultaneous coronary artery bypass grafting (CABG).

• • •

The names and numbers of patients who underwent mitral valve operations from January 1, 1991, to October 1, 1996, were obtained from a computer registry from the Department of Cardiovascular Surgery, Baylor University Medical Center. A total of 360 patients were found to have had mitral valve operations during this 69-month period, and the medical records of all 360 patients were reviewed to find those who had MVR because of ischemic MR and who underwent simultaneous CABG (Figure 1). Of the 360 patients, 329 were eliminated from further analysis for the following reasons: 84 had mitral stenosis; 89 had pure MR without angiographic evidence for coronary arterial narrowing; 70 had undergone a previous cardiac operation; 49 had ≥1 cardiac valves replaced in addition to the mitral valve; 2 had MVR associated with a left ventricular aneurysm; 31 had both MVR and CABG but the cause of MR was mitral valve prolapse; 3 had MVR and angioplasty rather than CABG; and 1 had mitral valve repair rather than MVR in addition to CABG. The remaining 31 patients had MVR and simultaneous CABG. This report focuses exclusively on these 31 patients.

The medical records, electrocardiographic, angiographic, operative, and morphologic (pathologic) reports were reviewed in detail in these 31 patients. The 31 patients included in this study were operated on by 12 different surgeons: 1 (ACH III) operated on 9 patients (29%); 1 (RFH) operated on 7 patients (23%); 5 different surgeons each operated on 2 patients; and 5 other surgeons each operated on 1 patient. Seventeen of the operatively excised valves were examined by WCR. In the remaining 14 valves, the status of the excised valves was determined from operative and pathologic reports. Of the 12 patients with ruptured papillary muscles, anterior and posterior leaflets were excised in 3 and only the anterior leaflet in the other 9; in the 19 patients without ruptured papillary muscles only the anterior leaflet was excised.

The Social Security Death Index (SSDI) was searched to learn how many of the 31 patients had died after hospital admission when the MVR and CABG had been performed. Each of the remaining patients whose names did not appear in the SSDI was contacted by telephone to determine their clinical status.

Pertinent findings in each of the 31 patients are provided in Table 1. The patients ranged in age at the time of MVR + CABG from 54 to 83 years (mean 69). AMI involved the anterior wall in 5 patients and the posterior (inferior) wall in 26 patients. All 31 patients were in New York Heart Association functional class III or IV just before MVR and CABG. The mean ejection fraction in the 31 patients was 49%. Ten patients (32%) were in shock preoperatively and 20 patients (64%) had intra-aortic balloon pumps inserted preoperatively. All 31 patients were followed at least 6 years, and 11 patients for at least 10 years. Twenty-six patients (83%) lived >30 days after combined MVR and CABG, 21 patients (65%) lived at least 1 year, and 18 patients (57%) lived at least 5 years. Of the 11 patients followed 10 years postoperatively, 4 (36%) are still alive. Survival in the 31 patients is graphically presented in Figure 2.

Twelve (39%) patients at operation had rupture of a portion of the left ventricular papillary muscle (Figure 3), and in each, the rupture was in the posteromedial papillary muscle (Table 1). In each, the electrocardiogram had indicated that the AMI involved the posterior wall. The interval from onset of AMI to MVR operation in 9 of these 12 patients ranged from 2 to 20 days (mean 7, median 4). The intervals from AMI to operation in the other 3 patients are unknown in 2 patients and was 6 months in the remaining patient. The left ventricular ejection fraction (from left ventriculography) was ≥45% in all 12 patients. Left ventricular cineangiography revealed 4+/4+ MR in 11 patients and 3+/4+ MR in the remaining patient. The left ventricular cavity in 6 patients was of normal size and was minimally dilated in another. Before operation, 9 of the 12 patients were in cardiogenic shock and each had an intra-aortic balloon pump inserted preoperatively. One additional patient also had an intra-aortic balloon pump inserted at operation.

TABLE 1 Observations in Each of the 31 Patients Who Underwent Coronary Artery Bypass Grafting (CABG) and Mitral Valve Replacement (MVR) for Pure Mitral Regurgitation (MR) Secondary to Myocardial Infarction

Case	Age (yr)/Sex	PMR	AMI Location	Interval (d) AMI to MVR	SH	DM	Pressures (mm Hg) LV (s/d)	SA (s/d)	PA (s/d)	PAW (mean)	EF (%)	MR by LV Cine (0 to 4+)	LV Dilated (0 to 4+)	Shock	IABP before MVR	No. CA >50%	No. CA A	Valve Inserted (size)	Interval (d) CC to MVR	Years Lived PO if Alive	Years Lived PO if Dead
1	59 M	+	Posterior	20	0	+	137/17	130/75	66/15	43	80	4+	0	0	0	2	1	SJM (29)	2	6	—
2	63 M	+	Posterior	4	0	+	73/0	77/55	37/24	19	46	4+	0	+	+	3	3	SJM (31)	1	—	7.4
3	63 M	+	Posterior	—	+	+	—	147/81	85/37	36	55	4+	3	0	+	3	4	SJM (27)	2	—	0.1
4	64 M	+	Posterior	4	0	0	100/21	93/68	33/18	15	64	4+	0	+	+	2	2	SJM (31)	2	9.6	—
5	64 F	+	Posterior	3	0	0	76/21	78/62	56/39	38	54	4+	0	+	+	1	1	SJM (27)	2	8.8	—
6	66 M	+	Posterior	8	+	0	78/28	77/62	60/34	42	64	4+	0	+	+	3	3	HPX (29)	7	—	0.2
7	66 F	+	Posterior	7	+	0	100/27	112/74	68/38	31	45	4+	4	+	+	1	1	SJM (25)	1	—	0.1
8	69 M	+	Posterior	11	0	0	76/17	83/47	44/21	22	49	4+	—	+	+	3	5	CE (27)	3	—	0.1
9	70 M	+	Posterior	—	+	0	115/17	97/63	47/22	25	50	3+	3	+	+	3	2	SJM (29)	3	—	0.1
10	71 F	+	Posterior	180	+	0	128/19	131/72	61/20	22	47	4+	4	0	0	3	4	CE (27)	1	—	11.3
11	79 M	+	Posterior	2	+	0	108/23	107/59	56/18	20	70	4+	0	+	+	3	5	HPX (29)	1	—	9.7
12	81 M	+	Posterior	2	0	0	62/9	62/45	50/16	20	50	4+	1	+	+	3	2	CE (31)	1	—	0.1
Subtotals	68 25%F	12	100% Posterior	24	6	3	96/18	100/64	55/25	28	56	3.9	1.4	9	10	2.5	2.8	7 mechanical	2.1	8.8 (3 alive)	3.2 (9 dead)
13	54 M	0	Posterior	720	0	0	—	128/80	21/10	—	55	4+	—	0	0	3	3	SJM (29)	—	9.3	—
14	54 F	0	Anterior	—	+	+	110/14	111/57	—	—	30	4+	1	0	+	3	3	SJM (27)	2	7.5	—
15	58 M	0	Posterior	60	+	0	101/12	101/58	49/17	22	49	3+	0	0	0	1	1	SJM (33)	30	10.3	—
16	63 F	0	Posterior	1710	0	+	132/28	131/71	63/7	37	41	4+	4	0	0	3	3	SJM (27)	11	—	10.8
17	64 M	0	Posterior	30	0	0	—	96/56	33/12	12	25	4+	1	0	+	3	3	CE (29)	1	10.4	—
18	64 M	0	Posterior	2	0	0	137/37	142/83	92/44	36	40	4+	2	0	+	3	3	SJM (31)	1	—	0.3
19	65 F	0	Posterior	—	+	0	101/20	99/49	40/19	26	50	4+	2	0	+	3	2	SJM (27)	1	—	7
20	66 M	0	Posterior	720	0	0	127/13	121/54	—	—	45	3+	0	0	0	3	5	HPX (29)	3	—	1.6
21	69 M	0	Posterior	360	0	0	142/19	143/83	37/16	18	45	4+	0	0	+	3	4	HPX (29)	1	9.6	—
22	70 M	0	Anterior	60	+	+	123/27	136/78	58/31	34	57	4+	2	0	+	3	4	SJM (29)	8	—	6.1
23	73 F	0	Anterior	1800	+	+	93/22	110/60	51/18	28	44	4+	1	0	+	3	3	CE (29)	5	—	0.7
24	73 F	0	Anterior	270	0	0	142/22	148/99	78/30	25	40	4+	4	0	+	2	1	SJM (29)	4	7.1	—
25	74 F	0	Anterior	1800	0	0	155/23	159/80	68/29	26	36	4+	3	0	0	3	3	CE (27)	3	9.7	—
26	76 F	0	Posterior	7	+	0	150/29	166/66	61/29	28	54	4+	0	0	+	3	3	HPX (25)	1	—	5.6
27	77 M	0	Posterior	12	+	+	197/24	198/98	—	—	51	4+	0	0	0	3	4	HPX (29)	11	—	4.6
28	77 F	0	Posterior	—	+	+	130/18	140/50	—	—	60	4+	—	0	+	3	3	SJM (27)	—	7.3	—
29	81 M	0	Posterior	13	+	↓	113/19	114/55	40/16	25	55	4+	1	0	0	3	4	CE (29)	3	—	0.3
30	81 F	0	Posterior	720	0	0	152/15	147/69	—	—	44	3+	3	0	0	2	1	CE (25)	28	—	2.6
31	83 F	0	Posterior	15	0	+	86/14	82/35	33/17	18	49	4+	0	+	0	3	1	CE (27)	13	—	0.9
Subtotals	70 53% F	19	74% Posterior	519	9	8	129/21	130/67	51/21	26	46	3.9	1.4	1	10	2.8	2.8	9 Mechanical	7.4	8.9 (8 alive)	4 (11 dead)
Totals	69 42% F	39% Rupture	84% Posterior	328	15	11	116/20	118/66	53/23	27	50	3.9	1.4	10	20	2.7	2.8	16 Mechanical	5.2	9.7 (11 Alive)	3.5 (20 dead)

A = anastamoses; AMI = acute myocardial infarction; CC = cardiac catheterization; CA = coronary artery; CE = Carpentier-Edwards bioprosthesis; Cine = cineography; DM = diabetes mellitus; EF = ejection fraction; HPX = Hancock porcine xenograft; bioprothesis; IABP = intra-aortic balloon pump; LV = left ventricle; MR = mitral regurgitation; MVR = mitral valve replacement; PA = pulmonary artery; PAW = pulmonary artery wedge pressure; PMR = papillary muscle rupture; PO = postoperative; SA = systemic artery; SH = systemic hypertension; SJM = St. Jude Medical prothesis; s/d = peak systole/end diastole; + = present or positive; 0 = absent or negative; — = no information available or not applicable; ↓ = narrowed in luminal diameter.

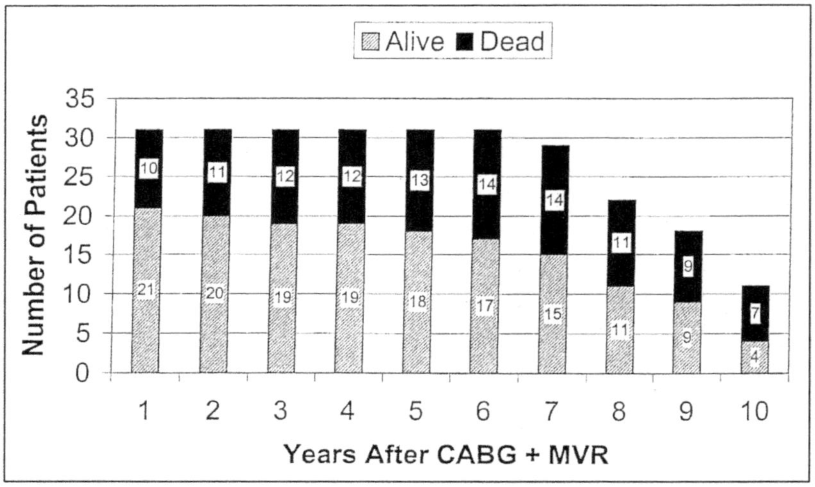

FIGURE 2. Survival in patients with combined CABG and MVR for severe MR secondary to myocardial infarction (n = 31). The column height represents the total number patients. The *striped portion* of the column represents the number of patients who are alive. The *black portion* of the column represents the number of patients who have died. All 31 patients were followed at least 6 years. Nineteen patients were followed at least 7 years, 22 were followed at least 8 years, 18 were followed at least 9 years, and 11 were followed at least 10 years.

Mechanical mitral valve prostheses were placed in 7 patients and bioprostheses were placed in the other 5 patients. Of these 12 patients, 5 patients died within 30 days of operation and another died within 60 days of operation. The other 6 all lived at least 7 years postoperatively.

Nineteen of the 31 patients had severe MR due to papillary muscle necrosis or fibrosis rather than papillary muscle rupture (Figure 4 and Table 1). The location of the myocardial infarct by electrocardiogram was posterior in 14 patients (74%) and anterior in 5 patients (26%). The interval from the onset of AMI to operation in 16 of the 19 patients ranged from 2 days to 5 years (mean 1.6 years, median 270 days). The mean left ventricular ejection fraction was 46%. All but 3 patients had left ventricular ejection fractions ≥40%. Four of the 19 patients (21%) had 3 or 4+ left ventricular cavity dilatation, 7 (37%) had 1 or 2+ left ventricular cavity dilatation, and 8 (42%) had no left ventricular cavity dilatation. Left ventricular cineography revealed 4+ MR in 16 patients and 3+ in 3 patients. One patient was in cardiogenic shock before operation and 10 had an intra-aortic balloon pump inserted preoperatively. Of these 19 patients, none died within 60 days of MVR; 2 died within 6 months and another 2 died within 1 year. Mechanical mitral valve prostheses were placed in 9 patients and bioprostheses were placed in the other 10 patients. Eleven patients (57%) have died since operation with a mean survival of 4.0 years. Eight patients (43%) are still alive with a mean survival of 8.9 years.

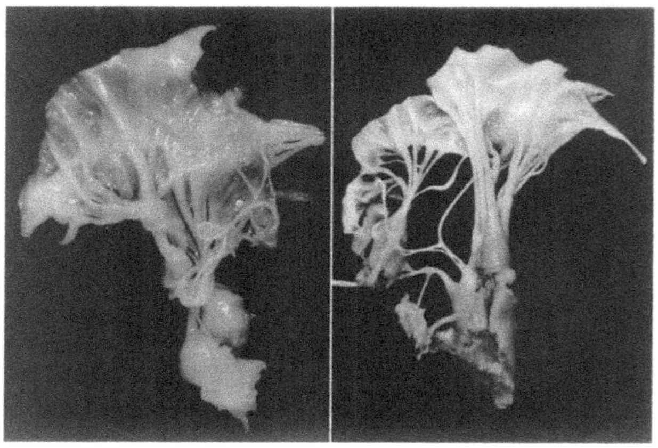

FIGURE 3. Photographs of the operatively-excised mitral valves in patient 1 *(left)* and in patient 8 *(right)*, respectively (Table 1). In both patients the posteromedial papillary muscle is ruptured. In patient 1, the chordae have twisted around the ruptured muscle.

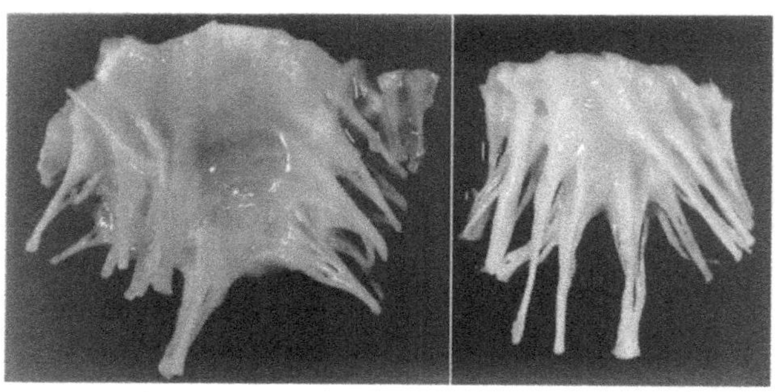

FIGURE 4. Photographs of anterior mitral leaflets excised in patients 14 *(left)* and 26 *(right)*, respectively (Table 1). Papillary muscle was not operatively excised in any of the 19 patients without papillary muscle rupture. Both leaflets have mildly thickened chordae, but otherwise are normal.

• • •

This analysis of 31 patients who had combined CABG and MVR for ischemic MR disclosed that the long-term outcome was good. Of the 26 patients who survived the early operative period, 17 (65%) lived >6 years postoperatively, and of the total group of 31 patients, 55% lived >6 years. Of the 18 patients followed at least 8 years, 9 (50%) are still alive. The 12 patients who had ruptured papillary muscles as the cause of the MR did not have as favorable an outcome as the 19 patients who had necrosis or fibrosis of a papillary muscle as the cause of the MR. Of the 12 patients with a ruptured papillary muscle, 6 died within 60 days of the operation; the other 6 lived >7 years. Of the 19 patients with papillary muscle dysfunction without rupture, none died within 60 days of the operation; 10 lived >6 years, and all but 2 of them are alive >7 years after operation.

Previous reports of combined MVR and CABG for ischemic MR with follow-up of ≥5 years are summarized in Table 2. Of the 401 patients analyzed in these 5 reports, 336 patients (84%) survived the early oper-

TABLE 2 Previously Reported Studies of Coronary Artery Bypass Grafting and Mitral Valve Replacement for Pure Mitral Regurgitation Secondary to Myocardial Infarction

First Author	Year of Publication	No. of Cases	Mean Age (years)	Female	AMI Within 30 Days	MR 3+ or 4+	EF (%)	IABP before MVR	CABG @ MVR	Mean No. CA A	Papillary Muscle Rupture	Mechanical Valves	Mean Aortic Cross Clamp Time (min)	Survival After MVR		
														>30 Days	>1 Year	>5 Years
Connolly[1]	1986	16	64	31%	38%	100%	40	19%	100%	2.3	44%	13%	79	81%	81%	81%
Kay[2]	1986	40	—	—	—	—	—	—	100%	—	—	10%	—	65%	58%	27%
Colin[3]	1995	56	69	52%	48%	100%	—	—	89%	2	39%	29%	—	91%	91%	91%
Hausmann[4]	1999	197	64	—	—	100%	40	13%	88%	2	—	53%	—	86%	80%	73%
Bouchard[5]	2001	92	65	42%	16%	—	—	34%	77%	—	38%	87%	88	84%	82%	70%
Totals (sum or mean)		401	65	73 (45%)	48 (29%)	269 (100%)	40	60 (20%)	350 (87%)	2	64 (39%)	213 (53%)	87	336 (84%)	320 (80%)	283 (71%)

Abbreviations as in Table 1.

ative period and 283 patients (70%) survived >5 years. In the present study of 31 patients, 26 patients (84%) survived the early operative period and 18 patients (58%) survived >5 years. In the previously reported studies, it was not always clear how many patients had ruptured versus nonruptured left ventricular papillary muscles. Furthermore, whether the MR in some of the previously reported cases was due to mitral valve prolapse rather than papillary muscle ischemia (with or without rupture) was also not always clear.

The positive features of the present study include the relatively long follow-up, the division of the cases into those with and without papillary muscle rupture, and the careful study of the operatively-excised mitral valves to rule out mitral valve prolapse as the cause of MR. The present study is limited by the relatively small number of cases included.

1. Connolly MW, Gelbfish JS, Jacobwitz IJ, Rose DM, Mendelsohn A, Cappabianca PM, Acinapura AJ, Cunningham JN Jr. Surgical results for mitral regurgitation from coronary artery disease. *J Thorac Cardiovasc Surg* 1985;91:379–388.

2. Kay GL, Kay JH, Zubiate P, Yokoyama T, Mendez M. Mitral valve repair for mitral regurgitation secondary to coronary artery disease. *Circulation* 1986; 74(suppl I):I88–I98.

3. Cohn LH, Rizzo RJ, Adams DH, Couper GS, Sullivan TE, Collins JJ Jr, Aranki SF. The effect of pathophysiology on the surgical treatment of ischemic mitral regurgitation: operative and late risks of repair versus replacement. *Eur J Cardiothorac Surg* 1995;9:568–574.

4. Hausmann H, Siniawski H, Hetzer R. Mitral valve reconstruction and replacement for ischemic mitral insufficiency: seven years' follow up. *J Heart Valve Dis* 1999;8:536–542.

5. Bouchard D, Pellerin M, Carrier M, Perrault LP, Pagé P, Hébert Y, Cartier R, Dyrda I, Pelletier LC. Results following valve replacement for ischemic mitral regurgitation. *Can J Cardiol* 2001;17:427–431.

Tumor Excision Versus Valve Replacement for Papillary Fibroelastoma Involving the Mitral Valve

Mohammad Zaim Nawaz, MD[†], Allison Richey Lander, MD[a], Jeffrey M. Schussler, MD[a], Paul Arthur Grayburn, MD[b], Baron Lloyd Hamman, MD[b], and William Clifford Roberts, MD*[c,d]

We recently encountered a young man who had 3 strokes and a mass found by echocardiography on his mitral valve, which as a consequence was replaced. The tumor both grossly and histologically was a classic papillary fibroelastoma (PF). The patient's condition stimulated a discussion regarding whether excision of the PF or replacement of the valve containing it might be the preferred procedure. In an attempt to answer the question posed, patients previously reported in an English publication since the first mitral valve operation for PF involving an otherwise normal valve were reviewed.

• • •

A 37-year-old previously healthy house painter noted right-sided weakness unassociated with headache shortly after arising at 7 A.M. It resolved within minutes, but at about 8:30 A.M. right hemiplegia appeared and it persisted. By 10:00 A.M. he had arrived at the emergency room and right-sided weakness in both arm and leg was still present. He was in no distress. He did not smoke, drink alcohol, or use drugs intravenously. His body mass index was 19 kg/m^2. His blood pressure was 145/90 mm Hg initially, but 3 hours later and thereafter was about 120/85 mm Hg. No precordial murmur was heard. Electrocardiogram disclosed no abnormalities. The heart rate was 75 beats/min, and he was in sinus rhythm. A computed tomogram disclosed a remote cerebral infarct but no acute cerebral lesions. Magnetic resonance imaging of the head disclosed an acute infarct involving the left internal capsule and total occlusion of the left middle cerebral artery about 1.5 cm from its origin. The carotid and vertebral arteries were normal. The serum total cholesterol was 253, low-density lipoprotein cholesterol 197, high-density lipoprotein cholesterol 30, and triglycerides 166 mg/dl. The platelet count, prothrombin time, partial thromboplastin time, antithrombin III, protein C, protein S, anti-cardiolipin antibody, antinuclear antibody, and homocystine levels were normal. Factor V Leiden, platelet nuclear antibody 20210, and rapid plasma reagin were negative. By 5 P.M., the right-sided weakness had disappeared.

Cerebral angiography performed within 24 hours disclosed a non-occlusive thrombus in the arterior division of the left middle cerebral artery. During recovery from the procedure, he again developed aphasia and right upper extremity weakness. A repeat angiogram showed that the thrombus (embolus) had migrated, totally obstructing flow. Intra-arterial thrombolysis (tissue-plaminogen activator) was performed with restoration of flow to the anterior division of the middle cerebral artery and full recovery of voice and strength.

A transesophageal echocardiogram revealed a 0.9 × 0.7 cm mass on the atrial aspect of the anterior mitral leaflet with slight mitral regurgitation (Figure 1). Blood cultures were negative. Coronary angiography disclosed normal epicardial coronary arteries. At cardiotomy, the anterior mitral leaflet with the mass was resected and a St. Jude Medical (27 mm) prosthesis inserted. Early postoperatively, he developed transient complete heart block (ventricular rate 45 beats/min). On postoperative day 1 he was dyspneic and weak, and found to have cardiac tamponade. A pericardial "window" was created. When seen months after operation, he was asymptomatic.

The operatively excised anterior mitral leaflet, its chordae, and the mass together weighed 0.88 g (Figure 2). The leaflet and chordae were normal. Histologic study of the mass on the anterior leaflet showed it to be a classic PF.

• • •

The described patient had a single PF on the atrial aspect of his anterior mitral leaflet, 3 transient strokes, an angiographically demonstrated embolus in a middle cerebral artery that was lysed by a thrombolytic agent, and operative excision of the anterior mitral leaflet followed by mitral valve replacement. It is presumed that the source of the cerebral embolus was a thrombus on the PF, which dislodged and migrated to a cerebral artery. At the mitral operation no thrombus was seen on the PF and gross and histologic examination of the PF disclosed no evidence of thrombus. Nevertheless, there is supporting evidence from previously reported cases that such a mechanism is the cause of the stroke in our patient as in others. Of the 45 previously published cases of PF involving the mitral valve,[1–42] at least 3 patients with an operatively excised PF on the mitral valve were shown by gross and histologic study to have a thrombus superimposed on the PF.[4,28,36] Additionally, a patient with

[a]Department of Internal Medicine, Baylor University Medical Center; [b]Department of Internal Medicine (Division of Cardiology) and [c]Department of Cardiothoracic Surgery, and [d]Department of Pathology, Baylor Heart & Vascular Institute, Baylor University Medical Center, Dallas, Texas. Manuscript received September 21, 2005; revised manuscript received and accepted November 15, 2005.

*Corresponding author: Tel: 214-820-7911; Fax: 214-820-7533.

E-mail address: wcroberts@BaylorHealth.edu (W.C. Roberts).

[†]Cardiovascular Medicine Fellow, Scott & White Hospital, Texas A & M University, Temple, Texas.

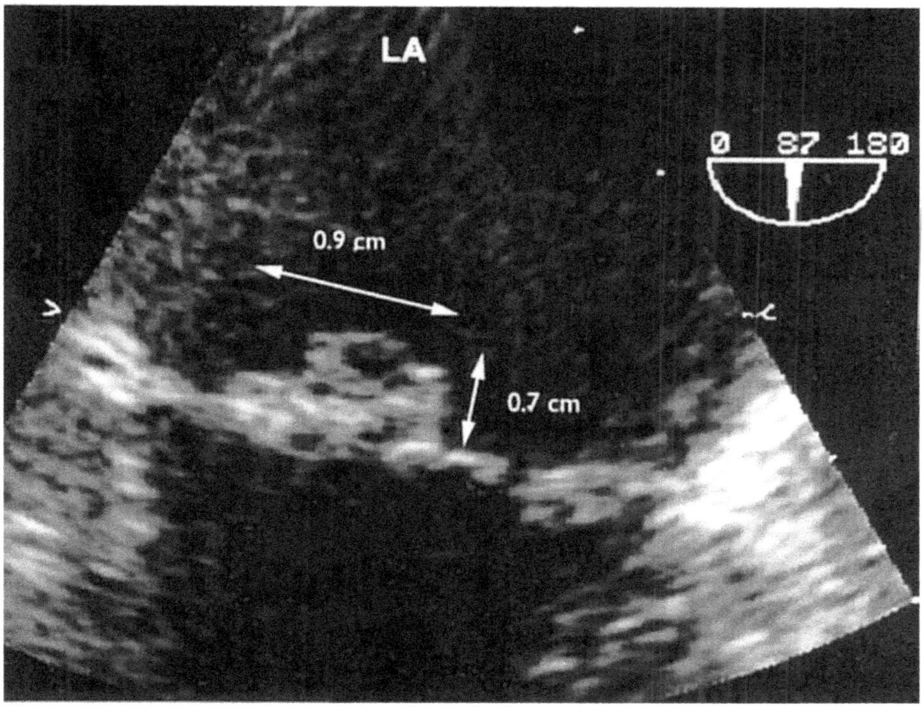

Figure 1. Transesophageal echocardiogram showing the elastofibroendothelioma on the atrial aspect of the anterior mitral leaflet. LA=left atrium.

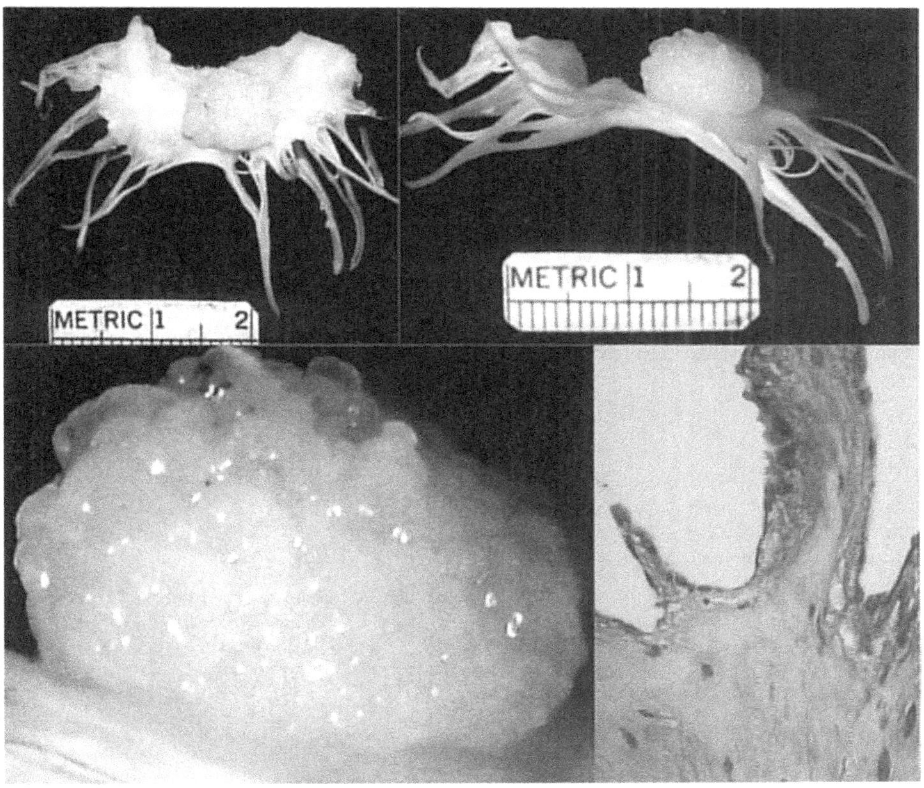

gure 2. Photographs of the operatively excised anterior mitral leaflet containing the elastofibroendothelioma (EFE) on its atrial aspect *(left upper, right and wer left)* and photomicrograph of a portion of the elastofibroendothelioma. The *upper right photograph* shows the extent of the protrusion of the EFE into e mitral orifice. The *lower left* is a very close up of the EFE. The photomicrograph is stained by the Movat method, and shows the endothelial cells lining e frons and the underlying fibrous and myxoid tissue. The photographs were taken by Ms. Jong Mi Ko.

Table 1
Reported patients having papillary fibroelastoma on the mitral valve and operative excision with or without leaflet repair

Case	Year of Report	First Author	Age (years) at MV Operation	Gender	TIA or Stroke	Cardiac Arrest	AMI	Largest Diameter (cm) of PF	Length of Follow-up After MV Operation (months)	Mitral Leaflet Involved	Chordae Tendineae Involved
1	1981	Shub[1]	55	F	0	0	0	1.0	—	Anterior	+
2	1983	Marvasti[2]	24	M	+	0	0	1.0	16	Posterior	+
3	1986	Topol[3]	27	M	+	0	0	1.5	6	Anterior	0
4	1987	McFadden[4]	41	F	+	0	0	0.5	—	Anterior	0
5	1988	Kasarskis[5]	43	F	+	0	0	1.8	—	Anterior	0
6	1988	Kasarskis[5]	52	M	+	0	0	1.3	36	Posterior	0
7	1989	Akagawa[6]	39	M	0	0	0*	2.5	—	Neither	+
8	1991	Mazzucco[7]	25	M	0	0	+	1.0	—	Anterior	0
9	1992	Valente[8]	31	M	0	0	+	1.7	—	Neither	+
10	1993	Gallo[9]	21	M	+	0	0	0.8	—	Anterior	+
11	1993	Thomas[10]	70	F	0	0	0*	1.5	—	Anterior	0
12	1993	Richard[11]	62	M	0	0	+	1.5	—	Anterior	0
13	1993	Braile[12]	15	M	0	0	0	2.6	6	Anterior	0
14	1993	Shapira[13]	73	F	0	0	0*	1.5	—	Posterior	0
15	1994	Zamora[14]	37	F	+***	0	0	0.8	—	Posterior	0
16	1994	Meyer[15]	38	M	0	0	0**	1.2	—	Posterior	0
17	1995	Pinelli[16]	27	F	+	0	0	0.7	6	Anterior	0
18	1995	Brown[17]	40	F	+	0	0	0.6	—	Anterior	+
19	1996	Hicks[18]	36	M	0	0	0*	0.6	—	Anterior	+
20	1996	Muir[19]	46	M	+	0	0	0.6	—	Anterior	0
21	1996	Menezes[20]	3	M	+	0	0	—	6	Anterior	+
22	1996	Ni[21]	31	F	+	0	0	1.0	—	Anterior	0
23	1997	Tkebuchava[22]	50	M	0	0	0**	1.0	5	Neither	+
24	1998	Moraes[23]	39	M	0	+	+	0.7	6	Anterior	0
25	1998	Al-Mohammad[24]	64	F	+	0	0	1.0	44	Anterior	+
26	1998	Mayer[25]	44	F	0	+	0	—	—	Anterior	0
27	1998	Conte[26]	40	F	+	0	0	1.5	12	Posterior	0
28	1998	Pacini[27]	72	F	+	0	0	4.0	12	Neither	+
29	1999	Grinda[28]	33	M	+	0	0	1.0	36	Anterior	0
30	1999	Sankar[29]	33	F	+	0	0	0.5	—	Anterior	0
31	1999	Howard[30]	39	M	0	+	+	0.7	3	Anterior	0
32	1999	DiMattia[31]	40	M	0	0	0	1.0	3	Anterior	+
33	1999	DiMattia[31]	50	M	0	0	+	1.2	—	Anterior	+
34	2000	Sastre-Garriga[32]	39	M	+	0	0	0.9	—	Posterior	0
35	2000	Sastre-Garriga[32]	32	F	+	0	0	1.5	—	Posterior	0
36	2000	Gölbasi[33]	32	M	+	0	0	1.0	—	Anterior	0
37	2000	Karaeren[34]	21	M	+	0	0	1.5	—	Anterior	0
38	2000	Toda[35]	78	F	+	0	0	0.8	4	Posterior	0

* Chest pain; ** palpitations; ***retinal artery occlusion.
AMI = acute myocardial infarction; MV = mitral valve; PF = papillary fibroelastoma; TIA = transient ischemic attack.

Table 2
Reported patients having papillary fibroelastoma on mitral valve and mitral valve replacement

Case	Year of Report	First Author	Age (years) at MV Operation	Gender	TIA or Stroke	Cardiac Arrest	AMI	Largest Diameter (cm) of PF	Length of Follow-up After MV Operation (months)	Mitral Leaflet Involved	Chorda[illegible] Tendinc[illegible] Involve[illegible]
1	1981	Fowles[36]	35	M	+	+	+	1.0	—	Posterior	0
2	1987	Dien[37]	25	M	+	+	0	—	81	Posterior	0
3	1989	Gorton[38]	77	F	+	0	0	2.0	9	Both	+
4	1994	Mann[39]	59	M	+	0	0	2.3	12	Neither	+
5	1995	Colucci[40]	66	F	+	0	0	1.5	12	Anterior	+
6	1998	Bailbé[41]	31	M	+	0	0	0.8	18	Unknown	+
7	2001	Shing[42]	34	M	+	0	0	1.0	6	Anterior	0

Abbreviation as in Table 2.

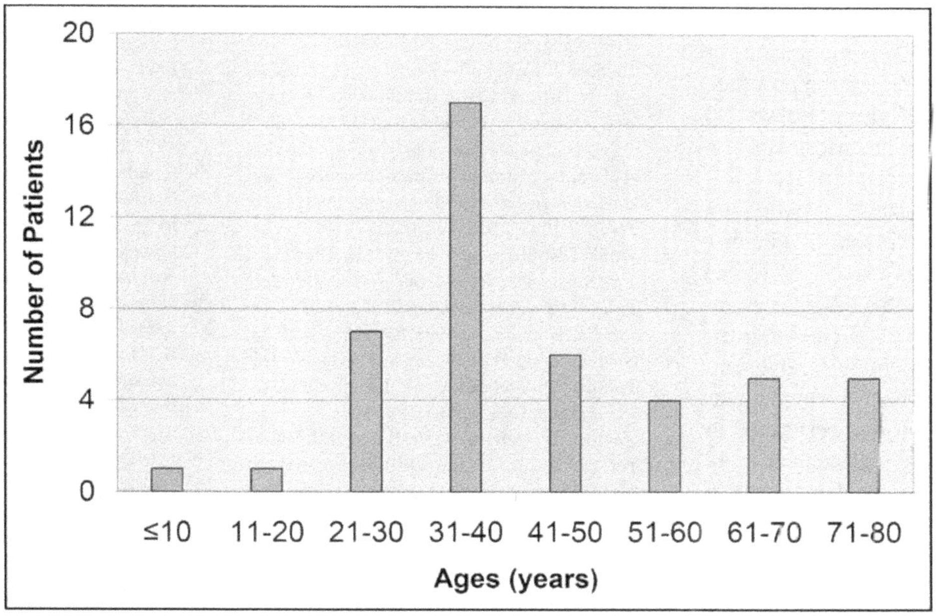

Figure 3. Ages (years) at time of mitral valve operations of 47 previously reported patients with papillary fibroelastoma involving the mitral valve.

PF involving a pulmonic valve also had superimposed thrombus on it.[43] In our patient and in the 45 previously reported patients with an PF on the mitral valve, no other source of embolism other than the PF could be demonstrated. Thus, it is reasonable to believe hat mitral PF was the source of sysemic embolism in our patient. It is not ragments of the PF which embolized, it s the thrombus superimposed on the PF.

Reports published in English of paients with PF involving an otherwise ormal (except for aging changes) mial valve with operative excision or mial replacement produced 45 individual eports.[1–42] Those having operative exision of the mitral PF are listed in Tale 1; those having mitral replacement re listed in Table 2, and the findings in oth groups are summarized in Figure . All but 3 of 45 patients presented with ther stroke and/or transient ischemic atck, and/or nonfatal cardiac arrest, and/or ute myocardial infarction. Although the atients ranged in age from 3 to 78 years, 3 (62%) were $<$40 years old (Figure 3). len were seen slightly more frequently an women (62% vs 38%). A precordial urmur was usually absent. The PFs on 1 both mitral leaflets, i.e., excluding the 5 cases in which the PF involved only the chordae tendineae, were usually small; of the 37 patients in whom the PF involved a mitral leaflet and the largest diameter was reported, the PF was $\leq$1.5 cm in 35 (95%), and the largest had a maximal diameter of 2.6 cm. In contrast, in 4 of the 5 patients in whom the PF spared a mitral leaflet and involved only its chordae tendineae, the maximal diameter of the PF was $>$1.7 cm (range 1.7 to 4.0). In only 1 of the 45 patients reported was the weight of the operatively excised PF recorded, and that was 0.29 g.

Of the 45 reported patients, 38 (84%) had PF excision and 7 (16%) had valve replacement. The argument for valve excision, of course, is that a mechanical prosthesis with its mandatory anticoagulation thereafter or a bioprosthesis with its inevitable degeneration is avoided. The argument for valve replacement is that worry of thrombus formation at the base of the excised PF and the potential regrowth of an PF on the valve are no longer possibilities. Recurrence, however, of an PF at the site of a previously excised PF has never been reported. Although all 45 previously reported cases presented as individual case reports (Tables 1 to 2; Figure 3) survived the operative period, follow-up information is scant at best. Of the 45 patients, follow-up information $>$1 month after the mitral operation was described in only 21 patients (47%) and ranged from 3 to 81 months (mean 16; median 9), and in 15 of the 21 patients (71%), the follow-up was $\leq$12 months. Thus, the preferred type of operative intervention remains unclear, but logic for most of these patients favors PF excision without valve replacement.

The data in the previously described cases came from individual case reports and included only cases where the PF was located on the mitral valve and was either excised or the mitral valve replaced. Two large collections[44,45] of cases of PF confirmed histologically after operative excision or at necropsy were not included in our analysis because both studies included all cases of cardiac PF irrespective of where the PF was located in the heart, and data on the cases involving only the mitral valve was limited.

Klarich and associates[44] included 4 cases of PF involving a mitral leafet among 12 cases of PF involving a cardiac valve having operative intervention: 3 had operative excision of the mitral PF and 1 had mitral replacement.

The latter patient had a flail anterior mitral leafet and that was the reason for the mitral replacement, not the presence of a PF on the mitral valve. Follow-up information on these 4 cases was not available.

Gowda and associates[45] reported on 725 cases of cardiac PF confirmed either at operation or autopsy, and 180 (25%) involved the mitral valve (223 cases involved the aortic valve, 65 cases the tricuspid valve, 43 the pulmonic valve, and the remainder presumably a non-valvular site). Surgical excision was performed in 325 patients and valve replacement in 42 patients. No recurrence of PF occurred in the patients having valve excision. It was not possible to separate data in the cases in whom the PF was located on the mitral valve from those involving other cardiac valves or only the mural endocardium.

1. Shub C, Tajik AJ, Seward JB, Edwards WD, Pruitt RD, Orszulak TA, Pluth JR. Cardiac papillary fibroelastoms. Two-dimensional echocardiographic recognition. *Mayo Clin Proc* 1981;56:629–633.
2. Marvasti MA, Obeid AI, Cohen PS, Giambartolomei A, Parker FB. Successful removal of papillary endocardial fibroma. *Thorac Cardiovasc Surg* 1983;31:254–255.
3. Topol EJ, Biern RO, Reitz BA. Cardiac papillary fibroelastoma and stroke. Echocardiographic diagnosis and guide to excision. *Am J Med* 1986;80:129–132.
4. McFadden PM, Lacy JR. Intracardiac papillary fibroelastoma: an occult cause of embolic neurologic deficit. *Ann Thorac Surg* 1987;43:667–669.
5. Kasarskis EJ, O'Connor W, Earle G. Embolic stroke from cardiac papillary fibroelastomas. *Stroke* 1988;19:1171–1173.
6. Akagawa H, Kawara T, Hirano A, Sugiwara S, Ogata M, Aoyagi S, Kosuga K, Ohishi K, Koga M. Excision of papillary endocardial tumor. *J Cardiovasc Surg* 1989;30:47–49.
7. Mazzucco A, Faggian G, Bortolotti U, Bonato R, Pittarello D, Centonze G, Thiene G. Embolizing papillary fibroelastoma of the mitral valve. *Tex Heart Inst J* 1991;18:62–66.
8. Valente M, Basso C, Thiene G, Bressan M, Stritoni P, Cocco P, Fasoli G. Fibroelastic papilloma: a not-so-benign cardiac tumor. *Cardiovasc Pathol* 1992;1:161–166.
9. Gallo R, Kumar N, Prabhakar G, Awada A, Maalouf Y, Duran CMG. Papillary fibroelastoma of mitral valve chorda. *Ann Thorac Surg* 1993;55:1576–1577.
10. Thomas MR, Jayakrishnan AG, Desai J, Monaghan MJ, Jewitt DE. Transesophageal echocardiography in the detection and surgical management of a papillary fibroelastoma of the mitral valve causing partial mitral valve obstruction. *J Am Soc Echocardiogr* 1993;6:83–86.
11. Richard J, Castello R, Dressler FA, Willman VL, Nashed A, Lewis B, Labovitz AJ. Diagnosis of papillary fibroelastoma of the mitral valve complicated by non-Q-wave infarction with apical thrombus: transesophageal and transthoracic echocardiographic study. *Am Heart J* 1993;126:710–712.
12. Braile DM, Rossi MA, Jacob JLB, Thevenard RS, Suzigan S, Ramos SG. Cystic fibroelastoma of the mitral valve:report of a case. *J Thorac Cardiovasc Surg* 1993;106:1228–1230.
13. Shapira OM, Williamson WA, Dugan JM. Papillary fibroelastoma of the mitral valve. *Cardiovasc Surg* 1993;1:599–601.
14. Zamora RL, Adelberg DA, Berger AS, Huettner P, Kaplan HJ. Branch retinal artery occlusion caused by a mitral valve papillary fibroelastoma. *Am J Ophthalmol* 1995;119: 325–329.
15. Meyer AH, Clements SD Jr., Sadel SM, Shanewise JS, Gravanis MB. Papillary fibroelastoma of the cardiac valves. *Heart Dis Stroke* 1994;3:318–319.
16. Pinelli G, Carteaux J-P, Mertes PM, Civit T, Trinh A, Villemot J-P. Mitral valve tumor revealed by stroke. *J Heart Valve Dis* 1995; 4:199–201.
17. Brown RD Jr., Khandheria BK, Edwards WD. Cardiac papillary fibroelastoma: a treatable cause of transient ischemic attack and ischemic stroke detected by transesophageal echocardiography. *Mayo Clin Proc* 1995;70: 863–868.
18. Hicks KA, Kovach JA, Frishberg DP, Wiley TM, Gurczak PB, Vernalis MN. Echocardiographic evaluation of papillary fibroelastoma: a case report and review of the literature. *J Am Soc Echocardiogr* 1996;9:353–360.
19. Muir KW, McNeish IBM, Grosset DG, Metcalfe M. Visualization of cardiac emboli from mitral valve papillary fibroelastoma. *Stroke* 1996;27:1133–1134.
20. de Menezes IC, Fragata J, Martins FM. Papillary fibroelastoma of the mitral valve in a 3-year-old child: case report. *Pediatr Cardiol* 1996;17:194–195.
21. Ni Y, von Segesser LK, Dirsch O, Schneider J, Jenni R, Turina M. Cardiac papillary fibroelastoma. *Thorac Cardiovasc Surg* 1996;44: 257–260.
22. Tkebuchava T, von Segesser LK, Gallino A, Dirsch O, Turina MI. Cardiac papillary fibroelastoma excision combined with reconstructive surgery. *Jpn Heart J* 1997;38:457–462.
23. Moraes D, Philippides GJ, Shapira OM. Papillary fibroelastoma of the mitral valve with systemic embolization. *Circulation* 1998;98: 1251–1252.
24. Al-Mohammed A, Pambakian H, Young C. Fibroelastoma: case report and review of literature. *Heart* 1998;79:301–304.
25. Mayer K, Niederhaeuser U, Jenni R. Cardiac papillary fibroelastoma with cerebral and coronary embolic events. *Heart* 1998;79:307.
26. Conte FJ, Katz AS. Fibroelastoma and embolic stroke. *Circulation* 1998;97:1648.
27. Pacini D, Farneti PA, Leone O, Galli R. Cardiac papillary fibroelastoma of the mitral valve chordae. *Euro J Cardiothorac Surg* 1998;13:322–324.
28. Grinda J-M, Couetil JP, Chauvaud S, D'Attellis N, Berrebi A, Fabiani J-N, Deloche A, Carpentier A. Cardiac valve papillary fibroelastoma: surgical excision for revealed or potential embolization. *J Thorac Cardiovasc Surg* 1999;117:106–110.
29. Sankar NM, Odayan MK, Morris M, Peterson H, Hanna WM. Cardiac valvular papillary fibroelastoma. A report of 2 cases. *Tex Heart Inst J* 1999;26:298–299.
30. Howard RA, Aldea GS, Shapira OM, Kasznica JM, Davidoff R. Papillary fibroelastoma: increasing recognition of a surgical disease *Ann Thorac Surg* 1999;68:1881–1885.
31. Di Mattia DG, Assaghi A, Mangini A, Ravagnan S, Bonetto S, Fundaro P. Mitral valve repai for anterior leaflet papillary fibroelastoma: tw case descriptions and a literature review. *Eur J Cardiothorac Surg* 1999;15:103–107.
32. Sastre-Garriga J, Molina C, Montaner J Mauleon A, Pujadas F, Codina A, Álvarez Sabin J. Mitral papillary fibroelastoma as cause of cardiogenic embolic stroke: report c two cases and review of the literature. *Eur J Neurol* 2000;7:449–453.
33. Gölbasi Z, Çiçek D, Aydogdu S, Can C. Papillary fibroelastoma of mitral valve. A rar cause of transient ischemic attack in th young. *Jpn Heart J* 2000;41:525–526.
34. Karaeren H, Ilgenli TF, Celik T, Deveci S Kuralay E, Barcin C, Uzun M, Genc C Demirtas E. Papillary fibroelastoma of th mitral valve with systemic embolizatio *Echocardiography* 2000;17:165–167.
35. Toda R, Iguro Y, Moriyama Y, Matsumo H, Taira A. Papillary fibroelastoma on th mitral valve. *Jpn J Thorac Cardiovasc Su* 2000;48:132–134.
36. Fowles RE, Miller DC, Egbert BM, Fitzgeald JW, Popp RL. Systemic embolizati from a mitral valve papillary endocardial broma detected by two-dimensional echocadiography. *Am Heart J* 1981;102:128–130
37. Dein JR, Frist WH, Stinson EB, Miller D Baldwin JC, Oyer PE, Jamieson S, Mitch RS, Shumway NE. Primary cardiac neplasms. Early and late results of surgi treatment in 42 patients. *J Thorac Cardiov Surg* 1987;93:502–511.
38. Gorton ME, Soltanzadeh H. Mitral va fibroelastoma. *Ann Thorac Su* 1989;47:605–607.
39. Mann J, Parker DJ. Papillary fibroelasto of the mitral valve: a rare cause of transi neurological deficits. *Br Heart J* 1994;71
40. Colucci V, Alberti A, Bonacina E, Gordini Papillary fibroelastoma of the mitral valve rare cause of events. *Tex Heart Inst J* 1995; 327–331.
41. Bailbé M, Coisne D, Babin P, Corbi P, M P, Rosier MP, Couderq C, Pouget Abadie

Gil R, Neau JP. Fibroélastome papillaire. Une étiologie rare des accidents vasculaires cérébraux du sujet jeune. *Rev Méd Interne* 1998;19:119–122.
42. Shing M, Rubenson DS. Embolic stroke and cardiac papillary fibroelastoma. *Clin Cardiol* 2001;24:346–347.
43. Fekete PS, Nassar VH, Talley JD, Boedecker EA. Cardiac papilloma. A case report with evidence of thrombotic origin. *Arch Pathol Lab Med* 1983;107:246–248.
44. Klarich KW, Enriquez-Sarano M, Gura GM, Edwards WD, Tajik AJ, Seward JB. Papillary fibroelastoma: echocardiographic characteristics for diagnosis and pathologic correlation. *J Am Coll Cardiol* 1997;30:784–790.
45. Gowda RM, Khan IA, Nair CK, Mehta NJ, Vasavada BC, Sacchi TJ. Cardiac papillary fibroelastoma: a comprehensive analysis of 725 cases. *Am Heart J* 2003;146:404–410.

Frequency of Atrial Fibrillation in Patients Having Mitral Valve Repair or Replacement for Pure Mitral Regurgitation Secondary to Mitral Valve Prolapse

Rafic Fouad Berbarie, MD[a,b], and William Clifford Roberts, MD[a,b,c,*]

Relatively little attention has been paid to the frequency of atrial fibrillation (AF) in patients with mitral regurgitation (MR) secondary to mitral valve prolapse (MVP). We reviewed clinical, electrocardiographic, echocardiographic, hemodynamic, and angiographic findings in 246 patients aged 21 to 84 years (mean 61) (66% men) who had mitral valve repair or replacement for MR secondary to MVP. Immediately before the mitral operation by electrocardiogram, only 37 patients (15%) had AF and the other 209 patients were in sinus rhythm. Of the latter, 32 had had a history of AF that had reverted to sinus rhythm spontaneously or with antiarrhythmic therapy. Thus, a total of 69 patients (28%) had AF at some time. In conclusion, the frequency of AF in patients with MR secondary to MVP and sick enough to warrant a mitral valve operation have a relatively low frequency of AF (persistent in 15%, paroxysmal in another 13%), percentages considerably lower than that seen in patients with mitral stenosis just before a mitral commissurotomy or replacement. **(Am J Cardiol 2006;97:1039–1044)**

Since its initial description in 1963, numerous articles on various aspects of mitral valve prolapse (MVP) have appeared.[1] Indeed, from 1966 to 2000, a total of 3,772 articles on MVP were cited on a Medline search. Although many articles mentioned atrial fibrillation (AF), few have focused on its frequency. This report focuses on the frequency of AF in a large group of patients having either mitral valve repair or replacement for mitral regurgitation (MR) secondary to MVP. The hypothesis was that the frequency of AF preoperatively would be relatively small despite the frequency of relatively large atrial cavities.

Methods

From March 1993 to January 2005, a total of 274 patients had mitral valve repair or replacement for pure, i.e., no element of mitral stenosis, MR secondary to MVP at Baylor University Medical Center. All of these operatively excised valves or portions of the valves were examined by 1 of us (WCR), and the etiology of the MR was determined by gross (and often histologic) examination of the operatively excised valve tissue plus examination of the medical record.[2] Of the 274 patients, 28 were eliminated from the present study because of a previous cardiac operation (10 patients), having a pacemaker (5 patients), having a proce dure performed simultaneously on the aortic valve (1 pa tient), or because the clinical chart was unavailable fo review (12 patients). The remaining 246 patients were in cluded in the present study. The mitral operation in thes patients was their first cardiac operation; all were >20 year of age, none had tricuspid valve replacement, or a procedur performed on the aortic valve.

The electrocardiogram immediately before the mitral op eration was reviewed in all 246 patients. Hemodynamic dat from cardiac catheterization was available in 143 patien (58%); coronary angiographic data were also available i 217 patients (88%); and echocardiographic data were avai able in 94 patients (38%).

Statistical analysis was completed using GB-STAT ve sion 10.0 (Dynamic Microsystems Inc., 2004). Variables a expressed as means, with corresponding ranges or freque cies, with corresponding percentages. Means and freque cies were compared with Student's *t* tests. The patients we divided and compared by preoperative rhythm, age, sex, ar whether mitral repair or replacement was done. A p valu <0.05 was considered statistically significant.

Results

The major findings in the 246 patients are listed in Table 1. T patients were divided into 2 groups: (1) those in whom t electrocardiogram immediately before the mitral valve ope tion disclosed sinus rhythm (n = 209; 85%); and (2) those whom the electrocardiogram immediately preoperative

From the [a]Baylor Heart & Vascular Institute, and the Departments of [b]Medicine (Division of Cardiology) and [c]Pathology, Baylor University Medical Center, Dallas, Texas. Manuscript received October 11, 2005; revised manuscript received and accepted November 4, 2005.

* Corresponding author: Tel: 214-820-7911; fax: 214-820-7533.

E-mail address: wc.roberts@baylorhealth.edu (W.C. Roberts).

Table 1
Preoperative clinical findings in 246 patients with and without pre-op atrial fibrillation by electrocardiogram immediately before mitral valve operation for mitral regurgitation secondary to mitral valve prolapse

Variable	Atrial Fibrillation		p Value
	No (n = 209) (85%)	Yes (n = 37) (15%)	
Age (years): range (mean)	21–81 (59)	34–84 (69)	<0.0001
White	191 (91%)	37 (100%)	<0.06
Men:women	143 (68%):66 (32%)	20 (54%):17 (46%)	0.10
Echocardiographic dimensions (mm) (mean)			
Left atrium	29–65 (50)	41–76 (54)	0.16
Left ventricular peak systole	13–48 (36)	17–50 (38)	0.53
Left ventricular end diastole	18–79 (60)	39–61 (56)	0.22
Pressures (mm Hg) (range) (mean)			
Pulmonary artery peak systole	17–87 (39)	41–76 (44)	0.12
Pulmonary artery mean	10–62 (25)	10–50 (29)	0.15
Left ventricular peak systole	68–198 (125)	89–190 (124)	0.92
Left ventricular end-diastole	3–36 (19)	9–39 (19)	0.99
Pulmonary artery wedge mean	3–43 (17)	5–31 (20)	<0.08
Right ventricular peak systole	12–83 (39)	20–71 (43)	0.14
Right ventricular end-diastole	2–24 (11)	4–25 (12)	0.52
Right atrial mean	1–35 (7)	1–20 (10)	<0.004
Aorta (peak systole)	68–200 (126)	87–199 (126)	0.90/0.67
(end diastole)	39–98 (70)	50–99 (71)	
Other hemodynamic			
Cardiac index (L/min/m^2)	1.4–5.4 (2.7)	1.5–4.1 (2.3)	<0.06
Ejection fraction (%)	30–75 (58)	25–70 (51)	0.0003
Body mass index (kg/m^2)(mean)	26	24	<0.006
≤25	109 (52%)	24 (65%)	0.15
26–30	77 (37%)	12 (32%)	0.56
>30	23 (11%)	1 (3%)	0.13
ystemic hypertension	106 (51%)	20 (54%)	0.74
lean New York Heart Association functional class (mean)	2.4	2.9	<0.002
I	38 (18%)	3 (8%)	
II	74 (35%)	6 (16%)	<0.002
III	76 (36%)	20 (54%)	
IV	21 (11%)	8 (22%)	<0.002
umber of major coronary arteries narrowed >50% in diameter:	(n = 182)	(n = 35)	
0	139 (77%)	24 (69%)	0.31
1	20 (11%)	3 (9%)	
2	11 (6%)	0 (0%)	
3	8 (4%)	5 (13%)	0.31
Left main	4 (2%)	3 (9%)	
oronary bypass	42 (20%)	10 (27%)	0.34

isclosed AF (n = 37; 15%). Of the 11 major variables nalyzed in the 2 groups, 5 showed significant differences. n contrast to the sinus rhythm group, preoperatively, the F patients were significantly older (69 vs 59 years), had a ower mean body mass index (24 vs 26 kg/m^2), had a higher ew York Heart Association functional class (2.9 vs. 2.4), higher mean right atrial pressure (10 vs 7 mm Hg), and ower mean ejection fraction (51% vs 58%).

Of the 209 patients with sinus rhythm by electrocardio-am immediately before the mitral valve operation, 32 5%) had had previous episodes of AF that had either onverted to sinus rhythm spontaneously or with use of tiarrhythmic drugs or electrical cardioversion. Thus, of e total 246 patients, 69 (28%) had had ≥1 episode of AF ersistent in 37 and paroxysmal in 32). Comparison of the rious variables depicted in Table 1 between the 37 pa-nts with persistent AF and the 32 patients with paroxysmal AF disclosed only 1 significant difference: the persistent group had a lower frequency of a history of systemic hypertension than the paroxysmal AF group (20 [54%] vs 23 [72%]; p = 0.01).

Comparison of 12 variables in the men versus the women are presented in Table 2. In contrast to the women, the men had significantly larger left ventricular cavities, lower left ventricular and aortic peak systolic pressures, lower ejection fractions, higher body mass indexes, more angiographic coronary arterial narrowing, and a higher frequency of simultaneous coronary arterial bypass grafting (at the time of the mitral operation).

Comparison of 13 variables in the 157 patients having mitral valve repair versus the 89 patients having mitral valve replacement are listed in Table 3; only 1 significant difference was found—the replacement group had a higher frequency of AF.

Table 2
Comparison of preoperative findings between the men and women who had mitral valve operations for mitral regurgitation secondary to mitral valve prolapse

Variable	Men (n = 163)	Women (n = 83)	p Value
Age (years)	21–84 (60)	27–84 (62)	0.21
White	156 (96%)	72 (87%)	<0.01
AF	20 (12%)	17 (20%)	0.095
Sinus rhythm + history of AF	22 (14%)	10 (12%)	0.66
Sinus rhythm − history of AF	121 (74%)	56 (68%)	0.32
Echocardiographic dimensions (mm)			
Left atrium	29–76 (51)	38–64 (49)	0.52
LV peak systole	13–48 (37)	17–50 (35)	0.36
LV end diastole	18–79 (61)	39–68 (56)	0.03
Pressures (mm Hg) (range)(mean)			
Pulmonary artery peak systole	17–87 (40)	17–86 (40)	0.99
Pulmonary artery mean	10–62 (26)	10–52 (26)	0.85
LV peak systole	68–163 (118)	94–198 (138)	<0.0001
LV end diastole	3–39 (19)	7–36 (18)	0.44
Pulmonary artery wedge mean	3–43 (18)	6–32 (16)	0.31
RV peak systole	12–71 (37)	22–83 (42)	0.05
RV end diastole	2–25 (11)	3–22 (11)	0.47
Right atrial mean	1–20 (7)	1–35 (7)	0.82
Aorta peak systole	68–177 (117)	91–200 (140)	<0.0001
Aorta end diastole	39–90 (67)	47–79 (74)	0.0001
Other hemodynamic data:			
Cardiac index (L/min/m^2)	1.5–5.4 (2.7)	1.5–4.6 (2.7)	0.98
Ejection fraction (%)	25–75 (55)	40–75 (60)	0.0007
Body mass index (kg/m^2) (mean)	26	25	<0.03
≤25	80 (49%)	53 (64%)	<0.03
26–30	65 (40%)	24 (29%)	0.09
>30	18 (11%)	6 (7%)	0.31
Systemic hypertension	79 (48%)	48 (58%)	0.14
Mean NYHA functional class (mean)	2.4	2.5	0.38
I	27 (17%)	14 (17%)	
II	58 (36%)	22 (27%)	0.18
III	60 (36%)	36 (43%)	
IV	18 (11%)	11 (13%)	0.18
No. of major coronary arteries narrowed >50% ↓ in diameter:	(n = 142)	(n = 75)	
0	99 (69%)	65 (80%)	
1	15 (11%)	7 (10%)	<0.004
2	11 (8%)	1 (1%)	
3	12 (8%)	1 (1%)	<0.004
Left main	5 (4%)	1 (1%)	
Coronary bypass	43 (26%)	8 (10%)	<0.004

AF = atrial fibrillation; LV = left ventricular; NYHA = New York Heart Association; RV = right ventricular.

Table 3
Comparison of preoperative findings between patients who had mitral valve repair versus replacement for mitral regurgitation secondary to mitral valve prolapse

Variable	Repair (n = 157)	Replacement (n = 89)	p Value
Age (years)	21–84 (59)	27–84 (62)	0.05
Men	106 (68%)	57 (64%)	0.52
White	147 (94%)	81 (91%)	0.38
AF	18 (11%)	19 (21%)	<0.04
Sinus rhythm + history of AF	26 (17%)	6 (7%)	<0.03
Sinus rhythm − history of AF	113 (72%)	64 (72%)	1.0
Echocardiographic dimensions (mm)			
Left atrium	38–65 (50)	27–76 (51)	0.58
LV peak systole	17–50 (38)	13–48 (34)	0.08
LV end diastole	39–79 (61)	18–79 (57)	0.12
Pressures (mm Hg)			
Pulmonary artery peak systole	17–77 (39)	18–87 (42)	0.15
Pulmonary artery mean	10–50 (25)	10–62 (27)	0.23
LV peak systole	94–83 (125)	68–198 (125)	0.83
LV end-systole	7–36 (19)	3–39 (18)	0.21
Pulmonary artery wedge mean	5–43 (17)	3–32 (18)	0.3
RV peak systole	12–71 (38)	22–83 (42)	0.1
RV end-diastole	3–25 (11)	2–22 (11)	0.7
Right atrial mean	1–35 (7)	1–20 (8)	0.3
Aorta peak systole	87–177 (126)	68–200 (125)	0.9
Aorta end diastole	39–97 (70)	49–99 (70)	0.9
Other hemodynamic data:			
Cardiac index (L/min/m^2)	1.4–4.7 (2.7)	1.5–5.4 (2.6)	0.8
Ejection fraction (%)	25–75 (57)	30–75 (57)	0.8
Body mass index (kg/m^2) (mean)	26	25	0.2
≤25	82 (52%)	50 (56%)	0.5
26–30	60 (38%)	30 (34%)	0.5
<30	15 (10%)	9 (10%)	1
Systemic hypertension	74 (47%)	53 (60%)	0.0
Mean NYHA functional class (mean)	2.4	2.5	0.4
I	26 (17%)	15 (17%)	
II	56 (36%)	24 (27%)	0.1
III	57 (36%)	39 (44%)	
IV	18 (11%)	11 (12%)	0.1
Major coronary arteries narrowed >50% ↓ in diameter:			
0	113/142 (79%)	54/75 (71%)	
1	14/142 (10%)	7/75 (9%)	0.1
2	7/142 (5%)	4/75 (5%)	
3	7/142 (5%)	6/75 (8%)	0.
Left main	1/142 (1%)	5/75 (7%)	
Coronary bypass	27 (17%)	24 (27%)	0.

Abbreviations as in Table 2.

Comparison of 13 variables in 3 different age groups (21 to 50 vs 51 to 70 vs >70 years) are listed in Table 4. In comparison to 1 or both of the younger age groups, the 59 patients >70 years of age had a higher frequency of AF, a higher percentage had mitral replacement (compared with repair), higher peak systolic and mean pulmonary arter pressures, higher left ventricular peak systolic pressur higher mean pulmonary arterial wedge pressures, hig right ventricular peak systolic pressures, higher peak s tolic aortic pressures, lower cardiac indexes, higher N

Table 4
Comparison of the findings by age in patients undergoing mitral valve operation for mitral regurgitation secondary to mitral valve prolapse

Variable	Age Groups (years)			p Values		
	21–50 (n = 57)	51–70 (n = 130)	>70 (n = 59)	1 vs 2	2 vs 3	1 vs 3
Men:women	40 (70%):17 (30%)	89 (68%):41 (32%)	34 (58%):25 (42%)	0.79	0.18	0.18
White	51 (89%)	120 (92%)	57 (97%)	0.51	0.20	<0.10
AF	3 (5%)	12 (9%)	22 (37%)	0.35	0.0001	0.0001
Sinus rhythm (ECG) + history of AF	3 (5%)	24 (18%)	5 (8%)	<0.02	<0.08	0.51
Sinus rhythm (ECG) − history of AF	51 (90%)	94 (72%)	32 (55%)	<0.01	<0.03	0.001
Mitral repair/replacement	40 (70%)/17 (30%)	88 (68%)/42 (32%)	29 (49%)/30 (51%)	0.79	<0.02	<0.03
Echocardiographic dimension (mm):						
Left atrium	39–63 (48)	29–65 (50)	34–76 (51)	0.24	0.92	0.32
LV peak systole	36–47 (40)	13–48 (36)	17–50 (35)	0.18	0.74	<0.07
LV end diastole	56–78 (64)	18–79 (59)	39–73 (57)	0.13	0.39	<0.008
Pressures (mm Hg)						
Pulmonary artery peak systole	17–61 (31)	17–18 (41)	21–86 (44)	<0.002	0.25	0.0001
Pulmonary artery mean	10–44 (21)	10–62 (26)	14–52 (28)	<0.02	0.27	0.0005
LV peak systole	76–167 (118)	68–183 (121)	89–198 (137)	0.50	<0.002	<0.003
LV end-diastole	7–30 (17)	3–39 (19)	7–32 (18)	0.26	0.41	0.70
Pulmonary artery wedge mean	5–28 (13)	3–43 (18)	6–31 (19)	<0.02	0.61	<0.003
RV peak systole	20–66 (33)	20–83 (39)	12–81 (43)	<0.04	0.18	<0.005
RV end-diastole	2–24 (11)	3–22 (11)	3–25 (12)	0.75	0.30	0.62
Right atrial mean	1–12 (6)	1–35 (7)	1–20 (8)	0.30	0.20	<0.03
Aorta peak systole	91–163 (119)	68–177 (122)	87–200 (137)	0.61	<0.002	<0.004
Aorta end-diastole	52–98 (73)	47–94 (69)	39–99 (69)	<0.07	0.84	0.20
Other hemodynamic data:						
Cardiac index (L/min/m^2)	1.9–4.7 (3.0)	1.4–4.3 (2.6)	1.5–5.4 (2.5)	<0.05	0.51	<0.04
Ejection fraction (%)	30–70 (57)	35–75 (58)	25–75 (56)	0.91	0.25	0.47
Body mass index (kg/m^2)	20–41 (25)	17–46 (26)	18–34 (24)	0.11	<0.02	0.50
Systemic hypertension	18 (32%)	71 (55%)	37 (65%)	<0.005	0.20	0.0006
Mean NYHA functional class	2.1	2.4	2.8	<0.02	<0.02	0.0001
I	16 (30%)	19 (15%)	5 (8%)			
II	21 (37%)	46 (35%)	13 (22%)	<0.04	<0.02	0.0001
III	15 (26%)	51 (39%)	30 (51%)			
IV	4 (7%)	14 (11%)	11 (19%)	<0.04	<0.02	0.0001
No. of major coronary arteries narrowed >50% in diameter:	(n = 43)	(n = 120)	(n = 54)			
0	37 (86%)	93 (77%)	34 (63%)	0.21	<0.06	<0.02
1	3 (7%)	13 (11%)	6 (11%)			
2	1 (2%)	8 (7%)	3 (6%)			
3	2 (5%)	5 (4%)	6 (11%)			
Left main	0 (0%)	1 (1%)	5 (9%)			
Coronary bypass	5 (9%)	28 (22%)	18 (31%)	<0.04	0.19	<0.004

ECG = electrocardiogram; other abbreviations as in Table 2.

York Heart Association functional classes, and greater coronary arterial narrowing.

Discussion

The heretofore described data in 246 patients having mitral valve repair or replacement for MR due to MVP disclosed that the frequency of AF preoperatively was relatively low, namely, 15%. Compared with the 209 patients with sinus rhythm preoperatively, the 37 patients with AF were significantly older, less likely to be men, more likely to be lean, more likely to have severe heart failure, to have higher right atrial pressures and lower left ventricular ejection fractions. The frequency of AF in previously published reports of patients with MVP is listed in Table 5.[2–13]

The frequency of AF among patients with MR from MVP severe enough to warrant a mitral operation might logically be expected to be >15% because the disease process would appear to be in a relatively late stage. Earlier stages of MVP, for example, in cases picked up by community screening programs (auscultation, echocardiography) among asymptomatic MVP patients or early symptomatic patients, have an even lower frequency of MVP. Indeed, Freed and colleagues[10] reviewed echocardiograms in 3491 offspring cohorts of the Framingham Heart Study, and found 84 subjects (2.4%) to have MVP. Only 1 (1.2%) had AF. The subjects with MVP were leaner than the subjects without MVP. None had a mitral valve operation. Grigioni and associates[12] analyzed 360 patients (aged 65 ± 13 years; 74% men in the local Rochester, Minnesota, community)

Table 5
Previous publications of patients with mitral valve prolapse showing frequency of atrial fibrillation and other variables

First Author	Year of Publication	Method of Diagnosis of MVP	No. of Patients With MVP	Age (years) Range (mean)	Men	AF	Angiographic Coronary Disease	Mitral Valve Operation
Waller[2]	1982	Surgical	60	36–73 (55)	29 (48%)	4 (7%)	3/23 (13%)	69 (100%)
Ranganathan[3]	1973	S or Autopsy	16	37–69 (—)	9 (56%)	11 (69%)	—	Most
Higgins[4]	1976	Echo	40*	50–90 (65)	40* (100%)	14 (35%)	—	—
Kolibash[5]	1983	Au, Echo, An	62	60–81 (—)	25 (40%)	13 (21%)	4/26 (15%)	21 (34%)
Tresch[6]	1985	Operation	30	25–72 (60)	20 (67%)	13 (43%)	3/29 (10%)	30 (100%)
Penkoske[7]	1985	Operation	31	— (63)	17 (55%)	18 (58%)	9 (29%)	31† (100%)
Kolibash[8]	1986	Operation	86	26–82 (60)	53 (62%)	48 (56%)	8 (9%)	76 (88%)
Naggar[9]	1986	Echo	145	≥60	71 (49%)	27 (18%)	—	22 (15%)
Freed[10]	1999	Echo	84‡	26–84 (56)	34 (41%)	1 (1%)	—	1 (1%)
Ohki[11]	2001	Echo	118	32–68 (50)	69 (58%)	29 (25%)	—	—
Grigioni[12]	2002	Echo	89§	52–78 (65)	59 (66%)	19 (21%)	—	35 (39%)
Avierinos[13]	2002	Echo	833‖	29–71 (50)	300 (36%)	67 (8%)	—	65 (8%)

* Studied at a Veterans-Administration Hospital.
† Mitral-valve repair in each.
‡ Diagnosed from a general population survey (Framingham).
§ Focused on patients with sinus rhythm at diagnosis of "degenerative" mitral regurgitation and percent who developed AF at 5 and 10 years of follow-up.
‖ Focused on patients with asymptomatic MVP in a community (Rochester).
An = angiography; Au = auscultation; MVP = mitral valve prolapse; S = surgery; other abbreviation as in Table 2.

with MR due to flail mitral leaflet (n = 360) and patients with grade 3 or 4 MR secondary to MVP (n = 89). All 449 patients were in sinus rhythm at diagnosis. By 10 years after diagnosis, however, nearly 50% had developed AF. The patients who developed AF were older and had larger left atria than did those who remained in sinus rhythm.

It is well known that MVP tends to be more frequent in women than in men. It has been estimated that MVP is present in about 8 million adults in the USA. The MVP patients who develop enough MR to warrant mitral valve operation, however, are more often men than women. In the present study, 163 (66%) of the 246 patients were men. The reason for the dominance of men in this circumstance is unclear.

The ages of the patients included in the present study ranged from 21 to 84 years (mean 61). The mean age of these patients places them, of course, in a category where coronary artery disease is relatively frequent. Surprisingly, however, only 54 (22%) had angiographic evidence of narrowing >50% in diameter of ≥1 epicardial coronary artery. A possible explanation for this relatively low frequency of angiographically demonstrated coronary arterial narrowing may be the relatively high frequency of body mass indexes of ≤25 kg/m^2. Of the 246 patients, 134 (54%) had this relatively low body mass index and, furthermore, only 24 (10%) were obese (body mass index >30 kg/m^2).

Why AF appears to be less frequent in adults with MR from MVP than in similar aged adults with mitral stenosis has received virtually no attention. Mitral stenosis in adults is virtually always of rheumatic origin, a process which affects the left atrial wall as well as the mitral valve with or without involvement of other valves.[14] In contrast, MVP has no direct effect on the atrial walls other than the secondary hemodynamic consequences. In other words, the atrial walls are histologically abnormal in patients with mitral stenosis, whereas these walls are histologically normal, except for myofiber hypertrophy in patients with MVP.

Like virtually all clinical investigations, this work has limitations. An important one is the lack of hemodynamic, angiographic, and echocardiographic data on all the patients included. Another limitation is almost certainly different standards regarding need for operative intervention among the multiple cardiologists referring these patients for cardiac operations. Additionally, some of the cardiac surgeons leaned more to mitral repair versus mitral replacement than did others.

1. Barlow JB, Pocock WA, Marchand P, Denny M. The significance late systolic murmurs. *Am Heart J* 1963;66:443–452.
2. Waller BF, Morrow AG, Maron BJ, Del Negro AA, Kent KM, McGrath FJ, Wallace RB, McIntosh CL Roberts WC. Etiology clinically isolated, severe, chronic, pure mitral regurgitation: analys of 97 patients over 30 years of age having mitral valve replaceme *Am Heart J* 1982;104:276–288.
3. Ranganathan N, Silver MD, Robinson TI, Kostuk WJ, Felderhof C Patt NL, Wilson JK, Wigle ED. Angiographic-morphologic correlati in patients with severe mitral regurgitation due to prolapse of posterior mitral valve leaflet. *Circulation* 1973;48:514–518.
4. Higgins CB, Reinke RT, Gosink BB, Leopold GR. The significance mitral valve prolapse in middle-aged and elderly men. *Am Hear* 1976;91:292–296.
5. Kolisbash AJ, Bush CA, Fontana MB, Ryan JM, Kilman J, Woo CF. Mitral valve prolapse syndrome: analysis of 62 patients aged years and older. *Am J Cardiol* 1983;52:534–539.
6. Tresch DD, Doyle TP, Boncheck LI, Siegel R, Keelan MH Jr, Olin GN, Brooks HL. Mitral valve prolapse requiring surgery. Clinical pathologic study. *Am J Med* 1985;78:245–250.

7. Penkoske PA, Ellis FH Jr, Alexander S, Watkins E Jr. Results of valve reconstruction for mitral regurgitation secondary to mitral valve prolapse. *Am J Cardiol* 1985;55:735–738.
8. Kolibash AJ Jr, Kilman JW, Bush CA, Ryan JM, Fontana ME, Wooley CF. Evidence for progression from mild to severe mitral regurgitation in mitral valve prolapse. *Am J Cardiol* 1986;58:762–767.
9. Naggar CZ, Pearson WN, Seljan MP, with the technical assistance of Mannock LK, Masrof S, Elwood DJ. Frequency of complications of mitral valve prolapse in subjects aged 60 years and older. *Am J Cardiol* 1986;58:1209–1212.
10. Freed LA, Levy D, Levine RA, Larson MG, Evans JC, Fuller DL, Lehman B, Benjamin EJ. Prevalence and clinical outcome of mitral-valve prolapse. *N Engl J Med* 1999;341:1–7.
11. Ohki R, Yamamoto K, Okayama M, Nonaka M, Suzuki C, Ikeda U, Shimada K. The site of mitral valve prolapse is a predictor of atrial fibrillation. *Am J Cardiol* 2001,88:811–813.
12. Grigioni F, Avierinos J-F, Ling LH, Scott CG, Bailey KR, Tajik AJ, Frye RL, Enriquez-Sarano M. Atrial fibrillation complicating the course of degenerative mitral regurgitation. Determinants of long-term outcome. *J Am Coll Cardiol* 2002;40:84–92.
13. Avierinos J-F, Gersh BJ, Melton LJ III, Bailey KR, Shub C, Nishimura RA, Tajik AJ, Enriquez-Sarano M. Natural history of asymptomatic mitral valve prolapse in the community. *Circulation* 2002;106:1355–1361.
14. Bailey GWH, Braniff BA, Hancock EW, Cohn KE. Relation of left atrial pathology to atrial fibrillation in mitral valve disease. *Ann Intern Med* 1968;69:13–20.

Some observations on mitral and aortic valve disease

William Clifford Roberts, MD, and Jong Mi Ko, BA

SOURCES FOR MORPHOLOGIC STUDIES

Before 1960, the only source for studying the heart was the autopsy. The early years of cardiac valve replacement provided a rich source of necropsy "material" until valve techniques and artificial heart valves became more refined. In the 1950s and 1960s, most physicians attributed valvular heart disease in adults to rheumatic heart disease. During the 1960s and 1970s, many thousands of patients with rheumatic heart disease underwent replacement of one or more cardiac valves. By the 1980s, most of this rheumatic heart disease pool of patients had undergone operation; in addition, the frequency of rheumatic fever and subsequently rheumatic heart disease had dropped dramatically. By the 1970s, the congenitally malformed aortic valve was found to be frequent in adults with aortic stenosis (AS), and mitral valve prolapse (MVP) was being recognized as a common cause of pure (no associated stenosis) mitral regurgitation (MR). By the 1990s, the frequency of autopsies in US hospitals had dropped enormously compared with the 1950s, and operatively excised cardiac valves were becoming the major source of anatomic study. Although established by the 1980s, cardiac transplantation was rarely performed in patients with valvular heart disease.

Table 1. Functional and anatomic classification of valvular heart disease in 1010 necropsy patients aged ≥15 years*

Functional class	Patients (%)	Anatomic class				
		AV	MV	MV-AV	TV-MV	TV-MV-A
1. Aortic stenosis (AS)	292 (29%)	256 (88%)	0	35 (12%)	0	1 (0.3%)
2. Mitral stenosis (MS)	189 (19%)	0	117 (62%)	40 (21%)	13 (7%)	19 (10%
3. MS + AS	152 (15%)	0	0	120 (79%)	0	32 (21%
4. Aortic regurgitation (AR)†	119 (12%)	107 (90%)	0	10 (8%)	0	2 (2%)
5. Mitral regurgitation (MR)	97 (10%)	0	85 (88%)	8 (8%)	1 (1%)	3 (3%)
6. MS + AR	65 (6%)	0	52 (80%)	0	0	13 (20%
7. MR + AR	45 (4%)	0	0	39 (87%)	0	6 (13%)
8. AS + MR	23 (2%)	0	0	21 (91%)	0	2 (9%)
9. Tricuspid stenosis + MS ± AS	28 (3%)	0	0	0	4 (14%)	24 (86%
Totals	1010 (100%)‡	363 (36%)	254 (25%)	273 (27%)	18 (2%)	102 (10

* Excludes patients with mitral regurgitation secondary to coronary heart disease (papillary muscle dysfunction), carcinoid heart dise hypertrophic cardiomyopathy, and those with infective endocarditis limited to one or both right-sided cardiac valves. Tricuspid v regurgitation was present in many patients in most of the nine functional groups. All patients were in functional class III or IV (York Heart Association), and more than half had one or more cardiac operations.

† In many patients, the aortic valve cusps were normal or nearly normal and the regurgitation was the result of disease of the a (the Marfan and Marfan-like syndrome, syphilis, systemic hypertension, healed aortic dissection).

‡ The hearts in all 1010 patients were examined and classified by WCR.

From Roberts WC, 1987 (1); reproduced with permission from Roberts WC, 1983 (39).

AV indicates aortic valve; MV, mitral valve; TV, tricuspid valve.

FREQUENCY OF VARIOUS VALVULAR DISORDERS IN NECROPSY STUDIES

Roberts (1) personally studied 1010 hearts at necropsy in patients with fatal valvular heart disease *(Table 1)*. All had died between 1955 and 1980 and the specimens were retrieved fr a number of different hospitals, most of which were locate the Washington, DC, area. As shown in Table 1, these cases v given both a *functional* (valve stenosis ± regurgitation or p regurgitation [no element of stenosis]) and an *anatomic* clas cation. A number of these patients had only one dysfunctic valve but in addition had one or more anatomically abnor valves (normal function). (A valve may be anatomically abnor yet function normally.) AS was the most common functic

From the Baylor Heart and Vascular Institute and the Departments of Path and Medicine (Cardiology), Baylor University Medical Center, Dallas, Texas.

Corresponding author: William C. Roberts, MD, Baylor Heart and Vas Institute, Baylor University Medical Center, 621 North Hall Street, Dallas, 75226 (e-mail: wc.roberts@BaylorHealth.edu).

Table 2. Type of valvular dysfunction in patients* having aortic valve replacement and/or mitral valve replacement or repair at Baylor University Medical Center at Dallas (1993–2006)

Valve dysfunction	Patients (%)
1. Aortic stenosis (AS)	985 (53%)
2. Mitral stenosis (MS)	129 (7%)
3. MS + AS	54 (3%)
4. Aortic regurgitation (AR)†	326 (17%)
5. Mitral regurgitation (MR)*	313 (17%)
6. MS + AR	10 (<1%)
7. MR + AR	28 (1%)
8. AS + MR	27 (1%)
9. Tricuspid stenosis + MS + AS	0
Totals	1872 (100%)‡

Excludes patients with mitral regurgitation secondary to coronary heart disease (papillary muscle dysfunction), carcinoid heart disease, hypertrophic cardiomyopathy, and those with infective endocarditis limited to one or both right-sided cardiac valves. Tricuspid valve regurgitation was present in many patients in most of the nine functional groups.

In many patients, the aortic valve cusps were normal or nearly normal and the regurgitation was the result of disease of the aorta (the Marfan and Marfan-like syndrome, syphilis, systemic hypertension, healed aortic dissection).

The operatively excised valves in the 1872 patients were examined and classified by WCR.

sorder (29%); in 35 (12%) of these 292 patients, the mitral aflets were diffusely thickened (rheumatic heart disease) but ere was no clinical evidence of mitral dysfunction. Most of e 256 patients with AS and anatomically normal mitral valves d congenitally unicuspid or bicuspid aortic valves.

Mitral stenosis (MS) was the next most common function- valve disease, but 72 (38%) of these 189 patients also had atomic involvement of one or more other cardiac valves. All tients with MS, whether isolated or associated with a func- nal disorder of another cardiac valve, had the valvular disease ributed to rheumatic heart disease.

Combined MS and AS was the third most common func- nal valvular disease (15%), and 32 (21%) of these 152 cases o had anatomic disease of the tricuspid valve leaflets. The rely regurgitant lesions (aortic regurgitation [AR], MR, both) were less common. Tricuspid stenosis of rheumatic ology occurred in only 3% of the 1010 cases, and all had ociated MS with or without associated AS. No other large ies of patients with valvular heart disease studied at necropsy been reported in the last 25 years, and it is unlikely that h a large series, all studied by a single physician, will be umulated in the future because of the low autopsy rates in st hospitals today and because few specimens are retained efinitely after autopsy.

ANGING FREQUENCY OF VARIOUS VALVULAR DISORDERS IN CENT DECADES IN THE WESTERN WORLD

Today the most frequently studied operatively excised valve ne stenotic aortic valve, followed by a portion of posterior mitral leaflet in patients with MR excised secondary to MVP (*Table 2*). Operatively excised purely regurgitant aortic valves with or without excision of portions of ascending aorta are also common. Purely regurgitant mitral valves that are replaced usually yield only anterior mitral leaflets as specimens; the posterior leaflet is usually not excised. Tricuspid valves are rarely excised today.

The remainder of this article discusses specific mitral and aortic valvular disorders.

AORTIC STENOSIS (± REGURGITATION)

Frequency and causes

If systemic hypertension is not considered, AS is the second most common potentially fatal or fatal heart disease after coronary heart disease. There are three major causes of AS: *atherosclerosis* (formerly called degenerative), *congenitally malformed valves*, and *rheumatic heart disease*.

That atherosclerosis is a cause of AS is derived primarily from five pieces of evidence:

1. Patients with familial homozygous hyperlipidemia (serum total cholesterol levels >800 mg/dL from birth) usually develop calcific deposits on the aortic aspects of their aortic valve cusps early in life, usually by the teenage years (2).
2. Progression of AS can be slowed by lowering total and low-density lipoprotein cholesterol levels by statins (3).
3. Patients >65 years of age with AS involving a three-cuspid aortic valve (unassociated with mitral valve disease) usually have extensive atherosclerosis involving the major epicardial coronary arteries and usually other systemic arterial systems (4).
4. Serum total cholesterol levels and concomitant coronary bypass grafting tend to be higher in patients with AS involving three-cuspid aortic valves than in patients of similar age and sex without AS or with congenitally bicuspid aortic valves (5).
5. Histologic study of three-cuspid stenotic aortic valves demonstrates features similar to those in atherosclerotic plaques (2).

The unicuspid aortic valve appears to be stenotic from birth (6, 7). The congenitally bicuspid valve, however, is infrequently stenotic at birth but becomes stenotic as calcific deposits form on the aortic aspects of the cusps (8). Rheumatic heart disease never involves the aortic valve anatomically without also involving the mitral valve (9). Although the mitral valve may be diffusely abnormal anatomically, its function can be normal. Consequently, a patient with rheumatic heart disease can present initially with only aortic valve dysfunction, and therefore rheumatic heart disease has to be considered a cause of functionally isolated AS (± AR) or pure AR (9).

Valve structure

In patients with isolated AS (± AR) (only cardiac valve anatomically abnormal) the aortic valve may be unicuspid, bicuspid, tricuspid, or quadricuspid. The congenitally *unicuspid valve* is of two types: acommissural and unicommissural (7, 10). The acommissural valve, which represents <10% of the unicuspid valves, has a central orifice and no distinct commissures. The

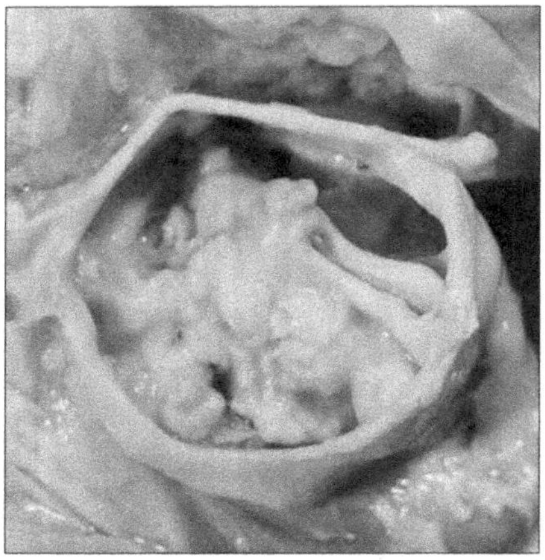

Figure 1. Aortic stenosis. *Congenitally unicuspid unicommissural aortic valve* in a 48-year-old man. The heart weighed 750 g. Reproduced with permission from Falcone MW et al, 1971 (7).

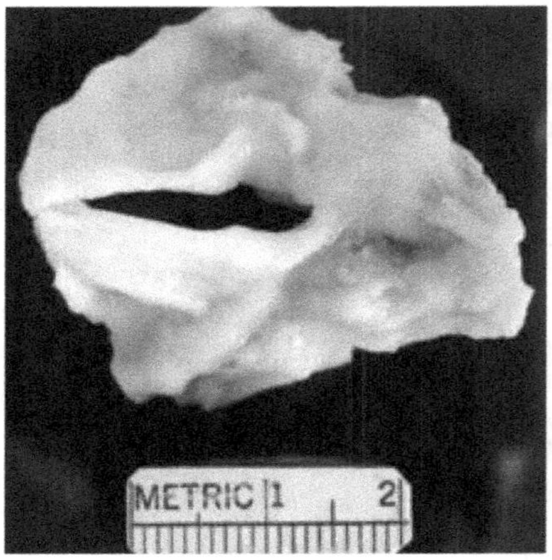

Figure 2. Aortic stenosis. Operatively excised *unicuspid unicommissural aortic valve* in a 41-year-old man. The valve weighed 5.42 g. The mean transvalvular pressure gradient was 51 mm Hg.

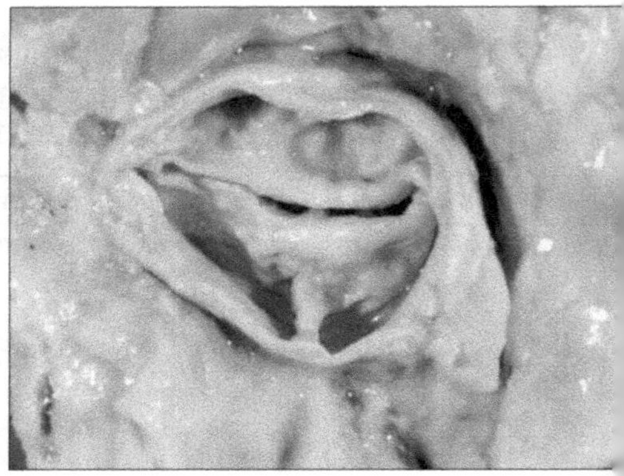

Figure 3. Aortic stenosis. *Congenitally bicuspid aortic va* in a 61-year-old man. At catheterization 2 years before h death, the peak systolic transvalvular pressure gradient w 45 mm Hg when the cardiac index was 2.6 L/min/m². He h complete heart block secondary to destruction of the atriove tricular bundle by calcium. The heart weighed 700 g.

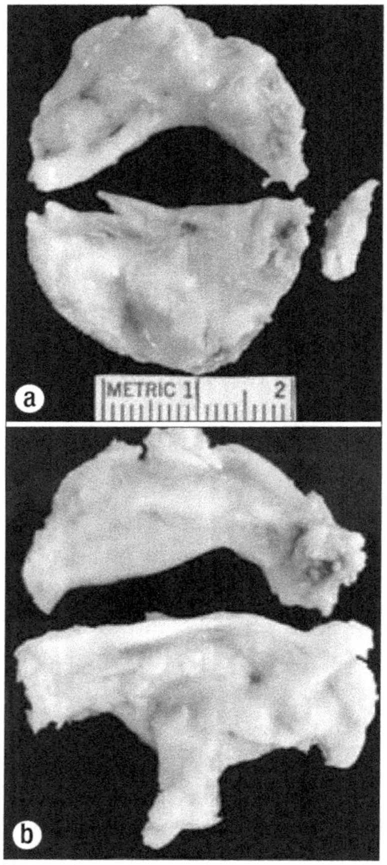

Figure 4. Aortic stenosis. Two operatively excised *congenitally bicuspid aortic valves.* **(a)** Valve in a 60-year-old man with severe heart failure. The valve weighed 4.65 g. **(b)** Valve in a 66-year-old man. The valve weighed 4.79 g and the peak systolic transvalvular gradient was 84 mm Hg.

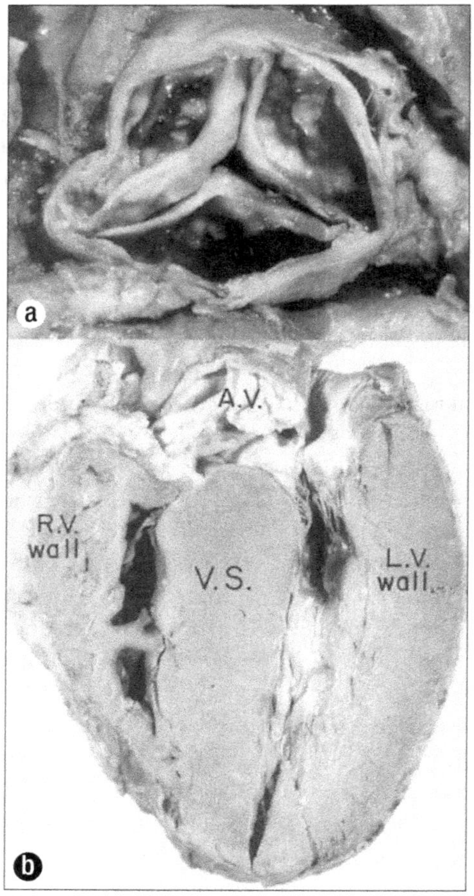

Figure 5. Aortic stenosis. **(a)** Three-cuspid aortic valve and **(b)** longitudinal section of the heart in an 89-year-old man whose heart weighed 440 g. None of the three aortic valve commissures are fused. The mitral annulus contains calcific deposits. Reproduced with permission from Roberts WC et al, 1971 (4).

unicommissural valve, which constitutes most of the unicuspid valves, has one commissure and usually two other rudimentary commissures (raphae) and a vertical orifice extending from the only true commissure *(Figures 1 and 2)* (9).

The *congenitally bicuspid valve (Figu 3 and 4)* of course has two cusps, and th are usually of slightly unequal size in bo cuspal surface area and weight. Usually o of the two cusps contains a raphe in its ce tral portion. Often the raphe cusp has fr margins that are V-shaped with the apex the V pointing to the raphe, producing concave configuration. The nonraphe cu in this circumstance commonly has a co vex configuration that fits nicely into t concave shape of the raphe cusp such th associated regurgitation is absent or mi mal. These bicuspid valves with a conca configuration of the raphe cusp and a conv appearance of free margin of the nonrap cusp are often confused with tricuspid val with fusion of one of three commissur In other bicuspid valves the free margins both cusps are relatively straight.

The *tricuspid aortic valve* is common older patients with AS (atherosclerotic c gin) and in patients in whom the AS is rheumatic etiology. (These latter patie always have mitral leaflets that are diffu fibrotic [with or without focal calcific dep its], or at least the margins of both leaflets everywhere thickened by fibrous tissue.) In tients with AS of rheumatic etiology, on more of the three commissures are often fu and the cusps may be either diffusely or foc fibrotic with or without commissural fusio calcific deposits. The stenotic tricuspid ao valve in older persons contains calcific dep on the aortic surfaces, usually involving the sites of cuspal att ments, and the commissures characteristically are not fused *(Fi 5)*. Thus, operative excision produces three cusps, none of whi attached to another *(Figure 6)*. Older patients with AS o

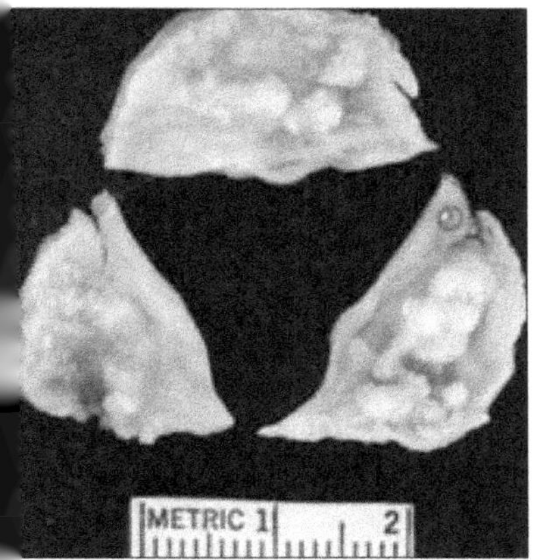

igure 6. Aortic stenosis. Operatively ex-sed aortic valve in a 70-year-old man. ıe valve weighed 1.69 g, the peak systolic ansvalvular gradient was 55 mm Hg, and ft ventricular function was normal (ejection ıction = 60%).

also have calcified mitral anomaly. *Figure 7* shows how calcium might develop in both the aortic valve and the mitral annulus.

The *quadricuspid aortic valve* is rare (12). When present and if dysfunctional, the dysfunction is usually pure AR. AS with a quadricuspid valve is exceedingly rare, seen by Roberts (13) in 1 of 1118 operatively excised stenotic aortic valves.

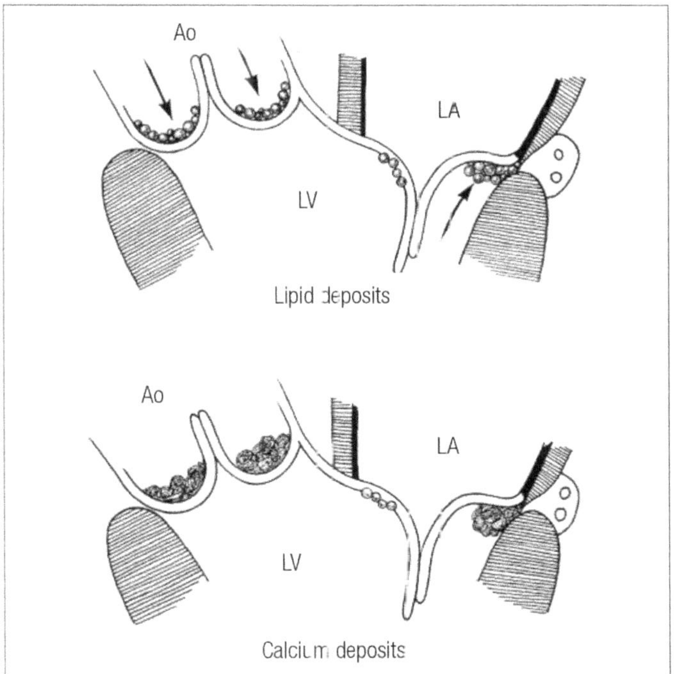

Figure 7. Aortic valve and mitral annular calcium. Commonly calcific deposits are present in the aortic valve cusps mitral annulus, and epicardial coronary arteries. Roberts has referred to this condition as "the senile cardiac calcification syndrome" (11). The cause of the deposits is speculative, but atherosclerosis seems to be the most reasonable. In younger individuals lipid deposits are usually present on the aortic aspects of the aortic valve cusps and on the ventricular aspects of the posterior mitral leaflet and, to a much lesser extent, on the ventricular aspect of the anterior mitral leaflet. The lipid in these locations is usually both intracellular and extracellular. Degeneration of the lipid probably leads to the calcific deposits in these locations.

ecropsy studies of patients with isolated aortic stenosis (± R) and never a cardiac operation—natural history

During a 32-year period at the National Institutes of Health JIH), Roberts collected (mainly from hospitals in the Wash-gton, DC, area) the hearts of 192 adults (aged 16–99 years) ith isolated AS; none of them had ever had a cardiac opera-ɔn (unpublished data). Of the 192 patients, 139 (72%) were en and 53 (28%) were women *(Table 3)*. The average age of e men was 61 years, and that of the women, 71 years, the same average ages of death as in coronary heart disease. The weight of the hearts was 610 ± 135 g (normal, <400 g) in the men and 486 ± 111 g (normal, <350 g) in the women. The aortic valve was congenitally unicuspid in 17 patients (9%), congenitally bicuspid in 89 patients (46%), and tricuspid in 86 (45%) *(Table 4)*. Other observations in these 192 patients are shown in Tables 3 and 4.

Table 3. Findings at necropsy in unoperated isolated aortic valve stenosis in men vs women (n = 192)

ɑriable	Men (n = 139)		Women (n = 53)	
ǝe (years): range (mean)	16–99 (61)		32–90 (71)	
ʼmptomatic	103/129 (80%)		41/49 (84%)	
ɫtal cholesterol (mg/dL)	206 ± 63		161± 26	
ʼverity of stenosis				
1+	24 (17%)		7 (13%)	
2+	22 (16%)		9 (17%)	
3+	93 (67%)		37 (70%)	
ronary narrowing				
0	73 (53%)		20 (38%)	
≥1	66 (47%)		33 (62%)	
tral annular calcium				
0	101 (73%)		23 (43%)	
1+–3+	38 (27%)		30 (57%)	
ɑrt weight (g)	610 ± 135		486 ± 111	
ʼtic valve				
Jnicuspid	16 (12%)	59%	1 (2%)	45%
Bicuspid	66 (47%)		23 (43%)	
Tricuspid	57 (41%)		29 (55%)	
t ventricular				
Fibrosis	57 (41%)		13 (25%)	
Necrosis	13 (9%)		5 (9%)	

Weights of operatively excised stenotic aortic valves

The weight of operatively excised stenotic aortic valves is useful in quantitating the severity of the stenosis because the weight is determined primarily by the quantity of calcific deposits and the larger the calcific deposits, the greater the transvalvular pressure gradient (13–24). Roberts and colleagues (22) reported weights in 1849 operatively excised stenotic valves in patients aged 21 to 91 years without concomitant mitral valve replacement or mitral stenosis. These authors found that the weight of the stenotic valves varied inversely with the number of aortic valve cusps (14). The unicuspid valves were the heaviest, the bicuspid valves the next heaviest, and the tricuspid aortic valves, the lightest. The men had heavier valves than did the women *(Figure 8)*, and the younger patients had heavier valves than did the older patients. The mean weights of the valves were similar in patients whose body mass index was <25, 25–30, and >30 kg/m^2. Mean valve weights also were heavier in the patients

Table 4. Underlying structure of the aortic valve in unoperated patients studied at necropsy with isolated aortic valve stenosis with or without associated aortic regurgitation (n = 192)

Variable	Unicuspid (n = 17) [9%]	Bicuspid (n = 89) [46%]	Tricuspid (n = 86) [45%]
Age (years): range (mean)	25–73 (46)	16–87 (62)	36–99 (64)
Males	16 (94%)	66 (74%)	57 (66%)
Symptomatic	15 (88%)	73/84 (87%)	57/78 (73%)
Total cholesterol (mg/dL)	216	203	173
Mode of death			
Sudden (outside hospital)	1 (6%)	15 (17%)	11 (13%)
Sudden (inside hospital)	1 (6%)	13 (15%)	6 (7%)
Nonsudden (cardiac)	14 (82%)	47 (53%)	45 (52%)
Vascular	0	2 (2%)	4 (5%)
Noncardiovascular	1 (6%)	12 (14%)	20 (23%)
Severity of stenosis			
1+	1 (6%)	11 (12%)	19 (22%)
2+	0	14 (16%)	17 (20%)
3+	16 (94%)	64 (72%)	50 (58%)
Coronary narrowing			
0	15 (88%)	57 (64%)	41 (48%)
≥1	2 (12%)	32 (36%)	45 (52%)
Mitral annular calcium			
0	12 (71%)	72 (81%)	40 (47%)
1+–3+	5 (29%)	17 (19%)	46 (53%)
Heart weight (g) (mean)	617	578	573
Left ventricular			
Fibrosis	8/15 (53%)	34/88 (39%)	28/85 (33%)
Necrosis	1/16 (6%)	8/87 (9%)	9/85 (11%)

who *did not* undergo simultaneous coronary artery bypass grafting than in those who did.

Table 5 shows various clinical findings in the 1849 patients whose stenotic aortic valves were studied by Roberts and colleagues (22). The patients underwent aortic valve replacement at three different institutions: NIH from 1963 to 1989, Georgetown University Medical Center (GUMC) from 1969 to 1992, and Baylor University Medical Center (BUMC) from 1993 to 2004. All 1849 operatively excised stenotic valves were examined and classified by WCR. Patients having simultaneous mitral valve replacement or mitral stenosis were excluded. The valves excised at NIH and at GUMC from 1963 to 1992 were heavier than the valves excised at BUMC from 1993 to 2004: men 4.05 ± 1.91 (NIH), 4.36 ± 1.83 (GUMC), and 3.11 ± 1.51 g (BUMC); women 2.80 ± 1.26 (NIH), 3.02 ± 1.26 (GUMC), and 1.89 ± 0.87 g (BUMC).

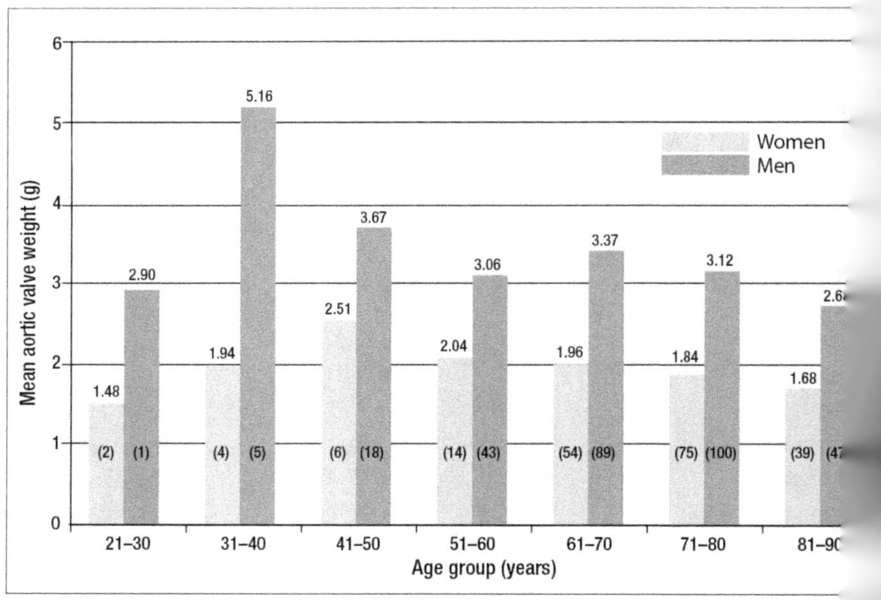

Figure 8. Aortic valve weights in men and women in each of 7 decades. All had aortic stenosis. Reproc with permission from Roberts WC and Ko JM, 2003 (14).

Not only did the valve weights vary according to valve struc ture (unicuspid > bicuspid > tricuspid), but often there was varia tion in individual cusps among patients with bicuspid valves an among patients with tricuspid valves (15, 16). Of 200 operativel excised stenotic congenitally bicuspid valves, the two cusps in 15 patients (76%) differed in weight by >0.2 g, and in 48 patien (24%) the cusps were of similar weight (≤0.2 g difference) (15 In 161 of the 200 patients, a raphe was present in one of the tw cusps: the raphe and nonraphe cusps differed in weight in 12 patients (74%) with the raphe cusps being heavier in 89 patien (55%), lighter in 31 patients (19%), and of similar weight in 4 (26%). Of the 39 patients without a raphe in one cusp, in 3 patients (82%) the two cusps were of different (>0.2 g) weig and in 7 patients (18%), similar in weight (≤0.2 g).

Of 260 operatively excised stenotic three-cuspid aort valves, all three cusps differed (by >0.1 g) in weight in 71 p tients (27%); all three cusps were similar (≤0.1 g difference) weight in 33 patients (13%), and in 156 patients (60%) o cusp differed from either of the other two cusps which we similar in weight (16).

Why might cusps of operatively excised stenotic valves d fer in weight? The most likely explanation seems to be th the cusps differ in size, that is, in surface area, from birth. T cusp with the largest surface area has, of course, a larger a on which calcium can be deposited, and the weight of a cu is determined primarily by the amount of calcium deposit on its aortic surface.

Relation of aortic valve weight to transvalvular peak systoli pressure gradient

The best determinant of the magnitude of obstruction patients with AS has been debated. Determinants conside have been aortic valve area or index, mean transvalvular syst gradient, and peak transvalvular systolic gradients. Roberts a Ko (17) compared the weights of operatively excised sten

Table 5. Data in patients having isolated aortic valve replacement for aortic stenosis (± aortic regurgitation) at three different medical centers

Variable	NIH (1963–1989)	GUMC (1969–1992)	BUMC (1993–2004)
Valve structure			
Unicuspid			
Men	84/342 (25%)	56/255 (22%)	36/601 (6%)
Women	14/110 (13%)	24/145 (17%)	12/356 (4%)
Bicuspid			
Men	158/342 (46%)	129/255 (50%)	316/601 (53%)
Women	53/110 (48%)	68/145 (47%)	153/356 (43%)
Tricuspid			
Men	47/342 (14%)	63/255 (25%)	242/601 (40%)
Women	28/110 (25%)	48/145 (33%)	186/356 (52%)
ndeterminate			
Men	53/342 (15%)	7/255 (3%)	7/601 (1%)
Women	15/110 (14%)	5/145 (3%)	5/356 (1%)
Age (years): range (mean ± SD)			
Men	21–82 (54 ± 12)	24–88 (64 ± 11)	25–91 (69 ± 12)
Men ≥65	62/331 (19%)	124/251 (49%)	424/601 (71%)
Women	33–86 (57 ± 11)	22–89 (67 ± 12)	27–91 (70 ± 11)
Women ≥65	27/104 (26%)	94/142 (66%)	273/356 (77%)
Gender			
Men	342/452 (76%)	255/400 (64%)	601/957 (63%)
Women	110/452 (24%)	145/400 (36%)	356/957 (37%)
Aortic valve weight (g): range (mean ± SD)			
Men	0.70–10.2 (4.05 ± 1.91)	1.20–11.0 (4.36 ± 1.83)	0.89–11.30 (3.11 ± 1.51)
Women	0.55–5.50 (2.80 ± 1.26)	0.40–6.70 (3.02 ± 1.26)	0.45–4.97 (1.89 ± 0.87)
Left ventricular to aortic peak systolic gradient (mm Hg): range (mean ± SD)			
Men	10–145 (69 ± 30)	10–160 (69 ± 25)	10–141 (52 ± 23)
Women	10–165 (76 ± 34)	30–170 (81 ± 32)	10–133 (54 ± 28)
Aortic valve area (cm^2): range (mean ± SD)			
Men	0.20–1.90 (0.66 ± 0.32)	0.27–1.97 (0.75 ± 0.31)	0.20–1.90 (0.78 ± 0.26)
Women	0.23–1.10 (0.53 ± 0.21)	0.20–1.30 (0.57 ± 0.21)	0.18–1.49 (0.67 ± 0.22)
Cardiac index (L/min/m^2): range (mean ± SD)			
Men	1.10–5.00 (2.58 ± 0.72)	1.00–7.30 (2.87 ± 0.93)	–
Women	1.60–4.50 (2.68 ± 0.69)	1.60–6.20 (2.79 ± 0.81)	–
Simultaneous coronary bypass			
Men	21/238 (9%)	77/198 (39%)	332/601 (55%)
Women	6/74 (8%)	29/118 (25%)	167/356 (47%)

oduced with permission from Roberts WC et al, 2005 (22).

C indicates Baylor University Medical Center; GUMC, Georgetown University Medical er; NIH, National Institutes of Health.

aortic valves to peak transvalvular systolic pressure gradient and to aortic valve area. The results of these studies in 201 men and in 123 women with isolated AS are shown in *Table 6*. In both men and women the weights of the stenotic aortic valves increased significantly as the peak left ventricular-to-aortic systolic gradient increased, but valve weight had essentially no relation to aortic valve area. Women had significantly lower valve weights, with peak gradients similar to those in men. In men with valve weights from 1 to 2 g, the peak transvalvular gradient averaged 36 mm Hg and the valve areas, 0.86 cm^2; in the men with valve weights >6 g, the peak gradients averaged 87 mm Hg, whereas the valve was 0.71 cm^2. In women with valve weights ≤1 g, the peak gradient averaged 28 mm Hg and valve area, 0.83 cm^2; in women whose valve weighed from >3 to 4 g, the peak gradients averaged 85 mm Hg, and the valve area, 0.51 cm^2 (Table 6).

Relatively few operatively excised aortic valves in adults with AS are ≥5 g, and those reaching that weight are usually congenitally malformed. Of unicuspid valves, 37 (30%) of 124 valves in men and 5 (11%) of 44 in women reached this weight; of bicuspid valves, 96 (18%) of 521 valves in men and 4 (2%) of 236 valves in women reached this weight (unpublished data). In contrast, only 15 (4%) of 361 tricuspid valves in men and only 2 (0.7%) of 281 valves in women reached this weight. Of 1038 operatively excised stenotic aortic valves in men, 161 (16%) were ≥5 g, and of 571 valves in women, only 13 (2%) reached this weight. Seven operatively excised stenotic valves weighed ≥10 g: all were in men and all seven were either unicuspid or bicuspid and the peak pressure gradient across them ranged from 80 to 143 mm Hg (average, 101) (unpublished data).

Associated coronary arterial narrowing

Patients with operatively excised congenitally unicuspid and bicuspid valves have significantly less epicardial coronary arterial narrowing than do patients with tricuspid aortic valves *(Table 7)*. Concomitant coronary artery bypass grafting also varies according to the era during which the aortic valve replacement was done and the institution where it was done. Also, criteria for performing coronary artery bypass grafting in patients having aortic valve replacement have changed with time.

Relation to left bundle branch block and/or complete heart block

At one time, patients with AS and left bundle branch block or complete heart block were believed to have these conduction disturbances because of associated severe coronary arterial narrowing from atherosclerosis. Study at necropsy, however, of many patients with combined AS and left bundle branch block or complete heart block has indicated that the conduction disturbance was due not to associated coronary narrowing but to destruction of the left bundle branches or the atrioventricular bundle by calcific deposits that had extended caudally from the aortic valve (Roberts, unpublished data). Most of these patients had congenitally malformed aortic valves—not tricuspid valves—and severe degrees of hemodynamic obstruction as a result of the heavy calcific deposits.

Table 6. Age, body mass index, concomitant coronary artery bypass, left ventricular to aortic peak systolic gradients, and aortic valve areas in seven aortic valve weight groups in men and in women

AV weight (g)	No. of patients	Age (years): range (average)	BMI (kg/m^2): range (average)	AV weights (g): range (average)	LV–aorta PSG (mm Hg): range (average)	AV area (cm^2): range (mean)	Coronary bypass	UAV or BAV	Ejection fraction (%) No.	Range (mean)	No. (%) ≤40	No. (%) >40
Men												
≤1	0	–	–	–	–	–	–	–	–	–	–	–
>1–2	41	47–90 (72)	19–37 (27)	1.16–2.00 (1.64)	11–81 (36)	0.27–1.43 (0.86)	27 (66%)	11 (27%)	37	15–78 (48)	13 (35%)	24 (65%
>2–3	60	29–87 (69)	20–43 (29)	2.01–3.00 (2.58)	15–97 (45)	0.42–2.25 (0.89)	32 (53%)	24 (40%)	52	10–85 (51)	14 (27%)	38 (73%
>3–4	50	37–84 (69)	17–40 (27)	3.03–4.00 (3.40)	20–100 (56)	0.20–1.63 (0.75)	26 (52%)	30 (60%)	44	15–80 (53)	7 (16%)	37 (84%
>4–5	29	42–87 (69)	18–45 (28)	4.01–4.84 (4.40)	20–108 (64)	0.32–1.06 (0.67)	11 (38%)	25 (86%)	26	15–70 (53)	5 (19%)	21 (81%
>5–6	12	49–90 (70)	24–36 (28)	5.03–5.93 (5.60)	50–116 (71)	0.40–0.88 (0.60)	3 (25%)	10 (83%)	10	20–65 (43)	4 (40%)	6 (60%
>6	9	38–84 (58)	21–38 (28)	6.24–11.30 (7.92)	35–141 (87)	0.39–1.23 (0.71)	2 (22%)	8 (89%)	8	15–70 (51)	2 (25%)	6 (75%
Women												
≤1	10	55–85 (74)	21–44 (30)	0.69–0.95 (0.83)	15–62 (28)	0.34–1.28 (0.83)	7 (70%)	2 (20%)	9	30–70 (47)	4 (44%)	5 (56%
>1–2	73	19–88 (71)	17–51 (29)	1.02–1.99 (1.46)	10–119 (49)	0.18–1.49 (0.72)	40 (55%)	14 (19%)	66	15–80 (56)	9 (14%)	57 (86
>2–3	29	30–87 (70)	18–50 (28)	2.04–3.00 (2.42)	26–113 (63)	0.27–1.09 (0.58)	15 (52%)	12 (41%)	23	30–80 (54)	4 (17%)	19 (83
>3–4	10	47–85 (73)	17–35 (26)	3.14–4.00 (3.42)	53–131 (85)	0.23–0.78 (0.51)	3 (30%)	9 (90%)	9	45–75 (53)	0	9 (100
>4–5	1	83	29	4.27	53	0.75	0	1 (100%)	1	50	0	1 (100
>5–6	0	–	–	–	–	–	–	–	–	–	–	–
>6	0	–	–	–	–	–	–	–	–	–	–	–

Reproduced with permission from Roberts WC and Ko JM, 2004 (17).
AV indicates aortic valve; BAV, bicuspid aortic valve; BMI, body mass index; LV, left ventricular; PSG, peak systolic gradient; UAV, unicuspid aortic valve.

PURE AORTIC REGURGITATION

There are two major causes of pure (no element of stenosis) AR: 1) conditions affecting primarily the valve, and 2) conditions affecting the aorta and only secondarily causing the valve to be incompetent. Roberts and Ko (25) recently reviewed the cause of pure AR in 268 patients having isolated aortic valve replacement at BUMC from 1993 to 2005. As shown in *Table 8*, conditions affecting primarily the valve were the cause of the AR in 122 patients (46%), and nonvalve conditions were the cause in 146 patients (54%). Among the former, the *congenitally bicuspid valve* unassociated with infective endocarditis was the problem in 59 patients, 22 (37%) of whom had resection of portions of the dilated ascending aorta. Eleven of the 22 patients with resected aortas had severe loss of medial elastic fibers. Infective endocarditis was the cause in 46 patients, 15 (33%) of whom had congenitally bicuspid aortic valves. Thus, of the 122 with valve conditions causing the AR, 74 (61%) had congenitally bicuspid aortic valves. Why one congenitally

Table 7. Frequency of concomitant coronary artery bypass grafting among patients having isolated aortic valve replaceme for aortic stenosis at three different institutions*

Valve structure	NIH (1963–1989) (n = 259)	GUMC (1969–1992) (n = 308)	BUMC (1993–2007) (n = 1351)
Unicuspid	2/61 (3%)	13/55 (24%)	13/83 (16%)
Bicuspid	13/140 (9%)	42/162 (26%)	280/646 (43%
Tricuspid	10/58 (17%)	47/91 (52%)	390/622 (63%

*Excludes cases in which the number of valve cusps was unclear (indeterminate).

BUMC indicates Baylor University Medical Center; GUMC, Georgetown University Me Center; NIH, National Institutes of Health.

bicuspid aortic valve becomes stenotic (8, 26), another pure regurgitation without superimposed infective endo ditis (27), another becomes severely dysfunctional only w

Table 8. Causes of aortic regurgitation in patients having isolated aortic valve replacement at Baylor University Medical Center (1993–2005)

Causes of aortic regurgitation	Total	Age (years) at operation: range (mean)	M	F	Acute	Chronic	SH	CABG	Portions of ascending aorta: Excised	Portions of ascending aorta: Examined histologically	Portions of ascending aorta: CMN (3+, 4+)	BAV	Calcium deposits on AV cusps	Aortic valve weight (g): range (mean): Men	Aortic valve weight (g): range (mean): Women
Valve (n = 122; 46%)															
ongenital nalformation vithout infective endocarditis															
Bicuspid	59 (22%)	22–77 (55)	49	10	0	59	39 (66%)	18 (31%)	22	22	11	59	31	0.52–2.99 (1.42)	0.68–1.80 (1.24)
Quadricuspid	2 (1%)	53, 79 (66)	0	2	0	2	0	1 (50%)	0	0	0	0	0	—	0.57, 1.13 (0.85)
Tricuspid	5 (2%)	33–48 (40)	3	2	0	5	2 (40%)	0	1	1	0	0	0	1.11–1.40 (1.23)	0.34, 0.66 (.050)
nfective ndocarditis	46 (17%)	21–82 (45)	31	15	27	19	29 (63%)	7 (15%)	6	4	0	15	8	0.77–2.31 (1.53)	0.44–2.50 (0.98)
heumatic?	8 (3%)	25–63 (47)	6	2	0	8	6 (75%)	2 (25%)	0	0	0	0	3	1.10–2.45 (1.81)	1.31, 1.83 (1.57)
iscellaneous	2 (1%)	24, 42 (33)	1	1	0	2	2 (100%)	1 (50%)	0	0	0	0	0	0.55	—
onvalve (n = 146; 54%)															
ortic ssection	28 (10%)	25–78 (58)	20	8	21	7	22 (79%)	5* (17%)	28	20	5	3	4	0.51–1.19 (0.81)	0.37–0.90 (0.59)
arfan or rme fruste	15 (6%)	21–71 (47)	9	6	0	15	10 (67%)	1† (7%)	15	13	13	0	2	0.73–1.01 (0.94)	0.35–0.85 (0.66)
ortitis	12 (4%)	35–82 (66)	5	7	0	12	10 (83%)	5 (42%)	12	12	12	0	2	0.63–0.79 (0.70)	0.35–0.70 (0.54)
ology unclear	91 (34%)	50–84 (66)	58	33	0	91	83 (91%)	46 (51%)	7	7	0	0	26	0.48–2.13 (1.08)	0.31–1.74 (0.73)
tal	268 (100%)	21–84 (57)	182 (68%)	86 (32%)	48 (18%)	220 (82%)	203 (76%)	86 (32%)	91 (34%)	76	41	77 (29%)	76/263 (29%)	0.48–2.99 (1.22) 151‡	0.31–2.50 (0.81) 75‡

ır other patients had CABG due to extension of the aortic dissection into a coronary artery.

e additional patient had CABG due to extension of the aortic dissection into a coronary artery.

mber of cases with aortic valve weight.

roduced with permission from Roberts WC et al, 2006 (25).

ndicates aortic valve; BAV, bicuspid aortic valve; CABG, coronary artery bypass grafting; CMN, "cystic medial necrosis" (magnitude of loss of elastic fibers in the aorta's media); male; M, male; SH, systemic hypertension.

ective endocarditis appears (28), and some function nor- lly an entire lifetime is unclear (8). Of 85 patients, aged 15 79 years, with congenitally bicuspid aortic valves studied utopsy by Roberts (8), 61 valves (72%) were stenotic, 2) had pure regurgitation without superimposed infective ocarditis, 9 (11%) had AR because of infective endocar- s, and 13 (15%) functioned normally during the patients' to 59 years of life (mean, 45).

Rheumatic heart disease is a relatively infrequent cause of pure in patients with normally functioning mitral valves (9). All patients (by our definition of rheumatic heart disease) have diffuse fibrosis of the mitral leaflets or at least diffuse thickening of the margins of these leaflets. In this circumstance mitral valve function would be normal despite the anatomic abnormality.

Infective endocarditis more commonly involves a three-cuspid aortic valve than a two-cuspid one because the tricuspid valve is so much more common than the bicuspid valve (28).

Rheumatoid arthritis is a rare cause of AR. The anatomic abnormality is specific for this condition and consists of rheumatoid nodules within the aortic valve cusps (29, 30).

Conditions affecting the ascending aorta and causing it to dilate cause AR more commonly than those conditions

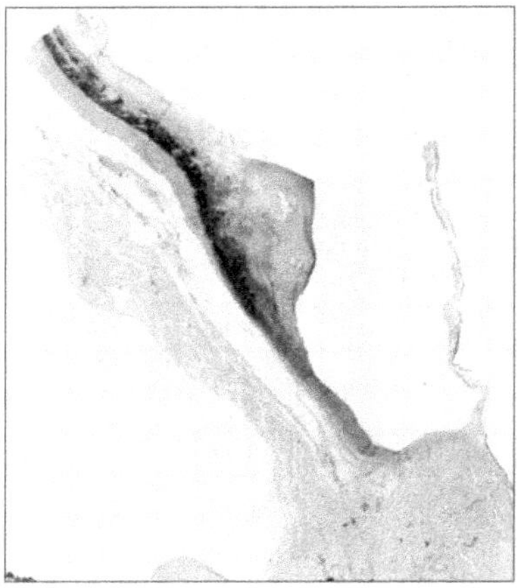

Figure 9. Cardiovascular syphilis. Photomicrographs of an aortic valve cusp, sinus portion of aorta (behind the cusp), and proximal tubular portion of ascending aorta, which is thickened by intimal and adventitial fibrous tissue. Many medial elastic fibers have been destroyed. The location of the process in the tubular portion of the aorta with sparing of the sinus portion of the aorta is characteristic of cardiovascular syphilis. Elastic tissue stain, ×4.5.

affecting primarily the aortic valve. Of 146 patients having pure AR and isolated aortic valve replacement, the cause of the AR was not determined after examination of the operatively excised aorta and aortic valve (25). Many of these patients had *systemic hypertension* but only mild dilation of the aorta, and all had normal or nearly normal three-cuspid aortic valves. It is likely that systemic hypertension in some way played a role in the AR (31, 32).

Aortic dissection usually produces acute AR due to the splitting of the aortic media behind the aortic valve commissures, resulting in prolapse of one or more cusps toward the left ventricular cavity (33).

Diffuse thickening of the tubular portion of the central ascending aorta with sparing of the aortic wall behind the sinuses is characteristic of *cardiovascular syphilis* (34). These patients generally undergo a cardiovascular operation because of diffuse aneurysmal dilatation of the tubular portion of ascending aorta, not as a rule because of severe AR. *Granulomatous (giant cell) aortitis* grossly mimics cardiovascular syphilis but is far less common. During the past 10 years, 15 patients have had resection of aneurysmally dilated syphilitic aortas with or without simultaneous aortic valve replacement at BUMC (unpublished). The characteristic histologic feature of cardiovascular syphilis is extensive thickening of the aortic wall due to fibrous thickening of the intima and adventitia *(Figure 9)*. The medial elastic fibers and smooth-muscle cells are also replaced focally by scars due to narrowings in the vasa vasora. Focal collections of plasma cells and lymphocytes are present in the adventitia. Giant cell aortitis is similar to syphilitic aortitis except for the presence of multinucleated giant cells.

The AR in patients with *the Marfan syndrome* and forme fruste varieties of it is the result of severe dilatation of the sinus portion and proximal tubular portion of the aorta (35). The consequence of the "aortic root" dilatation is stretching of the aortic valve cusps in roughly a straigh line between the commissures, leading to a wide-open centr regurgitant stream. In contrast to cardiovascular syphilis, th aortic wall in the Marfan syndrome is thinner than norm due to the massive loss of medial elastic fibers and lack o thickening of either the intima or the adventitia.

Ankylosing spondylitis causes AR by involving both the valv cusps and the portion of aorta behind and adjacent to th lateral attachments of the aortic valve cusps (36, 37). Abo 5% of patients with this form of arthritis develop AR. Th bases of the aortic valve cusps become densely thickened b fibrous tissue, which is also present on the ventricular aspect the anterior mitral leaflet and on the left ventricular aspect the membranous ventricular septum. Varying degrees of hea block may result from this subaortic deposit of dense fibro tissue. The AR associated with ankylosing spondylitis is usual severe, with diastolic pressures in both the aorta and the le ventricle often being similar. The histologic appearance of t aorta in ankylosing spondylitis is similar to that in syphilit but the syphilitic process never extends onto the aortic val cusps or into the subvalvular area and rarely involves the w of aorta behind the sinuses.

A diagram of the various conditions affecting the aor valve is shown in *Figure 10*.

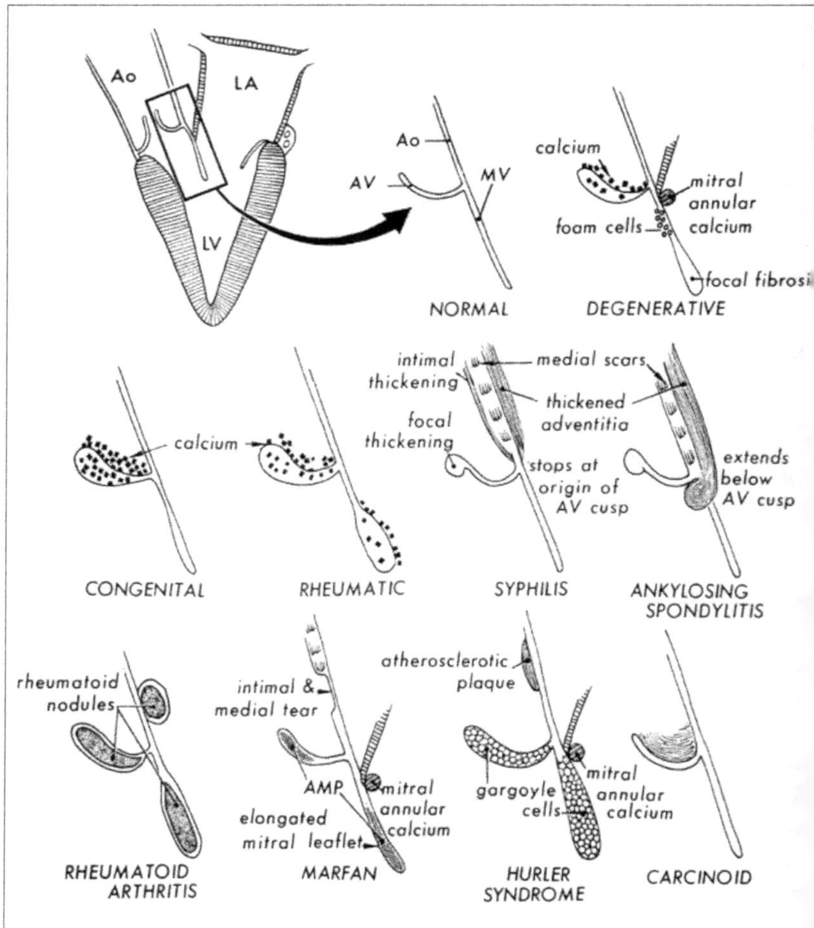

Figure 10. Some of the conditions affecting the aorta or aortic valve or mitral valve. Reproduce permission from Roberts WC and Perloff JK, 1972 (38).

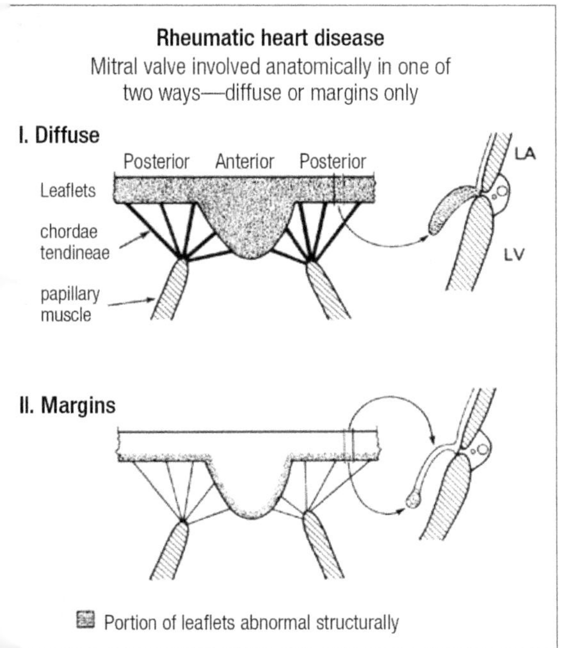

gure 11. The two types of anatomic involvement of the mitral lve in rheumatic heart disease.

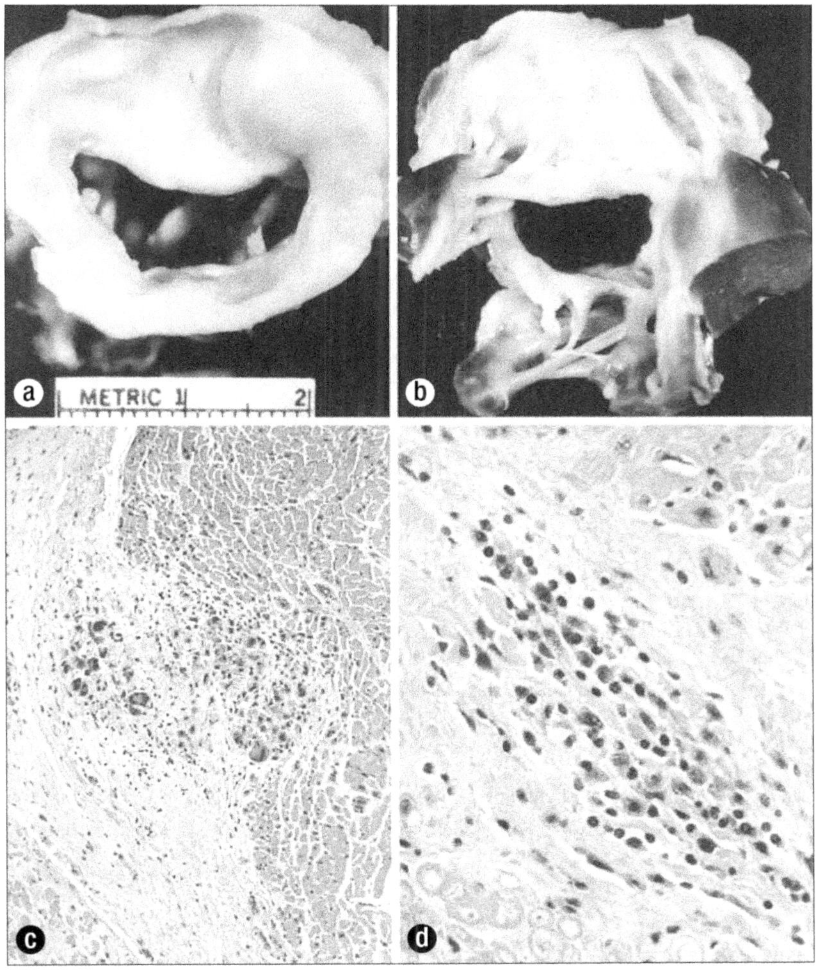

Figure 12. Acute rheumatic fever and mitral stenosis Excised mitral valve in a 23-year-old Indian woman with mitral stenosis (13 mm Hg mean diastolic pressure gradient between pulmonary artery wedge and left ventricle) and regurgitation. She had had acute rheumatic fever initially at age 7 years and recurrence of migratory polyarthritis at age 22. During the early postoperative course after mitral valve replacement, she had swelling and pain in one knee and one ankle and erythema about two joints. Shown are the excised valves viewed from **(a)** the left atrium and **(b)** the left ventricle and **(c, d)** Aschoff bodies, which were numerous in both excised left ventricular papillary muscles. Hematoxylin and eosin stain, ×110 (c), ×400 (d). Reproduced with permission from Virmani R and Roberts WC, 1977 (41).

ITRAL STENOSIS

Of the 1010 patients aged ≥15 years with nctionally severe valvular cardiac disease stud-d at necropsy by Roberts up to 1980, 434 4%) had MS (1). MS occurred alone in 189 4%) patients and in combination with other nctional valve lesions in the other 245 patients 6%). MS was of rheumatic etiology in all 434 tients.

Rheumatic heart disease may be viewed as a sease of the mitral valve; other valves also may involved both anatomically and functionally, t anatomically the mitral valve is always in-lved (38, 39) *(Figure 11)*. *Aschoff bodies* have ver been reported in hearts without anatomic ease of the mitral valve (39). Of the first 543 tients with severe valvular heart disease that Roberts and rmani (40) studied at necropsy, 11 (2.7%) had Aschoff bod-, and all had anatomic mitral valve disease. The 11 patients nged in age from 18 to 68 years (mean, 38), and 9 had a tory of acute rheumatic fever; 9 had MS with or without sfunction of one or more other cardiac valves; 1 had isolated ; and 1 had both AR and MR. All 11 had diffuse fibrous ckening of the mitral leaflets, and all but one had diffuse atomic lesions of at least two other cardiac valves. Thus, ong patients with chronic valve disease, Aschoff bodies, only anatomic lesion pathognomic of rheumatic heart ease, usually indicate diffuse anatomic lesions of one or re cardiac valves, and the most common hemodynamic on is MS ± MR.

Although rare at necropsy in patients with fatal chronic ve disease, Aschoff bodies are fairly common in the heart patients having mitral commissurotomy for MS. Among 481 patients having various valve operations, Aschoff bodies were found by Virmani and Roberts (41) in 40 (21%) of 191 operatively excised left atrial appendages, in 4 (2%) of 273 operatively excised left ventricular papillary muscles, and in 1 (6%) of 17 patients in whom both appendage and papillary muscle were excised. Of these 45 patients with Aschoff bodies, 44 had MS *(Figure 12)* and only one, a 10-year-old boy, had pure MR. Sinus rhythm was present preoperatively in 38 (84%), and atrial fibrillation in 7 (16%).

Not only is rheumatic heart disease a disorder of the cardiac valves, it may also affect mural endocardium, epicardium, and myocardium. The atrial walls virtually always have increased amounts of fibrous tissue in both the myocardial interstitium and in the mural endocardium, atrophy of some and hypertrophy of other myocardial cells, and hypertrophy of smooth muscles in the mural endocardium. In all patients with rheumatic MS, the leaflets are diffusely thickened either by fibrous

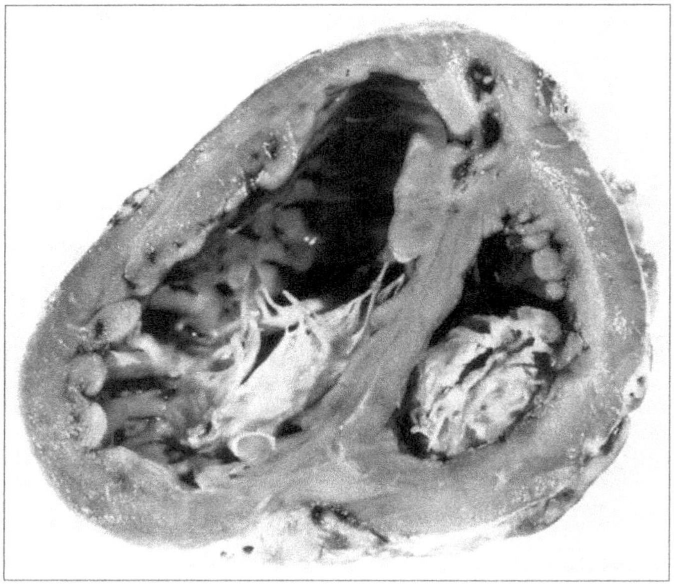

Figure 13. Mitral stenosis. Heart in a 16-year-old boy who had acute rheumatic fever at age 6 years and chronic heart failure beginning at age 10. He had severe mitral stenosis and tricuspid valve regurgitation. At cardiac catheterization 10 hours before death, the right ventricular pressure was 100/20 and the left ventricular pressure, 100/10 mm Hg. By left ventricular angiogram, the left ventricular cavity was of normal size and there was no mitral regurgitation. At necropsy, the heart weighed 450 g (patient weight, 43 kg). The right ventricular cavity was greatly dilated, and both ventricular walls were of similar thickness. Both mitral and tricuspid valve leaflets were diffusely thickened and free of calcific deposits. No Aschoff bodies were found. Reproduced with permission from Roberts WC, 1983 (39).

tissue or calcific deposits or both, the two commissures are usually fused, and the chordae tendineae are usually (but not always) thickened and fused *(Figures 13 and 14).*

The amount of calcium in the leaflets of stenotic mitral valves varies considerably *(Figure 15).* Generally, the calcific deposits are more frequent and in larger quantities in men than in women, in older than in younger patients, and in those with higher vs those with lower pressure gradients between the left atrium and left ventricle (Figure 14). The rapidity with which calcium develops also varies considerably: it is present at a younger age in men than in women. Lachman and Roberts (42) determined the presence or absence and the extent of calcific deposits in operatively excised stenotic mitral valves in 164 patients aged 26 to 72 years. The amount of calcific deposits in the stenotic mitral valves correlated with *sex* and the *mean transvalvular pressure gradient (Figure 16),* but it did not correlate with the patients' age (after 25 years), cardiac rhythm, pulmonary arterial or pulmonary arterial wedge pressure, previous mitral commissurotomy, presence of thrombus in the body or appendage of left ventricle, or the presence of disease in one or more other cardiac valves. Of the 164 patients, radiographs of the operatively excised valve showed no calcific deposits in 14 and only minimal deposits in 43. Of these 57 patients, however, 37 had moderate or severe MR. The remaining 20 in an earlier era would have been ideal or nearly ideal candidates for mitral commissurotomy (43).

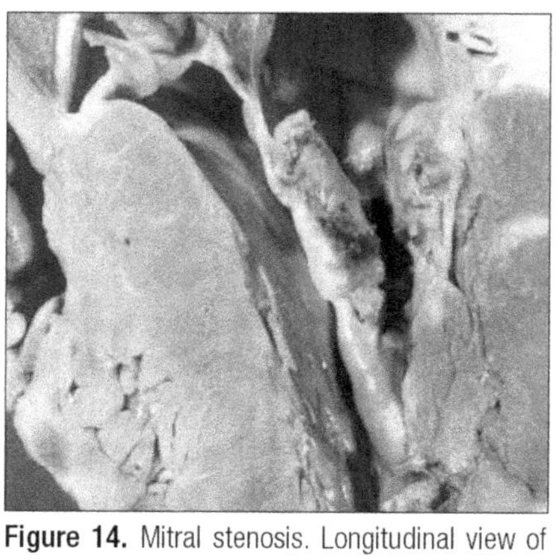

Figure 14. Mitral stenosis. Longitudinal view of a very narrow and thickened mitral valve in a 55-year-old man with equal peak systolic pressures in the right and left ventricles and no associated mitral regurgitation during cannulation of the aorta for planned mitral valve replacement. Both anterior and posterior mitral leaflets are heavily calcified. Reproduced with permission from Roberts WC, 1983 (39).

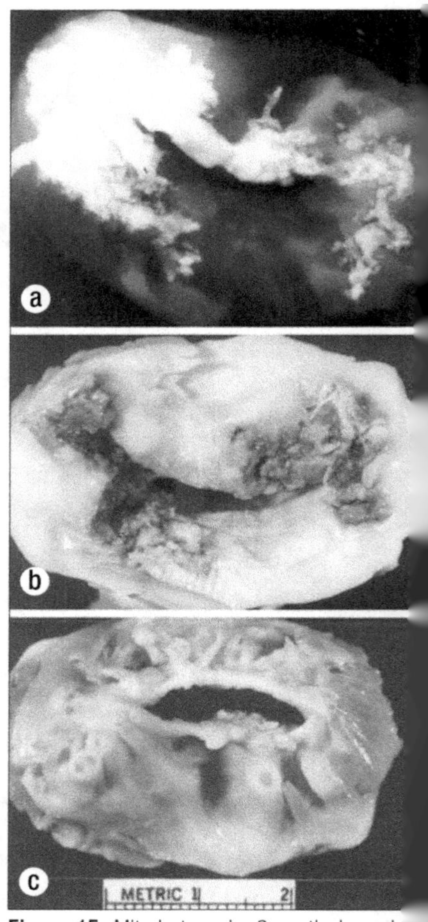

Figure 15. Mitral stenosis. Operatively excis heavily calcified stenotic mitral valve in a 57-ye old man with combined mitral stenosis (12 mm mean transvalvular diastolic gradient) and ao stenosis. **(a)** Radiograph of the excised valve. View of valve from the left atrial aspect. Thro are present near and at the commissures. **(c)** V from the left ventricular aspect. The orifice is verely narrowed.

A major complication of MS is *thrombus formation in left atrial cavity.* The thrombus may be limited to the at appendage (by far most common) or be located in both appendage and body of the left atrium. Left atrial "bo thrombus was observed in 5% of the 1010 necropsy patie with fatal valvular heart disease studied by Roberts, and all severe MS (unpublished data). Left atrial "body" throm was not found in any of the 165 patients with pure MR. patients with left atrial "body" thrombus had atrial fibrillati In contrast, of 46 patients with MS who had cardiotomy at National Heart, Lung, and Blood Institute and had throm in the left atrial "body," 42 (91%) had atrial fibrillation an (9%) had sinus rhythm. *Thrombus appears to occur in the b of the left atrium only in patients with MS, and atrial fibr tion in the absence of MS is incapable of forming thromb the left atrial body.*

Calcific deposits on the mural endocardium of the left atr almost certainly are indicative of previous organization of

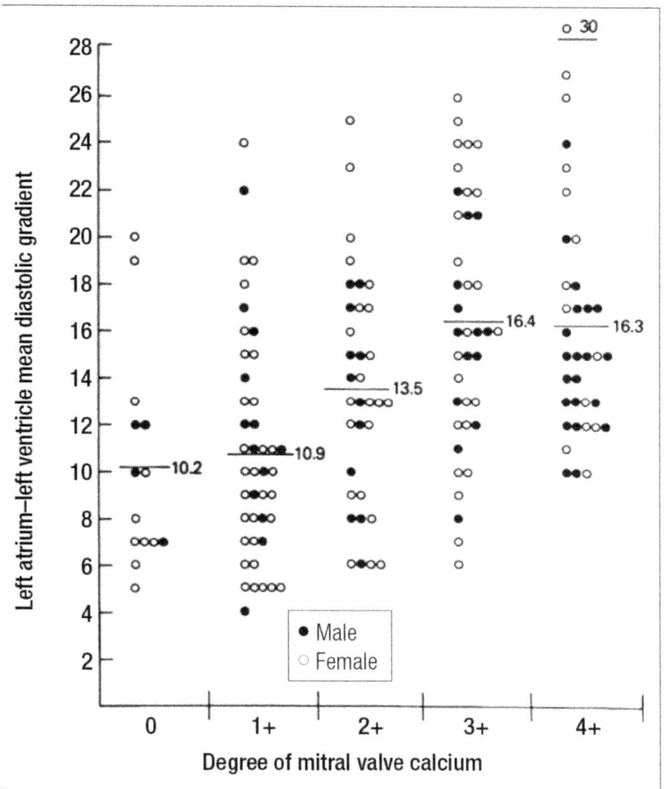

...ure 16. Mitral stenosis. Comparison of the relation of the mean left atrial–left ...ntricular diastolic gradient to the quantity of mitral valve calcium graded by ...diograph of the operatively excised mitral valve. The greater the quantity of ...tral calcium, the greater the transvalvular gradient. Reproduced with permission ...m Lachman AS and Roberts WC, 1978 (42).

...ial thrombi (44). Histologically, the "calcific thrombi" also ...ntain cholesterol clefts and are identical to atherosclerotic ...aques. The observation that left atrial thrombi can organize ...o lesions identical to atherosclerotic plaques supports the view ...at atherosclerotic plaques may in part be the result of organiza...n of thrombi.

Nonrheumatic causes of MS include *congenital anomalies* ..., 39); *large mitral annular calcific deposits associated with left ...ntricular outflow obstruction* (45, 46) *(Figure 17); neoplasms* ...articularly myxoma) protruding through the mitral orifice ...); *large vegetations from active infective endocarditis* (48); and ...course a mechanical prosthesis or bioprosthesis used to replace ...ative mitral valve (49).

Histologic examination of sections of stenotic mitral valves ...en stained for elastic fibers shows the mitral leaflet to have lost ...st or all of its spongiosa element such that the leaflet itself con...s entirely or nearly entirely of the fibrosa element. The leaflet ...are the chordae) is outlined by an elastic fibril (which stains ...ck by an elastic tissue stain), and covering it on both atrial ... ventricular aspects is dense fibrous tissue containing focally ...e vascular channels. Similar dense fibrous tissue surrounds ... chordae, and the chordae themselves appear normal.

Patients with MS usually have distinct pulmonary vascular ...nges secondary to the pulmonary venous and arterial hy...tension. These anatomic changes consist of thickening of ... media of the muscular and elastic pulmonary arteries and focal intimal fibrous plaques. Plexiform lesions never occur in the lungs as a result of MS. The alveolar septa also thicken due to dilatation of the capillaries, proliferation of lining alveolar cells, and some increase of alveolar septal fibrous tissue.

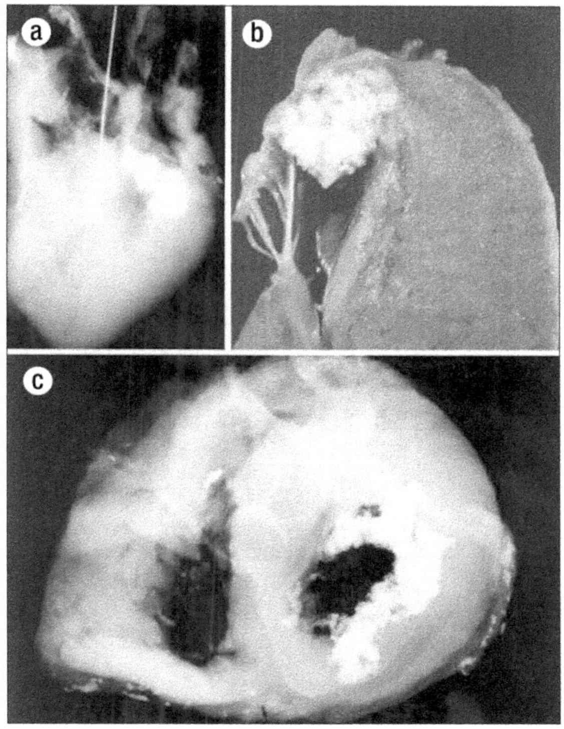

Figure 17. Mitral annular calcium. Heavily calcified mitral annulus in a 71-year-old woman with previous second-degree heart block and a pacemaker for 23 months. She died of acute myocardial infarction complicated by rupture of the left ventricular free wall. **(a)** Radiograph of the heart at necropsy showing mitral annular calcium and the pacemaker leads. **(b)** Longitudinal section showing heavy calcific deposits behind the posterior mitral leaflet. **(c)** Radiograph of the base of the heart (after removing its apical one-half) showing the circumferential extent of the mitral annular calcific deposits. Reproduced with permission from Roberts WC et al, 1973 (34).

PURE MITRAL REGURGITATION

Pure MR (no element of MS) is the most common dysfunctional cardiac valve disorder, and, in contrast to MS, it has many different causes. If patients with MR due to left ventricular dilatation from any cause (ischemic cardiomyopathy, idiopathic dilated cardiomyopathy, anemia, etc.) are excluded, the most common cause of MR treated operatively in the Western world today is *MVP (Figures 18 and 19).* This condition, which was described initially in the 1960s by Barlow and colleagues (50) and by Criley and colleagues (51), is now recognized to occur in approximately 5% of adults, and, if one considers this condition a congenital deficiency of mitral tissues—which we do—it is the most common congenital cardiovascular disease. Among 97 patients having mitral valve replacement for pure MR from 1968 to 1981 at the National Heart, Lung, and Blood Institute, MVP was responsible in 60 patients (62%), papillary muscle dysfunction from coronary heart disease in 29 (30%), infective endocarditis in 5 (5%), and possibly rheumatic disease in 3 (3%) (52).

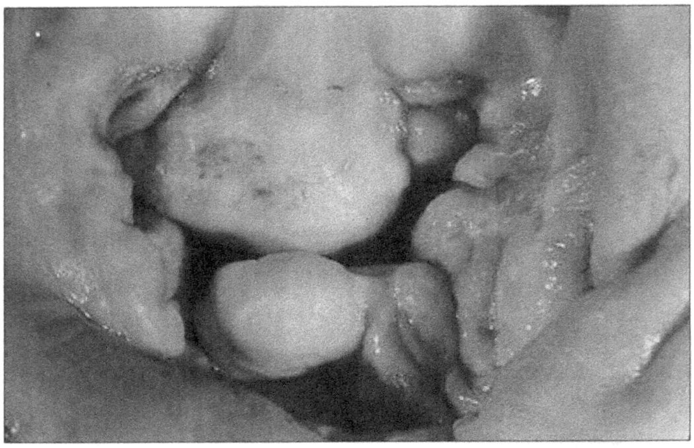

Figure 18. Mitral valve prolapse. View from above shows prolapse of both anterior and posterior cusps in a man who died from consequences of an acute myocardial infarction.

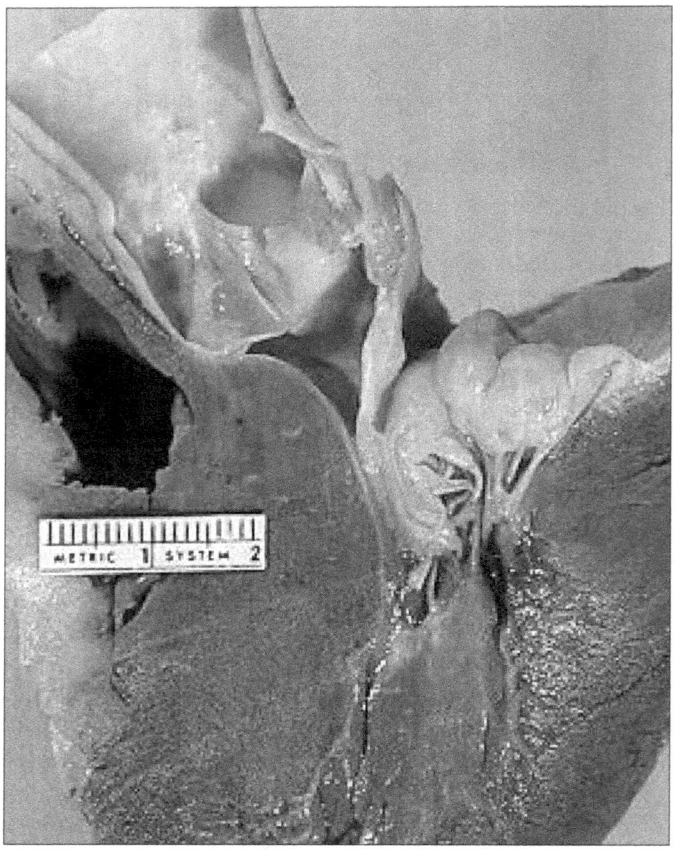

Figure 19. Mitral valve prolapse. View of prolapsed posterior leaflet in a 74-year-old woman who during life was found to have a precordial murmur but never had symptoms of cardiac dysfunction.

Although several authors have attempted to do so, defining MVP has not been easy (1). The following have proved useful in separating the valve affected by MVP from mitral valves affected by other conditions:

1. *Focal lengthening of the posterior and/or anterior mitral leaflets from their site of attachment to their distal margins.* Normally, the length of the posterior leaflet from its attachment to distal margin is about 1 cm. In MVP, this leaflet focally is often as long as the anterior leaflet (52).
2. *Elongation and thinning of chordae tendineae.*
3. *Focal thickening of the posterior and/or anterior leaflet.* Thi finding is particularly prominent on the portion of leaflet th prolapses toward or into the left atrium during ventricul systole. The atrial surface is uniformly smooth. The thickenin of the leaflet produces a spongy feel.
4. *Increase in area, either focally or diffusely, of one or both mitr leaflets* (52).
5. *Loss of chordae tendineae on the ventricular aspect of the post rior mitral leaflet.* It is rare to actually see a ruptured chord but what is seen are areas where chordae should be attache but none are there. They presumably ruptured in the pa and with time were matted down on the leaflets' ventricul aspect, giving this surface a "bumpy" appearance and fe Chordae are nearly uniformly missing (previously ruptured) portions of posterior mitral leaflet excised during mitral valve rep or during replacement. Indeed, MVP appears to be by far t most common cause of ruptured chordae tendineae. Infecti endocarditis is the next most frequent cause (53).
6. *Dilatation of the mitral annulus.* Annular dilatation is pro ably the major cause of development of severe MR in t presence of MVP (52, 54). (The other is rupture of chord tendineae.) Normally, the mitral annulus in adults averag about 9 cm in circumference. In patients with left ventricu dilatation from any cause, with or without MR, the mit circumference usually dilates slightly, usually to about cm or <25% above normal (55). Among patients with M associated with severe MR, this annular circumference gen ally increases >50% to 12 to 18 cm. Acute rupture of chor tendineae may occur in patients with MVP in the absence mitral annular dilatation.
7. *An increase in the transverse dimension of the mitral leaf such that the length of the mitral circumference measured o line corresponding to the distal margin of the posterior leafl much larger than the circumference measured at the level of mitral annulus* (52). In the normal mitral valve, the two the same. It is analogous to a skirt gathered at the waist. leaflets of the opened normal mitral valve are flat or smo on the atrial aspect (like the mucosa of the ileum) whe those of the opened floppy mitral valve are undulating (those of the duodenum or jejunum).
8. *Focal thickening of mural endocardium of the left ventricle be the posterior mitral leaflet.* Salazar and Edwards (56) called t fibrous thickenings "friction lesions" to indicate that they believed to result from friction between the overlying lea and chordae and the underlying left ventricular wall. L and Edwards (57) observed these "friction lesions" in 77 (7 of 102 necropsy cases of MVP, and Dollar and Roberts found them in 23 (68%) of 34 necropsy cases of MVP.
9. *Fibrinous deposits on the atrial surface of the prolapsed por of mitral leaflet and particularly at the angle formed bet the prolapsed leaflet and left atrial wall* (mitral valve–left a angle). These fibrin deposits may be a source of embol

Histologically, the MVP valve is distinctive. Elastic ti stains reveal that the mitral leaflet and chordae are surrour by a single thick elastic fibril. The underlying leaflet general

Table 9. Reported necropsy cases of mitral valve prolapse

First author, year (reference)	Number with MVP	Age (years)	Male/female	MVP cause of death	No. of mitral leaflets prolapsed 1/2	MR	RCT	IE	SD	MS	ASD*	MAC	HW increased	DMA
Pomerance, 1969 (60)	35†	51–98 (mean 74)	23/12	4	12/23	8	2‡	2	1	0	1	9	13	–
Davies, 1978 (61)	90§	<40–100	44/46	6	69/21	23	–	9	13	0	0	3	8ǁ	6
Lucas, 1982 (57)	102¶	69 ± 12	62/40	4	34/68	18	7‡	7	0	1	3	–	–	–
Lucas, 1982 (57)	69**	–	–	–	–	–	19‡	7	16	20	9	–	–	–
Dollar, 1991 (58)	56**	16–70 (mean 48)	33/23	29	50/6	32	18‡	0	15	2	4	12	30††	40

ecundum type atrial septal defect.
hirty cases from a single hospital (1% of autopsies).
nassociated with infective endocarditis.
ases acquired from four different hospitals (4.5% of autopsies).
eart weight >300 g.
ases seen in a single community hospital (7% of autopsies).
Cases "whose hearts had been sent to Edwards or Roberts for his opinion and interest."
Heart weight >350 g in women and >400 g in men.
D indicates atrial septal defect; DMA, dilated mitral annulus; HW, heart weight; IE, infective endocarditis; MAC, mitral annular calcium; MR, mitral regurgitation; MS, the Marfan ndrome; MVP, mitral valve prolapse; RCT, ruptured chordae tendineae; SD, sudden death; –, no information available.

ut not always—contains an excessive amount of the spongiosa ement, and this causes the leaflet itself to be a bit thicker than ormal. Most of the leaflet thickening, however, is due to superposed fibrous tissue on both its atrial and ventricular aspects. he covering on the atrial side of the leaflet contains numerous astic fibrils, whereas that on the ventricular aspect contains few no elastic fibrils. Often on the ventricular aspect, previously ptured and now "matted" chordae tendineae are covered by rous tissue. The spongiosa element within the leaflet itself pears normal—just increased in amount—and therefore the rase "mucoid degeneration" appears inappropriate.

Ultrastructural studies of mitral valves grossly characteristic MVP have disclosed alterations of the collagen fibers in the flets and in the chordae tendineae (59). These changes have cluded fragmentation, splitting, swelling, and course granuity of the individual collagen fibers, and also spiraling and isting of the fibers. These alterations in the structure of the llagen are probably far more important than the excess acid ucopolysaccharide material in the leaflet in that they lead to cal weakness of the leaflets and chordae and their subsequent ngation. The left ventricular systolic pressure exerted against se weakened areas may account for the prolapse.

Just as the frequency of MVP varies clinically depending on age and sex group being examined and in the clinical criteria ployed for diagnosis (auscultatory, echocardiographic, angiophic), its frequency at necropsy is quite variable and the varia- is determined by several factors: 1) age and sex group of the ulation being examined; 2) type of institution where necropsy erformed (general hospital, referral hospital for cardiovascular ease, or medical examiner's [coroner's] office); 3) expertise in diovascular disease of the physician performing the necropsy or orting the findings; 4) percentage of total deaths having autop- at the particular hospital; 5) presence or absence of evidence of cardiac disease before death; 6) whether the patient underwent mitral valve replacement or repair; and 7) whether the percentage of patients being examined had a high frequency of the Marfan syndrome, infective endocarditis, atrial septal defect, and so on.

No study shows better how bias alters the finding in necropsy studies than the one performed by Lucas and Edwards *(Table 9)* (57). These investigators, in one portion of their study, determined the frequency of and complications of floppy mitral valves observed at necropsy in one community (nonreferral) hospital for adults. Of 1376 autopsies performed, 7% or 102 patients had morphologically floppy mitral valves at necropsy. Their mean age at death was 69 ± 12 years; 62 (61%) were men and 40 (39%) were women. Of the 102 patients, MVP was the cause of death in only four. Of the 102 patients, one leaflet had prolapsed in 34 patients and two leaflets in 68. Only 18 had anatomic evidence of previous MR; 7 had infective endocarditis; 7 had ruptured chordae tendineae (without infection); 1 had the Marfan syndrome; and 3 had secundum atrial septal defect. No patient died suddenly. In contrast, in the other portion of their study, these authors described complications in 69 necropsy patients whose hearts had been sent to Edwards for his opinion and interest. Among these 69 patients, 16 (23%) had died suddenly and unexpectedly; 19 (28%) had ruptured chordae tendineae (without infection); 7 (10%) had infective endocarditis; 20 (29%) had the Marfan syndrome; and 9 (13%) had secundum-type atrial septal defect. Thus, in contrast to their infrequency in their community hospital series, most cases submitted to their cardiovascular registry from other institutions had ruptured chordae, infective endocarditis, sudden unexpected and unexplained death, or the Marfan syndrome.

The earlier studies by Pomerance (60) and by Davies and colleagues (61) can also be compared to the community hospital series of Lucas and Edwards (57) *(Table 9)*. The study by

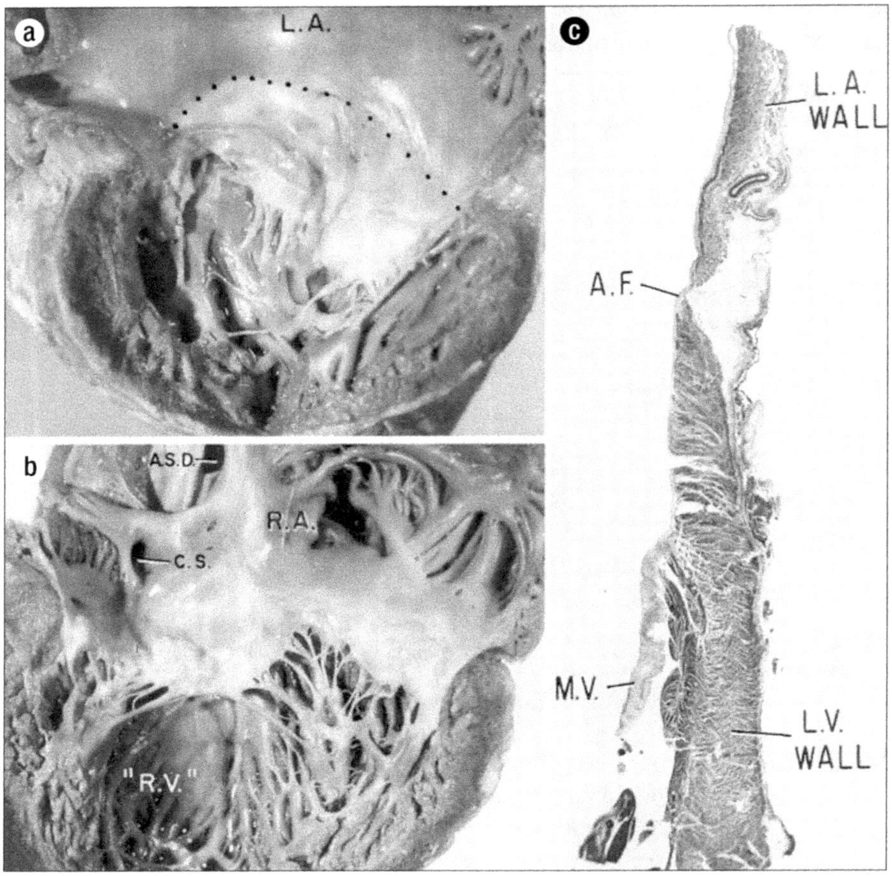

Figure 20. Corrected transposition of the great arteries and Ebstein's anomaly of the left-sided atrioventricular valve in a 38-year-old woman who was cyanotic from birth and in heart failure periodically all of her life. She also had severe pulmonic valve stenosis and ventricular septal defect. She died shortly after operative insertion of a conduit between the left subclavian and left main pulmonary arteries. **(a)** Opened left atrium (LA) and anatomic right ventricle. The normal annulus is shown by the dotted line. **(b)** Opened right atrium (RA) and anatomic left ventricle (RV). ASD indicates atrial septal defect; CS, ostium of coronary sinus. **(c)** Histologic section of left atrial and left ventricular (LV) walls showing the normal annulus fibrosis (AF) and insertion of the mitral valve (MV) considerably caudal to the annulus and directly across from the ventricular wall. Verhoeff-von Gieson stain, ×4. Reproduced with permission from Berry WB et al, 1964 (67).

Dollar and Roberts (58) is comparable to the study of Lucas and Edwards and their selected cases. These authors studied at necropsy 56 patients, aged 16 to 70 years (mean, 48), and compared findings in the 15 who died suddenly and unexpectedly with the other 41 who did not. Compared with the 34 patients without associated congenital heart disease and with non-MVP conditions capable in themselves of being fatal, the 15 patients who died suddenly with isolated MVP were younger (mean age, 39 vs 52 years), were more often women (67% vs 26%), had a lower frequency of MR (7% vs 38%), and were less likely to have ruptured chordae tendineae (29% vs 67%).

The frequency of atrial fibrillation is different in patients with MVP and those with MS immediately before a mitral valve replacement or "repair." Among 246 patients aged 21 to 84 years (mean, 61; men, 66%) who had mitral valve repair or replacement for MR secondary to MVP, Berbarie and Roberts (62) found only 37 patients (15%) (mean age, 60) with atrial fibrillation and 209 patients (88%) with sinus rhythm. In contrast, of 104 patients aged 33 to 80 years (12% men) with rheumatic MS severe enough or symptomatic enough to warrant mitral valve replacement, Sims and Roberts (63) foun[d] atrial fibrillation by electrocardiogram im[-] mediately preoperatively in 47 (45%) an[d] sinus rhythm in 57 (55%).

Other causes of pure mitral regurgitation

Cleft anterior mitral leaflet. Partial atrio[-] ventricular "defect" includes a spectrum of five anatomic anomalies (64). Som[e] patients have all five and others have onl[y] one or two. The five are the following: 1 defect in the lowermost portion of the atri[al] septum, so-called primum atrial septal de[-] fect; 2) defect in, or absence of, the posterc basal portion of the ventricular septum; 3 cleft anterior mitral leaflet; 4) anomalou chordae tendineae from the anterior mitr[al] leaflet to the crest of the ventricular se[p-] tum; and 5) partial or complete absenc of the septal tricuspid valve leaflet. The are at least four potential functional cons[e-] quences of these five anatomic anomalie 1) shunt at the atrial level, 2) shunt at th ventricular level, 3) MR, and 4) obstru[c-] tion to left ventricular outflow. Well ov 95% of patients with partial atrioventric[u-] lar defect have a primum-type atrial sept defect, and most of those without a pr[i-] mum defect have a shunt at the ventricul level. The occurrence of MR from a cl[eft] in the anterior mitral leaflet unassociat with a defect in either atrial or ventricul septa is rare, but such has been the case several reported patients (65).

Left-sided atrioventricular valve regur[gi-] tation associated with corrected transpositi[on] of the great arteries. Corrected transposition is an entity that h produced much confusion (66, 67). Corrected transpositi and complete transposition are quite different; the only thi they have in common is the word "transposition." Compl transposition is essentially one defect: the great arteries transposed, so that the aorta arises from the right ventri and the pulmonary trunk from the left ventricle. In correc transposition, the great arteries also are transposed, but in dition, the ventricles, atrioventricular valves, epicardial co nary arteries, and conduction system are inverted. Patie with complete transposition die because they have inadequ communications between the two circuits. Patients with c rected transposition theoretically should be able to live a lifespan, but usually this is not the case because associa defects—namely, ventricular septal defect or regurgitatior the left-sided atrioventricular valve or both—cause the he to function abnormally. The left-sided valve anatomically tricuspid valve (in the case of the situs solitus heart), and most frequent abnormality is the Ebstein-type abnorma *(Figure 20).* Although most patients with corrected trans

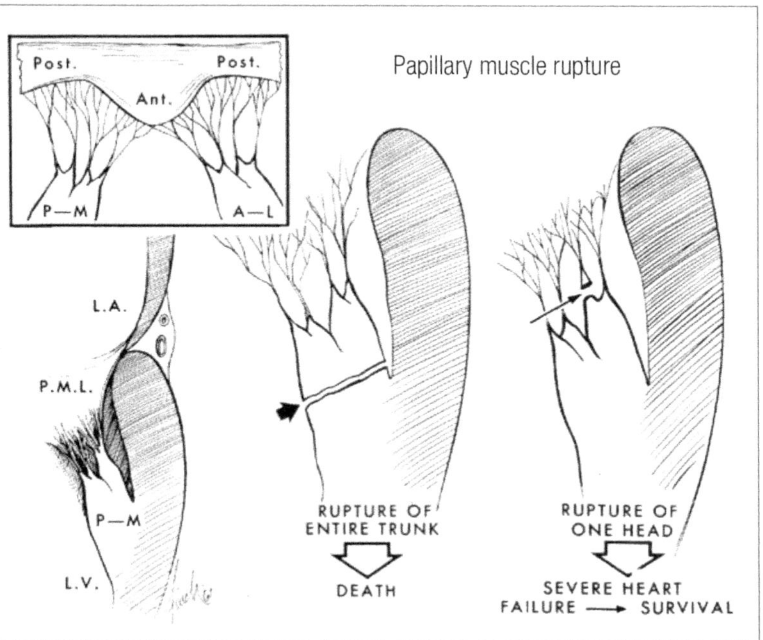

gure 21. Papillary muscle rupture secondary to acute myocardial infarction. Representation the possible consequences of papillary muscle rupture during acute myocardial infarction. pture of the entire trunk is incompatible with survival (left). With rupture of an apical "head" ght), survival depends on the extent to which function of the left ventricle has been impaired the infarct. With severely impaired left ventricular function, the additional burden of even odest MR may be intolerable. If the left ventricle is less severely compromised, survival is ssible for weeks or months, but heart failure will almost invariably develop. Modified with rmission from Morrow AG et al, 1968 (72).

ion present with excessive pulmonary blood flow because the left-to-right shunt via the ventricular septal defect, an casional patient with corrected transposition has no defect in e cardiac septa and has evidence of pure "MR," occasionally staken for other causes of MR (68).

Infective endocarditis. The most common cardiac valve afted by infective endocarditis is the aortic valve, and the mitral ve is most commonly affected by vegetations growing down anterior mitral leaflet from the regurgitant aortic valve caus- mitral leaflet damage and chordal rupture (69, 70). Infection lated to the mitral valve is far less common, and when this uation occurs the vegetations are on the atrial aspects of the tral leaflets (71).

Coronary heart disease. The MR in patients with coronary rt disease is due to myocardial infarction, which may tely cause necrosis of one or more left ventricular papil- muscles (usually the posteromedial one) with or without ture of the entire muscle or, far more commonly, rupture a portion of the "tip" of the papillary muscle (38, 72, 73) *gure 21).* Rupture, either partial or complete, of a papil- muscle during acute myocardial infarction is a far less nmon cause of acute MR than is necrosis of a papillary scle and the free wall beneath it. When it occurs late after te myocardial infarction, the MR is usually the result of tation of the left ventricular cavity and severe scarring of a illary muscle, which tends to pull the mitral leaflets later- preventing proper coaptation of the two mitral leaflets ing ventricular systole.

Cardiomyopathy. Most patients with idiopathic dilated cardiomyopathy (74), ischemic cardiomyopathy (75, 76), and hypertrophic cardiomyopathy (77) have MR at some time in their course. The first two conditions of course are associated with dilatation of the left ventricular cavity primarily in a lateral or right-to-left direction—not in a caudal-cephalad direction—and the consequence is abnormal papillary muscle "pull" on the mitral leaflets during ventricular systole with resulting incomplete coaptation of the mitral leaflets. Evidence that mitral annular dilatation is the prime cause of MR in patients with dilated cardiomyopathy is lacking (55). The cause of MR in patients with hypertrophic cardiomyopathy is entirely different from that in patients with dilated cardiomyopathy and results at least in part in anterior movement of the anterior mitral leaflet toward the ventricular septum during ventricular systole (77). Patients with chronic anemia, e.g., sickle cell anemia, usually also have MR from papillary muscle fibrosis and left ventricular cavity dilatation (78).

1. Roberts WC. Congenital cardiovascular abnormalities usually silent until adulthood. In Roberts WC, ed. *Adult Congenital Heart Disease*. Philadelphia: FA Davis, 1987:631–691.
2. Sprecher DL, Schaefer EJ, Kent KM, Gregg RE, Zech LA, Hoeg JM, McManus B, Roberts WC, Brewer HB Jr. Cardiovascular features of homozygous familial hypercholesterolemia: analysis of 16 patients. *Am J Cardiol* 1984;54(1):20–30.
3. Moura LM, Ramos SF, Zamorano JL, Barros IM, Azevedo LF, Rocha-Gonçalves F, Rajamannan NM. Rosuvastatin affecting aortic valve endothelium to slow the progression of aortic stenosis. *J Am Coll Cardiol* 2007;49(5):554–561.
4. Roberts WC, Perloff JK, Costantino T. Severe valvular aortic stenosis in patients over 65 years of age. A clinicopathologic study. *Am J Cardiol* 1971;27(5):497–506.
5. Stephan PJ, Henry AC 3rd, Hebeler RF Jr, Whiddon L, Roberts WC. Comparison of age, gender, number of aortic valve cusps, concomitant coronary artery bypass grafting, and magnitude of left ventricular-systemic arterial peak systolic gradient in adults having aortic valve replacement for isolated aortic valve stenosis. *Am J Cardiol* 1997;79(2):166–172.
6. Roberts WC, Morrow AG. Congenital aortic stenosis produced by a unicommissural valve. *Br Heart J* 1965;27:505–510.
7. Falcone MW, Roberts WC, Morrow AG, Perloff JK. Congenital aortic stenosis resulting from a unicommissural valve. Clinical and anatomic features in twenty-one adult patients. *Circulation* 1971;44(2):272–280.
8. Roberts WC. The congenitally bicuspid aortic valve. A study of 85 autopsy cases. *Am J Cardiol* 1970;26(1):72–83.
9. Roberts WC. Anatomically isolated aortic valvular disease. The case against its being of rheumatic etiology. *Am J Med* 1970;49(2):151–159.
10. Roberts WC, Ko JM. Clinical and morphologic features of the congenitally unicuspid acommissural stenotic and regurgitant aortic valve. *Cardiology* 2007;108(2):79–81.
11. Roberts WC. The senile cardiac calcification syndrome. *Am J Cardiol* 1986;58(6):572–574.
12. Hurwitz LE, Roberts WC. Quadricuspid semilunar valve. *Am J Cardiol* 1973;31(5):623–626.
13. Roberts WC, Ko JM, Filardo G, Henry AC, Hebeler RF Jr, Cheung EH, Matter GJ, Hamman BL. Valve structure and survival in *sexagenarians* having aortic valve replacement for aortic stenosis (± aortic regurgitation) with versus without coronary artery bypass grafting at a single US medical center (1993 to 2005). *Am J Cardiol* 2007;100(8):1286–1292.

14. Roberts WC, Ko JM. Weights of operatively-excised stenotic unicuspid, bicuspid, and tricuspid aortic valves and their relation to age, sex, body mass index, and presence or absence of concomitant coronary artery bypass grafting. *Am J Cardiol* 2003;92(9):1057–1065.
15. Roberts WC, Ko JM. Weights of individual cusps in operatively-excised congenitally bicuspid stenotic aortic valves. *Am J Cardiol* 2004;94(5):678–681.
16. Roberts WC, Ko JM. Weights of individual cusps in operatively-excised stenotic three-cuspid aortic valves. *Am J Cardiol* 2004;94(5):681–684.
17. Roberts WC, Ko JM. Relation of weights of operatively excised stenotic aortic valves to preoperative transvalvular peak systolic pressure gradients and to calculated aortic valve areas. *J Am Coll Cardiol* 2004;44(9):1847–1855.
18. Roberts WC, Ko JM. Frequency by decades of unicuspid, bicuspid, and tricuspid aortic valves in adults having isolated aortic valve replacement for aortic stenosis, with or without associated aortic regurgitation. *Circulation* 2005;111(7):920–925.
19. Roberts WC, Ko JM, Matter GJ. Isolated aortic valve replacement without coronary bypass for aortic valve stenosis involving a congenitally bicuspid aortic valve in a nonagenarian. *Am J Geriatr Cardiol* 2006;15(6):389–391.
20. Roberts WC, Ko JM, Garner WL, Filardo G, Henry AC, Hebeler RF Jr, Matter GJ, Hamman BL. Valve structure and survival in *octogenarians* having aortic valve replacement for aortic stenosis (± aortic regurgitation) with versus without coronary artery bypass grafting at a single US medical center (1993 to 2005). *Am J Cardiol* 2007;100(3):489–495.
21. Roberts WC, Ko JM, Filardo G, Henry AC, Hebeler RF Jr, Cheung EH, Matter GJ, Hamman BL. Valve structure and survival in *septuagenarians* having aortic valve replacement for aortic stenosis (± aortic regurgitation) with versus without coronary artery bypass grafting at a single US medical center (1993 to 2005). *Am J Cardiol* 2007;100(7):1157–1165.
22. Roberts WC, Ko JM, Hamilton C. Comparison of valve structure, valve weight, and severity of the valve obstruction in 1849 patients having isolated aortic valve replacement for aortic valve stenosis (with or without associated aortic regurgitation) studied at 3 different medical centers in 2 different time periods. *Circulation* 2005;112(25):3919–3929.
23. Roberts WC, Ko JM, Filardo G, Henry AC, Hebeler RF Jr, Cheung EH, Matter GJ, Hamman BL. Valve structure and survival in *quinquagenarians* having aortic valve replacement for aortic stenosis (± aortic regurgitation) with versus without coronary artery bypass grafting at a single US medical center (1993 to 2005). *Am J Cardiol* 2007;100(10):1584–1591.
24. Roberts WC, Ko JM, Filardo G, Kitchens BL, Henry AC, Hebeler RF Jr, Cheung EH, Matter GJ, Hamman BL. Valve structure and survival in *quadragenarians* having aortic valve replacement for aortic stenosis (± aortic regurgitation) with versus without coronary artery bypass grafting at a single US medical center (1993 to 2005). *Am J Cardiol* 2007;100(11):1683–1690.
25. Roberts WC, Ko JM, Moore TR, Jones WH 3rd. Causes of pure aortic regurgitation in patients having isolated aortic valve replacement at a single US tertiary hospital (1993 to 2005). *Circulation* 2006;114(5):422–429.
26. Roberts WC. The structure of the aortic valve in clinically isolated aortic stenosis: an autopsy study of 162 patients over 15 years of age. *Circulation* 1970;42(1):91–97.
27. Roberts WC, Morrow AG, McIntosh CL, Jones M, Epstein SE. Congenitally bicuspid aortic valve causing severe, pure aortic regurgitation without superimposed infective endocarditis. Analysis of 13 patients requiring aortic valve replacement. *Am J Cardiol* 1981;47(2):206–209.
28. Roberts WC, Oluwole BO, Fernicola DJ. Comparison of active infective endocarditis involving a previously stenotic versus a previously nonstenotic aortic valve. *Am J Cardiol* 1993;71(12):1082–1088.
29. Carpenter DF, Golden A, Roberts WC. Quadrivalvular rheumatoid heart disease associated with left bundle branch block. *Am J Med* 1967;43(6):922–929.
30. Roberts WC, Kehoe JA, Carpenter DF, Golden A. Cardiac valvular lesions in rheumatoid arthritis. *Arch Intern Med* 1968;122(2):141–146.
31. Waller BF, Zoltick JM, Rosen JH, Katz NM, Gomes MN, Fletcher RD, Wallace RB, Roberts WC. Severe aortic regurgitation from systemic hypertension (without aortic dissection) requiring aortic valve replacement: analysis of four patients. *Am J Cardiol* 1982;49(2):473–477.
32. Waller BF, Kishel JC, Roberts WC. Severe aortic regurgitation from sy temic hypertension. *Chest* 1982;82(3):365–368.
33. Roberts WC. Aortic dissection: anatomy, consequences, and causes. *A Heart J* 1981;101(2):195–214.
34. Roberts WC, Dangel JC, Bulkley BH. Nonrheumatic valvular cardi disease: a clinicopathologic survey of 27 different conditions causi valvular dysfunction. *Cardiovasc Clin* 1973;5(2):333–446.
35. Roberts WC, Honig HS. The spectrum of cardiovascular disease in t Marfan syndrome: a clinico-morphologic study of 18 necropsy patien and comparison to 151 previously reported necropsy patients. *Am He J* 1982;104(1):115–135.
36. Bulkley BH, Roberts WC. Ankylosing spondylitis and aortic regurgitatic Description of the characteristic cardiovascular lesion from study of eig necropsy patients. *Circulation* 1973;48(5):1014–1027.
37. Roberts WC, Hollingsworth JF, Bulkley BH, Jaffe RB, Epstein S Stinson EB. Combined mitral and aortic regurgitation in ankyl ing spondylitis. Angiographic and anatomic features. *Am J M* 1974;56(2):237–243.
38. Roberts WC, Perloff JK. Mitral valvular disease. A clinicopathologic surv of the conditions causing the mitral valve to function abnormally. *A Intern Med* 1972;77(6):939–975.
39. Roberts WC. Morphologic features of the normal and abnormal mit valve. *Am J Cardiol* 1983;51(6):1005–1028.
40. Roberts WC, Virmani R. Aschoff bodies at necropsy in valvular he disease. Evidence from an analysis of 543 patients over 14 years of that rheumatic heart disease, at least anatomically, is a disease of the mi valve. *Circulation* 1978;57(4):803–807.
41. Virmani R, Roberts WC. Aschoff bodies in operatively excised at appendages and in papillary muscles. Frequency and clinical significan *Circulation* 1977;55(4):559–563.
42. Lachman AS, Roberts WC. Calcific deposits in stenotic mitral val Extent and relation to age, sex, degree of stenosis, cardiac rhythm, pr ous commissurotomy and left atrial body thrombus from study of operatively-excised valves. *Circulation* 1978;57(4):808–815.
43. Roberts WC, Lachman AS. Mitral valve commissurotomy versus repla ment. Considerations based on examination of operatively excised sten mitral valves. *Am Heart J* 1979;98(1):56–62.
44. Roberts WC, Humphries JO, Morrow AG. Giant right atrium in rh matic mitral stenosis. Atrial enlargement restricted by mural calcificat *Am Heart J* 1970;79(1):28–35.
45. Hammer WJ, Roberts WC, deLeon AC. "Mitral stenosis" secondar combined "massive" mitral anular calcific deposits and small, hyper phied left ventricles. Hemodynamic documentation in four patients. *J Med* 1978;64(3):371–376.
46. Theleman KP, Grayburn PA, Roberts WC. Mitral "annular" calc forming a complete circle "O" causing mitral stenosis in association a stenotic congenitally bicuspid aortic valve and severe coronary a disease. *Am J Geriatr Cardiol* 2006;15(1):58–61.
47. Roberts WC. Neoplasms involving the heart, their simulators, and ad consequences of their therapy. *Proc (Bayl Univ Med Cent)* 2001;14(4): 376.
48. Roberts WC, Ewy GA, Glancy DL, Marcus FI. Valvular stenosis prod by active infective endocarditis. *Circulation* 1967;36(3):449–451.
49. Roberts WC, Bulkley BH, Morrow AG. Pathologic anatomy of ca valve replacement: a study of 224 necropsy patients. *Prog Cardiovas* 1973;15(6):539–587.
50. Barlow JB, Pocock WA, Marchand P, Denny M. The significance o systolic murmurs. *Am Heart J* 1963;66:443–452.
51. Criley JM, Lewis KB, Humphries JO, Ross RS. Prolapse o mitral valve: clinical and cine-angiocardiographic findings. *Br H* 1966;28(4):488-496.
52. Waller BF, Morrow AG, Maron BJ, Del Negro AA, Kent KM, Mc FJ, Wallace RB, McIntosh CL, Roberts WC. Etiology of clinically iso severe, chronic, pure mitral regurgitation: analysis of 97 patients ov years of age having mitral valve replacement. *Am Heart J* 1982;104 1):276–288.

53. Roberts WC, Braunwald E, Morrow AG. Acute severe mitral regurgitation secondary to ruptured chordae tendineae: clinical, hemodynamic, and pathologic considerations. *Circulation* 1966;33(1):58–70.
54. Roberts WC, McIntosh CL, Wallace RB. Mechanisms of severe mitral regurgitation in mitral valve prolapse determined from analysis of operatively excised valves. *Am Heart J* 1987;113(5):1316–1323.
55. Bulkley BH, Roberts WC. Dilatation of the mitral anulus. A rare cause of mitral regurgitation. *Am J Med* 1975;59(4):457–463.
56. Salazar AE, Edwards JE. Friction lesions of ventricular endocardium. Relation to chordae tendineae of mitral valve. *Arch Pathol* 1970;90(4):364–376.
57. Lucas RV Jr, Edwards JE. The floppy mitral valve. *Curr Probl Cardiol* 1982;7(4):1–48.
58. Dollar AL, Roberts WC. Morphologic comparison of patients with mitral valve prolapse who died suddenly with patients who died from severe valvular dysfunction or other conditions. *J Am Coll Cardiol* 1991;17(4):921–931.
59. Rentería VG, Ferrans VJ, Jones M, Roberts WC. Intracellular collagen fibrils in prolapsed ("floppy") human atrioventricular valves. *Lab Invest* 1976;35(5):439–443.
60. Pomerance A. Ballooning deformity (mucoid degeneration) of atrioventricular valves. *Br Heart J* 1969;31(3):343–351.
61. Davies MJ, Moore BP, Braimbridge MV. The floppy mitral valve. Study of incidence, pathology, and complications in surgical, necropsy, and forensic material. *Br Heart J* 1978;40(5):468–481.
62. Berbarie RF, Roberts WC. Frequency of atrial fibrillation in patients having mitral valve repair or replacement for pure mitral regurgitation secondary to mitral valve prolapse. *Am J Cardiol* 2006;97(7):1039–1044.
63. Sims JB, Roberts WC. Comparison of findings in patients with versus without atrial fibrillation just before isolated mitral valve replacement for rheumatic mitral stenosis (with or without associated mitral regurgitation). *Am J Cardiol* 2006;97(7):1035–1038.
64. Braunwald E, Ross RS, Morrow AG, Roberts WC. Differential diagnosis of mitral regurgitation in childhood: clinical pathological conference at the National Institutes of Health. *Ann Intern Med* 1961;54:223–242.
65. Barth CW 3rd, Dibdin JD, Roberts WC. Mitral valve cleft without cardiac septal defect causing severe mitral regurgitation but allowing long survival. *Am J Cardiol* 1985;55(9):1229–1231.
66. Schiebler GL, Edwards JE, Burchell HB, Dushane JW, Ongley PA, Wood EH. Congenital corrected transposition of the great vessels: a study of 33 cases. *Pediatrics* 1961;27(5 Suppl):849–888.
67. Berry WB, Roberts WC, Morrow AG, Braunwald E. Corrected transposition of the aorta and pulmonary trunk: clinical, hemodynamic and pathologic findings. *Am J Med* 1964;36:35–53.
68. Roberts WC, Ross RS, Davis FW Jr. Congenital corrected transposition of the great vessels in adulthood simulating rheumatic valvular disease. *Bull Johns Hopkins Hosp* 1964;114:157–172.
69. Buchbinder NA, Roberts WC. Left-sided valvular active infective endocarditis. A study of forty-five necropsy patients. *Am J Med* 1972;53(1):20–35.
70. Arnett EN, Roberts WC. Active infective endocarditis: a clinicopathologic analysis of 137 necropsy patients. *Curr Probl Cardiol* 1976;1(7):2–76.
71. Fernicola DJ, Roberts WC. Clinicopathologic features of active infective endocarditis isolated to the native mitral valve. *Am J Cardiol* 1993;71(13):1186–1197.
72. Morrow AG, Cohen LS, Roberts WC, Braunwald NS, Braunwald E. Severe mitral regurgitation following acute myocardial infarction and ruptured papillary muscle. Hemodynamic findings and results of operative treatment in four patients. *Circulation* 1968;37(4 Suppl):II124–II132.
73. Barbour DJ, Roberts WC. Rupture of a left ventricular papillary muscle during acute myocardial infarction: analysis of 22 necropsy patients. *J Am Coll Cardiol* 1986;8(3):558–565.
74. Roberts WC, Siegel RJ, McManus BM. Idiopathic dilated cardiomyopathy: analysis of 152 necropsy patients. *Am J Cardiol* 1987;60(16):1340–1355.
75. Virmani R, Roberts WC. Quantification of coronary arterial narrowing and of left ventricular myocardial scarring in healed myocardial infarction with chronic, eventually fatal, congestive cardiac failure. *Am J Med* 1980;68(6):831–838.
76. Ross EM, Roberts WC. Severe atherosclerotic coronary arterial narrowing and chronic congestive heart failure without myocardial infarction: analysis of 18 patients studied at necropsy. *Am J Cardiol* 1986;57(1):51–56.
77. Klues HG, Maron BJ, Dollar AL, Roberts WC. Diversity of structural mitral valve alterations in hypertrophic cardiomyopathy. *Circulation* 1992;85(5):1651–1660.
78. Berezowski K, Mautner GC, Roberts WC. Scarring of the left ventricular papillary muscles in sickle-cell disease. *Am J Cardiol* 1992;70(15):1368–1370.

Gross and Histological Features of Excised Portions of Posterior Mitral Leaflet in Patients Having Operative Repair of Mitral Valve Prolapse and Comments on the Concept of Missing (= Ruptured) Chordae Tendineae

William C. Roberts, MD,*†‡ Travis J. Vowels, BBA,* Jong M. Ko, BA,* Robert F. Hebeler, Jr, MD§
Dallas, Texas

Objectives The aim of the study is to describe gross and histological features of operatively excised portions of mitral valves in patients with mitral valve prolapse (MVP).

Background Although numerous articles on MVP (myxomatous or myxoid degeneration, billowing or floppy mitral valve) have appeared, 2 virtually constant histological features have been underemphasized or overlooked: 1) the presence of superimposed fibrous tissue on both surfaces of the leaflets and surrounding many chordae tendineae; and 2) the absence of many chordae tendineae on the ventricular surfaces of the leaflets as the result of their being hidden (i.e., covered up) by the superimposed fibrous tissue.

Methods We examined operatively excised portions of prolapsed posterior mitral leaflets in 37 patients having operative repair.

Results Histological study of elastic-tissue stained sections disclosed that the leaflet thickening was primarily due to the superimposed fibrous tissue. All leaflets had variable increases in the spongiosa element within the leaflet itself with some disruption and/or loss of the fibrosa element and occasionally complete separation of it from the spongiosa element. Both the leaflet and chordae were separated from the superimposed fibrous tissue by their black-staining elastic membranes.

Conclusions These findings demonstrate that the posterior leaflet thickening in MVP is mainly due to the superimposed fibrous tissue rather than to an increased volume of the spongiosa element of the leaflet itself. The superimposed fibrous tissue on both leaflet and chordae is likely the result of subsequent abnormal contact of the leaflets and chordae with one another. Chordal rupture (i.e., missing chordae) occurred in all 37 patients, but finding individual ruptured chords was rare. (J Am Coll Cardiol 2014;63:1667–74) © 2014 by the American College of Cardiology Foundation

Although numerous publications have appeared describing auscultory, angiographic, echocardiographic, and morphological features of mitral valve prolapse (MVP) (myxomatous or myxoid degeneration), surprisingly, none have reproduced the various histological features of the operatively excised mitral valves or parts thereof in color after staining for elastic fibers, an absolute necessity for proper evaluation, because a black-staining elastic membrane separates the leaflet and chordae from the superimposed fibrous tissue, a constant feature of MVP. In this report, we focus on the contribution of the superimposed fibrous tissue to the leaflet and chordal thickening, and second, we introduce the concept that missing or hidden chords (those lying beneath the superimposed fibrous tissue) are equivalent to ruptured chords.

From the *Baylor Heart and Vascular Institute, Baylor University Medical Center, Dallas, Texas; †Department of Internal Medicine (Division of Cardiology), Baylor University Medical Center, Dallas, Texas; ‡Department of Pathology, Baylor University Medical Center, Dallas, Texas; and the §Department of Cardiothoracic Surgery, Baylor University Medical Center, Dallas, Texas. The study was funded by the Baylor Health Care System Foundation, Dallas, Texas. The authors have reported that they have no relationships relevant to the contents of this paper to disclose.

Manuscript received August 31, 2013; revised manuscript received November 7, 2013, accepted November 12, 2013.

Methods

Since March 1993, all specimens excised at operation by cardiac surgeons at Baylor University Medical Center a

Abbreviations and Acronyms

MR = mitral regurgitation

MVP = mitral valve prolapse

Dallas have been submitted to the surgical pathology division of the pathology department, and all such specimens have been described by one of us (W.C.R.) who submitted the pathology report. Most gross specimens were photographed. After describing the submitted specimen, clinical, echocardiographic, and hemodynamic data were retrieved online via the Baylor University Medical Center at the Dallas Electronic Medical Records and the Apollo Cardiovascular Database. A total of 500 mitral valves or portions thereof were received from January 2005 through June 2013 (Fig. 1). Of this number, 140 patients underwent mitral valve repair or replacement for severe mitral regurgitation (MR) secondary to MVP. After excluding those patients where preoperative echocardiograms (n = 71) were not available to us or histological sections of the excised valves were not prepared or retrievable (n = 14) or the patients had chronic renal failure (n = 4), 51 patients were available for study: 14 had mitral valve replacement and were then excluded from the present study; 37 had mitral valve repair, and in each, portions of the posterior leaflet were studied. Sections of the posterior leaflets were cut from the margin of attachment to the free margin and submitted for histological preparation. After processing in alcohol and xylene, 2 sections were cut from each paraffin block: one was stained by hematoxylin/eosin, and the other, by elastic van Geison.

Results

Pertinent data from the 37 patients are summarized in Table 1. (Data on the 14 patients having mitral valve replacement for MVP are shown in the table simply for comparison.) The operative report in all 37 patients indicated "prolapse" of a portion of posterior mitral leaflet and that the prolapsed segment was the one almost always excised. None of the 37 had calcific deposits in the operatively excised specimens. All 37 patients also had an annular ring inserted.

Examination of the posterior mitral leaflet in the 37 patients disclosed several consistent features (Figs. 2 to 9, Table 2). All 37 operatively excised portions of posterior mitral leaflet had "missing" (i.e., ruptured) chordae tendineae on gross examination. Histologically, the leaflet itself and the chordae tendineae were clearly demarcated by an elastic membrane (elastic van Geison stain). Both atrial and ventricular aspects of the leaflet in all 37 patients contained superimposed fibrous tissue, thicker on the atrial side than on the ventricular side. Additionally, numerous elastic fibers were present in the superimposed fibrous tissue on the atrial aspect, whereas few if any were present in the superimposed fibrous tissue on the

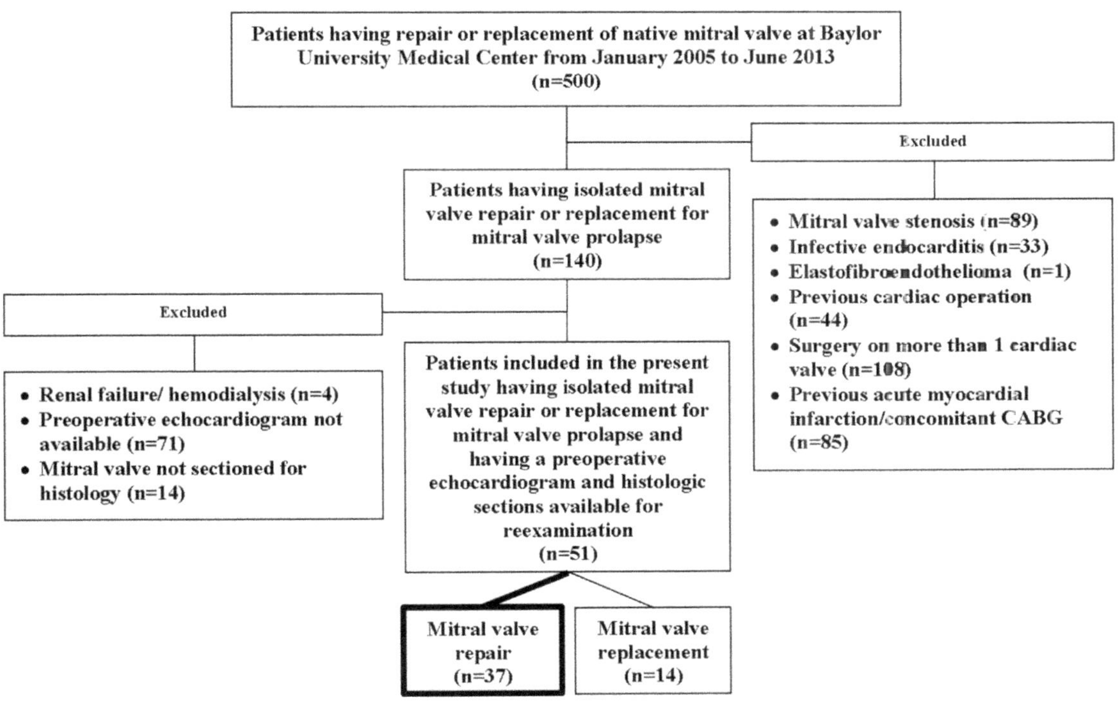

Figure 1 Flow Chart

Chart showing the origin of the 37 patients included in the present study. CABG = coronary artery bypass grafting.

Table 1 **Comparison of Various Variables Among Patients Having Isolated MV Repair or Replacement for Mitral Valve Prolapse**

Variable	MV Repair (n = 37) (73%)	MV Replacement* (n = 14) (27%)
Age (yrs)	56 ± 13 [59] (31–78)	59 ± 15 [56] (34–79)
Sex		
M	31 (84%)	7 (50%)
F	6 (16%)	7 (50%)
Ethnicity		
W	32 (86%)	11 (79%)
B	2 (5%)	3 (21%)
H	2 (5%)	0
A	1 (3%)	0
Atrial fibrillation	13 (35%)	7 (50%)
Pressures (mm Hg)		
Pulmonary arterial wedge (n = 29)	15 ± 5 [15] (7–27)	21 ± 10 [21] (6–39)
RV		
Peak systole (n = 32)	39 ± 13 [34] (16–70)	44 ± 15 [41] (18–66)
End diastole (n = 32)	11 ± 4 [11] (2–19)	14 ± 6 [14] (3–23)
Right atrial mean (n = 31)	7 ± 4 [5] (0–16)	11 ± 8 [11] (0–21)
LV		
Peak systole (n = 34)	120 ± 19 [118] (90–162)	115 ± 16 [111] (99–144)
End diastole (n = 36)	18 ± 6 [18] (6–31)	19 ± 8 [16] (12–35)
Aorta		
Peak systole (n = 34)	117 ± 19 [115] (79–147)	121 ± 19 [120] (95–155)
End diastole (n = 34)	66 ± 15 [69] (19–93)	73 ± 15 [69] (56–101)
Cardiac index (l/min/m^2) (n = 27)	2.66 ± 0.48 [2.63] (1.97–3.71)	2.25 ± 0.68 [2.34] (1.38–3.35)
EF (%) (n = 30) (by catheterization)	60 ± 10 [65] (30–75)	55 ± 20 [60] (25–80)
MV regurgitation		
3+	3 (8%)	2 (14%)
4+	34 (92%)	12 (86%)
MV weight (g)	0.70 ± 0.46 [0.51] (0.20–1.94)	1.52 ± 1.18 [1.50] (0.04–4.07)
MV size (mm)		
Ring	31 ± 3	—
Prosthesis	—	29 ± 3

Values are mean ± SD, [median], (range), or n (%). *These cases are included here simply for quick comparison with the patients having mitral valve (MV) repair.

A = Asian; B = black; EF = ejection fraction; H = Hispanic; LV = left ventricle; RV = right ventricle; W = white; + = positive or present; 0 = negative or absent.

ventricular aspect. The fibrous tissue surrounding the chordae tendineae was similar to that on the ventricular aspect of the leaflet. Within the mitral leaflet itself—enclosed by the elastic membrane—the spongiosa element seemed increased in quantity in all patients, more so in the distal one-half than in the proximal one-half of the leaflet; and the fibrosa element was interrupted focally and/or decreased in quantity or both.

Discussion

Examination of operatively excised portions of posterior mitral leaflet in each of the 37 patients having mitral repair for MVP produced 2 major findings: 1) the leaflet and chordal thickening in patients with MVP is due in large part to superimposed fibrous tissue on both the atrial and ventricular surfaces of the leaflets and surrounding the chordae tendineae; and 2) rupture of posterior leaflet chordae tendineae is a nearly universal finding in patients with MVP, and MR is severe enough to warrant operative repai but that seeing 1 or more ruptured chordae is infrequent because they are covered ("hidden") by the superimpose fibrous tissue on the ventricular surface of the leaflet. I essence, the absence of chordae (missing chordae) is syn onymous with earlier rupture of chordae.

We surmise that the superimposed fibrous tissue on bot leaflet and chordae is entirely due to abnormal contact of th leaflets with one another over many years or decades. Tha the underlying leaflet and chordae are essentially intac suggests that the basic process in MVP is a slow, gradual los and/or interruption of collagen fibers (in the fibrosa elemen of the leaflet and in the chordae tendineae, which are devoi of a spongiosa element). The loss and/or interruption c collagen fibers within the leaflet and chordae seems to b responsible for the gradual elongation of the leaflets an chordae in MVP, which in turn leads to inappropriate leafl contact and to the superimposed fibrous tissue ("callu formation) (Fig. 10).

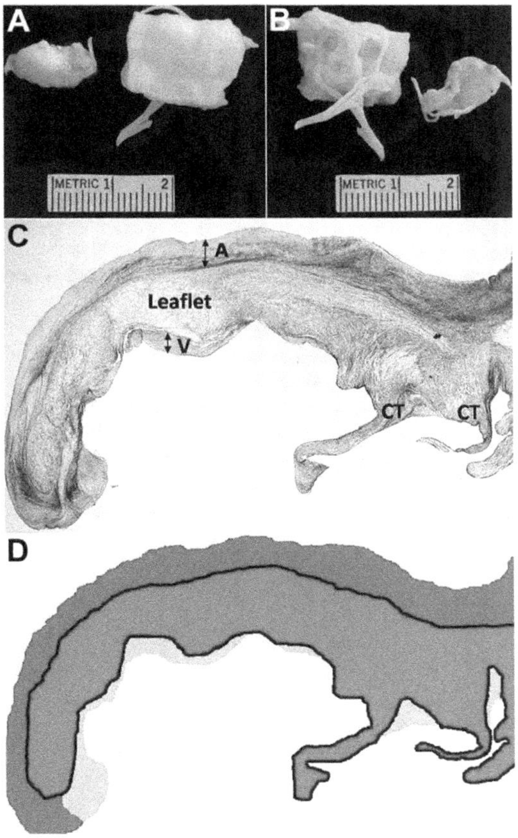

Figure 2 Patient #1 in Table 2

Photographs of the atrial (A) surface **(A)** and ventricular (V) surface **(B)** of a portion of excised posterior mitral valve leaflet. Most chordae are missing from the V surface shown in **B. (C)** Photomicrograph showing superimposed fibrous tissue on both the A and V surfaces and increased spongiosa element within the leaflet itself outlined by its black-staining elastic membrane (elastic van Geison, 20×). **(D)** Rendering of the same valve with **red** representing the leaflet itself, **green** representing the superimposed fibrous tissue on the A surface, and **yellow** representing the superimposed fibrous tissue on the V surface. CT = chordae tendineae.

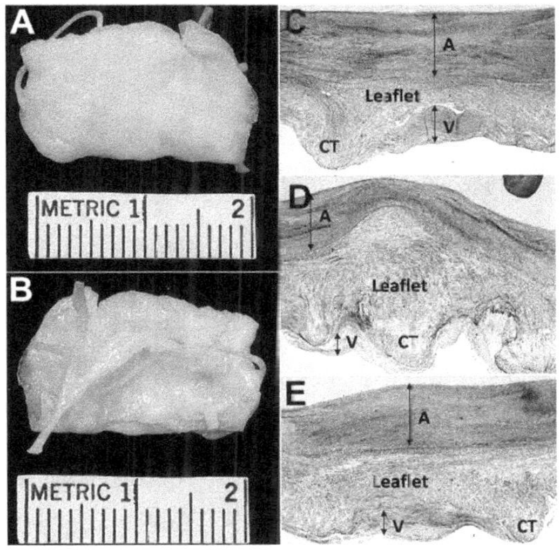

Figure 3 Patient #2 in Table 2

Photographs of the A surface **(A)** and V surface **(B)** of a portion of excised posterior leaflet. Most chordae are missing from the V surface shown in **B. (C to E)** Photomicrographs showing superimposed fibrous tissue on both the A and V surfaces and increased spongiosa element within the leaflet itself outlined by its black-staining elastic membrane (elastic van Geison, 40×). Abbreviations as in Figure 2.

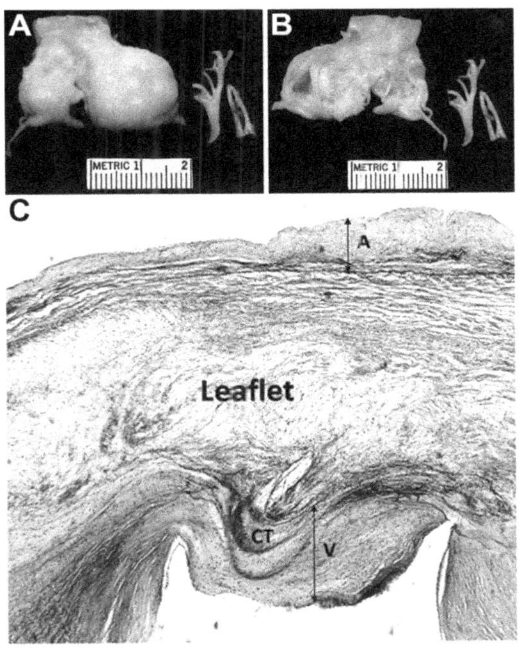

Figure 4 Patient #3 in Table 2

Photographs of the A surface **(A)** and V surface **(B)** of a portion of posterior leaflet. Most chordae are missing from the V surface shown in **B. (C)** Photomicrograph showing superimposed fibrous tissue on both the A and V surfaces and severely increased spongiosa element within the leaflet itself outlined by its black-staining elastic membrane (elastic van Geison, 40×). Abbreviations as in Figure 2.

The superimposed fibrous tissue on the atrial and ventricular aspects of the posterior mitral leaflet is quite different histologically. On the atrial aspect, the surface is usually smooth, and the fibrous tissue is dense and contains numerous parallel-lying elastic fibers, simulating in a way the media of an elastic artery. By contrast, the superimposed fibrous tissue on the ventricular surface and surrounding the chordae tends to have an irregular surface, the collagen is less dense, and it contains few, if any, elastic fibers. The atrial surfaces, of course, are the ones making abnormal leaflet contact; the ventricular surfaces are receiving the impact of the left ventricular systolic pressure. The reason for the structural difference between the 2 surfaces is unclear.

That the identification of a ruptured chord is infrequent but that covered (by fibrous tissue) chordae are nearly

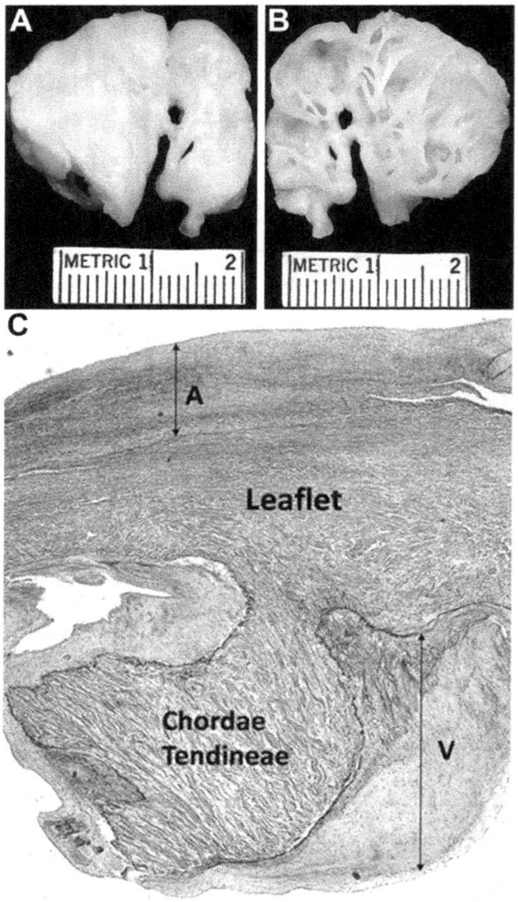

Figure 5 Patient #4 in Table 2

Photographs of the A surface **(A)** and V surface **(B)** of a portion of excised posterior leaflet. Most chordae are missing from or tangled on the V surface shown in **B. (C)** Photomicrograph showing superimposed fibrous tissue on both the A and V surfaces and no or minimal increase in the spongiosa element within the leaflet itself, which is outlined by its black-staining elastic membrane (elastic van Geison, 40×). Abbreviations as in Figure 2.

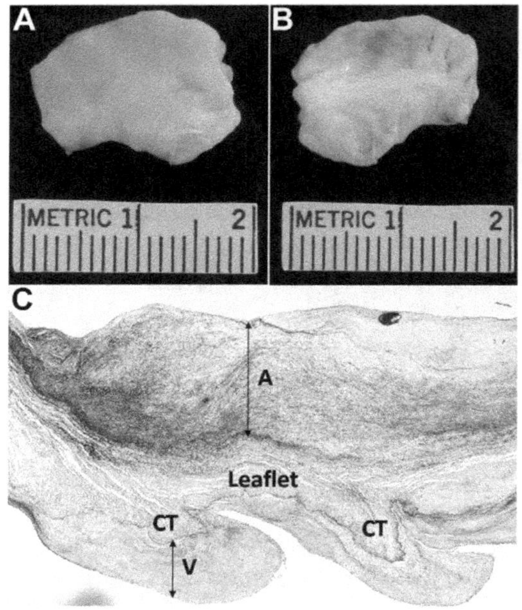

Figure 6 Patient #5 in Table 2

Photographs of the A surface **(A)** and V surface **(B)** of a portion of excised posterior leaflet. All chordae are missing from the V surface shown in **B. (C)** Photomicrograph showing superimposed fibrous tissue on both the A and V surfaces and only mildly increased spongiosa element within the leaflet itself, outlined by its black-staining elastic membrane (elastic van Geison, 40×). Abbreviations as in Figure 2.

universal in patients with MVP and MR severe enough to warrant operative repair strongly suggest that most chordal ruptures are clinically silent and occur possibly multiple times through the years. Also, the patients having acute heart failure might have ruptured a primary chord (i.e., one arising from a papillary muscle itself and not one actually attached to the mitral leaflet, as would be the case with a tertiary chord, which would unlikely lead to MR or to a sudden worsening of MR).

This article, of course, follows numerous ones discussing gross and histological features of prolapsed mitral valves examined at either necropsy or after operative excision (1–20). Few, however, mentioned the superimposed fibrous tissue on the leaflet and chordae, probably because elastic-tissue stains were not used, a requirement to see the outline of the underlying leaflet and chordae. Additionally, none mentioned hidden—previously ruptured—chordae by the overlying fibrous tissue. Thus, chordal rupture in MVP is far more common than previously appreciated (10,13,14,16,21–23).

Elastic-tissue stains were prepared on all histological sections of the operatively excised posterior mitral leaflets, a requirement to separate the superimposed fibrous tissue from the underlying leaflet itself. In all cases, the operative specimen and histological sections of it were studied and described by the same individual (namely, W.C.R.) and not by a variety of persons with varying knowledge of and interest in cardiovascular disease. All patients included had pre-operative echocardiograms described by the reader to be characteristic of MVP. The present report excluded all patients with angiographic evidence of significant coronary narrowing and any patient having coronary artery bypass grafting; all patients with a dysfunctioning aortic valve or aortic valve repair or replacement and all patients with associated mitral stenosis or prior infective endocarditis at any time were also excluded. All these exclusions were an attempt to make certain the patients included herein were a group with "pure" MVP.

Study limitations. We studied only patients with MVP who had MR severe enough to warrant mitral valve repair. Whether our observations hold true for younger patients

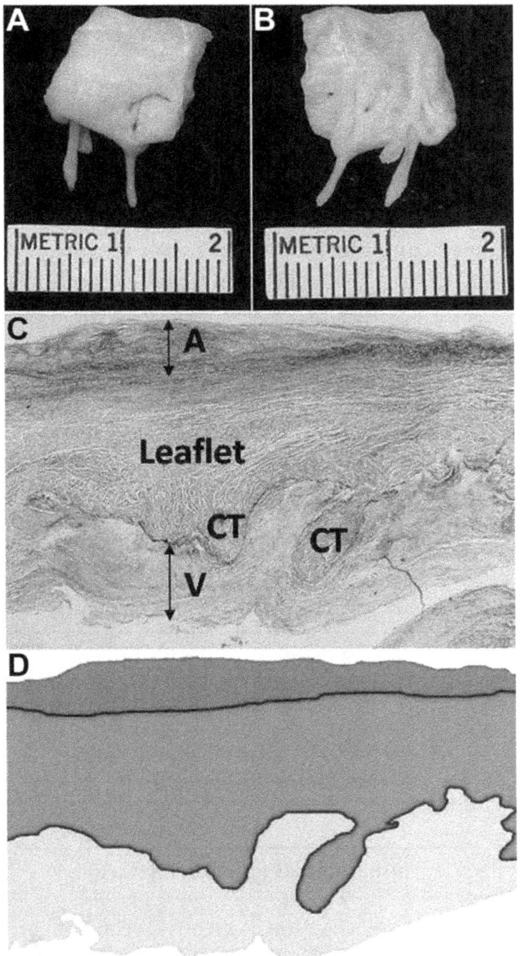

Figure 7 Patient #6 in Table 2

Photographs of the A surface **(A)** and V surface **(B)** of a portion of excised posterior leaflet. Most chordae are missing from the V surface. **(C)** Photomicrograph showing superimposed fibrous tissue on both the A and V surfaces and mildly increased spongiosa element within the leaflet itself, which is outlined by its black-staining elastic membrane (elastic van Geison, 40×). **(D)** Rendering of the same valve with **red** representing the leaflet itself, **green** representing the superimposed fibrous tissue on the A surface, and **yellow** representing the superimposed fibrous tissue on the V surface. Abbreviations as in Figure 2.

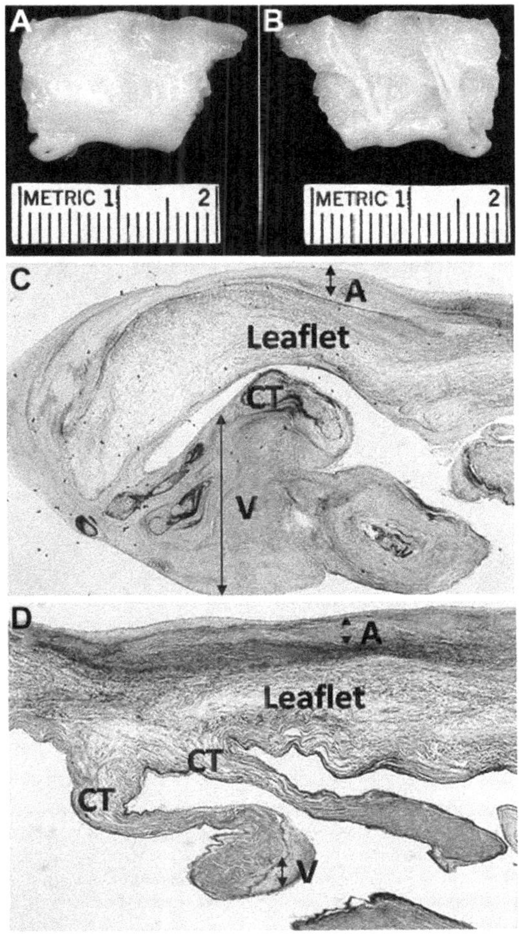

Figure 8 Patient #7 in Table 2

Photographs of the A surface **(A)** and V surface **(B)** of a portion of excised posterior leaflet. Most chordae are missing from the V surface shown in **B**. **(C)** Photomicrograph distally at the free margin showing a large amount of superimposed fibrous tissue on both the A and V surfaces and almost complete replacement of the fibrosa element by the spongiosa element within the leaflet itself outlined by its black-staining elastic membrane (elastic van Geison, 40×). **(D)** Photomicrograph of the same valve to the annulus showing less superimposed fibrous tissue on the A and V surfaces and only a moderate increase in the spongiosa element within the leaflet (elastic van Geison, 40×). Abbreviations as in Figure 2.

e.g., with mild MR from MVP) is unclear. Additionally, he amount of mitral leaflet tissue available to examine varied rom patient to patient. Although all 37 patients had pre-:ordial systolic murmurs recorded in the medical record, vhether the murmur was pansystolic or late systolic only or ccompanied by 1 or more systolic clicks was not recorded. The echocardiograms were interpreted by a number of lifferent echocardiographers. Details of the thickness of the nitral leaflets were not recorded in any echocardiographic eport and not by any surgeon at operation.

Conclusions

This study of operatively-excised posterior mitral leaflets in patients with MR secondary to MVP indicates that the leaflet thickening is the result primarily of superimposed fibrous tissue on both surfaces of the leaflet and that previously ruptured chordae, nearly universal, are usually covered by the superimposed fibrous tissue on the ventricular surface by the time of operative intervention.

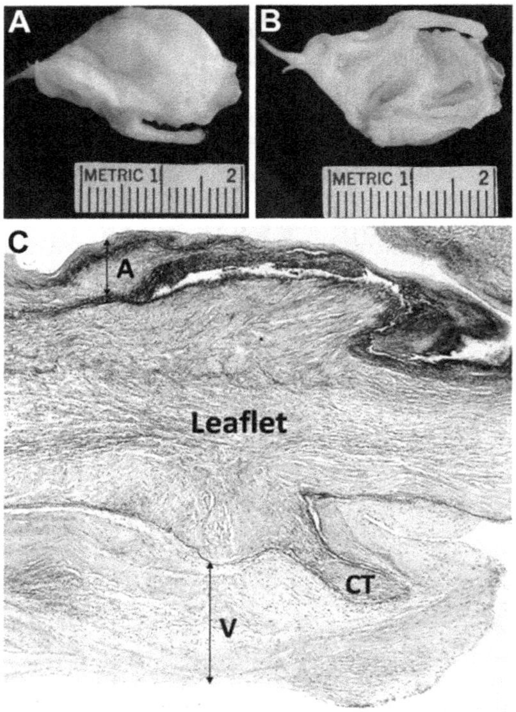

Figure 9 Patient #8 in Table 2

Photographs of the A surface **(A)** and V surface **(B)** of a portion of excised posterior leaflet. Most chordae are missing from the V surface. **(C)** Photomicrograph showing superimposed fibrous tissue on both the A and V surfaces and increased spongiosa element within the valve leaflet itself, outlined by its black-staining elastic membrane (elastic van Geison, 40×). Abbreviations as in Figure 2.

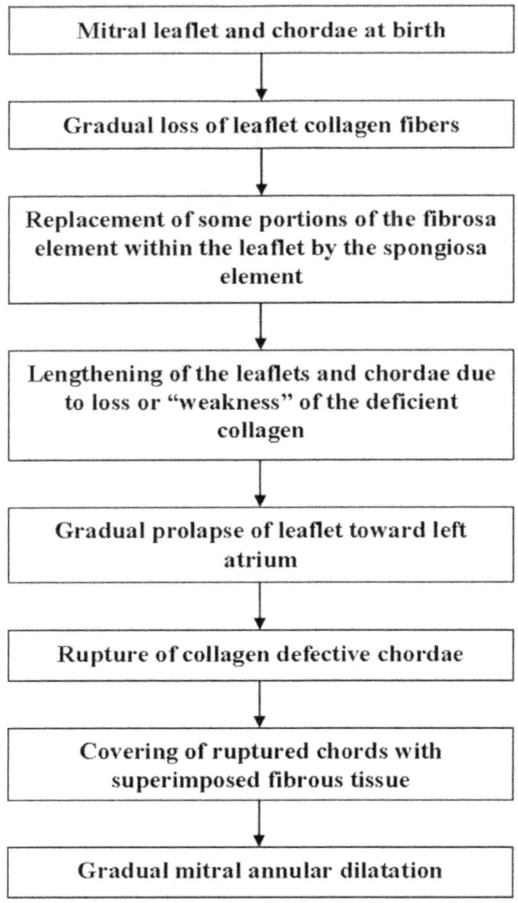

Figure 10 Chart Showing Likely Mechanism of Mitral Valve Prolapse

Mitral valve prolapse going from initial loss of collagen, to partial replacement by the spongiosa element, to leaflet elongation and chordal rupture with focal leaflet prolapse, and gradual thickening due to superimposed fibrous tissue.

Table 2 Comparison of Various Variables Among 8 Patients Having Isolated MV Repair for MV Prolapse Whose Valves Are Illustrated Both Grossly and Histologically

					Pressures (mm Hg)				
Patient #	Figure #	Age (yrs)	Sex	Race	RV (s/d)	LV (s/d)	Aorta (s/d)	EF (%)	MV Weight (g)
1	2	43	M	W	34/15	112/12	111/74	70	1.02
2	3	46	F	W	26/10	101/13	104/55	40	0.64
3	4	48	M	W	38/14	102/23	106/67	65	1.94
4	5	54	M	W	31/11	—	120/55*	65	1.61
5	6	54	F	W	—	—	100/55*	—	0.33
6	7	55	M	W	34/10	137/19	135/80	70	0.31
7	8	59	M	A	41/9	116/14	121/85	30	0.47
8	9	66	M	W	16/2	92/6	96/69	—	0.81

*Indirect blood pressure measurement.
s/d = systole/diastole; other abbreviations as in Table 1.

Reprint requests and correspondence: Dr. William C. Roberts, Baylor Heart and Vascular Institute, Baylor University Medical Center at Dallas, 3500 Gaston Avenue, Dallas, Texas 75246. E-mail: wc.roberts@baylorhealth.edu.

REFERENCES

1. Fernex M, Fernex C. Mucoid degenerescence of the mitral valve; functional repercussions. Helv Med Acta 1958;25:694–705.
2. Read RC, Thal AP, Wendt VE. Symptomatic valvular myxomatous transformation (the floppy valve syndrome). A possible forme frusta of the Marfan syndrome. Circulation 1965;32:897–910.
3. Bittar N, Sosa JA. The billowing mitral valve leaflet. Report on fourteen patients. Circulation 1968;38:763–70.
4. Trent JK, Adelman AG, Wigle ED, Silver MD. Morphology of a prolapsed posterior mitral valve leaflet. Am Heart J 1970;79:539–43.
5. McCarthy LJ, Wolf PL. Mucoid degeneration of heart valves: "blue valve syndrome". Am J Clin Pathol 1970;54:852–6.
6. Shappell SD, Marshall CE. Ballooning posterior leaflet syndrome. Syncope and sudden death. Arch Intern Med 1975;135:664–7.
7. Davies MJ, Moore BP, Braimbridge MV. The floppy mitral valve. Study of incidence, pathology, and complications in surgical, necropsy, and forensic material. Br Heart J 1978;40:468–81.
8. Olsen EGJ, Al-Rufaie HK. The floppy mitral valve. Study on pathogenesis. Br Heart J 1980;44:674–83.
9. Rippe J, Fishbein MC, Carabello B, et al. Primary myxomatous degeneration of cardiac valves. Clinical, pathological, haemodynamic, and echocardiographic profile. Br Heart J 1980;44:621–9.
10. Hickey AJ, Wilcken DEL, Wright JS, Warren BS. Primary (spontaneous) chordal rupture: relation to myxomatous valve disease and mitral valve prolapse. J Am Coll Cardiol 1985;5:1341–6.
11. van der Bel-Kahn J, Duren DR, Becker AE. Isolated mitral valve prolapse: chordal architecture as an anatomic basis in older patients. J Am Coll Cardiol 1985;5:1335–40.
12. Hanson TP, Edwards BS, Edwards JE. Pathology of surgically excised mitral valves. Arch Pathol Lab Med 1985;109:823–8.
13. Olson LJ, Subramanian R, Ackermann DM, Orszulak TA, Edwards WD. Surgical pathology of the mitral valve: a study of 712 cases spanning 21 years. Mayo Clin Proc 1987;62:22–34.
14. Roberts WC, McIntosh CL, Wallace RB. Mechanisms of severe mitral regurgitation in mitral valve prolapse determined from analysis of operatively excised valves. Am Heart J 1987;113:1316–23.
15. Virmani R, Atkinson JB, Forman MB. The pathology of mitral valve prolapse. Herz 1988;13:215–26.
16. Turri M, Thiene G, Bortolotti U, Mazzucco A, Gallucci V. Surgical pathology of disease of the mitral valve, with special reference to lesions promoting valvular incompetence. Int J Cardiol 1989;22:213–9.
17. Dollar AL, Roberts WC. Morphologic comparison of patients with mitral valve prolapse who died suddenly with patients who died from severe valvular dysfunction or other conditions. J Am Coll Cardiol 1991;17:921–31.
18. Agozzino L, Falco A, de Vivo F, de Vinventiis C, de Luca L, Esposito S, Cotrufo M. Surgical pathology of the mitral valve: gross and histological study of 1288 surgically excised valves. Int J Cardiol 1992;37:79–89.
19. Shirani J, Roberts WC. Clinical and morphologic features of mitral valve prolapse in octogenarians. Am J Cardiol 1993;72:1316–9.
20. Butany J, Privitera S, David TE. Mitral valve prolapse: an atypical variation of the anatomy. Can J Cardiol 2003;19:1367–73.
21. Cooley DA, Gerami S, Hallman GL, Wukasch DC, Hall RJ. Mitral insufficiency due to myxomatous transformation: "floppy valve syndrome". J Cardiovasc Surg 1972;13:346–9.
22. Chadraratna PA, Aronow WS. Incidence of ruptured chordae tendineae in mitral valve prolapse syndrome. An echocardiographic study. Chest 1979;75:334–9.
23. Grenadier E, Alpan G, Keidar S, Palant A. The prevalence of ruptured chordae tendineae in the mitral valve prolapse syndrome. Am Heart J 1983;105:603–10.

Key Words: mitral regurgitation ▪ mitral valve prolapse ▪ mitral valve repair.

Lipoma of the Mitral Valve

William C. Roberts, MD[a,b,c,d,*], Paul A. Grayburn, MD[a,b,c,d], and Baron L. Hamman, MD[a,b,c,d]

Described herein is a 67-year-old morbidly obese man who had a lipoma excised from his posterior mitral leaflet after it was found by echocardiogram. Findings in 6 other previously reported cases are reviewed. **(Am J Cardiol 2017;119:1121−1123)**

Every human heart contains some adipose tissue. It is most commonly located in the subepicardial regions, right ventricular free wall, and atrial septum. These fatty infiltrates are not localized or encapsulated but simply invade the subepicardial spaces or the spaces between the myocardial cells. On rare occasion, the adipose tissue cells are encapsulated forming distinct masses and then they can be called lipomas. They have been reported to occur in the

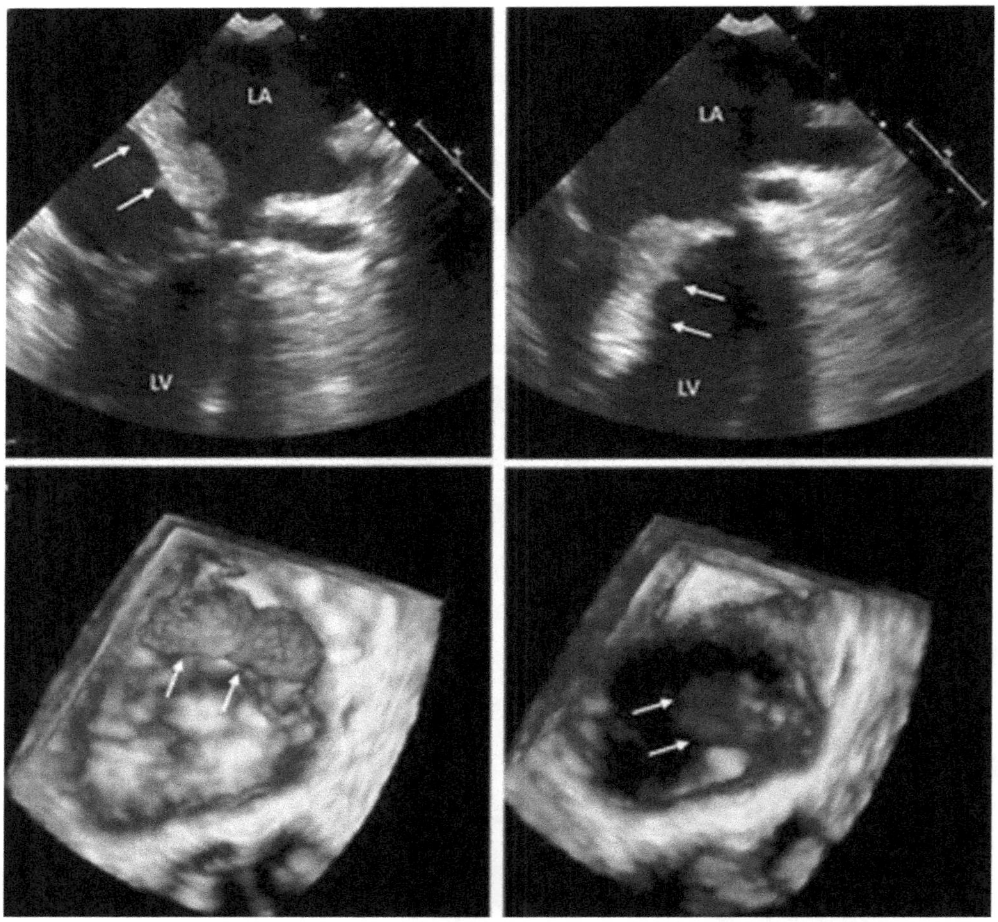

Figure 1. Transesophageal images of a large echo-dense mass attached to the medial scallop *(arrows)* of the posterior mitral leaflet. *Upper left*: End-systolic frame showi the mass extending cephalad into the left atrium (LA). *Upper right*: End-diastolic frame showing the mass extending into the left ventricle (LV). *Bottom left*: End-systolic dimensional "surgeon's view" showing the mass from the left atrial aspect. *Bottom right*: End-diastolic 3-dimenional "surgeon's view" showing the mass in the LV

atrial and ventricular cavities and walls [1−12] and in tl atrioventricular valves.[13−18] Risk factors for these cardi lipomas have not been delineated. This report was prompt by finding a mass on the mitral valve by echocardiogra and that led to its operative excision and morpholog examination.

[a]Baylor Heart and Vascular Institute, [b]Division of Cardiology, Department of Internal Medicine, [c]Department of Pathology, and [d]Department of Cardiothoracic Surgery, Baylor University Medical Center, Dallas, Texas. Manuscript received November 24, 2016; revised manuscript received and accepted November 29, 2016.

See page 1123 for disclosure information.

*Corresponding author: Tel: (214) 820-7911; fax: (214) 820-7533.

E-mail address: william.roberts1@BSWHealth.org (W.C. Roberts).

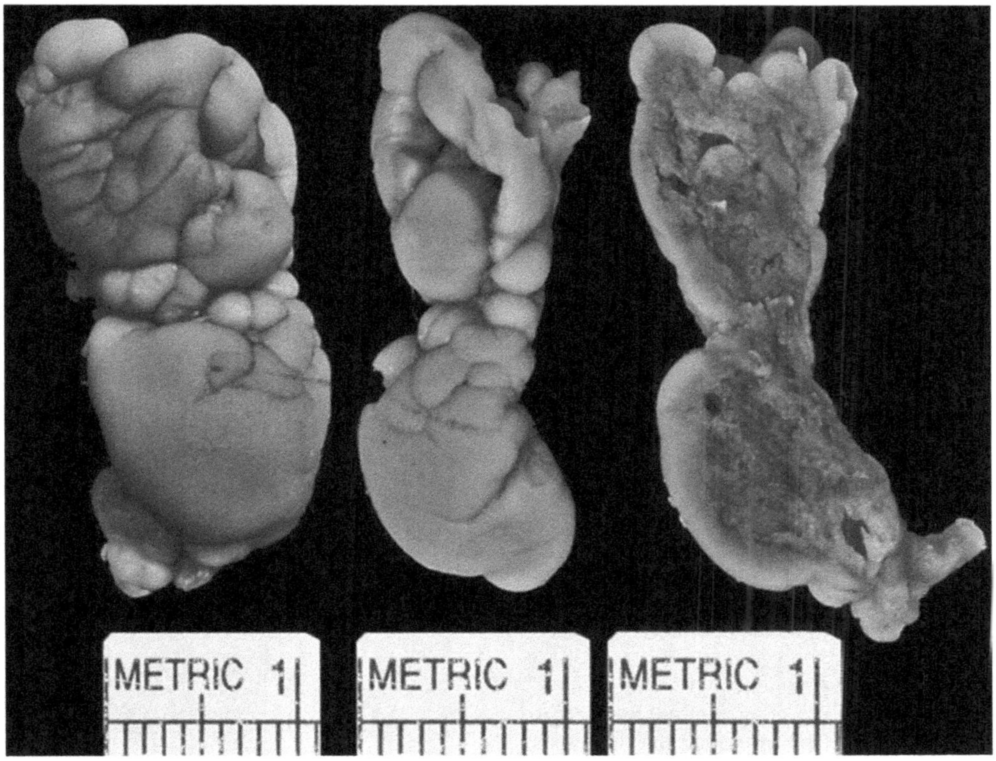

Figure 2. Photograph of the lipoma excised at operation. The *left* and *center* photos are exterior views showing the lumpy fatty deposits. The *right view* shows the necrotic interior of the lipoma.

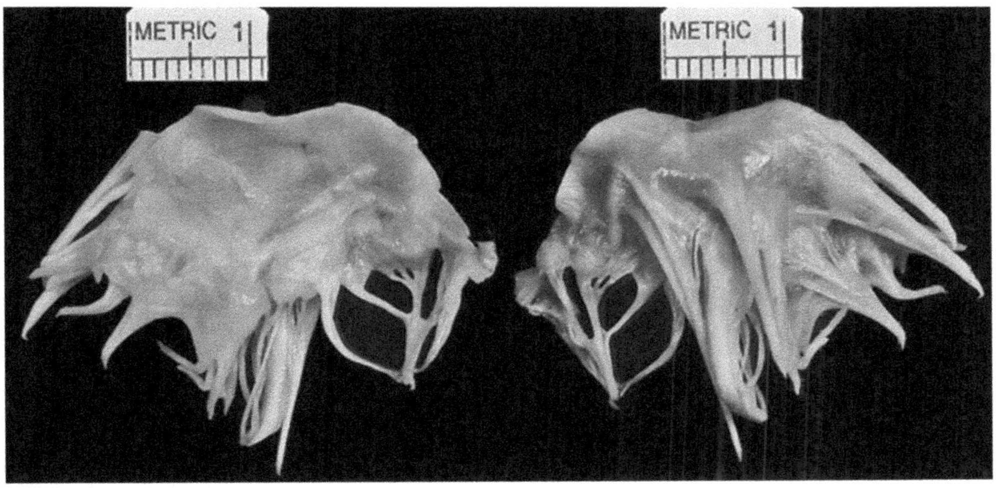

Figure 3. Operatively excised mitral valve. The *left photograph* shows the atrial aspect and the *right photograph*, the ventricular aspect.

Case Description

A 67-year-old man was hospitalized because of generalized weakness and exertional dyspnea for 3 weeks. In times past he had had periodic atrial fibrillation and had received a pacemaker. In the hospital, he was found to have pre-existing pneumonia and was treated accordingly. Because his symptoms could also have resulted from cardiac disease, an echocardiogram was performed and a mobile mass attached to the posterior mitral leaflet was found (Figure 1). The patient weighed 320 pounds and stood 74 inches in height (body mass index 41 kg/m^2). A precordial murmur was not present. At operation, the mass was attached by a single stalk to the posterior mitral leaflet. It was excised intact by incising the stalk and then the mitral valve was replaced by a metallic (ON-X 31/33) mechanical prosthesis. The mass weighed 2.30 g and histologically was a lipoma (Figure 2). Most of the interior of the mass consisted of necrotic adipose tissue cells. His postoperative course was uneventful. The excised anterior mitral leaflet is shown in Figure 3.

Table 1
Previously reported cases of lipomas involving the mitral valve

First Author (Year) [Reference]	Age (Yrs) at Excision	Sex	Leaflet Location on MV	Weight (g) of Lipoma	Operatively Excised	Symptoms Before Excision	Method of Diagnosis	MVR	MV Leaflet	Reason for Echo	MR	BMI (Kg/m^2)
1. Barberger-Gateau (1978) [13]	12	M	Posterior	4	+	0	Echo	+	Normal	Murmur	+	
2. Behnam (1983) [14]	16	F	Posterior	—	+	0	Echo	+	Normal	Murmur	+	
3. Anderson (1988) [15]	54	M	Posterior	—	+/−	+	Echo	+	Normal	Dizziness	+	
4. Dollar (1989) [16]	66	F	Posterior	2	+	+	Echo	+	Normal	Dyspnea	+	33
5. Vadmal (1998) [17]	5	M	Anterior	—	+	0	Echo	0	Normal	Murmur*	+	
6. Harth (2003) [18]	56	F	Anterior	3	+	0	Echo	0	Normal	"Thud"	+	
7. Present Case	67	M	Posterior	2.3	+	+	Echo	+	Normal	Dyspnea	+	41

BMI = body mass index; Echo = echocardiography; F = female; M = male; MR = mitral regurgitation; MV = mitral valve; MVR = mitral valve replacement.

— = no information available.

* This patient was known to have a perimembraneous ventricular septal defect.

Discussion

At least 6 reports have appeared (Table 1), each describing a single patient with a lipoma involving the mitral valve and in each the lipoma was operatively excised. In each of the 6 patients either the presence of a precordial murmur or abnormal sound (4 patients) or symptoms (2 patients) suggesting cardiac disease prompted the performance of an echocardiogram which provided the diagnosis. The lipoma involved the posterior mitral leaflet only in 4 patients and the anterior leaflet in 2. In 4 patients, the lipoma was firmly attached to the mitral leaflet with or without entangling the chordae tendineae and the valve was replaced; in 2 patients, the lipoma was attached to the anterior leaflet by a stalk, as in our patient, or by a small attachment and in both of these patients the valve was preserved. The fact that the interior of the lipoma in our patient was necrotic suggests that the lipoma had been in place for years. In only 1 previously reported patient was body weight or height or body mass index mentioned and that patient was obese. The presently described patient was morbidly obese (body mass index 41 kg/m^2). Both anterior and posterior leaflets in all 6 patients, as in the present patient, appeared to be normal in areas where the lipoma was not attached. In only 3 of the 6 patients was the operatively excised lipoma weighed (2 to 4 g). In the present patient it weighed 2.3 g. All patients survived the operative procedure without complications.

Disclosures

The authors have no conflicts of interest to disclose.

1. Crockett JE, Decker D, Reed W, Dunn M, Leger L. Lipoma of the heart. *Am J Cardiol* 1964;14:394–398.
2. Bradford JH, Nomeir AM, Watts LE. Left ventricular lipoma: echocardiographic and angiographic features. *South Med J* 1980;73:663–665.
3. Harada K, Seki I, Kobayashi H, Okuni M, Sakurai I. Lipoma of the heart in a child: clinical, echocardiographic, angiographic, and pathological features. *Jpn Heart J* 1980;21:903–910.
4. Zingas AP, Carrera JD, Murray CA III, Kling GA. Lipoma of the myocardium. *J Comput Assist Tomogr* 1983;7:1098–1100.
5. Hananouchi GI, Goff WB II. Cardiac lipoma: six-year follow-up with MRI characteristics, and a review of the literature. *Magn Reson Imaging* 1990;8:825–828.
6. Steger CM. Intrapericardial giant lipoma displacing the heart. *ISRN Cardiol* 2011;2011:243637.
7. Zhu SB, Zhu J, Liu Y, Wang RP. Surgical treatment of a giant symptomatic cardiac lipoma. *J Thorac Oncol* 2013;8:1341–1342.
8. Patris V, Argirious M, Lama N, Sakellaridis T, Charitos C. Trans-aortic excision of intraventricular lipoma with the assistance of arthroscopi camera. *J Thorac Dis* 2013;5:E140–E143.
9. Ismail I, Al-Khafaji K, Mutyala M, Aggarwal S, Cotter W, Hakim H, Khosia S, Arora R. Cardiac lipoma. *J Community Hosp Intern Me Perspect* 2015;5:28449.
10. Barbuto L, Ponsiglione A, Del Vecchio W, Altiero M, Rossi G, D Rosa D, Pisani A, Imbriaco M. Humongous right atrial lipoma: correlative CT and MR case report. *Quant Imaging Med Surg* 2015;5 774–777.
11. Saikia MK, Kalita JP, Kapoor M, Phukon P, Malviya A Padmanabhan A. Surgical resection of giant lipoma of interventricul septum presenting as RVOTO: a case report. *J Cardiovasc Dis Re* 2015;6:152–155.
12. Zhang HW, Zhong MH, Meng W, Zhang EY, Gu J, Hu J. Imag section: intramuscular lipoma as an unusual cause of right ventricul outflow tract obstruction. *Echocardiography* 2016;33:328–329.
13. Barberger-Gateau P, Paquet M, Desaulniers D, Chenard J. Fibrolipom of the mitral valve in a child: clinical and echocardiographic feature *Circulation* 1978;58:955–958.
14. Behnam R, Williams G, Gerlis L, Walker D, Scott O. Lipoma of th mitral valve and papillary muscle. *Am J Cardiol* 1983;5 1459–1460.
15. Anderson DR, Gray MR. Mitral incompetence associated with lipor infiltrating the mitral valve. *Br Heart J* 1988;60:169–171.
16. Dollar AL, Wallace RB, Kent KM, Burkhart MW, Roberts WC. Mit valve replacement for mitral lipoma associated with severe obesity. *A J Cardiol* 1989;64:1405–1407.
17. Vadmal MS, Hajdu SI. Lipoma of the mitral valve in a child. *Ann C Lab Sci* 1998;28:242–245.
18. Harth M, Ruemmele P, Knuechel-Clarke R, Elsner D, Riegger Sclerosed lipoma of the mitral valve. *J Heart Valve Dis* 2003;12(722–725.

Mitral Valve Repair for Pure Mitral Regurgitation Followed Years Later by Mitral Valve Replacement for Mitral Stenosis

Tiffany M. Becker, BS[a], Paul A. Grayburn, MD[a,b], and William C. Roberts, MD[a,b,c,*]

We describe herein 2 patients who developed severe mitral stenosis (MS) approximately two decades after a mitral valve repair operation for pure mitral regurgitation (MR) secondary to mitral valve prolapse. This report's purpose is to point out that use of a circumferential mitral annular ring during the repair has the potential to produce a transmitral pressure gradient just like that occurring after mitral valve replacement utilizing a mechanical prosthesis or a bioprosthesis in the mitral position. **(Am J Cardiol 2017;120:160–166)**

Recently, we reported findings in 29 patients who had undergone mitral valve repair operations for pure MR with insertion of an annular ring and later underwent mitral valve replacement for either recurring MR or development of MS or obstruction to left ventricular outflow.[1] The present report was prompted by study of 2 additional patients who developed severe MS many years (≈20) after the repair operation for pure MR due to mitral valve prolapse. Because of the late development of well-documented MS, an infrequently reported occurrence after a repair operation for pure MR, we believe that this additional report is worthwhile.

Patients Described

Pertinent features in each of the 2 patients are summarized in Table 1. At the first operation, patient #1 had a quadrangular resection of a portion of posterior mitral leaflet and ring insertion; patient #2 had the ring insertion but whether a portion of the posterior leaflet was resected is uncertain. The interval between the 2 mitral valve operative procedures was 19 years in patient #1 and 21 years in patient #2. Just before the replacement operation the mean transmitral gradient by echocardiogram was 10 mm Hg in patient #1 and 12 mm Hg in patient #2 (Figures 1 to 3). Computed tomographic imaging in patient #1 showed focal calcific deposits in the mitral leaflets, something not present before the repair operation 19 years earlier (Figure 4). Certain morphologic features of the operatively excised mitral valves and rings are shown in Figures 5 and 6. At early postoperative follow-up both patients were asymptomatic (case #1 four months and case #2 one month postoperatively, respectively).

Table 1
Pertinent clinical and morphologic features in the 2 patients having mitral valve repair for mitral valve prolapse and approximately 20 years later mitral valve replacement for mitral stenosis

Variable	Case #1	Case #2
1. Age (years) at the mitral repair operation	21	32
2. Age (years) at mitral valve replacement	40	53
3. Interval (years) between the 2 operations	19	21
4. Sex	Man	Woman
5. Atrial Fibrillation	0	+
6. Ventricular arrhythmia	0	+
7. Body mass index (Kg/m^2)	29	35
8. Degree of mitral regurgitation (0-4$^+$)	1$^+$	1$^+$
9. Transvalvular mean gradient (mmHg)*	10	12
10. Mitral area (cm^2) just before mitral replacement*	1.1	1.2
11. Right ventricular peak systolic pressure (mmHg)*	46	--
12. Left ventricular ejection fraction (%)*	55	45
13. Left atrial cavity size (cm)*	4.7	5.0
14. Left ventricular cavity size*	Normal	Normal
15. Type of mitral ring	Duran (31mm)	Carpentier-Edwards
16. Area (cm^2) enclosed by the operatively excised mitral ring	2.8	3.5
17. Substitute valve inserted (mitral position)	Bioprosthesis (#27)	Mechanical (SJM) (#29)

-- = no information available; SJM = St. Jude Medical.
* By echocardiogram just before the mitral valve replacement operation.

Discussion

Development of MS after a mitral valve repair operation for pure MR using an annular ring may not be a rare occurrence. Indeed, 16 of the 29 patients described in the previously mentioned study developed some degree of MS before the replacement operation.[1] Although nearly

[a]Baylor Heart and Vascular Institute, [b]Division of Cardiology, Department of Internal Medicine, and [c]Department of Pathology, Baylor University Medical Center, Dallas, Texas. Manuscript received January 3, 2017; revised manuscript received and accepted March 20, 2017.
See page 163 for disclosure information.
*Corresponding author: Tel: (214) 820-7911; fax: (214) 820-7533.
E-mail address: william.roberts1@bswhealth.org (W.C. Roberts).

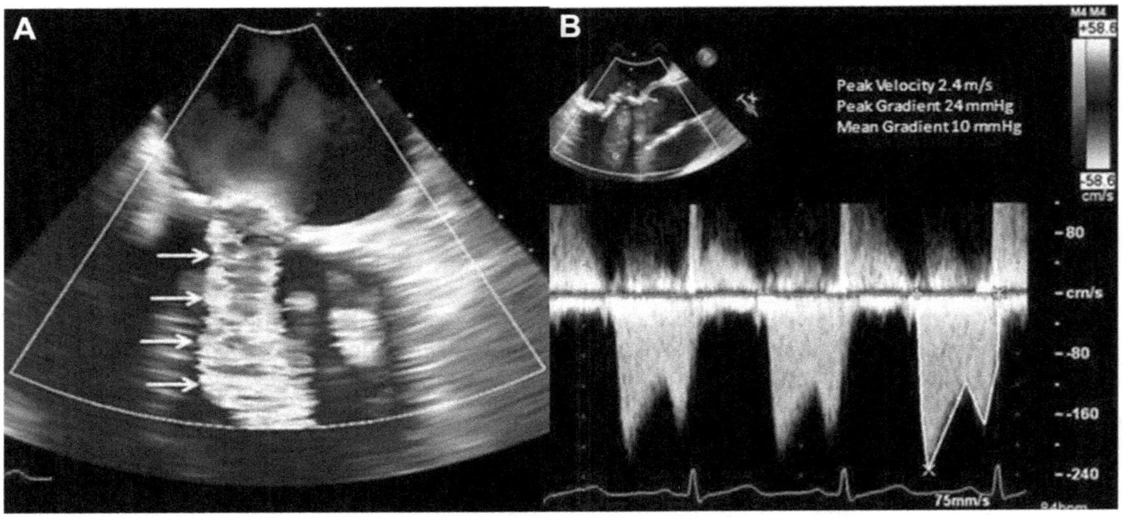

Figure 1. (Case #1) *(A)* Four-chamber view showing markedly turbulent diastolic flow into the left ventricle, characterized by a mosaic color Doppler pattern *(arrows)*. *(B)* Continuous-wave Doppler profile of mitral inflow showing elevated velocities/gradients.

all prosthetic and bioprosthetic substitute valves utilized for mitral valve replacement have an inherent gradient, the 2 patients described herein developed MS many years later, due presumably primarily to late thickening of the valve leaflets and chords. Measurement of the area enclosed by the ring excised at the time of mitral valve replacement, however, indicated that the area was much smaller than that of a normal mitral valve, suggesting at

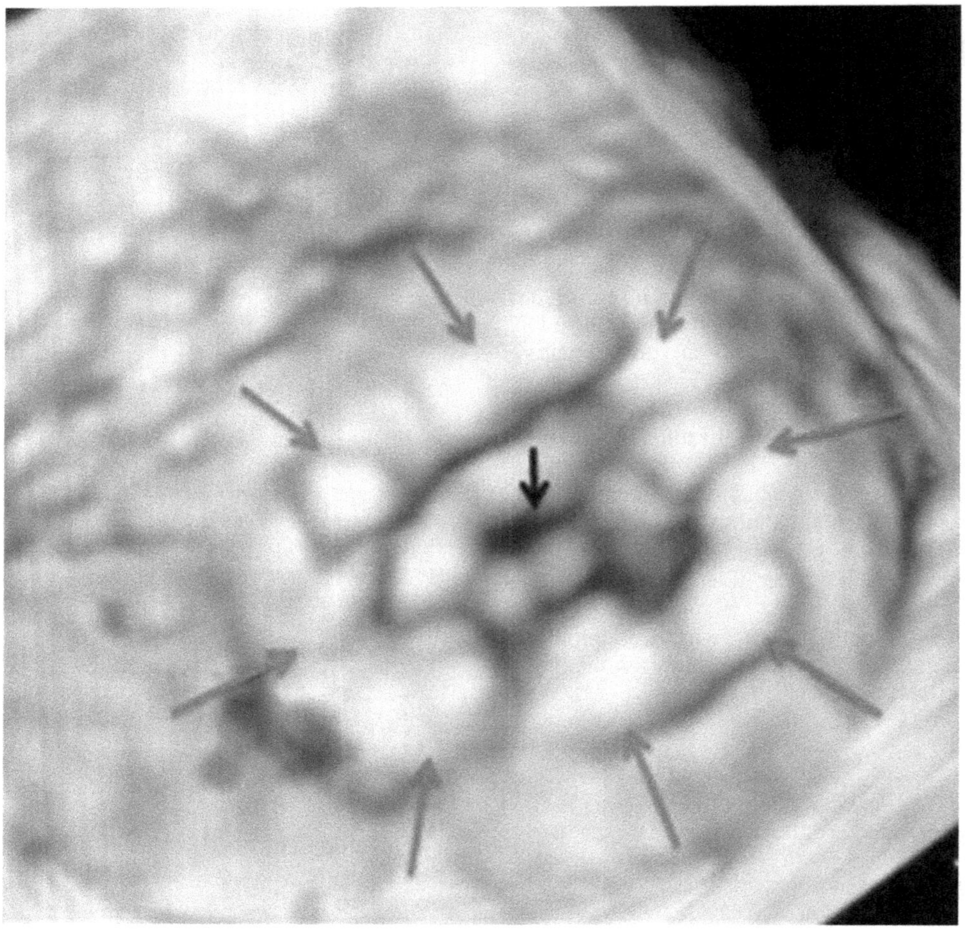

Figure 2. (Case #1) 3D "Surgeon's view" from early diastole showing mitral ring *(blue arrows)*. Within the ring, there is thickened leaflet and subvalvu tissue with a small orifice *(black arrow)*.

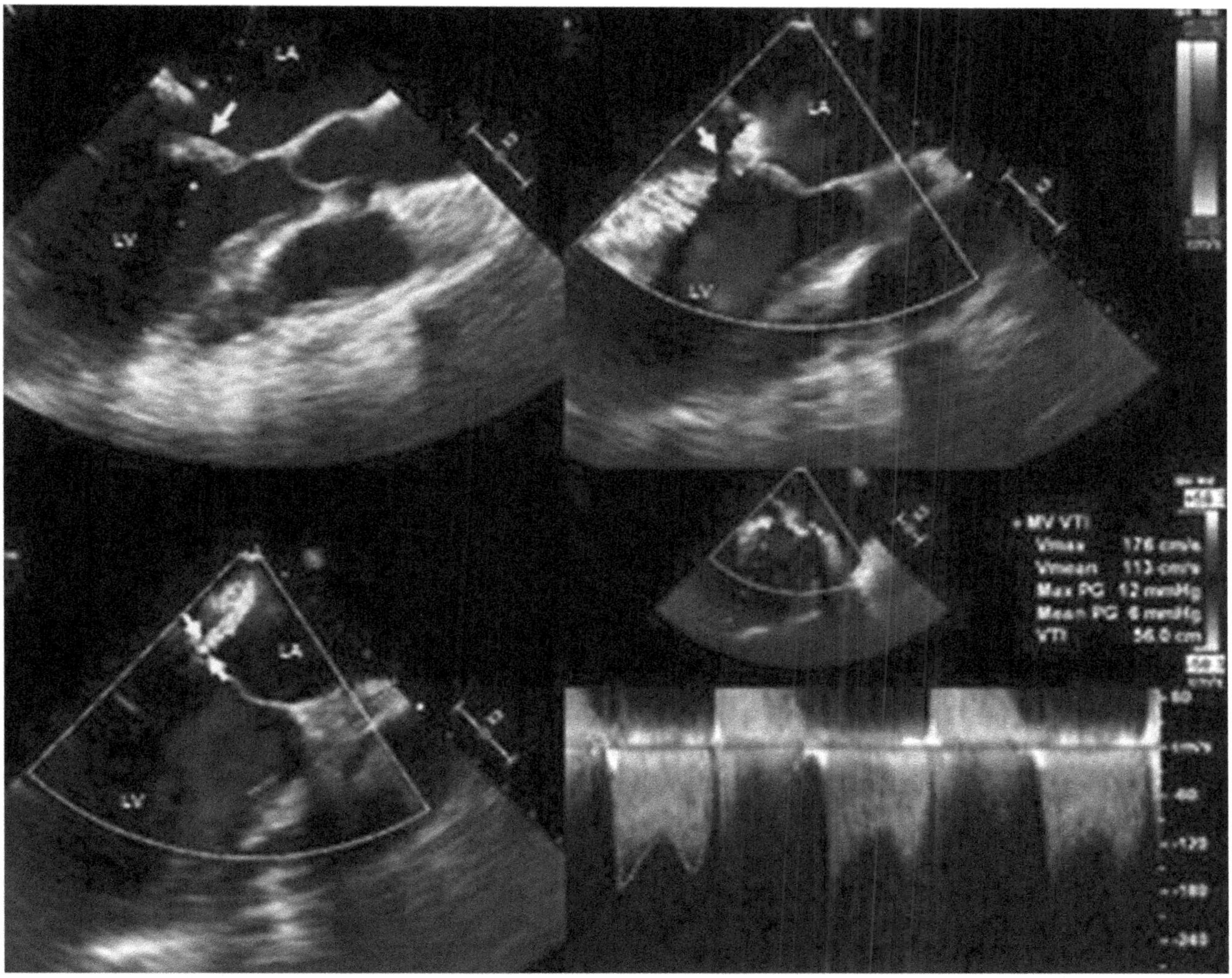

'igure 3. (Case #2) Intraoperative TEE images from the patient. *Top left:* long-axis view showing thickened anterior mitral leaflet *(arrow)*. *Top right:* diastolic rame showing mitral stenosis jet *(arrow)*. *Bottom left:* systolic frame showing mild mitral regurgitation with vena contracta width 3 mm *(arrows)*. *Bottom ight:* continuous-wave Doppler velocity profile across the mitral valve showing peak gradient 12 mm Hg and mean gradient 6 mm Hg under anesthesia.

east the possibility that the ring inserted at the time of nitral repair may have been a bit too small for the long erm. In both patients after the repair operation the mitral eaflets appeared to "gather" within the ring area, like the athering at the waist of a woman's skirt, causing focal brous thickening of the leaflets due to constant abnormal ontact over nearly 20 years. Both patients described ere asymptomatic for over 15 years after the repair rocedure. Had these 2 patients had the repair operation age 55 years, the average age of the repair procedure in e previously mentioned report,[1] both may well have ed before developing symptoms of mitral dysfunction gain.

A number of articles have appeared providing follow- after a mitral valve repair operation for pure MR, ainly mitral valve prolapse.[2–23] Several of them have entioned the development of MS after the mitral valve pair operation[3–5,14–17,21–23] (Table 2). The frequency of development of MS according to these published reports is very uncommon. The average age of the mitral repair, however, was in the 50s or 60s such that long follow-up, as in our 2 described patients, may not have been possible. Additionally, echocardiograms are not performed routinely in all these patients, suggesting that the actual frequency of MS perhaps will be much more common than suggested by these reports. In addition to these reports,[3–5,14–17,21–23] which included many patients, at least 5 case studies in adults have appeared in patients developing MS several years after mitral valve repair for pure MR (Table 3).[24–28]

How can the development of MS after mitral repair for pure MR be avoided? One might be to use an annular ring which is not too small. A second might be to use a partial annuloplasty band rather than a circumferential ring. These opinions of course need to be proven to be right or wrong.

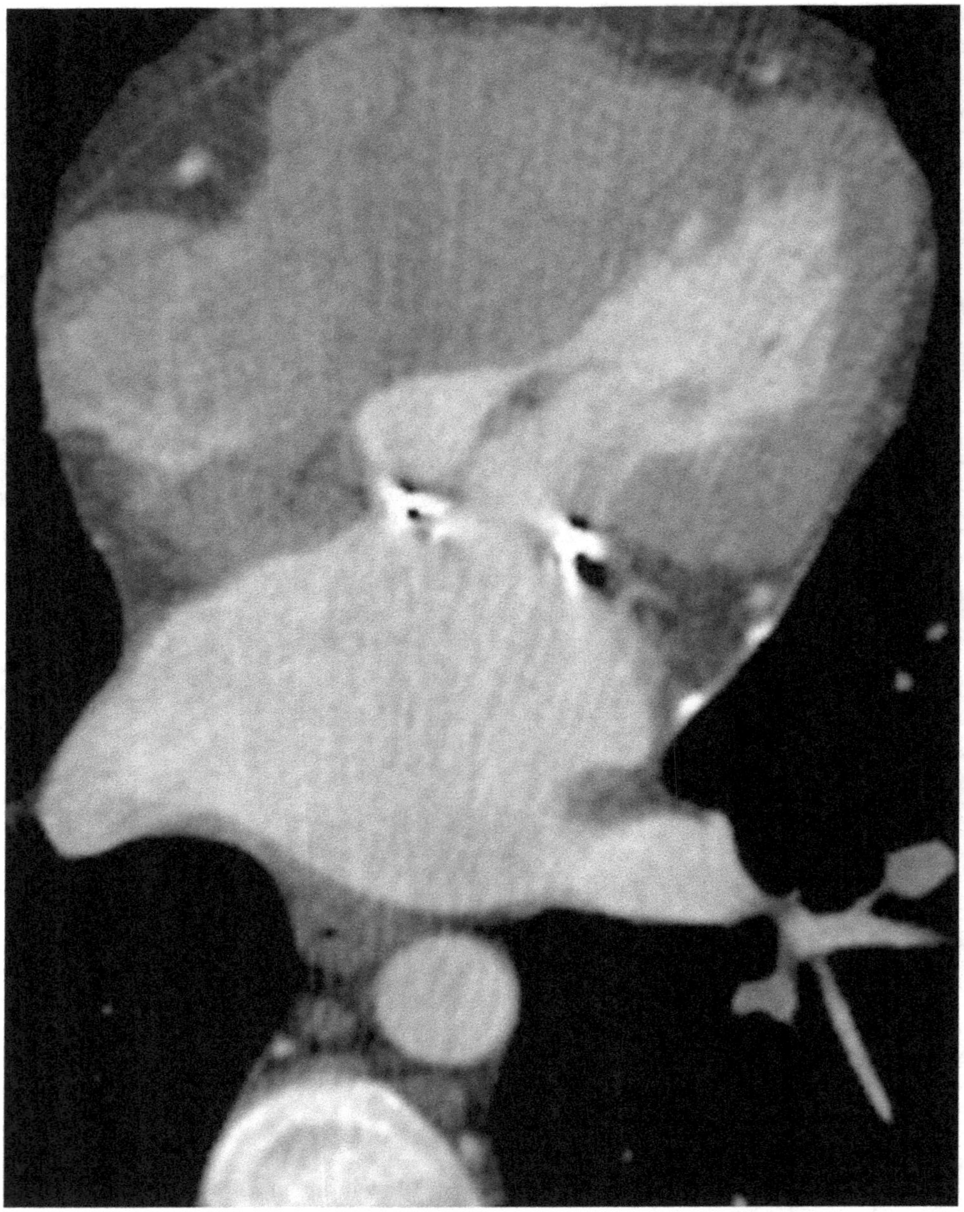

Figure 4. (Case #1) Computed tomographic image in the patient described. Shown here is the left atrium, the calcific deposits behind the mitral ring, and the l ventricular cavity. The orifice of the mitral valve is quite narrow. LA = left atrium; LV = left ventricle.

Disclosures

The authors have no conflicts of interest to disclose.

1. Roberts WC, Moore M, Ko JM, Hamman BL. Mitral valve replacement after failed mitral ring insertion with or without leaflet/chordal repair for pure mitral regurgitation. *Am J Cardiol* 2016;117:1790–1807.
2. Marwick TH, Stewart WJ, Currie PJ, Cosgrove DM. Mechanisms of failure of mitral valve repair: an echocardiographic study. *Am Heart J* 1991;122:149–156.
3. El Asmar B, Perier P, Couetil JP, Carpentier A. Failures in reconstructive mitral valve surgery. *J Med Liban* 1991;39:7–11.
4. Fernandez J, Joyce DH, Hirschfeld K, Chen C, Laub GW, Adkins MS, Anderson WA, Mackenzie JW, McGrath LB. Factors affecting mitral valve reoperation in 317 survivors after mitral valve reconstruction. *Ann Thorac Surg* 1992;54:440–448.
5. Niederhäuser U, Carrel T, von Segesser LK, Laske A, Turina Reoperation after mitral valve reconstruction: early and late results. *E J Cardiothorac Surg* 1993;7:34–37.
6. Cohn LH, Couper GS, Aranki SF, Rizzo RJ, Kinchla NM, Collins JJ Long-term results of mitral valve reconstruction for regurgitation of myxomatous mitral valve. *J Thorac Cardiovasc Surg* 1994;1 143–151.
7. Carpentier AF, Lessana A, Relland JYM, Belli E, Mihaileanu Berrebi AJ, Palsky E, Loulmet DF. The "Physio-ring": an advan concept in mitral valve annuloplasty. *Ann Thorac Surg* 1995; 1177–1186.
8. Gillinov AM, Cosgrove DM, Lytle BW, Taylor PC, Stweart R McCarthy PM, Smedira NG, Muehrcke DD, Apperson-Hansen Loop FD. Reoperation for failure of mitral valve repair. *J Tho Cardiovasc Surg* 1997;113:467–475.
9. David TE, Omran A, Armstrong S, Sun Z, Ivanov J. Long-term res of mitral valve repair for myxomatous disease with and without cho

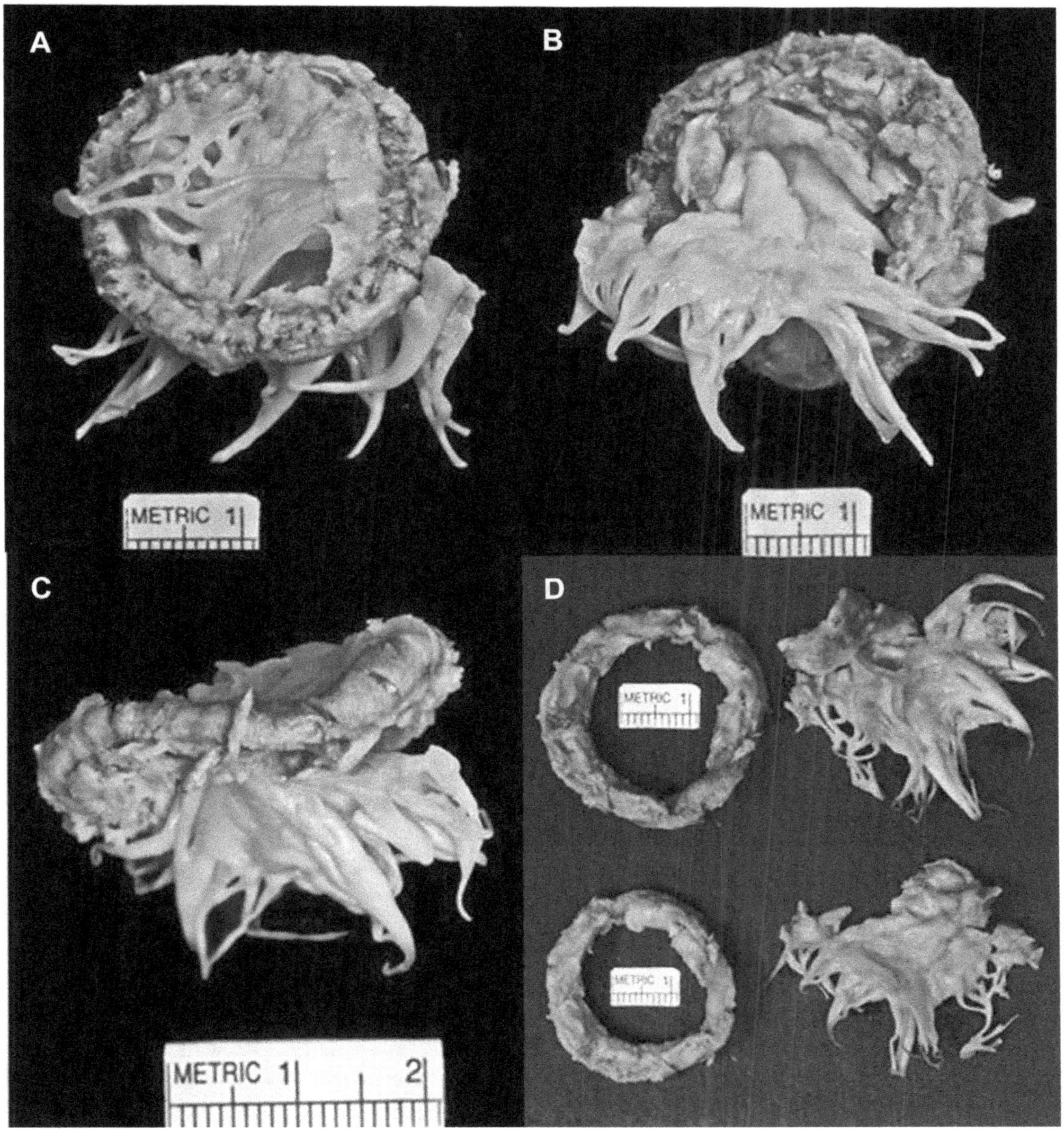

Figure 5. (Case #1) Shown here is the mitral valve with the circumferential ring attached *(A to C)* and after excision of the mitral valve from the circumferential ring *(D)*. *(A)* A view from what would be the left atrium showing the very small orifice of the mitral valve. *(B)* A view of the mitral valve within the mitral annular ring. *(C)* A side view of the mitral leaflets attached to the ring. *(D)* A view of the ring after detachment of the mitral valve. The top one shows the ring from what would be atrial side and the atrial aspect of the anterior mitral leaflet. A calcific fragment is attached to the anterior leaflet. The lower portion shows the ring from the ventricular aspect and the anterior mitral leaflet from the ventricular aspect.

replacement with expanded polytetrafluoroethylene sutures. *J Thorac Cardiovasc Surg* 1998;115:1279–1286.

10. Gillinov AM, Cosgrove DM, Blackstone EH, Diaz R, Arnold JH, Lytle BW, Smedira NG, Sabik JF, McCarthy PM, Loop FD. Durability of mitral valve repair for degenerative disease. *J Thorac Cardiovasc Surg* 1998;116:734–743.
11. Totaro P, Tulumello E, Fellini P, Rambaldini M, La Canna G, Coletti G, Zogno M, Lorusso R. Mitral valve repair for isolated prolapse of the anterior leaflet: an 11-year follow-up. *Eur J Cardiothorac Surg* 1999;15:119–126.
12. Smolens IA, Pagani FD, Deeb M, Prager RL, Sonnad SS, Bolling SF. Prophylactic mitral reconstruction for mitral regurgitation. *Ann Thorac Surg* 2001;72:1210–1216.
13. Braunberger E, Deloche A, Berrebi A, Fayssoil A, Celestin JA, Meimoun P, Chatellier G, Chauvaud S, Fabiani JN, Carpentier A. Very long-term results (more than 20 years) of valve repair with Carpentier's techniques in nonrheumatic mitral valve insufficiency. *Circulation* 2001;104:I8–I11.
14. Ibrahim MF, David TE. Mitral stenosis after mitral valve repair for non-rheumatic mitral regurgitation. *Ann Thorac Surg* 2002;73:34–36.
15. David TE, Ivanov J, Armstrong S, Rakowski H. Late outcomes of mitral valve repair for floppy valves: implications for asymptomatic patients. *J Thorac Cardiovasc Surg* 2003;125:1143–1152.
16. David TE, Ivanov J, Armstrong S, Christie D, Rakowski H. A comparison of outcomes of mitral valve repair for degenerative disease with posterior, anterior, and bileaflet prolapse. *J Thorac Cardiovasc Surg* 2005;130:1242–1249.
17. Suri RM, Schaff HV, Dearani JA, Sundt TM III, Daly RC, Mullany CJ, Enriquez-Sarano M, Orszulak TA. Recurrent mitral regurgitation after

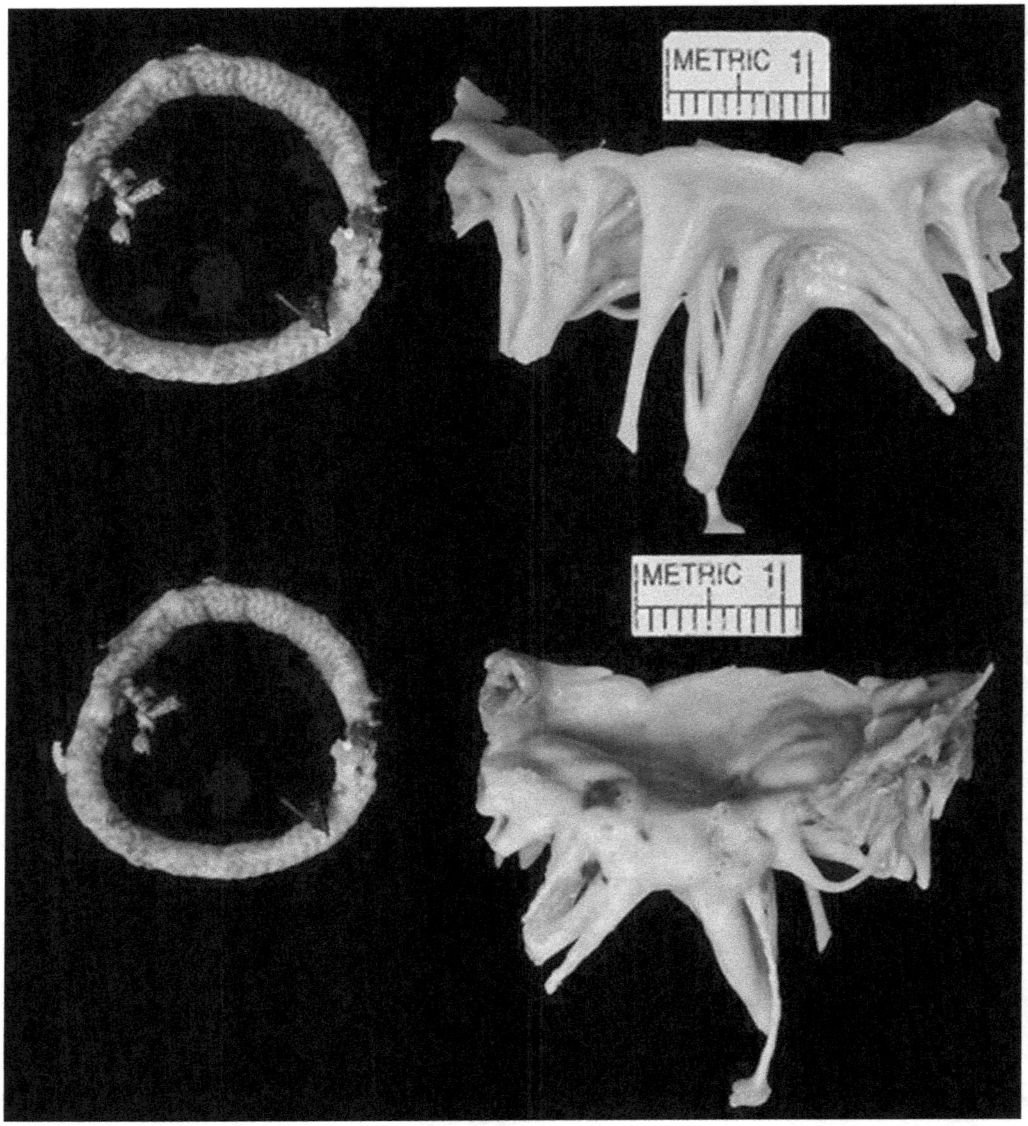

Figure 6. (Case #2) Operatively excised mitral ring *(left)* and anterior mitral leaflet *(right)* from the ventricular aspect *(upper)* and atrial aspect *(lower)*. Th distal third of the leaflet is thickened by fibrous tissue and focal calcific deposits. Likewise, most chordae tendinae are thickened by fibrous tissue.

Table 2
Previously published reports describing frequency of mitral valve reoperation late for mitral stenosis after mitral valve repair for pure mitral regurgitation

Last Name of First Author (Year)	No. of Patients with MV Repair	MV Ring Inserted	Age at Original MV Repair (Years) Range (Mean)	Male: Female	Follow-up Time (Years) Range (Mean)	Reoperation	Interval between Operations (Years) Range (Mean)	MVR	No. developing MS following MV Repair	No. wit MS havi MVR
Asmar (1991)	1705	–	–	–	0-16 (_)	72 (4%)	0-13 (5.0±3.5)	61 (3%)	12 (0.7%)	12 (0.7%
Fernandez (1992)	313	4 (1%)	9-81 (57)	110:203	1-20 (7)	63 (20%)	1-15 (6)	–	8 (3%)	–
Niederhäuser (1993)	346	5 (1%)	_ - _ (47±16)	–	_ - _ (5)	68 (20%)	_ - _ (7)	62 (18%)	17 (5%)	17 (5%)
Ibrahim (2002)	478	405 (85%)	51-61 (56)	–	1-11 (4.1±2.8)	–	4-9 (6)	3 (0.6%)	4 (0.8%)	3 (0.6%
David (2003)	488	488 (100%)	_ - _ (58±13)	347:71	3-19 (7)	22 (5%)	_ - _ (_)	18 (4%)	2 (0.4%)	2 (0.4%
David (2005)	701	668 (95%)	18-88 (58±13)	512:189	0-23 (6.9±4.0)	27 (4%)	5-8 (_)	–	3 (0.4%)	–
Suri (2006)	145	–	_ - _ (66±12)	102:43	_ - _ (3.3±4.1)	145 (100%)	_ - _ (4.1±5.1)	81 (56%)	1 (1%)	0
Chung (2007)	294	294 (100%)	_ - _ (53±13)	175:119	(3.0±1.9)	7 (2%)	(1-7) (_)	–	14 (5%)	3 (1%)
Chan (2016)	829	829 (100%)	_ - _ (64±13)	567:262	_ - _ (4.3±3.5)	21 (3%)	_ - _ (8.2)	14 (2%)	3 (0.4%)	0
Lazam (2017)	1709	–	_ - _ (65±12)	1265:444	4-18 (9)	95 (5%)	–	–	4 (0.2%)	–

MS = mitral stenosis; MV = mitral valve; MVR = mitral valve replacement; – = no information available.

Table 3
Previously published case reports describing the late development of mitral stenosis following mitral valve repair

Last Name of First Author (year)	Sex	Age at repair (years)	Cause of the MR	Quadrangular Resection of PML	Duran Ring Inserted (Size: mm)	Interval between repair and presentation of mitral stenosis (years)	Mitral valve area (cm^2)	Mean mitral valve gradient by echocardiogram (mmHg)	MVR	Interval between initial repair and MVR or PBMV or second operation (years)
Tanaka (2003)	Woman	50	MVP	+	+ (25)	3	–	–	+	3
Nishida (2005)	Woman	43	MVP	+	+ (27)	3	0.67*	22	+	4
Song (2010)	Woman	57	MVP	+	+ (25)	7	–	10	0†	7
Sachpekidis (2012)	Man	60	IC	0	+ (27)	5	1.29	10	0‡	–‡
Salenger (2016)	Woman	22	IC	0	+ (25)	12	0.6	28	0§	12

IC = ischemic cardiomyopathy; MR = mitral regurgitation; MVP = mitral valve prolapse; MVR = mitral valve replacement; PBMV = percutaneous balloon mitral valvuloplasty; PML = posterior mitral leaflet.
* At cardiac catheterization.
† At the second operation the ring and pannus tissue were excised and a commissurotomy was performed.
‡ Refused operation.
§ The patient underwent PBMV.

repair: should the mitral valve be re-repaired? *J Thorac Cardiovasc Surg* 2006;132:1390–1397.

18. De Bonis M, Lorusso R, Lapenna E, Kassem S, De Cicco G, Torracca L, Maisano F, La Canna G, Alfieri O. Similar long-term results of mitral valve repair for anterior compared with posterior leaflet prolapse. *J Thorac Cardiovasc Surg* 2006;131:364–370.
19. Suri RM, Schaff HV, Dearani JA, Sundt TM III, Daly RC, Mullany CJ, Enriques-Sarano M, Orszulak TA. Survival advantage and improved durability of mitral repair for leaflet prolapse subsets in the current era. *Ann Thorac Surg* 2006;82:819–827.
20. Dumont E, Gillinov AM, Blackstone EH, Sabik JF III, Svensson LG, Mihaljevic T, Houghtaling PL, Lytle BW. Reoperation after mitral valve repair for degenerative disease. *Ann Thorac Surg* 2007;84: 444–450.
21. Chung CH, Kim JB, Choo SJ, Kim KS, Song H, Song MG, Song JK, Kang DH, Lee JW. Long-term outcomes after mitral ring annuloplasty for degenerative mitral regurgitation: Duran ring versus Carpentier-Edwards ring. *J Heart Valve Dis* 2007;16: 536–545.
22. Chan V, Elmistekawy E, Ruel M, Hynes M, Mesana TG. How does mitral valve repair fail in patients with prolapse?-Insights from longitudinal echocardiographic follow-up. *Ann Thorac Surg* 2016;102: 1459–1465.
23. Lazam S, Vanoverschelde JL, Tribouilloy C, Grigioni F, Suri RM, Avierinos JF, de Meester C, Barbieri A, Rusinaru D, Russo A, Pasquet A, Michelena HI, Huebner M, Maalouf J, Clavel MA, Szymanski C, Enriquez-Sarano M. Twenty-year outcome after mitral repair versus replacement for severe degenerative mitral regurgitation: analysis of a large, prospective, multicenter, international registry. *Circulation* 2017;135:410–422.
24. Tanaka K, Makuuchi H, Naruse Y, Kobayashi T, Hayashi I, Takayama T, Namifusa Y. Mitral stenosis due to fibrous tissue overgrowth after mitral valve repair. *J Cardiovasc Surg* 2003;44:59–60.
25. Nishida H, Takahara Y, Takeuchi S, Mogi K. Mitral stenosis after mitral valve repair using the Duran flexible annuloplasty ring for degenerative mitral regurgitation. *J Heart Valve Dis* 2005;14:563–564.
26. Song S, Cho SH, Yang JH, Park PW. Repair for mitral stenosis due to pannus formation after Duran ring annuloplasty. *Ann Thorac Surg* 2010;90:93–94.
27. Sachpekidis V, Agatzoglis M, Styliadis I, Mosialos L, Kaprinis I, Monaghan MJ, Adamopoulos C. Three-dimensional imaging of pannus overgrowth after mitral valve repair. *Echocardiography* 2012;29: 210–213.
28. Salenger R, Diao X, Dawood MY, Herr DL, Sample GA, Pichard A, Gammie JS. Percutaneous rescue for critical mitral stenosis late after mitral valve repair. *Ann Thorac Surg* 2016;102:417–418.

The Mitral Valve 16 Months After Operative Insertion of the Alfieri Stitch

Samreen Fathima, MD, Shelley A. Hall, MD, Paul A. Grayburn, MD, and William C. Roberts, MD*

We describe considerable fibrous thickening of the mitral leaflets 16 months after insertion of an Alfieri stitch in a previously anatomically normal but functionally regurgitant mitral valve. Whether this type of mitral thickening will occur after percutaneous insertion of the mitral clip for pure mitral regurgitation remains to be determined. **(Am J Cardiol 2019;123:695–696)**

In the early 1990s, Alfieri et al[1] introduced what became known as "The Alfieri Stitch," a bowtie procedure or edge-to-edge mitral valve repair for patients with pure mitral regurgitation. The operation usually decreased the severity of the mitral regurgitation and it usually reduced the pulmonary arterial pressure. The procedure, however, was not without complications, a major one being the conversion of the previous mitral regurgitation to mitral stenosis. Subsequently, of course, percutaneous transcatheter mitral valve repair has proved to be effective and has replaced the operative approach.[2–5] Only 1 published photo late after insertion of "the stitch" has been found.[6] The present report describes another patient who had "the stitch" operatively inserted months earlier.

Case Description

A 19-year-old man, who was born in January 1998, had heart failure (HF) shortly after birth. The degree of HF waxed and waned during the next 15 or so years. By June 2016 (age 17), the HF had reached the point that a left ventricular assist device was inserted and at the same procedure an Alfieri stitch was placed on the mitral leaflets to decrease the degree of functional mitral regurgitation. Neither the left ventricular assist device nor the Alfieri stitch proved to be beneficial. The patient gained 40 pounds during the next several months because of worsening HF. An echocardiogram 6 months before the heart transplant showed mild mitral regurgitation, thickening of the distal third of the mitral leaflets, severe dilatation of both ventricular cavities, and severe tricuspid valve regurgitation (Figure 1). Echocardiographic findings before and after placement of the Alfieri stitch are summarized in Table 1. In October 2017 (age 18), heart transplantation was performed. Examination of the native heart showed it to be typical of idiopathic dilated cardiomyopathy. It weighed 330 g. The mitral leaflets, which had been anatomically normal at the time of insertion of the Alfieri stitch, were now quite thickened by fibrous tissue, particularly in their distal halves (Figure 2). When contacted in November 2018, 13 months after the heart transplant, the patient was asymptomatic and working.

Discussion

Described in this report is considerable fibrous thickening of the mitral leaflets after insertion of an Alfieri stitch 16 months earlier. Today, the Alfieri stitch operation is infrequently performed but the insertion of the mitral clip by the percutaneous route is now frequently performed.[2–4] Whether the percutaneous approach will also cause the leaflets to thicken and potentially convert an occasional patient from pure mitral regurgitation to mitral stenosis remains to be seen.

Disclosures

The investigators have no conflicts of interest to disclose.

1. Alfieri O, Maisano F, De Bonis M, Stefano PL, Torracca L, Oppizzi M, La Canna G. The double-orifice technique in mitral valve repair: a simple solution for complex problems. *J Thorac Cardiovasc Surg* 2001;122:674–681.
2. Feldman T, Kar S, Rinaldi M, Fail P, Hermiller J, Smalling R. Percutaneous mitral repair with the MitraClip system: safety and midterm durability in the initial EVEREST (endovascular valve edge-to-edge repair study) cohort. *J Am Coll Cardiol* 2009;54:686–694.
3. Maisano F, La Canna G, Colombo A, Alfieri O. The evolution from surgery to percutaneous mitral valve interventions: the role of the edge-to-edge technique. *J Am Coll Cardiol* 2011;58:2174–2182.
4. Feldman T, Foster E, Glower DD, Glower DG, Kar S, Rinaldi MJ, Fail P, Smalling RW, Siegel R, Rose GA, Engeron E, Loghin C, Trento A, Skipper ER, Fudge T, Letsou GV, Massaro JM, Mauri L. EVEREST II Investigators. Percutaneous repair or surgery for mitral regurgitation. *N Engl J Med* 2011;364:1395–1406.
5. Stone GW, Lindenfeld JA, Abraham WT, Kar S, Lim DS, Mishell JM, Whisenant B, Grayburn PA, Rinaldi M, Kapadia SR, Rajagopal V, Sarembock IJ, Brieke A, Marx SO, Cohen DJ, Weissman NJ, Mack MJ, for the COAPT Investigators. Transcatheter mitral-valve repair in patients with heart failure. *N Engl J Med* 2018;379:2307–2318.
6. Privitera S, Butany J, Cusimano RJ, Silversides C, Ross H, Leask R. Alfieri mitral valve repair clinical outcome and pathology. *Circulation* 2002;106:173–174.

Baylor Scott & White Heart and Vascular Institute, the Departments of Pathology and Internal Medicine (Division of Cardiology), Baylor University Medical Center, Dallas, Texas. Manuscript received August 7, 2018; revised manuscript received and accepted November 12, 2018.

See page 695 for disclosure information.

*Corresponding author: Tel: (214) 820-7911; fax: (214) 820-7533.

E-mail address: William.Roberts1@bswhealth.org (W.C. Roberts).

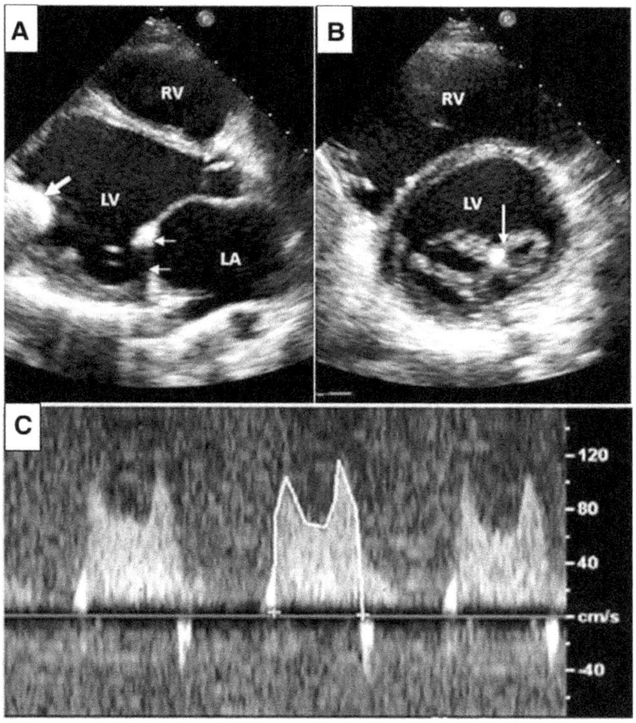

Figure 1. Echocardiographic images after insertion of a left ventricular assist device (LVAD) and Alfieri stitch. (*A*) Parasternal long-axis view showing thickened mitral leaflets with restricted diastolic excursion (*small arrows*). Both ventricular cavities and the left atrium are dilated (left ventricle at end-diastole = 6.2 cm, and at peak systole = 5.9 cm). The LVAD cannula is seen at lower left (*large arrow*). (*B*) Parasternal short-axis view showing Alfieri stitch (*arrow*) with double orifice mitral valve. (*C*) Mean transmitral gradient is 3 mm Hg by continuous wave Doppler.

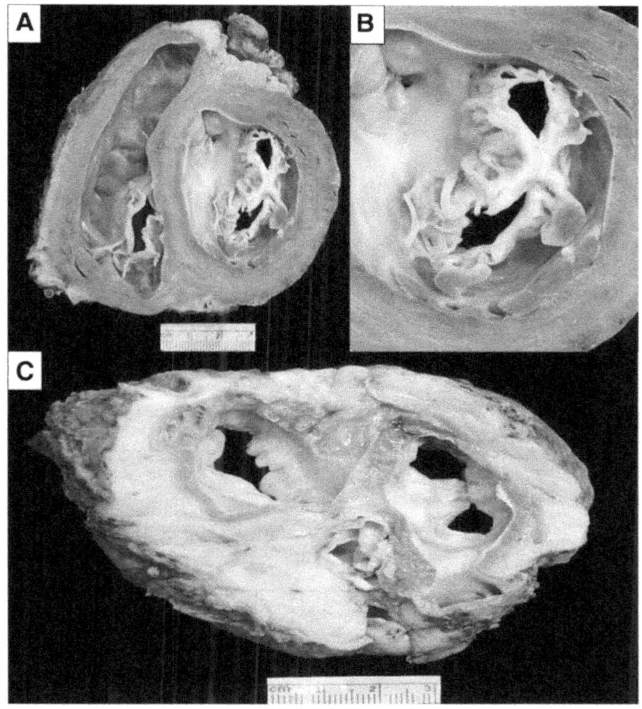

Figure 2. Photographs of the heart of patient described. (*A*). Cross section of the ventricles at the level of tricuspid and mitral valves showing the ventricular aspect of the Alfieri stitch. (*B*) A close-up of the mitral valves from the ventricular aspect. (*C*) View of the tricuspid and mitral valves after "deroofing" the atrial walls. The quantity of adipose tissue in the atrioventricular sulci is excessive.

Table 1
Echocardiographic data before and after placement of the Alfieri stitch

Variable	Pre-OP (days)	Post-OP (days)	
	−10	+1	+330
Peak velocity in early diastolic transmitral flow (m/s)	1.8	1.1	1.0
Decel time (m/s)	230	89	282
Mean gradient (mm Hg)	0	6	3
Mitral regurgitation (0-3+)	3+	1+	3+
Left ventricular internal diameter end diastole (mm)	83	74	62
Left ventricular posterior wall, peak systole (mm)	69	–	59
Left ventricular posterior wall, end diastole (mm)	7	8	6
Left ventricular ejection fraction (%)	37	34	10

www.ingramcontent.com/pod-product-compliance
Lightning Source LLC
LaVergne TN
LVHW062145200926
848484LV00007B/1865

* 9 7 9 8 8 8 8 6 2 1 5 6 1 *